Handbook of Treatment for Eating Disorders

HANDBOOK OF TREATMENT FOR EATING DISORDERS

Second Edition

Edited by

David M. Garner, PhD
Toledo Center for Eating Disorders
Bowling Green State University
University of Toledo

and

Paul E. Garfinkel, MD
Clarke Institute of Psychiatry
University of Toronto

THE GUILFORD PRESS
New York   London

To Maureen, and our children, Kyle and Sarah
—D. M. G.

To Dorothy, and our children,
Jonathan, Stephen, and Joshua
—P. E. G.

© 1997 The Guilford Press
A Division of Guilford Publications, Inc.
72 Spring Street, New York, NY 10012

Printed in the United States of America

This book is printed on acid-free paper.

Last digit is print number: 9   8   7   6   5   4   3   2   1

Library of Congress Cataloging-in-Publication Data

Handbook of treatment for eating disorders / edited by David M. Garner
   and Paul E. Garfinkel. — 2nd ed.
       p.   cm.
     Rev. ed. of: Handbook of psychotherapy for anorexia nervosa and
   bulimia. © 1985
     Includes bibliographical references and indexes.
     ISBN 1-57230-186-4
     1. Eating disorders—Treatment.   I. Garner, David M., 1947–   .
   II. Garfinkel, Paul E., 1946–   .   III. Handbook of psychotherapy
   for anorexia nervosa and bulimia.
     [DNLM: 1. Eating Disorders—therapy.   2. Eating Disorders—
   psychology.   WM 175 H2364 1997]
   RC552.E18H67   1997
   616.85′2606—DC21
   DNLM/DLC
   for Library of Congress   97-3395
                                                          CIP

Contributors

David E. Adson, MD, Adult Psychiatry Division, University of Minnesota, Minneapolis, Minnesota

W. Stewart Agras, MD, Department of Psychiatry, Stanford University, Palo Alto, California

Arnold E. Andersen, MD, Department of Psychiatry, University of Iowa, Iowa City, Iowa

Claire Cynara Beumont, BA, Alfred Hospital, Camperdown, New South Wales, Australia

Pierre J. V. Beumont, MB ChB, MSc, MPhil, FRCP (Edin), PRACP, FRPsych, FRANZCP, Department of Psychiatry, University of Sydney, New South Wales, Australia; Alfred Hospital, Camperdown, New South Wales, Australia

C. Laird Birmingham, MD, Eating Disorders Program, St. Paul's Hospital, Vancouver, British Columbia, Canada

Wayne Bowers, PhD, Eating Disorders Program, Department of Psychiatry, University of Iowa, Iowa City, Iowa

Rachel Bryant-Waugh, MA, Department of Psychological Medicine, Hospital for Sick Children, London, England

Jacqueline C. Carter, MA, Department of Psychiatry, University of Oxford, Warneford Hospital, Oxford, England

Authur H. Crisp, MD, DSc, FRCP, FRCPsych, Department of Psychological Medicine, St. George's Hospital Medical School, University of London, London, England (retired); Psychiatric Research Unit, Atkinson Morley's Hospital, Wimbledon, London, England

Janis H. Crowther, PhD, Department of Psychology, Kent State University, Kent, Ohio

Christopher Dare, MD, Section of Psychotherapy, Institute of Psychiatry, DeCrespigny Park, London, England

Amy Baker Dennis, PhD, Department of Psychiatry, Wayne State University, Detroit, Michigan

Karen Edmonson, MA, MALP, Department of Psychiatry, University of Minnesota, Minneapolis, Minnesota

Ivan Eisler, MA, Section of Psychotherapy, Institute of Psychiatry, DeCrespigny Park, London, England

Kay Evans, RN, MS, Eating Disorders Unit, Department of Psychiatry, Univerity of Iowa, Iowa City, Iowa

Christopher G. Fairburn, DM, MPhil, FRCPsych, Department of Psychiatry, University of Oxford, Warneford Hospital, Oxford, England

Patricia Fallon, PhD, Private Practice, Seattle, Washington

Ingrid Federoff, MA, Department of Psychology, University of Toronto, Toronto, Ontario, Canada

Paul E. Garfinkel, MD, Clarke Institute of Psychiatry, Department of Psychiatry, University of Toronto, Toronto, Ontario, Canada

David M. Garner, PhD, Toledo Center for Eating Disorders, Toledo, Ohio; Department of Psychology, Bowling Green State University, Bowling Green, Ohio; Women's Studies Program, University of Toledo, Toledo, Ohio

Elliot M. Goldner, MD, Eating Disorders Program, St. Paul's Hospital, Vancouver, British Columbia, Canada

Alan Goodsitt, MD, Department of Psychiatry, MacNeal Hospital, Berwyn, Illinois

Allan S. Kaplan, MD, FRCPsych, Program for Eating Disorders, Toronto Hospital, Department of Psychiatry, University of Toronto, Toronto, Ontario, Canada

Ann Kearney-Cooke, PhD, Institute for Psychotherapy, Cincinnati, Ohio

Bryan Lask, MD, Department of Psychological Medicine, Hospital for Sick Children, London, England

Marsha D. Marcus, PhD, Western Psychiatric Institute and Clinic, Pittsburgh, Pennsylvania

James E. Mitchell, MD, Department of Neuroscience, University of North Dakota, Fargo, North Dakota

Lawrence D. Needleman, PhD, Department of Psychology, Ohio State University, Columbus, Ohio

Marion P. Olmsted, PhD, Program for Eating Disorders, Toronto Hospital, University of Toronto, Toronto, Ontario, Canada

Kathleen M. Pike, PhD, Department of Psychiatry, College of Physicians and Surgeons, Columbia University, New York, New York

Janet Polivy, PhD, Department of Psychology, University of Toronto, Toronto, Ontario, Canada

Claire Pomeroy, MD, Department of Medicine, University of Minnesota, Minneapolis, Minnesota; Department of Veterans Affairs Medical Center, Minneapolis, Minnesota

Pauline S. Powers, MD, Department of Psychiatry and Behavioral Medicine, College of Medicine, University of South Florida, Tampa, Florida

James C. Rosen, PhD, Department of Psychology, University of Vermont, Burlington, Vermont

Gerald F. M. Russell, MD, Institute of Psychiatry, University of London, London, England (retired); Eating Disorders Unit, Hayes Grove Priory Hospital, Hayes, Kent, England

Randy A. Sansone, MD, Department of Psychiatry, College of Medicine, University of Oklahoma, Tulsa, Oklahoma

Nancy E. Sherwood, PhD, Department of Psychology, Kent State University, Kent, Ohio

Joseph A. Silverman, MD, Department of Pediatrics, Columbia University College of Physicians and Surgeons, New York, New York

Victoria Smye, MHSc, RN, Eating Disorders Program, St. Paul's Hospital, Vancouver, British Columbia, Canada

Sheila Specker, MD, Department of Psychiatry, University of Minnesota, Minneapolis, Minnesota

Ruth Striegel-Moore, PhD, Department of Psychology, Wesleyan University, Middletown, Connecticut

Michael Strober, PhD, Eating Disorders Program, Department of Psychiatry, Neuropsychiatric Institute and Hospital, University of California at Los Angeles, Los Angeles, California

Stephen W. Touyz, PhD, Department of Psychology, University of Sydney, Sydney, New South Wales, Australia

Kelly M. Vitousek, PhD, Department of Psychology, University of Hawaii, Honolulu, Hawaii

B. Timothy Walsh, MD, Department of Psychiatry, College of Physicians and Surgeons, Columbia University, New York, New York

Hazel Williams, Department of Psychiatry, University of Sydney, Royal Prince Alfred Hospital, Sydney, New South Wales, Australia

G. Terence Wilson, PhD, Graduate School of Applied and Professional Psychology, Rutgers University, Piscataway, New Jersey

Stephen A. Wonderlich, PhD, Department of Neuroscience, University of North Dakota, Fargo, North Dakota

Preface

In the 12 years since the publication of our original *Handbook of Psychotherapy for Anorexia Nervosa and Bulimia*, we have witnessed a dramatic surge of research on and clinical interest in the treatment of eating disorders. There have been major advancements in the areas of assessment, epidemiology, diagnosis, complications, identification of psychological and biological factors important in pathogenesis, and empirical research on treatment outcome. Binge eating disorder had not yet emerged in the psychiatric nomenclature at the time of the first handbook. A second generation of pyschological and drug treatment studies has led to refinement of the viable options for interventions. The rapid expansion in the knowledge-base in the field of eating disorders, in addition to changes in the health care environment, has led to new theoretical formulations as well as to thoughtful debate regarding the traditional models of clinical care. We felt the time was right for an authoritative compendium of the major treatment approaches for eating disorders.

A primary goal of this book is to present the main approaches to treatment in sufficient detail—when possible to even follow a manual-type format—to give clinicians a step-by-step blueprint for the conduct of therapy. Emphasis was placed on keeping the accounts practical, with case illustrations and examples of therapist–client dialogue. At the same time, we wanted the description of approaches to be both authoritative and well grounded in research. To achieve this balance, we chose prominent clinicians who also have been on the cutting edge of the treatment research literature. To our delight, virtually all of those asked generously agreed to participate, and the result has met our ambitious aspiration for a text that can be used to improve teaching, training, and the quality of clinical care.

The 30 chapters that comprise the book are organized into five major sections. The first, "The Context for Treatment," sets the stage for discussion of the various approaches and includes chapters on the history of the main eating disorders, diagnostic issues, assessment, and the sequencing and integration of treatment approaches. The chapters provide fascinating examples of the changes in our understanding of treatment, as well as the remarkable clinical insights that have been preserved from the earliest descriptions. For more than a hundred years, recognition of the family's role has led to suggestions for family members' involvement in and their exclusion from the treatment process. Details of nutritional rehabilitation and the profound role of feeding on psychological state were observed by Marce in 1860, and many of the major details of modern treatment were described by Ryle more than 50 years ago.

The second section of the book, "Cognitive-Behavioral and Educational Approaches," contains comprehensive chapters on approaches most widely supported by a steady stream of research over the last decade—at least when applied to bulimia nervosa. Empirical support for their application to anorexia nervosa has been slow to develop; however, several controlled trials are currently under way that should shed light on treatment efficacy. The elaboration of these approaches to anorexia nervosa has exposed both broad areas of consensus, as well as some key points of debate. For example, earlier accounts emphasized the overlap between cognitive-behavioral treatments for bulimia nervosa and anorexia nervosa; the chapters in this section underscore some important differences in content and style of the cognitive-behavioral approach when applied to these two eating disorders. The economy and effectiveness of psychoeducation have generated increasing interest in the last decade, and two chapters in this section describe approaches with somewhat different goals and points of emphasis. This section concludes with an exceptional chapter on a cognitive-behavioral approach to body image disturbance, paralleling another excellent chapter in the following section describing body image treatment from a feminist–psychodynamic perspective.

The next section, "Psychodynamic, Feminist, and Family Approaches," contains chapters by preeminent clinicians who have shaped much of the thinking in the eating disorders field. The dynamic approaches do not simply reiterate the traditional views of etiology; they provide rich and compelling formulations as well as practical details for blending psychotherapy and medical management to meet the special needs of eating disorder patients. Interpersonal psychotherapy has gained empirical support in recent years, and the chapter describing this approach is an extension of the manual used in a number of controlled research studies. Feminist approaches to treatment have played a major role in shaping current thinking about therapy regardless of orientation, and the chapter on feminist–psychodynamic treatment is both thoughtful and practical in covering key points on the conduct of therapy. Finally, family therapy has had a long and honored history in the treatment of eating disorders. Its presentation in this volume represents the distilla-

tion of years of work at the Maudsley Hospital and advances the understanding of family therapy to a new level.

The next section, "Hospital and Drug Treatments," includes chapters detailing the hospital and medical management of eating disorders. Hospital treatment remains the mainstay of management when patients suffer from serious medical complications. The inpatient chapter is a well-established protocol based on years of clinical experience. The discussion of partial treatment follows with many of the same components, but in a format that is very appealing because of its implications for cost savings. The specific technology for promoting weight gain is detailed next. Pharmacological treatments have been a major source of empirical study in the last decade, and the major advancements are distilled in the next chapter.

The last section, "Special Topics in Treatment," contains shorter chapters that represent some the the most important advances in the area of eating disorders. As the field has evolved, it has become clear that standard treatments must be altered to address the special needs of certain patient populations. Anorexia nervosa has a mortality rate higher than that of any other psychiatric disorder, and the chapter on managing medical complications provides a thorough overview of the potential problems as well as the practical recommendations for mitigating their pernicious influence. A series of chapters on other special topics provide the clinician with stategies for adapting treatment to deal with sexual abuse, substance abuse, concurrent medical conditions, personality disorders. prepubertal eating disorders, and binge-eating disorder, as well as addressing patients who refuse to engage in therapy. This section also includes chapters on group therapy and self-help for eating disorders. These chapters tackle difficult questions, such as the specific adaptations needed in therapy to address dual diagnoses with substance abuse, personality disorders, and sexual abuse. The chapter on sexual abuse combines a scholarly review of this area with very practical recommendations for treatment, informed by feminist thinking. The chapter on eating disorder patients with concurrent medical conditions reveals the special steps that must be taken to disentangle the complex issues facing these patients.

We are grateful for the assistance, support, and encouragement of a number of key people in producing this volume. At Central Behavioral

Healthcare of Toledo, Ohio, we appreciate the support of Drs. Stanley Zupnick, Dennis Kogut, Wayne Graves, Norman Giddan, and Rebecca Yager, and their staff. From the Psychiatry Section of the Toledo Hospital, we thank Drs. Lurley Archambeau, Ilze Sturis, Judy Cutsinger, Marcia Young, and Julie Welshans. The dedication of Julie Desai of the Toledo Center for Eating Disorders, dedication was invaluable. We are grateful to Drs. Aaron Beck, Harriet Adams, Jaime Vazquez, Lionel Rosen, Sam Plyler, and Maureen Garner for ongoing support and stimulation. We wish to thank the staff of The Guilford Press, and in particular Editor in Chief Seymour Weingarten, for outstanding guidance and incredible efficiency in all stages of the project. We are especially indebted to copy editor Marie Sprayberry, whose valuable comments and suggestions reflected both technical expertise and extraordinary knowledge of the content area. Thanks also to Barbara Chernow for an excellent job in coordinating the production process.

It has been a particular pleasure for both of us to edit this volume together. It has given us an opportunity to extend a rewarding collaboration that began almost 25 years ago when we were both completing our postgraduate training. During the intervening years, our patients and our colleagues have continued to provide us with insights and opportunities that have allowed us to remain dedicated to our interest in finding ways to improve the quality of clinical care. Finally, we are very grateful to our distinguished contributors who individually and collectively have been the major forces in improving the quality of care that eating disorder patients can expect to receive today. Their efforts in creating this volume have matched our highest expectations for clinical insight and scholarship.

DAVID M. GARNER
PAUL E. GARFINKEL

Contents

I

THE CONTEXT
FOR TREATMENT

CHAPTER 1

Anorexia Nervosa: Historical Perspective on Treatment

JOSEPH A. SILVERMAN

The aim of this chapter is to recount the most important events in the history of anorexia nervosa, particularly as they pertain to treatment.

THE EARLY LITERATURE

Early religious literature contains many descriptions of what was probably anorexia nervosa, but these descriptions of holy people who repudiated the pleasures of the flesh did not contain mention of treatment (Beumont, Al-Alami, & Touyz, 1987). In 1689, Richard Morton published a magnum opus, *Phthisiologia, seu Exercitationes de Phthisi,* which is considered the first medical account of anorexia nervosa—a condition that he referred to as "a Nervous Consumption" caused by "Sadness, and anxious Cares." In his book, which was translated into English in 1694 as *Phthisiologia, or, a Treatise of Consumptions,* Morton outlined in painstaking detail the many disease processes that cause wasting of body tissue (see Bliss & Branch, 1960, pp. 8–11). He described anorexia nervosa in two patients. One was a young woman called "Mr. Duke's daughter," who was afflicted at age 18 and suffered for 2 years before seeking Morton's help. The other was a boy, described as "The Son of Reverend Minster Steele, my very good Friend." This young man became ill at age 16 and also suffered for

about 2 years before seeking Morton's assistance.

In each case, Morton used what would today be called "pharmacotherapy." To help Mr. Duke's daughter, he employed "aromatic bags" and "Stomach Plaisters" externally, and prescribed for internal use "bitter Medicines, Chalybeates and Juleps made of Cephalick and Antihysterick Waters, sufficiently impregnated with Spirit of salt Armoniack, and Tincture of Castor, and other things of that Nature." Unfortunately, shortly thereafter his female patient died. Mr. Steele's son was treated similarly with the use of "Antiscorbutick, Bitter, and Chalybeate Medicines," but his treatment was "without any benefit." Morton then advised a change of milieu, presumably to get the boy away from a home that was in constant turmoil because his father was repeatedly arrested and charged for activities related to his nonconformist religious beliefs. The boy was advised to "abandon his studies, to go into the Country Air, and to use Riding and a Milk Diet (and especially to drink Asses milk) for a long time." We do not know, regrettably, whether this treatment was helpful (Morton, 1694).

Similar cases were described in 1767 by Robert Whytt, professor of the theory of medicine at the University of Edinburgh, and in 1768 by De Valangin, of the Royal College of Physicians in London. De Valangin reported successful treatment with advice from a physician: "A young lady who was . . . advised to reduce her fat . . . lived only upon tea, with the smallest quantity of bread and butter, till at last prevailed upon by her physician to take more nourshing food, to increase the quantity daily, without too much distending her contracted stomach at first, and to drink a lettle generous wine, she soon recovered a perfect state of health" (quoted in Beumont et al., 1987, p. 107; original spelling preserved).

DEVELOPMENTS IN THE 19TH CENTURY

Almost 100 years would pass before another truly significant article pertaining to the treatment of anorexia nervosa would appear in the medical literature. It came from the hand of Dr. Louis-Victor Marcé of the Hôpital Biçetre of Paris. Marcé was a prominent alienist in Paris, a trainee of Charcot, and a veritable dynamo of productivity. During the 8 years before his premature death at age 36, he published 8 books and 17 manuscripts on various psychiatric subjects. One of these reports was entitled "Note sur une Forme de Délire Hypochondriaque Consécutive aux Dyspepsies et Caractérisée Principalement par le Refus d'Aliments." He presented this paper at the October 31, 1859 meeting of the Société Médico-Psychologique in Paris. About 2 months later, the report was published in France (Marcé, 1860a); soon thereafter, an abbreviated English translation appeared in London (Marcé, 1860b).

In this report, Marcé clearly depicted the syndrome that would in less than 15 years be called "anorexia nervosa." He made it clear that the illness was psychiatric and not physical in nature, and that the psychopathology was profound. His treatment regimen included the following recommendations:

> This hypochondriacal delirium, then, cannot be advantageously encountered so long as the subjects remain in the midst of their own family and their habitual circle: the obstinate resistance which they offer, the sufferings of the stomach, which they enumerate with incessant lamentation, produce too vivid emotion to admit of the physician acting with full liberty and obtaining the necessary moral ascendancy. It is therefore indispensable to change the habitation and surrounding circumstances, and to entrust the patients to the care of strangers. If the refusal of food continues notwithstanding these efforts, it becomes necessary to employ intimidation, and even force. If by this last method a satisfactory result be not obtained, I would not hesitate to recommend the use of the oesophagus sound. But it is necessary to proceed progressively and by degrees. Each day and at each repast the nourishment, be it liquid or solid, should be gradually increased, and it would be even well to weigh the food, in order to proceed with greater sureness and confidence without relinquishing a single step.
>
> Adjunct means should not be neglected, and bitters, as well as steel medicine, combined with sufficient alimentation, may render good service. As to exercise and gymnastics, which are commonly recommended, they have the inconvenience of occasioning a great expenditure of strength, which the daily alimentation is unable to withstand; these should therefore be reserved until convalescence is well established, and should be used with great caution.
>
> When, by the aid of these precautions, the amount of nourishment has been raised to proper proportions, the patients will be seen to undergo a great change, their strength and condition to return, and their intellectual state to be modified in a most striking manner. It will be prudent, however, for a long time to exercise rigorous watchfulness, and to combat energetically the retrograde tendency, should such appear. Relapses are in these cases easy; and besides, this form of hypochondria is the index of a nervous predisposition which cannot be noticed without a feeling of uneasiness as to the intellectual future of the subject. (Marcé, 1860b, pp. 264–266)

Two prominent physicians separately described anorexia nervosa in 1873, and this was the year that the disorder received its current name. One of these medical giants was Charles Lasègue, professor of clinical medicine in the Faculty of Medicine of Paris and physician to La Pitié Hospital. The other was Sir William W. Gull, physician at Guy's Hospital, and arguably London's greatest clinician. Lasègue's (1873a) paper, "De l'Anorexie Hystérique," was published in Paris in April 1873. An English translation (Lasègue, 1873b, 1873c), "On Hysterical Anorexia," was printed in London in two parts in September of that year. Twenty-seven days after the latter publication, Gull presented his own case reports entitled "Anorexia Nervosa (Apepsia Hysterica, Anorexia Hysterica)" to the Clinical Society of London, which published them the next year (Gull, 1874).

Lasègue's contribution was more profound, in that he delved deeply into the psychopathology of the illness and attempted to understand it. He did not recommend any therapeutic maneuvers, medications, or shortcuts. In fact, he literally did not discuss therapy as such. What he did do was to issue a set of caveats. He wrote:

Woe to the physician who, misunderstanding the peril, treats as a fancy without object or duration an obstinacy which he hopes to vanquish by medicines, friendly advice or by the still more defective resource, intimidation. With hysterical subjects, a first medical fault is never reparable. Ever on the watch for the judgments concerning themselves, especially such as are approved by the family, they never pardon. . . . At this initial period, the only prudent course is to observe, to keep silent, and to remember that when voluntary inanition dates from several weeks it has become a pathological condition, having a long course to run. (1873b, pp. 265–260)

He added:

The most active gastric stimuli, purgatives, whether mild or drastic, produce no effect good or bad, the same may be said of diffusible stimuli, fetid gums, valerian, hydrotherapeutics, douches at different temperatures, as also of tonics, preparations of iron, cutaneous derivatives, etc. Laxatives alone are of use by removing constipation, none of the other agents even producing a diminution of the anorexia. (1873b, pp. 265–266)

Lasègue recommended quiet, watchful waiting on the part of the physician. As a patient deteriorated, she would develop amenorrhea, wasting, dryness of skin, a heart murmur, debility, anemia, and fatigue. All these signs would cause great anxiety among her relatives and friends, causing them to feel that the situation was desperate. When the patient herself became anxious "from the sad appearance of those who surrounded her . . . her self-satisfied indifference receives a shock. The moment has now arrived when the physician, if he has been careful in managing the case with a prevision of the future, resumes his authority" (Lasèque, 1873c, p. 68).

Gull's important 1874 paper was quite brief. In it, he described three starving teenage patients, the Misses A, B, and C. He recommended that "food should be administered at intervals varying inversely with the exhaustion and emaciation. The inclination of the patient must be in no way consulted . . . experience has shown plainly the danger of allowing the starvation process to go on. . . . By warmth, and steady supplies of food and stimulants, the strength may be gradually resuscitated, and recovery completed." He added that "the want of appetite is, I believe, due to a morbid mental stage." Finally he wrote, "the treatment is obviously that which is fitted for persons of unsound mind. The patients should be fed at regular intervals and surrounded by persons who would have moral control over them; relations and friends being generally the worst attendants." The diet recommended by Gull consisted of feedings of milk, cream, soup, eggs, fish, and chicken every 2 hours (Gull, 1874, pp. 22–26).

In 1888, in the course of 63 days, 11 articles about anorexia nervosa appeared in the *Lancet*. Included were three reports, an editorial, six letters, and one note.

The first report was by Sir William Gull and would be his last publication. His 42-line note described the illness and recovery in a 14-year-old girl. He stated now that the cause of most cases of anorexia nervosa was "perversions of the ego." His patient was treated with "light food every few hours," administered by a nurse from Guy's (Gull, 1988, pp. 516–517).

Soon thereafter, *Lancet* printed a report from a prominent physician who insisted that the patients "must be removed entirely from their usual domestic surroundings, involving, as they always do, much that is unwholesome for the patient and tending directly to foster perversion of the ego." He recommended rest, massage, and abundant overfeeding, and stated categorically that without isolation, treatment would fail. He labeled the illness "neurasthenia." Another report belittled the need for isolation and scorned the use of massage, referring to is as "that most fashionable . . . humbug." The writer concluded that the subject of anorexia nervosa is more sinned against than sinning, and can be cured without imprisonment. Hovell (1888a, 1888b) similarly emphasized that patients should be treated firmly but with kindness and compassion. However, forcible alimentation, consisting variously of milk, beef-tea, puddings, and brandy, was recommended by several physicians. Others proposed rectal feeds. No one any longer used medications, and psychotherapy was never considered (quoted in Silverman, 1988, pp. 928–930).

Descriptions of anorexia nervosa became common in the last years of the 19th century, particularly in the German and French literature. Jean-Martin Charcot (1889) followed the advice of Lasègue that a patient should be isolated from the family and that visitation should only occur if the patient made progress. Gilles de la Tourette (1895) emphasized the psychological nature of anorexia nervosa and distinguished subtypes based on whether or not food refusal was due to voluntary abstention or gastric spasms.

THE FIRST HALF OF THE 20TH CENTURY: VARYING VIEWS

Pierre Janet (1911/1929) considered anorexia nervosa a purely psychological disorder and distinguished two subtypes: obsessional and hysterical. Patients of the obsessional type refused to eat because of a fear of becoming fat and of achieving psychosexual maturity. Janet emphasized the loathing that these patients felt about their bodies, and their food refusal in spite of intense hunger. The hysterical form of anorexia nervosa was considered less common and resulted from a complete loss of appetite.

In 1914, the history of anorexia nervosa took an abrupt turn away from a psychogenic interpretation: A landmark paper by Morris Simmonds described pituitary insufficiency as leading to the severe weight loss in some patients. This formulation captured widespread interest, and until about 1930 anorexia nervosa was largely attributed to pituitary pathology. Simmonds's work had a lasting impact and set the stage for endocrinological approaches to understanding and treating anorexia nervosa. Patients were given pituitary extracts and implants in subsequent years, with little appreciation of the psychological variables that had led to their emaciation. It was not until the writings of Berkman (1930), who reported on a series of 117 patients, that a psychogenic interpretation was again applied to anorexia nervosa. Berkman was clear in describing the physiological disturbances seen in the disorder as secondary to the psychological disturbance and as reversible with psychotherapy. In the same year, Venables (1930) posited a psychological etiology in describing nine cases of anorexia nervosa.

On October 15, 1936, John A. Ryle, Regius Professor of Physic at the University of Cambridge and a consulting physician to Guy's Hospital, delivered the Schorstein Memorial Lecture at the London Hospital; it was published 2 days later in the *Lancet.* In what is perhaps one of the best clinical accounts ever written on the subject, Ryle (1936) described in definitive and microscopic detail the clinical picture found in anorexia nervosa. The clinical sagacity of his understanding of the disorder is evident in the following extended excerpts from his section on treatment:

> The first essential, after diagnosis, is to explain to the patient and the parents separately the nature of the disease in the simplest and most direct terms. A strong assurance should be given that recovery will take place when the starvation habit is corrected and the appetite restored by giving the stomach a sufficient intake of nourishing food to maintain, not only the general bodily requirements, but also its own efficiency, of which appetite is a normal expression. The absence of "organic disease" must be confidently stressed. Parent and daughter must both be allowed to see that the physician has a complete grasp of the situation. In a few cases I have been told that the patient proceeded to get well from the time of the consultation, a reminder of the value of simple emphatic statement and reassurance. If home surroundings or maternal psychology are unsatisfactory of if the programme initiated at home is not proceeding satisfactorily, treatment is better carried out in a nursing-home. Doctor and nurse must obtain early and full control over the patient and from the beginning ensure that the food provided is eaten. In some cases, it may be necessary to sit with the patient until each meal is finished. Firmness, kindness, and tact must be employed in just proportions, and the nurse must never let herself be wheedled into concessions. A mixed dietary from the beginning is preferable, and sloppy, invalid diets are to be avoided. Extra milk and glucose can, however, be employed if so given as not to interfere with a returning appetite at the proper mealtimes. It should be remembered that some patients are capable not only of declining food but also of hiding or disposing of it, and even of inducing vomiting in the lavatory when the nurse's back is turned. Treatment should be started in bed and be continued there until very definite physical and psychological improvements, with a gain of a stone or more if more than a stone has been lost, are registered. Gull stressed the importance of warmth. Cold and the restless activity of body and mind manifest in these cases both tend to interfere with weight recovery. Visitors and particularly near relatives who are likely to cause tears or other emotional reactions should be disallowed or strictly "rationed" at first. A hospital ward is an unsuitable place for treatment.

Ryle cautioned against the use of thyroid or ovarian hormones; he reminded his readers of Gull's admonition that the "want of appetite is . . . due to a morbid mental state." He went on to say:

> Psycho-analytical methods are also unwise and may do harm. Direct inquiries into motive and difficulties are better avoided, at any rate in the earlier stages and in the youthful cases. Explanation, reassurance, distraction, and firm treatment of the starvation are usually adequate, and will secure a steady and approximately parallel improvement in the mental and physical states. Not uncommonly a waywardness of periodic emotionalism or a subdued or alternatively a "bossy" attitude of mind persists after physical recovery, but this is hardly to be regarded as a continuance of the disease. With the return of regular periods, which may not follow for some weeks, months, or even a year or two after the restitution of weight, recovery can usually be regarded as complete. Relapses are not common. Partial recoveries with partial restitution of weight sufficient to allow a return to active life are more so. (Ryle, 1936, pp. 893–899)

In 1940, Waller, Kaufman, and Deutsch described the symptoms of anorexia nervosa as the results of symbolic or unconscious fantasies stemming from fears of oral impregnation. These oral impregnation fantasies were presumed to be associated with marked guilt, against which the weight loss of anorexia nervosa was thought to be a defense. Symbolic interpretations reemerged to form the basis for subsequent drive-related psychoanalytic formulations by Thoma (1967), who theorized that anorexia nervosa results from "oral ambivalence" and abandonment at the genital stage of development.

MODERN PIONEERS: BRUCH, CRISP, AND RUSSELL

Although there have been many notable contributions to the literature on psychotherapy for anorexia nervosa, the penetrating formulations of Hilde Bruch, Arthur Crisp, and Gerald Russell have been perhaps most influential in providing insights regarding the conduct of psychotherapy (Garner, 1985). Many of the developments in treatment over the past 20 years have been recapitulations or refinements of the observations of these modern pioneers.

Bruch (1962, 1973, 1978) proposed that the self-starvation in anorexia nervosa represents a struggle for autonomy, competence, control, and self-respect. According to this view, the mother's failure to recognize and confirm the child's expression of independent needs results in inner confusion, expressed in three overlapping areas of perceptual/conceptual disturbance pathognomonic in anorexia nervosa. These are (1) body image disturbance, characterized by the tendency to overestimate body size; (2) interoceptive disturbance, reflected by an inability to accurately identify and respond to internal sensations, such as hunger, satiety, affective states, and sexual feelings; and (3) all-pervasive feelings of ineffectiveness, reflected by feelings of loss of control. Mara Selvini Palazzoli (1974) independently proposed a similar theory regarding the genesis of anorexia nervosa. Her object relations view holds that an anorexia nervosa patient experiences the body as "the maternal object, from which the ego wishes to separate itself at all costs" (Selvini Palazzoli, 1974, p. 90).

Bruch (1973) proposed a "fact-finding" approach to psychotherapy that involves the gradual but deliberate relabeling of misconceptions and errors in thinking resulting from faulty developmental experiences. Such therapy is aimed at helping a patient discover a "genuine self" by encouraging and confirming authentic expressions of thoughts and feelings. Bruch offered specific advice to the psychotherapist, who "must pay minute attention to the discrepancies in the patient's recall of the past and to the way she perceives or misinterprets current events, to which she will respond inappropriately. The therapist must be honest in confirming or correcting what the patient communicates" (1978, p. 136). Bruch went on to comment on the process of therapy, "during which erroneous assumptions and attitudes are recognized, defined, and challenged so that they can be abandoned. It is important to proceed slowly and use concrete small events as episodes for illustrating certain false assumptions or illogical deductions. The whole work needs to be done by reexamining actual aspects of living, by using relatively small events as they come up" (1978, pp. 143–144). Bruch's emphasis on the patient's beliefs and assumptions in the conduct of psychotherapy served as a springboard for modern cognitive therapy for the disorder (Garner & Bemis, 1982).

Crisp (1967, 1980) has made a compelling

case for the importance of a developmental model, in which the central psychopathology of anorexia nervosa is rooted in the biological and psychological experiences accompanying the attainment of an adult weight. According to this view, anorexia nervosa is an attempt to cope with fears and conflicts associated with psychobiological maturity. The dieting and consequent starvation become the mechanisms by which the patient regresses to a prepubertal shape, hormonal status, and experience (Crisp, 1980; see also Chapter 13, this volume). Crisp has consistently emphasized the meaning of the subpubertal weight in developmental terms. The implication for psychotherapy has been on the need for renourishment to allow patients to confront the dynamic issues that have led to their "phobic fear" of adult body weight as part of the process of mastering alternative coping strategies.

Russell (1970; see also Chapter 2, this volume) has recognized the variable presentation of anorexia nervosa and emphasized the morbid fear of fatness as the central psychopathology of the disorder. He has emphasized the need to correct the starvation state in order to correct the self-perpetuating nature of the syndrome. Russell also stresses the role of experienced nursing staff in the hospital management of anorexia nervosa.

THE EMERGENCE OF BINGE EATING AS A SYMPTOM

Anorexia nervosa has always been most noted for the symptom of self-imposed starvation; however, part of the evolutionary history of the disorder involves the emergence of binge eating as part of the clinical picture. In his classic paper on anorexia nervosa, Gull (1874) described occasional bouts of overeating in one patient: "for a day or two the appetite was voracious, but this was rare and exceptional." Binge eating was identified as a symptom in early reports on anorexia nervosa (Berkman, 1930; Bruch, 1962; Crisp, 1967; Dally, 1969; Guiora, 1967; King, 1963; Meyer & Weinroth, 1957; Nemiah, 1950; Theander, 1970; Russell, 1970). Berkman (1930) reported binge eating in two-thirds of his anorexia nervosa patients in response to a sensation of fullness. In later reports, binge eating has been described in approximately one-half of anorexia nervosa patients presenting for treatment (Casper, Eckert, Halmi, Goldberg, &

Davis, 1980; Garfinkel, Moldofsky, & Garner, 1980; Hsu, Crisp, & Harding, 1979).

Casper (1983) has traced the history of binge eating in anorexia nervosa, highlighting the small number of cases reported in the literature prior to the 20th century. She suggests that the symptom of binge eating has become a more common theme in anorexia nervosa, and that this represents a change in the expression of the underlying psychopathology. Russell (1985) considers this change in presentation as reflecting an actual shift over the years in the central psychopathology in anorexia nervosa. In early case reports, there was an emphasis either on starvation as a defense against sexuality or on the theme of asceticism, with food restriction representing such spiritual ideals as self-sacrifice and control over bodily urges (Bell, 1985; Casper, 1983; Rampling, 1985). In the past century, the ascetic motif has become less prominent, replaced by a "drive for thinness" or a "morbid dread of fatness" as the more common motivational themes (Casper, 1983; Russell, 1985).

According to Russell (1985), the increased appearance of binge eating, both in patients with anorexia nervosa and in patients who are not emaciated, is the most dramatic evidence for a transformation in the psychopathology of anorexia nervosa. However, the actual extent to which binge eating has become more common in anorexia nervosa is unclear, owing to the fact that the symptom may have been identified less reliably in earlier reports. The fact that binge eating is more easily concealed than emaciation may account for underreporting in early writings.

The original rationale for subtyping anorexia nervosa came from studies in which "bulimic" patients were contrasted with patients who did not engage in binge eating, referred to as "fasters" (Casper et al., 1980) or "restricters" (Garfinkel et al., 1980). In a review of 14 studies in which anorexia nervosa patients were subclassified into bulimic and nonbulimic subtypes, DaCosta and Halmi (1992) found that the bulimic anorexia nervosa patients were older than the nonbulimic patients at the time of presentation. The duration of illness was consistently longer for bulimic anorexia nervosa patients across the six studies in which these data were reported. Perhaps of greatest significance in most studies comparing bulimic and nonbulimic anorexia nervosa patients is the finding that the bulimic patients report greater impulsivity, social involvement, sexual activity, family dysfunction, and depression, and more conspicuous emotional disturbance in general (DaCosta & Halmi, 1992).

More recently, it has been argued that the compensatory behaviors frequently associated with binge eating (i.e., self-induced vomiting and/or laxative abuse), rather than binge eating per se, are the most relevant markers for subclassifying anorexia nervosa (Garner, 1993; Garner, Garner, & Rosen, 1993). Garner et al. (1993) have found that anorexia nervosa patients who purge, regardless of whether or not they report objective binge episodes, may be meaningfully distinguished from nonpurging patients in terms of psychopathology. Thus, many of the characteristics previously thought to distinguish bulimic anorexia nervosa patients also apply to patients who do not experience objective episodes of binge eating, but who control their weight at least in part through purging. These results, combined with the medical risks associated with purging behaviors, have highlighted the need for psychotherapy to address purging as well as binge-eating behavior.

CONCLUSION

In a period of over 300 years, we have traveled a long distance from Morton's cases who were treated with "pharmacotherapy" and country air. Marcé (1860b) felt that it was "indispensable to change the habitation and surrounding circumstances, and to entrust the patients to the care of strangers" (p. 265). He also believed in forced feedings if necessary. He used some form of pharmacotherapy as well, but only as an adjunct to treatment. Lasègue, writing in 1873, believed in seizing control over the patient after a period of careful, watchful waiting. Gull (1874) recommended rest, warmth, and the regular and frequent introduction of food in the utter disregard of the anorexia of the patient. Later in the 19th century, forced feedings either by mouth, by tube, or by rectum became the vogue. Simmonds (1914) caused a brief interlude in which psychological approaches were replaced by a focus on the pituitary. Ryle's 1936 paper signified a return to psychological formulations, and his recommendations included proper diet and a "gradual and sensible readjustment of the mental outlook." He stated finally that "the advancement of practical medi-

cine, both physical and psychological, still lies largely with earlier diagnosis and rational preventive treatment" (p. 899). This was followed by the application of psychoanalytic theory to anorexia nervosa, which provided a rich understanding of the patient but relatively little practical advice regarding treatment. Bruch, in particular, broke with this tradition and offered sensible and pragmatic suggestions for the conduct of therapy. Her sage advice and the views of Crisp and Russell have continued to have an impact on treatment today.

REFERENCES

Bell, R. (1985). *Holy anorexia.* Chicago: University of Chicago Press.

Berkman, J. M. (1930). Anorexia nervosa: Anorexia, inanition and low basal metabolic rate. *American Journal of Medical Science, 180,* 411–424.

Beumont, P. J. V., Al-Alami, M. S., & Touyz, S. W. (1987). The evolution of the concept of anorexia nervosa. In P. J. V. Beumont, G. D. Burrows, & R. C. Casper (Eds.), *Handbook of eating disorders: Part 1. Anorexia and bulimia nervosa* (pp. 105–116). New York: Elsevier.

Bliss, E. L., & Branch, C. H. H. (1960). *Anorexia nervosa: Its history, psychology, and biology.* New York: Hoeber.

Bruch, H. (1962). Perceptual and conceptual disturbances in anorexia nervosa. *Psychosomatic Medicine, 24,* 187–194.

Bruch, H. (1973). *Eating disorders: Obesity, anorexia nervosa and the person within.* New York: Basic Books.

Bruch, H. (1978). *The golden cage.* Cambridge, MA: Harvard University Press.

Casper, R. C. (1983). On the emergence of bulimia nervosa as a syndrome: A historical view. *International Journal of Eating Disorders, 2,* 3–16.

Casper, R. C., Eckert, E. D., Halmi, K. A., Goldberg, S. C., & Davis, J. M. (1980). Bulimia: Its incidence and clinical importance in patients with anorexia nervosa. *Archives of General Psychiatry, 37,* 1030–1034.

Charcot, J. M. (1889). *Clinical lectures on diseases of the nervous system* (Vol. 3). London: New Sydenham Society.

Crisp, A. H. (1967). The possible significance of some behavioral correlates of weight and carbohydrate intake. *Journal of Psychosomatic Research, 11,* 117–131.

Crisp, A. H. (1980). *Anorexia nervosa: Let me be.* London: Academic Press.

DaCosta, M., & Halmi, K. A. (1992). Classification of anorexia nervosa: Question of subtypes. *International Journal of Eating Disorders, 11,* 305–313.

Dally, P. J. (1969). *Anorexia nervosa.* New York: Grune & Stratton.

Garfinkel, P. E., Moldofsky, H., & Garner, D. M. (1980). The heterogeneity of anorexia nervosa. *Archives of General Psychiatry, 37,* 1036–1040.

Garner, D. M. (1985). Individual psychotherapy for anorexia nervosa. *Journal of Psychiatric Research, 19,* 423–433.

Garner, D. M. (1993). Binge eating in anorexia nervosa. In C. G. Fairburn & G. T. Wilson (Eds.), *Binge eating: Na-*

ture, assessment, and treatment (pp. 50–76). New York: Guilford Press.

Garner, D. M., & Bemis, K. M. (1982). A cognitive-behavioral approach to anorexia nervosa. *Cognitive Therapy and Research, 6,* 123–150.

Garner, D. M., Garner, M. V., & Rosen, L. W. (1993). Anorexia nervosa "restrictors" who purge: Implications for subtyping anorexia nervosa. *International Journal of Eating Disorders, 13,* 171–185.

Gilles de la Tourette, G. A. E. B. (1895). *Traité clinique et thérapeutique de l'hystérie* (p. 246). Paris: E. Plou, Nourriet.

Guiora, A. Z. (1967). Dysorexia: A psychopathological study of anorexia nervosa and bulimia. *American Journal of Psychiatry, 124,* 391–393.

Gull, W. W. (1874). Anorexia nervosa (apepsia hysterica, anorexia hysterica). *Transactions of the Clinical Society of London, 7,* 22–28.

Gull, W. W. (1888). Anorexia nervosa. *Lancet, i,* 516–517.

Hovell, D. D. (1888a). Editorial. *Lancet, i,* 583.

Hovell, D. D. (1888b). Letter to editor. *Lancet, ii,* 949.

Hsu, L. K. G., Crisp, A. H., & Harding, B. (1979). Outcome in anorexia nervosa. *Lancet, i,* 61–65.

Janet, P. (1929). *The major symptoms of hysteria* (2nd ed.). New York: Macmillan. (Original work published 1911)

King, A. (1963). Primary and secondary anorexia nervosa syndromes. *British Journal of Psychiatry, 109,* 470–479.

Lasègue, C. (1873a). De l'anorexie hystérique. *Archives Générales de Médecine, 1,* 384–403.

Lasègue, C. (1873b). On hysterical anorexia. *Medical Times and Gazette, 2,* 265–266.

Lasègue, C. (1873c). On hysterical anorexia. *Medical Times and Gazette, 2,* 367–369.

Marcé, L.-V. (1860a). Note sur une forme de délire hypochondriaque consécutif aux dyspepsies et caractérisée principalement par le refus d'aliments. *Annales Médico-Psychologiques, 6,* 15–28.

Marcé, L.-V. (1860b). On a form of hypochondriacal delirium occurring consecutive to dyspepsia, and characterized by refusal of food. *Journal of Psychological Medicine and Mental Pathology, 13,* 264–266.

Meyer, B. C., & Weinroth, L. A. (1957). Observations on psychological aspects of anorexia nervosa. *Psychosomatic Medicine, 19,* 389–398.

Morton, R. (1689). *Phthisiologia, seu exercitationes de phthisi.* London: S. Smith.

Morton, R. (1694). *Phthisiologia, or, a treatise of consumptions.* London: Smith & Walford.

Nemiah, J. C. (1950). Anorexia nervosa: A clinical psychiatric study. *Medicine, 29,* 225–268.

Rampling, D. (1985). Ascetic ideals and anorexia nervosa. *Journal of Psychiatric Research, 19,* 89–94.

Russell, G. F. M. (1970). Anorexia nervosa: Its identity as an illness and its treatment. In J. H. Price (Ed.), *Modern trends in psychological medicine* (Vol. 2, pp. 131–164). London: Butterworths.

Russell, G. F. M. (1985). The changing nature of anorexia nervosa: An introduction to the conference. *Journal of Psychiatric Research, 19,* 101–109.

Ryle, J. A. (1936). Anorexia nervosa. *Lancet, ii,* 893–899.

Selvini Palazzoli, M. P. (1974). *Self-starvation.* London: Chaucer.

Silverman, J. (1988). Anorexia nervosa in 1888. *Lancet, i,* 928–930.

Simmonds, M. (1914). Ueber embolische Prozesse in der Hypophysis. *Archives of Pathology and Anatomy, 217,* 226–239.

Theander, S. (1970). Anorexia nervosa: A psychiatric investigation of 94 female patients. *Acta Psychiatrica Scandinavica* (Suppl. 214), 1–194.

Thoma, H. (1967). *Anorexia nervosa.* New York: International Universities Press.

Venables, J. F. (1930). Anorexia nervosa: A study of the pathogenesis and treatment of nine cases. *Guy's Hospital Report, 80,* 213–216.

Waller, J. V., Kaufman, M. R., & Deutsch, F. (1940). Anorexia nervosa: A psychosomatic entity. *Psychosomatic Medicine, 2,* 3–16.

Whytt, R. (1767). *Observations on the nature, causes, and cure of those disorders which have been commonly called nervous, hypochondriac or histeric: To which are prefixed some remarks on the sympathy of the nerves.* (3rd ed.). London: T. Beckert, P. A. De Hondt, & J. Balfour.

CHAPTER 2

The History of Bulimia Nervosa

GERALD F. M. RUSSELL

It is not possible to write a truly historical account of bulimia nervosa. This diagnostic term was coined as recently as 1979, and there is therefore no true historical era available for study. But it is not only for linguistic reasons that my task is well-nigh impossible. The clinical description of this disorder is highly specific. First, it is necessary to meet a set of three diagnostic criteria: episodic overeating, vomiting and/or laxative abuse, and fear of fatness. Second (and this is important), the typical illness must be shown to have close links with its parent condition, anorexia nervosa. Bulimia nervosa was, after all, first described as a variant of anorexia nervosa (Russell, 1979). Thus, it does not suffice to search the literature for accounts of psychiatric disorders with the set of diagnostic criteria embodied in diagnostic manuals. Finally, we should consider the likelihood that bulimia nervosa is an illness more or less limited to contemporary times, in contrast with the historical era of anorexia nervosa (see Silverman, Chapter 1, this volume). For all these reasons, an exploration of the history of bulimia nervosa may be like looking for a will-o'-the-wisp.

In spite of these difficulties, enterprising scholars have studied the psychiatric literature—mainly from the time of the classical accounts of anorexia nervosa by Charles Lasègue (1873) and William Gull (1874). Regina Casper (1983) was the first pioneer to search accounts of patients with anorexia nervosa for the additional behaviors of overeating and vomiting, so as to identify patients whose case histories might resemble those of contemporary bulimia nervosa. Habermas (1989) followed a similar approach, searching the psychiatric literature for patients who had expressed fears of being overweight, in addition to having overeaten and induced vomiting. Van Deth and Vandereycken (1995) modified the diagnostic criteria for bulimia nervosa so as to make them suitable for the retrospective identification of bulimic disorders. They thought this necessary, for the compelling reasons that the modern diagnostic criteria for bulimia nervosa are too "time- and culture-bound" (p. 335). In doing this, they changed the focus of the search from bulimia nervosa to bulimic disorders in general. They nevertheless retained a criterion of dissatisfaction with feeling overweight, but only as an optional criterion. Another major difference in this study was that patients diagnosed as examples of hysterical vomiting were studied, rather than patients diagnosed as examples of anorexia nervosa.

This chapter begins with a brief survey of the practices of overeating and vomiting mentioned in the literature of antiquity and the lives of the Christian saints. This survey is brief because the findings are probably of no relevance to modern bulimia nervosa. Next, the observations by the scholars listed above are examined in some detail. Then a few detailed case histories from the psychiatric literature are examined for the light they may throw on modern bulimia nervosa. Finally, after a brief description of events in the 1970s leading to the definition of bulimia nervosa as a new disorder, there is a discussion of two important recent studies aimed at estimating the incidence of true bulimia nervosa during the 1960s and

1970s (according to the post-1979 diagnostic criteria for the disorder).

OVEREATING AND INDUCED VOMITING IN THE OLDER HISTORICAL LITERATURE (FROM ANTIQUITY TO THE 18TH CENTURY)

It is essential to avoid jumping to the conclusion that overeating (bulimia) or vomiting in ancient accounts is equivalent to the disorder we now know as bulimia nervosa. This is a trap into which even modern writers may fall. This is not altogether surprising when one considers the long period of confusion that followed the diagnostic criteria for so-called "bulimia," published in the *Diagnostic and Statistical Manual of Mental Disorders,* third edition (DSM-III; American Psychiatric Association [APA], 1980). At that time, at least in North America, bulimia was simply equated with recurrent episodes of binge eating, including elaborations of its behavioral characteristics and some psychological accompaniments. More specifically, the important criterion of a morbid fear of fatness was omitted, and even the criterion of attempted weight loss by self-induced vomiting was optional. This period of confusion was not corrected until the publication of DSM-III-R (APA, 1987). During these years, and to a smaller extent thereafter, writers were prone to use the terms "bulimia" and "bulimia nervosa" interchangeably, especially when searching through the older literature for preceding examples of bulimia nervosa. For this reason, brief accounts in the ancient historical literature are generally unhelpful, and we must concentrate our attention on the more detailed accounts in the psychiatric literature commencing during the early part of the 20th century.

Overeating and Induced Vomiting in Antiquity

In a brief but interesting historical account of induced vomiting and catharsis, Nasser (1993) has examined these practices in ancient Egypt, Greece, Rome, and Arabia. We learn that the ancient Egyptians purged themselves every month for 3 days in succession, using emetics and clysters to preserve health. This was because they supposed that the diseases to which human beings are prone proceeded from food itself. Nasser points out that much of the re-

sponsibility for advocating vomiting lay with the ancient physicians. Purgation was also a popular remedy, and its use increased in Europe by the Middle Ages. By the 17th century both emetics and purgatives were the commonest forms of treatment. Nasser concedes that the history of vomiting and catharsis may have no bearing on modern eating disorders, except inasmuch as the lavish self-administration of emetics and purgatives currently observed may be related to the fact that they were once prescribed by physicians.

Everyone is aware of the time-worn stories of the vomitorium in ancient Rome, to which people sometimes resorted for the purpose of swallowing an emetic. Seneca is said to have observed "Men eat to vomit and vomit to eat" (quoted in Pullar, 1972, p. 20). This story would remain a historical curiosity, were it not for a recent suggestion by Crichton (1996) that the Roman Emperors Claudius and Vitellius were bulimic. He provides an interesting account of the preoccupation of both these men with lavish and extravagant feasting. Vitellius displayed disgusting gluttony and was obese; both men drank heavily; and both are said to have resorted to habitual vomiting. Crichton does not claim that the excesses of these two emperors could be considered as early examples of modern bulimia nervosa, for the reason that there was no evidence of a drive for thinness on their part. On the other hand, he considers that their excesses might be viewed as "an historical variant of bulimia nervosa" (p. 205). There is doubt whether their eating excesses should be considered an eating disorder because, in the author's own words, such behavior "was practiced intermittently by some members of a prosperous and pampered elite" (p. 207) during the early Roman Empire.

There have also been arguments about the relevance of ancient accounts in the Babylonian Talmud of a condition called *boolmot* (Hebrew). This is translated as "ravenous hunger," or *bulimy* in Greek (Kaplan & Garfinkel, 1984). These authors considered that the condition described in the Talmud might be a *forme fruste* of DSM-III bulimia. This communication was rightly criticized by Vandereycken (1985), who detected that the term "bulimia" has several different meanings and may be associated with different forms of behavioral and even organic pathology. He further pointed out that "bulimia" as defined in DSM-III is confusing, merely signifies excessive hunger, and has been used in medicine for many centuries. "Bulimia nervosa" is preferable to denote the modern syndrome, which has much wider clinical connotations. A brief note on the meaning and origin of these terms is justified. "Bulimia" is derived from the Greek word *limos* ("hunger") with the prefix *bou* from *bous* ("bull," "ox"). Bulimia has at least two meanings: "hunger as great as that of an ox," or "sufficient to consume an entire ox" (Parry-Jones & Parry-Jones, 1991). Its other meanings are fully discussed by Ziolko and Schrader (1985). The addition of "nervosa" to denote the broad syndrome of bulimia nervosa served the purpose of denoting its clinical and etiological relationship with anorexia nervosa (Russell, 1979).

Bulimic Behavior among the Saints

Casper's (1983) method of seeking the additional behaviors of overeating and vomiting in the case histories of anorexic patients may be applied to the recorded lives of the saints. Bell (1985) put forward the thesis that some of the saints developed anorexia nervosa as a consequence of their lives of asceticism and spiritual fulfillment in order to achieve sanctity. If we assume the validity of his thesis, evidence may first be sought for the occurrence of overeating in the accounts of the saints' lives. According to Bell's own work, it would seem that Saint Mary Magdalen de Pazzi and Saint Veronica (born Orsola Giuliani) both displayed bulimic behavior in the course of their fasts. Saint Mary Magdalen de Pazzi lived from 1566 to 1607. Her early death was the result of self-mortification, including physical self-torture, and an unhealthy diet. Her sanctity was largely recognized because of her spiritual strength in the face of illness. She subsisted on bread and water for long periods. Nevertheless, she was observed by other sisters in the cloister to break her strict diet on at least one occasion, when she was tormented by cravings for food and gobbled it down. This was attributed to the work of the devil, who tempted her by opening the pantry cabinet, displaying before her the delicacies stored therein. Saint Veronica lived from 1660 until 1727, and her life is well documented through her autobiographies, as well as the observations of other sisters. The following is quoted from Bell (1985, p. 75):

In the time that she made her rigorous fast of five years . . . , the sisters sometimes found Sister Veronica in the kitchen, the refectory, or the dispensary, where she ate everything there was, and what is more, at other times they found her eating before the hour of Communion. . . .

This behavior was then attributed to a time-worn deception in Lucifer's arsenal of tricks. Bell's own interpretation is that Sister Veronica's behavior was that of "the repetitive binge eating/vomiting pattern, typical of acute anorexic behavior" (p. 76).

A strong case has been made by scholars for considering that Saint Catherine of Siena, who lived in the 14th century, developed anorexia nervosa in the course of her pursuit of asceticism leading to mystical experiences and spiritual fulfillment. The most remarkable feature of her asceticism was her prolonged abstinence from food and drink. There are no records that she was ever tempted to overeat. She regarded her inability to eat as a punishment for her sins, and a method of expiation. "The function of reparation was served by her vomiting. She felt compelled 'to let a fine straw or some such thing be pushed far down her throat to make her vomit'" (Rampling, 1985, p. 91), quoting her confessor, Raymond de Capua). Catherine became emaciated and died from starvation in 1380 at the age of 33 (Bell, 1985).

The well-documented stories of these pious women are in keeping with the diagnosis of anorexia nervosa. The only reason for mentioning them is that, following the method of Casper, the occurrence of overeating or self-induced vomiting should alert one to the possibility of bulimia nervosa. This can be safely dismissed in the case of these three saints, but a stickler for detailed psychiatric classification might consider them as examples of the "binge-eating/purging" subtype of anorexia nervosa, as defined in DSM-IV (APA, 1994).

THE SEARCH FOR BULIMIA NERVOSA IN THE PRE-1979 CLINICAL LITERATURE

As previously mentioned, a number of scholars have searched the literature for clinical case histories describing patients who would satisfy the modern criteria for bulimia nervosa. The pioneer in this search was Casper (1983), who was followed by Habermas (1989) and Van Deth and Vandereycken (1995). Mention should also be made of Parry-Jones and Parry-Jones (1991).

Casper used as her point of departure descriptions of patients with anorexia nervosa sufficiently detailed to identify symptoms resembling modern bulimia nervosa, such as overeating and vomiting. She also looked for the third criterion, the fear of fatness (or the desire for thinness). She remarked that it was not until about 1940 that comments such as "teased about being fat," "desire to be thin," and "bothered by excess weight" were recorded with frequency. She was perspicacious in identifying the one sentence in William Gull's 1874 article of relevance to her thesis: "Occasionally for a day or two, the appetite was voracious, but this was very rare and exceptional" (Gull, 1874, p. 23). Thereafter, there were only isolated references to case histories describing relevant behaviors such as self-induced vomiting. In general, the behaviors of overeating (bulimia) and/or vomiting are mentioned more in passing. For example, the article by Waller, Kaufman, and Deutsch (1940) is best known for their hypothesis that anorexia nervosa is an "acting out" of a specific fantasy—namely, the wish to be impregnated through the mouth. These authors recognized that the patients' behavior results at times in "compulsive eating" and at other times in guilt and rejection of food. In a detailed clinical analysis of anorexia nervosa, Nemiah (1950) described 14 patients. Four of them had episodes described as compulsive eating or orgies of stuffing themselves with food, leading the author to conclude that "anorexia nervosa should be considered, then, as not just the loss of appetite, but rather as a disturbance in eating, ranging from true anorexia at one extreme to bulimia at the other, frequently associated with nausea and vomiting" (Nemiah, 1950, p. 266).

In the first comprehensive monograph on anorexia nervosa, Bliss and Branch (1960) described several patients with "food binges" in whom "unrestricted gluttony may be followed by self-induced vomiting or starvation" (p. 67). In most of the patients so far reported, there were exceedingly few for whom any mention was made of a fear of fatness. Accordingly, few of them resembled cases of modern bulimia nervosa. Among the exceptions, two were recognized by Casper—Nadia (Janet, 1903), and Ellen West (Binswanger, 1944–1945). Habermas added the patients described by Wulff (1932).

Habermas (1989) adopted the same method as Casper, but used as his point of departure reports on patients of normal body weight who experienced bulimia and expressed a fear of obesity. Apart from the article by Wulff, that by Stähelin (1943) deserves mention, if only because it illustrates the dissimilarity between the patient he described and a typical case of modern bulimia nervosa. Stähelin's patient was a 20-year-old woman who, after a sudden suicide attempt, began to devour loaves of bread and sweet foods. This was followed by attempts to vomit. The patient described herself as addicted to food and said that eating provided a form of spiritual numbness as an alternative to suicide. Her periods had ceased for a while, but shortly after their resumption she became hypomanic. She subsequently developed catatonic schizophrenia. Habermas agrees with Casper that the medical literature refers to binge eating, self-induced vomiting, and the abuse of laxatives only seldom before the 1930s. He takes issue, however, with Casper's view that anorexic patients seldom expressed a fear of fatness before the 1960s. He believes that weight concerns occurred in anorexia nervosa from its beginning, but were overlooked by German and British medical writers. However, he gives credit to French physicians—Charcot and Janet in particular—for the observation that the anorexic patient was deeply concerned about her body size. Habermas's thesis is incorrect, as can be seen from Janet's later writings (1920) in which he dismisses the view that anorexic patients were fearful of fatness.

In another attempt to detect early variants of bulimia nervosa, Van Deth and Vandereycken (1995) took as their starting point accounts of hysterical vomiting from the 19th-century medical literature. Aware that the modern diagnostic criteria for bulimia nervosa are probably time- and culture-bound, they concentrated first on the behavioral aspects of bulimia nervosa (overeating and self-induced vomiting or laxative abuse). As noted earlier, they adopted modified criteria for the retrospective identification of bulimic disorders, whereby they deduced the presence of a serious concern about body weight by observing self-induced vomiting or weight unexpectedly remaining within normal limits in spite of episodes of overeating. These authors also found no references to patients' expressing concerns about their weight in 19th-century reports. They concluded that 19th-century hysterical or neurotic vomiting differed from modern forms of bulimia nervosa in several respects. For example, hysterical vomiting was seldom associated with overeating, and they thought it unlikely that such episodes would simply be unnoticed in the majority of vomiting patients. Moreover, clinicians only seldom reported hysterical vomiting that was manifestly self-induced or associated with the abuse of laxatives. They concluded that the sociocultural setting for the development of anorexia nervosa during the 19th century was not a fertile ground for its sister condition, bulimia nervosa.

A search for possible precursors of bulimia nervosa was also undertaken from a review of archives spanning the 17th to the late 19th century (Parry-Jones & Parry-Jones, 1991). The authors conceded that both the lay and medical commentators they studied sometimes indulged in anecdotal sensationalism, but they concluded that pathological voracity had been described consistently for centuries. On the other hand, only 3 of their 12 cases displayed "bulimia emetica," meaning vomiting after having ingested a great quantity of food. There was no evidence of self-induced vomiting, abuse of laxatives or diuretics, or use of dieting or exercise to prevent weight gain. No concern for body shape or weight was revealed in their historical data. They too concluded that the disorders described in their historical cases bore little resemblance to the modern syndrome of bulimia nervosa.

THE MORE CONVINCING FORERUNNERS OF MODERN BULIMIA NERVOSA

The Case of Nadia (Janet, 1903)

From an early age, Nadia expressed shame of her body. At the age of 4, she felt she was too tall; at 8, she said her hands were long and ridiculous; at 11, she felt that everyone looked at her legs. She then wore long skirts but still felt ashamed of her feet, her hips, and her muscular arms. The arrival of her puberty drove her to distraction. She removed her pubic hair because she was convinced that no one but a savage would be burdened with this monstrosity. When her breasts grew, she began to refuse food and to dress in such a manner as to conceal her femininity. Nadia was referred to Janet at the age of 22 with the diagnosis of anorexia nervosa (*anorexie hystérique*). For several years already she had imposed on herself a strict daily regimen: two helpings of clear soup, one egg yolk, one dessert spoon of vinegar, and one cup of very strong tea with the juice of a whole lemon. Although her weight was not mentioned, Janet described her as thin. She gave several reasons for her insistence on remaining thin. She feared becoming fat or appearing muscular or losing her pale complexion; this was not merely a question of vanity, for to become fat would be shameful and immoral. She was also ashamed to be seen or heard eating. Moreover, she believed her face was so ugly that she was reluctant to be seen in the street, and even when indoors she tended to sit in a dark corner. Nadia felt she was extremely brave to resist the temptation to eat, as she often felt ravenous. She spent several hours thinking of food and reading about large meals and banquets. From time to time, she succumbed to her great hunger and ate everything she could with gluttony. Sometimes she ate biscuits in secret. She confessed with guilt that she had allowed herself to taste some of the chocolates she was sending to her friends as Christmas presents. But there was no mention of vomiting.

Janet described repetitive thoughts and actions in his patient. She repeatedly sought reassurance from him: *"M'avez-vous trouvée aussi maigre que les autres fois? Faites-moi le plaisir de me dire que je serai toujours maigre.* [Do you think I'm as thin as the last time? Give me pleasure by saying that I will always be thin.]" (Janet, 1903, p. 37; my translation). When she tasted the chocolates intended as Christmas presents, she wrote more than 10 letters to Janet, as if confessing to a crime and expressing regret for her greed. She asked for reassurance when it appeared to her that the horse could not draw the coach in which she rode, because she had followed Janet's advice to eat some meat cutlets.

It is important to heed Janet's own diagnosis and his interpretation of the psychological mechanisms he elicited in Nadia. First, he was somewhat scathing about the diagnostic concept of anorexia nervosa (*anorexie hystérique*), which he described as superficial and in great need of elucidation. He added that typical anorexia nervosa was not as common as was generally believed. It was partly because of Nadia's extreme hunger and feelings for food that he rejected the diagnosis of anorexia nervosa in her. Instead, he concluded that she suffered primarily from an elaborate obsessional idea.

This idea went beyond a fear of fatness, which he considered too superficial to do justice to Nadia's illness. Its ramifications were wider, including sexual modesty (*craintes de la pudeur*), guilt, and shame of the entire body (*la honte du corps*). Janet's description of an obsessional shame of one's body has found a recent echo in the concept of "body disparagement" (Hsu & Sobkiewicz, 1991). In his exploration of Nadia's psychopathology, Janet elicited her reasons for her obsessional body shame: She wanted to remain a little girl for ever. And why? Nadia answered, *"Parce-que j'avais peur d'être moins aimée.* [Because I was afraid of not being loved as much]" (Janet, 1903, p. 40; my translation).

Janet's Nadia has been judged to be a worthy early example of bulimic attacks by Habermas (1989) and a true early description of bulimia by Pope, Hudson and Mialet (1985), meaning bulimia as defined in DSM-III.

The Case of Patient D (Wulff, 1932)

Wulff reported on four young women who experienced irresistible cravings for food, describing his fourth patient (Patient D) in greatest detail. This patient was first seen by Wulff when she was in her middle 20s, but he traced her obsessional neurosis (his primary diagnosis) to her earliest years. Her mother had died during her birth, and she was brought up by her father, together with her brother (who was older by 2 years). The father, a doctor, imposed a tyrannical dietary regimen to which Wulff attributed the first signs of obsessional behavior—a compulsion to collect dolls and dolls' clothing. During her play, the 5-year-old child imposed on her dolls the same orderly regimen as she suffered at the hands of her father. When she was aged 13, her world fell apart through the remarriage of her father. She acquired a string of young admirers who were expected to prove their devotion with presents of sweets and fruit. At 16 she married in spite of her father's opposition, but sought to impose on her husband a sexless marriage. When this failed, the couple separated and she once again acquired a string of admirers. Following the final separation from her husband, she went through periods of powerful cravings for food lasting 3 weeks, alternating with shorter periods of complete fasting. When overeating she consumed huge amounts of food, including pounds of confectionery, chocolate, and pastries. Her abdomen would swell, and the overeating often ended with abdominal pains and vomiting. She took castor oil to "cleanse" herself. During the phases of overeating she experienced deep depression, neglected herself, and slept a great deal. She expressed disgust with herself and slept in her dirty clothes so as to avoid catching sight of her body, which she considered disgustingly fat. When the overeating ceased, she fasted for about 3 days and rapidly lost weight Then she felt a return of happiness and inner cleanliness.

Wulff's diagnoses and interpretations were multiple and complex. In all four of his patients, he considered that he had come across a "symptom complex" that was not tied to any established psychiatric disorder, but could appear in a wide range of neuroses and represented a peculiar pathological alteration of biological function. He compared and contrasted the eating disorder with melancholic depression, and concluded that the patient's disgust with her own body was the direct result of her overeating. He saw a close relationship between the craving for food and other addictions, and described it as *"Ess sucht"* ("craving for eating") (Wulff, 1932, pp. 291, 293). Wulff believed that the disorder had been initiated by a loss of love, leading to depression and cravings for food and sleep. When the cravings for food were gratified, there arose strong feelings of self-disgust and despair. He also proposed a sexual symbolism for the eating disorder: He believed that the eaten objects (especially sweets, bread, and meat) had an unconscious association with the forbidden penis.

Patient D (like two of Wulff's other three patients) had had sexual experiences with her older brother during her earliest childhood. This and other family experiences, in Wulff's view, led to a disposition to oral regression.

Wulff's account is not often quoted, but Habermas (1989) and Stunkard (1990) considered that his patients shared many features of bulimia nervosa: binge eating alternating with fasting, a strong disgust with one's body, and (in the case of Patient D) frequent vomiting.

The Case of Ellen West (Binswanger, 1944–1945)

The story of Ellen West was told by Binswanger (1958) in a detailed biographical account, extending from her early life until her death at the age of 33. From the age of 10 Ellen lived in Switzerland, the daughter of Jewish parents who probably came from North America. She was intelligent, read widely, and wrote poetry. Entries in her diary expressed doubts about the purpose of life. She was fascinated with the sentence "Those whom the Gods love die young." Her early poems already revealed a marked variability of mood. Ellen had a strongly positive family history of depression and suicide on both sides of her family.

It was in her 20th year, after a second trip overseas, that Ellen lost the capacity to eat unconcernedly. While on a holiday she gained some weight, and her girlfriends teased her for being fat. That same year she developed a dread of becoming fat, avoided food, and went on long hikes. Her family expressed concern at her appearance on her return home. For the next 3 years, she experienced severe mood swings closely associated with eating disturbances. At 23, her dread of becoming fat was accompanied by an intense longing for food, especially sweets. At 24, she became severely depressed and became more determined to become thin, again taking long hikes and swallowing 36–48 thyroid tablets daily; this indeed led her to become thin, with trembling limbs. The next year she was treated for hyperthyroidism with bed rest, which led her to regain weight to 75 kg. At the age of 28 she married her cousin. On her wedding day she weighed 73 kg. She dieted during her honeymoon and again took thyroid periodically. Her periods ceased for a while, but at the age of 29 she had a miscarriage, followed again by the cessation of menstruation.

It was from her 30th year that Ellen became frankly ill, with increased eating disturbances. She became a vegetarian, increased her dosage of laxatives, and vomited every night. At the age of 31 she was still able to work, but studied calorie charts and recipes incessantly. When her weight had dropped to 45 kg, she agreed to enter a sanatorium for metabolic diseases. At first she gained weight to 50 kg, but was later found to be dropping food into her handbag and carrying weights on her person when she was weighed. By the age of 32 she had deteriorated further. She took 60–70 laxative tablets daily, which caused vomiting at night and diarrhea during the day. Her weight had fallen to 42 kg. She expressed her concern about her body size: "As soon as I feel a pressure at my waist, I mean the pressure of my waistband—my spirit sinks" (p. 251). She was prone to miss meals, but each day she consumed several pounds of tomatoes and 20 oranges. Soon after her 33rd birthday,

she developed severe depression with weeping, dread, and agitation. There followed drug overdoses and suicide attempts, such as throwing herself in front of a car. She was admitted to a medical clinic. At first she agreed to eat everything put before her, and her weight increased slowly to 52 kg in 2 months, but later she resumed repeated vomiting and occasional use of laxatives. After a brief improvement she relapsed into deeper depression and was seen by Kraepelin, who diagnosed melancholia.

The following month she was admitted to a psychiatric sanatorium at Kreuzlingen. During her 2½-month stay, disturbances of eating were prominent. She was described as devouring food like a wild animal, and yet her weight had fallen to 47 kg by the date of discharge. This was presumably because of continued vomiting, as it was observed that her salivary glands were much enlarged. (Binswanger was unaware that swollen salivary glands could result from vomiting; he thought that this sign indicated an endocrine disturbance [p. 360].) She continued to take laxatives. Her basic mood was one of despair. She expressed physical emptiness and longed for death. Shortly before her discharge she made serious suicidal threats. Binswanger obtained two further independent opinions, including that of Eugen Bleuler. The three psychiatrists thought that no reliable therapy was possible, and they acceded to Ellen's request to be discharged home. On her third day at home, Ellen ate more freely—so much so that for the first time in 13 years she felt satisfied and really full. In the afternoon she ate coffee creams and Easter eggs. In the evening she went for a walk with her husband and read poetry. She appeared cheerful. Later that evening, however, she took a lethal dose of poison, and on the following morning she was dead.

An attempt is made here to convey the flavor of Binswanger's existential analysis, his psychopathological analysis, and his approach to the diagnosis of Ellen West. These cover some 90 pages. What did he deduce from his existential analysis of two of the salient clinical features—the patient's "gluttony" (his term for "bulimia" [p. 343]) and her "dread of becoming fat" (the patient's own expression) (p. 280)? He discussed whether the gluttony should be considered an addiction. He viewed the gluttony as "an existential craving, a need to fill up an existential vacuum" (p. 346). He went on to say that his analysis had revealed the dread of becoming fat as a concretization of "a severe existential dread—the dread of withering whereby the world of the self becomes a tomb, a hole" (p. 349). He further discussed whether the dread of becoming fat might be a compulsion, a phobia, an overvalued idea, or a delusional idea. On the whole, he rejected all these psychopathological categories. When he approached the diagnosis of Ellen West's illness, he began by rejecting Kraepelin's opinion that she suffered from a manic–depressive psychosis, mainly because she did not go through phasic manic–depressive upsets. He argued further that the case history did not fit into a pathological personality development, because he did not believe that it could be understood as a remodeling of the patient's personality interacting with her environment. He finally concluded that Ellen West's illness consisted of a disease process (in the Jasperian sense)—namely, a special form of schizophrenia. In reaching this diagnosis, he had the support of Eugen Bleuler. Binswanger described it as the "polymorphous form of schizophrenia simplex" (p. 356) (meaning neurosis-like, with vague and multiple symptoms).

Binswanger referred to anorexia nervosa only in an oblique manner. He briefly mentioned "a form of pituitary cachexia," (p. 361) only to dismiss it because Ellen West's loss of weight was intentional and she displayed no true anorexia. A glimpse into his diagnostic leanings is provided by this quotation: "Much too often neuroses are diagnosed when we should already speak of a psychosis, and I still side with E. Bleuler when he declares that he 'regards the concepts of the neuroses as artefacts if they are not to count merely as symptom-complexes'" (p. 362).

It is also necessary to comment on Binswanger's therapeutic nihilism, which led him to allow Ellen West's discharge from the Kreuzlingen clinic, even though he felt certain that the patient would kill herself (p. 266). His reasoning stemmed from having diagnosed a progressive schizophrenic psychosis; hence he "could offer the husband very little hope." He added that "no definitely reliable therapy is possible" (p. 266). I have to conclude that although Binswanger was a careful clinical observer, this quality was not matched by the necessary qualities of compassion and therapeutic imagination. In mitigation, I should point out that Ellen West's final illness must have occurred well before 1926 (i.e., about 20 years before the publication of Binswanger's monograph). As he pointed out, this was a time when electroshock and cardiazol shock were unavailable. He mentioned that such treatment might have been attempted, although his pessimism led him to add that: "it could have been merely a question of postponing the final catastrophe" (p. 362).

Were Nadia, Patient D, and Ellen West Examples of Bulimia Nervosa?

If we simply consider the three basic diagnostic criteria of bulimia nervosa, they are amply satisfied by the case histories of Nadia (Janet, 1903), Patient D (Wulff, 1932), and Ellen West (Binswanger, 1944–1945). The requisite clinical features are summarized in the left-hand column of Table 2.1. The occurrence of a phase of anorexia nervosa, judged by weight loss during a stage of the illness, strengthens the view that the patient indeed had a disorder resembling bulimia nervosa. Nadia had first been diag-

TABLE 2.1. Evidence That Three Well-Described Patients Were True Forerunners of Bulimia Nervosa Patients

Clinical features	Janet (1903): Nadia	Wulff (1932): Patient D	Binswanger (1944–1945): Ellen West
Overeating	Great hunger	Periodic craving for eating	Gluttony
Compensatory behaviors	Fasting	Vomiting Castor oil Fasting	Thyroid tablets Laxatives Vomiting Fasting
Dread of fatness	Shame of body (*honte du corps*)	Disgust with fat body (*Ekelhafter Leib*)	Dread of becoming fat (*Angst*)
Phase of anorexia nervosa	In early course	No	In late course
Primary diagnosis	Obsessional neurosis	Obsessional neurosis	?schizophrenia,[a] ?melancholia[b]

[a]Diagnosis by Binswanger and Bleuler.
[b]Diagnosis by Kraepelin.

nosed as having anorexia nervosa, though Janet was not impressed. Ellen West was amenorrheic during the last 4 years of her illness, and during the last 18 months of her life she became severely underweight. Thus she is an interesting example of anorexia nervosa's appearing late in the course of an eating disorder that commenced with a protracted bulimic phase. So far, all three case histories fit reasonably well into the modern syndrome of bulimia nervosa. But there is a major reservation: In all three patients, there was a primary diagnosis of a severe psychiatric illness that more or less eclipsed the eating disorder. This was least so in Wulff's Patient D, who had an obsessional illness intertwined with periodic overeating. In the case of Janet's Nadia, her severe body disparagement began in early childhood and led to a more general limitation of her life than is usual in bulimia nervosa. Of the three, Ellen West probably suffered the most; the illness severely limited her activities, assumed the form of a psychosis (even if one questions Binswanger's diagnosis), and cost her her life. These are unusual associations and outcomes in bulimia nervosa.

DESCRIPTION OF BULIMIA NERVOSA IN THE 1970s

During the 1970s, there appeared clinical case reports in the literature closely resembling those that subsequently earned the diagnostic label of bulimia nervosa. Brusset and Jeammet (1971) carefully described three young patients in whom overeating alternated with undereating in the course of anorexia nervosa. One patient vomited and the other two took laxatives; two of them expressed bodily shame or fear of fatness. Boskind-Lodahl (1976) provided some clinical sketches selected from 138 "binger–starvers" or "bulimarexics" who responded to an advertisement placed in a university newspaper. These subjects reported "fasting, habitual forced vomiting, amphetamine and laxative abuse" (Boskind-Lodahl, 1976, p. 351). A distorted concept of body size was also mentioned. These two articles had but little influence on the conceptualization of eating disorders or their classification. Apart from the usual caprices that influence the recognition of significant observations in medical writings, there may have been other reasons for the relative lack of impact of these two articles. They were less concerned with the presentation of clinical data and more with etiological explanations—a psychoanalytic interpretation by Brusset and Jeammet, and a psychodynamic feminist perspective by Boskind-Lodahl.

My own series of 30 patients (Russell, 1979) was obtained between 1972 and 1978 from referrals to the psychiatric department of a general hospital. The most dramatic disturbance was often the patients' self-induced vomiting, but it was soon observed that this was a compensatory reaction to episodes of overeating. The patients disclosed that they vomited in order to mitigate the fattening effects of the food they ingested in large amounts. Three sets of disturbances were thus revealed: (1) intractable urges to overeat; (2) avoidance of the fattening effects of food by vomiting and/or abusing purgatives; and (3) a morbid fear of becoming fat. These disturbances were considered to be interdependent, with the fear of fatness fueling the other abnormal behaviors. The three disturbances were put forward as the diagnostic criteria of a new syndrome, differing in several respects from anorexia nervosa, but linked to it by virtue of sharing the same morbid fear of fatness. The other link was the observation that in cases of bulimia nervosa there had often been a previous episode of anorexia nervosa, albeit of mild severity. The close relationship with anorexia nervosa was enshrined in the name given to the new disorder—"bulimia nervosa" (Russell, 1979).

When DSM-III was published (APA, 1980), it included a new disorder termed "bulimia." In many ways this was an important landmark, but "bulimia" differed in important respects from "bulimia nervosa." First, insufficient emphasis was given to the specific psychological disturbance of the disorder—namely, the patient's pervasive dread of fatness. Second, the diagnosis excluded patients in whom the bulimic episodes were attributable to anorexia nervosa. Thus there was a failure to allow for the relationship between the two disorders. These criticisms were subsequently met in DSM-III-R (APA, 1987) and in the 10th revision of the *International Classification of Diseases* (ICD-10, World Health Organization, 1992), since when there has been broad international agreement on the status of bulimia nervosa as a diagnostic entity.

THE APPEARANCE OF BULIMIA NERVOSA AS A NEW DISORDER

From the evidence that has been presented, it is clear that bulimia nervosa, as it is recognized by today's clinicians, was virtually unknown until the latter half of the 20th century. The exceptions to this statement might be the patients described by Wulff (1932), Binswanger (1944–1945), and Janet (1903), in that order of credibility. Patients appeared in the 1970s, and thereafter the disorder became relatively common. The statement that bulimia nervosa was rare before the 1970s needs to be qualified, as it is correct when the full disorder is being considered. For a long time, there had been observations from reputable sources that overeating and self-induced vomiting may have been common practices among otherwise normal young female students at North American universities (A. J. Stunkard, cited in Russell, 1979). (Then, as now, the individuals in whom these behaviors were observed were nearly always female.) The subjects recruited by Boskind-Lodahl through an advertisement for "bingers–purgers" may have been examples of this less serious condition. But there is no doubt that the incidence of true bulimia nervosa increased during the 1980s and came to exceed that of anorexia nervosa (Fairburn & Beglin, 1990; Hoek, 1991; Hall & Hay, 1991).

It is important to adduce further evidence that bulimia nervosa has only occurred during comparatively recent times, because skeptics all too readily suppose that the disorder was overlooked by clinicians prior to its description in 1979. Two studies within recent years have indeed given evidence to this effect, and they are now summarized.

The first study was by Kendler et al. (1991), who interviewed 2,163 female subjects from a population-based twin register in Virginia. (The fact that they were twins is unimportant to the present argument.) Within this population, 60 subjects were given a definite or probable diagnosis of bulimia nervosa according to DSM-III-R criteria. The "lifetime prevalence" of bulimia nervosa was calculated as the proportion of individuals who merited the diagnosis at some time in their lives. The lifetime cumulative risk for definite or probable bulimia nervosa is shown in Figure 2.1 and is represented by three curves: for patients born before 1950, for those born between 1950 and 1959, and for those born after 1959. The three curves are clearly separated, thus demonstrating a cohort effect. The older subjects (born before 1950) were much less likely to have had bulimia nervosa than the younger subjects (born after 1959). The subjects of intermediate age had an intermediate risk for the disorder. The conclusions of Kendler and his colleagues were extremely cautious, and they were uncertain whether

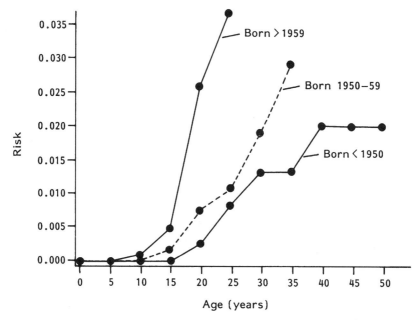

FIGURE 2.1. The lifetime cumulative risk for definite or probable bulimia nervosa in three cohorts in Virginia. From Kendler et al. (1991). Copyright 1991 by the American Psychiatric Association. Reprinted by permission.

their observation of a lower rate among the older subjects was attributable to an artifact (the older subjects might have been less aware of bulimia as a disorder, or they might have forgotten their bulimia). These cautious explanations are possible, but it is more credible that the older subjects reported less bulimia nervosa precisely because the disorder was uncommon before the 1970s, when they would have been at the age of risk for the disorder. In conclusion, this study has demonstrated a true cohort effect, confirming the relative rarity of bulimia nervosa before the 1970s.

The second study was that of Lucas and Soundy (1993) and was based on the Mayo Clinic Epidemiological Archives. These are probably the best clinical records in the world, and provide medical data for the entire population residing in Rochester, Minnesota (population 60,000 in 1985). The notes were searched for clinical descriptions of patients who would have merited a diagnosis of bulimia nervosa according to modern criteria. The findings are shown schematically in Figure 2.2; the solid curve shows the documented incidence of bulimia nervosa among the female population. The following should be noted:

1. Before 1980 a very small number of cases

were identified, and they were unusual (e.g., overweight men or infants who had been overfed). After the description of bulimia nervosa in 1979 and of bulimia in DSM-III in 1980, there was a sharp rise in detected cases. The curve in Figure 2.2 reaches a plateau indicating an incidence of 26.5 cases per year per 100,000 of the female population (Soundy, Lucas, Suman, & Melton, 1995). This is twice the incidence of anorexia nervosa.

2. The peak in 1983 is partly an artifact resulting from a drug trial that led the researchers to "solicit" for patients with bulimia nervosa.

This research confirms that bulimia nervosa appeared suddenly in the late 1970s, but several of the patients interviewed by Lucas and Soundy (1993) gave long histories, so that they must have acquired their illness some time previously. The dotted curves in Figure 2.2 are speculative, indicating the growing incidence of bulimia nervosa before it was recognized formally. The lower dotted curve corresponds approximately with the rates of detection of my own patients, beginning in 1972. However, it is more likely that the speculative upper curve is applicable, suggesting a slowly rising incidence several years before the appearance of cases in the 1970s.

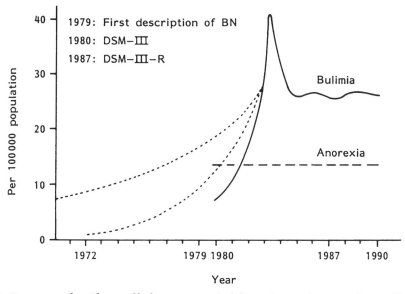

FIGURE 2.2. Documented incidence of bulimia nervosa (solid curve), speculative incidence of bulimia nervosa (dotted curves), and documented incidence of anorexia nervosa (dashed line) in the Mayo Clinic Epidemiological Archives. Adapted from Soundy, Lucas, Suman, & Melton (1995). Reprinted by permission from Russell (1995). Copyright 1995 by John Wiley & Sons, Ltd.

In conclusion, cases of bulimia nervosa probably occurred before the 1970s, but in far smaller numbers than are seen today.

DISCUSSION AND CONCLUSIONS

Bulimia, meaning simply overeating, has been known since antiquity. From a medico-historical point of view, it is of little interest. The history of bulimia nervosa is a different matter. In the introduction, I have referred to the annoying fact that the term "bulimia nervosa" cannot be applied, strictly speaking, to case histories published before 1979, as this was when the term was coined and applied to patients with a distinctive disorder. This linguistic objection has not deterred writers from searching for earlier descriptions of patients who might have been afflicted with conditions resembling post-1979 bulimia nervosa. This is entirely reasonable, so long as they can distinguish this specific disorder from nonspecific conditions such as bulimia. The present review has been mainly confined to case histories with some claim that they resemble modern bulimia nervosa. They raise legitimate questions. Is bulimia nervosa a new disorder? Can its history be traced back to earlier historical times? When Stunkard (1990) summarized in English the case reports by Wulff (1932), he concluded that "bulimia is not exclusively a modern disorder" (p. 268), so convinced was he that these patients closely resembled patients with the modern disorder. Incidentally, Stunkard studiously avoided any reference to bulimia nervosa, using the word "bulimia" throughout, and thereby failing to distinguish between the symptom and the disorder. In spite of this limitation, Stunkard makes this important historical point: "Unlike anorexia nervosa, for which a rich history has been traced to the Middle Ages, bulimia seems to have burst from the blue upon modern society, and it has achieved widespread recognition in a very short period of time" (p. 263).

When one is searching the literature for case histories resembling bulimia nervosa, it is as well to apply a set of strict requirements to justify a distinctive disorder. Apart from the three diagnostic criteria identified in 1979, it is necessary to establish that the illness is primarily an eating disorder, with a previous history of anorexia nervosa or at least intensive dieting behavior. Moreover, the illness should not be secondary to, or even associated with, another severe psychiatric illness. When these strict requirements are used, the only early descriptions of patients who pass the test are those by Wulff (1932), Binswanger (1944–1945), and Janet (1903), in that order of credibility. A larger series of case histories was put forward by Casper (1983) and especially by Habermas (1989, 1992). Credit must go to Casper, who in 1983 was the first to pose the important historical questions: Was bulimia (nervosa) observed and had it existed as a clinical entity before 1960? What kind of factors could have contributed to its recent rise? She observed that hardly any comments on overeating in the course of anorexia nervosa appeared between 1890 and 1940. She also noted that later on, Bruch (1962) and Thomä (1967) were both aware of overeating among anorexia nervosa patients; yet both considered this behavior to be a variant in the eating pattern of anorexic patients, rather than a distinct syndrome. As regards the etiological factors giving rise to the upsurge of bulimia nervosa, Casper put forward two compelling ideas. First, the increase of bulimia nervosa has probably been dependent on the greater frequency of patients' expressing their concern about their body shape in case reports written after 1940. The same argument has also been put forward to validate the view that anorexia nervosa has gradually changed over recent decades (Russell, 1984, 1985, 1993, 1995; Russell & Treasure, 1989). Casper's second idea was that bulimia nervosa recruits a "psychologically different type of girl or woman from the traditional anorexia nervosa patient" (p. 13). She suggested that they have more affective instability, more extroversion, greater interpersonal sensitivity, and greater impulse dyscontrol. There is indeed increasing evidence that different personality disorders are associated with bulimia nervosa, compared with anorexia nervosa (Halmi, 1995). The tendency to impulsivity in some of these patients finds its expression in the severe form of multi-impulsive bulimia nervosa, delineated by Lacey (1993).

My own view is that bulimia nervosa is indeed a new illness, notwithstanding its emergence from anorexia nervosa, and the very occasional description of similar patients in the pre-1979 literature (Russell, 1979, 1985, 1993, 1995). This view is endorsed by Casper (1983), by Van Deth and Vandereycken (1995), and, more grudgingly, by Habermas (1990, p. 216). My views about the causation of the upsurge of bulimia nervosa must remain tentative and could be seen as an extension of Casper's thesis, inasmuch as an all-pervasive preoccupation with body size is a relatively new phenomenon in patients with both anorexia nervosa and bulimia nervosa. It is precisely these morbid preoccupations that are most congruent with today's social "cult of thinness," pervasive in Westernized societies (Russell, 1993). The dangers of the resulting social pressures have been widely recognized (Garner, Garfinkel, Schwartz, & Thompson, 1980; Brumberg, 1988). Women respond to them by experimenting with weight-reducing diets. Anorexia nervosa is arguably an extension of extreme dietary behaviors, and bulimia nervosa can also be viewed as an escape or rebound from dietary restraint to binge eating (Blundell, 1990). To such partial explanations should be added the likelihood that Casper is correct in supposing that women prone to bulimia nervosa are "psychologically different" from those vulnerable to anorexia nervosa. Different genetic predispositions to the two disorders have also been proposed by Treasure and Holland (1995).

SUMMARY

1. Bulimia (meaning simply, episodic overeating) has been recognized since antiquity. It is not relevant to the important historical issues regarding the origins or newness of the syndrome bulimia nervosa.
2. Bulimia nervosa is a distinctive disorder that was identified in the late 1970s but presumably commenced at some uncertain period between the 1940s and 1960s. At first, bulimia nervosa was closely associated with anorexia nervosa, but gradually the two disorders became partly separate.
3. Bulimia nervosa is a new disorder. Very few case histories resembling modern bulimia nervosa before the 1940s have come to light, although the descriptions by Wulff, Binswanger, and Janet are close approximations.
4. The description of bulimia nervosa must have facilitated the recognition of the characteristic phenomena by clinicians, but this provides only a partial explanation for the sudden rise of the disorder.
5. The modern "cult of thinness" has exerted powerful and harmful effects on young women and has determined the frequency, clinical form, and psychological con-

tent of both anorexia and bulimia nervosa. Additional etiological factors are considered to be responsible for the differences between the two disorders.

REFERENCES

American Psychiatric Association (APA). (1980). *Diagnostic and statistical manual of mental disorders* (3rd ed.). Washington, DC: Author.

American Psychiatric Association (APA). (1987). *Diagnostic and statistical manual of mental disorders* (3rd ed., rev.). Washington, DC: Author.

American Psychiatric Association (APA). (1994). *Diagnostic and statistical manual of mental disorders* (4th ed.). Washington, DC: Author.

Bell, R. M. (1985). *Holy anorexia.* Chicago: University of Chicago Press.

Binswanger, L. (1944–1945). Der Fall Ellen West. *Schweizer Archiv für Neurologie und Psychiatrie, 53,* 255–277 (1944); *54,* 69–117 (1944); *55,* 16–40 (1945).

Binswanger, L. (1958). The case of Ellen West: An anthropological–clinical study (W. M. Mendel & J. Lyons, Trans.). In R. May, E. Angel, & H. F. Ellenberger (Eds.), *Existence: A new dimension in psychiatry and psychology* (pp. 237–364). New York: Basic Books. (The page numbering in the chapter is in accord with the translated text.)

Bliss, E. L., & Branch, C. H. (1960). *Anorexia nervosa: Its history, psychology and biology.* New York: Hoeber.

Blundell, J. E. (1990). How culture undermines the biopsychological system of appetite control. *Appetite, 14,* 113–115.

Boskind-Lodahl, M. (1976). Cinderella's stepsisters: A feminist perspective on anorexia nervosa and bulimia. *Journal of Women in Culture and Society, 2,* 342–356.

Bruch, H. (1962). Perceptual and conceptual disturbances in anorexia nervosa. *Psychosomatic Medicine, 24,* 187–194.

Brumberg, J. J. (1988). *Fasting girls: The emergence of anorexia nervosa as a modern disease.* Cambridge, MA: Harvard University Press.

Brusset, B., & Jeammet, P. (1971). Les périodes boulimiques dans l'évolution de l'anoréxie mentale de l'adolescente. *Revue de Neuropsychiatrie Infantile, 19,* 661–690.

Casper, R. A. (1983). On the emergence of bulimia nervosa as a syndrome: A historical view. *International Journal of Eating Disorders, 2*(3), 3–16.

Crichton, P. (1996). Were the Roman emperors Claudius and Vitellius bulimic? *International Journal of Eating Disorders, 19,* 203–207.

Fairburn, C. G., & Beglin, S. J. (1990). Studies of the epidemiology of bulimia nervosa. *American Journal of Psychiatry, 147,* 401–408.

Garner, D. M., Garfinkel, P. E., Schwartz, D., & Thompson, M. (1980). Cultural expectations of thinness in women. *Psychological Reports, 47,* 483–491.

Gull, W. W. (1874). Anorexia nervosa (apepsia hysterica, anorexia hysterica). *Transactions of the Clinical Society of London, 7,* 22–28.

Habermas, T. (1989). The psychiatric history of anorexia nervosa and bulimia nervosa: weight concerns and bulimic symptoms in early case reports. *International Journal of Eating Disorders, 8,* 259–273.

Habermas, T. (1990). *Heisshunger: Historische Bedingungen der Bulimia Nervosa.* Frankfurt: Fischer Taschenbuch.

Habermas, T. (1992). Further evidence on early case descriptions of anorexia and bulimia nervosa. *International Journal of Eating Disorders, 11,* 351–359.

Hall, A., & Hay, P. J. (1991). Eating disorder patient referrals from a population region, 1977–1986. *Psychological Medicine, 21,* 697–701.

Halmi, K. A. (1995). Current concepts and definitions. In G. Szmukler, C. Dare, & J. Treasure (Eds.), *Handbook of eating disorders: Theory, treatment and research* (pp. 29–42). Chichester, England: Wiley.

Hoek, H. W. (1991). The incidence and prevalence of anorexia nervosa and bulimia nervosa. *Psychological Medicine, 21,* 455–460.

Hsu, L. K. G., & Sobkiewicz, T. A. (1991). Body image disturbance: Time to abandon the concept for eating disorders? *International Journal of Eating Disorders, 10,* 15–30.

Janet, P. (1903). *Les obsessions et la psychasthénie: Vol. 1, Section 5. L'obsession de la honte du corps.* Paris: Germer Baillière.

Janet, P. (1965). Lecture XI. In *The major symptoms of hysteria* (2nd enlarged ed. [facsimile of 1st ed.], pp. 227–244). New York: Hafner.

Kaplan, A. S., & Garfinkel, P. E. (1984). Bulimia in the Talmud. *American Journal of Psychiatry, 141,* 721.

Kendler, K. S., Maclean, C., Neale, M. Kessler, R., Heath, A., & Eaves, L. (1991). The genetic epidemiology of bulimia nervosa. *American Journal of Psychiatry, 148,* 1627–1637.

Lacey, J. H. (1993). Self-damaging and addictive behaviour in bulimia nervosa: A catchment area study. *British Journal of Psychiatry, 163,* 190–194.

Lasègue, C. (1873). De l'anoréxie hystérique. *Archives Générales de Médecine, 21,* 385–403.

Lucas, A. R., & Soundy, T. J. (1993). The rise of bulimia nervosa. *World Psychiatric Association Book of Abstracts: Ninth World Congress of Psychiatry, Rio de Janeiro, Brazil, 6–12 June* (Abstract 544, p. 139).

Nasser, M. (1993). A prescription of vomiting: Historical footnotes. *International Journal of Eating Disorders, 13,* 129–131.

Nemiah, J. C. (1950). Anorexia nervosa: A clinical psychiatric study. *Medicine, 29,* 225–268.

Parry-Jones, B., & Parry-Jones, W. L. (1991). Bulimia: An archival review of its history in psychosomatic medicine. *International Journal of Eating Disorders, 10,* 129–143.

Pope, H. G., Hudson, J. I., & Mialet, J.-P. (1985). Bulimia in the late nineteenth century: The observations of Pierre Janet. *Psychological Medicine, 15,* 739–743.

Pullar, P. (1972). *Consuming passions: A history of English food and appetite.* London: Sphere Books.

Rampling, D. (1985). Ascetic ideals and anorexia nervosa. *Journal of Psychiatric Research, 19,* 89–94.

Russell, G. F. M. (1979). Bulimia nervosa: An ominous variant of anorexia nervosa. *Psychological Medicine, 9,* 429–448.

Russell, G. F. M. (1984). The modern history of anorexia nervosa. *Aktuelle Ernährungsmedizin, 9,* 3–7.

Russell, G. F. M. (1985). The changing nature of anorexia nervosa: An introduction to the conference. *Journal of Psychiatric Research, 19,* 101–109.

Russell, G. F. M. (1993). Social psychiatry of eating disorders. In D. Bhugra & J. Leff (Eds.), *Principles of social psychiatry* (pp. 273–297). Oxford: Blackwell Scientific.

Russell, G. F. M. (1995). Anorexia nervosa through time. In G. Szmukler, C. Dare, & J. Treasure (Eds.), *Handbook of eating disorders: Theory, treatment and research* (pp. 5–17). Chichester, England: Wiley.

Russell, G. F. M., & Treasure, J. (1989). The modern history of anorexia nervosa: An interpretation of why the illness has changed. *Annals of the New York Academy of Sciences, 575,* 13–30.

Soundy, T. J., Lucas, A. R., Suman, V. J., & Melton, L. J. (1995). Bulimia nervosa in Rochester, Minnesota from 1980 to 1990. *Psychological Medicine, 25,* 1065–1071.

Stähelin, J. E. (1943). Ueber präschizophrene Somatose. *Schweizerische Medizinische Wochenschrift, 39,* 1213–1215.

Stunkard, A. (1990). A description of eating disorders in 1932. *American Journal of Psychiatry, 147,* 263–268.

Thomä, H. (1967). *Anorexia nervosa* (G. Brydone, Trans.). New York: International Universities Press.

Treasure, J., & Holland, A. (1995). Genetic factors in eating disorders. In G. Szmukler, C. Dare, & J. Treasure (Eds.), *Handbook of eating disorders: Theory, treatment and research* (pp. 65–81). Chichester, England: Wiley.

Vandereycken, W. (1985). "Bulimia" has different meanings [Letter]. *American Journal of Psychiatry, 142,* 141–142.

Van Deth, R., & Vandereycken, W. (1995). Was late 19th century nervous vomiting an early variant of bulimia nervosa? *History of Psychiatry, vi,* 333–347.

World Health Organization. (1992). *The ICD-10 classification of mental and behavioural disorders: Clinical descriptions and diagnostic guidelines.* Geneva: Author.

Waller, J. V., Kaufman, M. R., & Deutsch, F. (1940). Anorexia nervosa: A psychosomatic entity. *Psychosomatic Medicine, 2,* 3–16.

Wulff, M. (1932). Ueber einen interessanten oralen symptomen-komplex und seine Beziehung zur Sucht. *Internationale Zeitschrift für Psychoanalyse, 18,* 281–302.

Ziolko, H. U., & Schrader, H. C. (1985). Bulimie. *Fortschrift Neurologie und Psychiatrie, 53,* 231–258.

CHAPTER 3

Diagnostic Issues

B. TIMOTHY WALSH
DAVID M. GARNER

Why should a chapter on diagnosis appear in a treatment-oriented handbook for eating disorders? Ideally, the process of diagnosis should go beyond simply describing a clinical entity. It should convey some understanding of the pathological process or the underlying cause of a disorder (Russell, 1988). Recent changes in the diagnostic nomenclature for eating disorders, such as the *Diagnostic and Statistical Manual of Mental Disorders,* fourth edition (DSM-IV; American Psychiatric Association [APA], 1994), and the *International Classification of Diseases,* 10th revision (ICD-10; World Health Organization [WHO], 1992), are evolutionary rather than revolutionary; however, they do convey improved understanding of clinical features. These diagnostic criteria are also relevant because they both formally define and distinguish the two major eating disorders, anorexia nervosa and bulimia nervosa. By drawing the boundaries for these eating disorders, the current criteria will have a substantial effect on clinical care and research.

DSM-IV also delineates a large and heterogeneous diagnostic category, "eating disorder not otherwise specified" (EDNOS), for individuals who have clinically significant eating disorders but who fail to meet all of the diagnostic criteria for anorexia nervosa or bulimia nervosa. Unfortunately, the term "not otherwise specified" could be interpreted as connoting eating problems of minor clinical significance. This assumption is incorrect, since the clinical picture for many individuals with EDNOS can be every bit as complicated and serious as that for persons with the two main eating disorders. Binge-

eating disorder is a specific example of an EDNOS included in DSM-IV (it appears in Appendix B as a criteria set "provided for further study"). This term has been proposed to apply to individuals who display a number of characteristics of bulimia nervosa, but who do not regularly engage in the inappropriate compensatory behaviors, such as self-induced vomiting, required for the diagnosis of bulimia nervosa. Other examples of EDNOS have received less attention but are of clear clinical importance. Terms such as "bulimia," "compulsive eating," and "normal weight bulimia," often used to describe eating disorders, do not appear in DSM-IV. Other diagnostic terms such as "anorexia nervosa, binge-eating/purging type," are new with the introduction of DSM-IV. Thus, a brief review of the current diagnostic terminology should be a helpful preface to the clinical chapters in this volume. A review of the diagnostic criteria for anorexia nervosa and bulimia nervosa is followed by a discussion of binge-eating disorder and other examples of EDNOS provided in DSM-IV.

ANOREXIA NERVOSA

A. Refusal to maintain body weight at or above a minimally normal weight for age and height . . .

Criterion A has two fundamental aspects. First, individuals with anorexia nervosa are required to be significantly underweight. Precisely what constitutes "significantly underweight" is left to the clinician's judgment, but DSM-IV provides, as a suggested guideline, weighing less than 85% of that expected. Although this guideline is a clinically useful one, it should not be interpreted rigidly. That is, if an individual meets all other criteria for anorexia nervosa, but weighs 90% of his or her expected weight, the clinician should still feel free to make the diagnosis of anorexia nervosa.

The ICD-10 diagnostic criteria for research provide a somewhat different guideline for the degree of underweight required for anorexia nervosa (WHO, 1992). The ICD-10 criterion is that the individual have a body mass index (the weight in kilograms divided by the height in meters squared) equal to or less than 17.5 kg/m^2. This guideline is a stricter one than the 85% of expected weight suggested by DSM-IV.

Most individuals with anorexia nervosa are of normal body weight prior to the onset of illness, and become underweight through a combination of strict dieting, exercise, and often the use of purging techniques, diuretics, or diet pills. Some individuals, however, develop anorexia nervosa during early adolescence; rather than losing weight, they simply fail to gain weight while their height increases, and thereby become significantly underweight (see Lask & Bryant-Waugh, Chapter 28, this volume).

The other essential aspect of Criterion A for anorexia nervosa is that the person wishes to be underweight and makes conscious attempts to avoid gaining weight. Individuals with anorexia nervosa typically skip meals and, when eating, avoid foods that they view as high in fat. They also often exercise excessively in an attempt both to burn calories and to improve their sense of well-being.

B. Intense fear of gaining weight or becoming fat, even though underweight.

Despite the fact that individuals with anorexia nervosa are by definition underweight, they are impressively concerned that they will become substantially overweight if they cease their vigorous efforts to remain in control of their eating and exercising. For most individuals with anorexia nervosa, the fear of actually becoming obese is not based on fact. Most have never been significantly overweight, and such individuals are not particularly likely to come from families with obesity. However, for many, "fat" does not actually mean "obese"; it simply means "fatter" than they feel they can tolerate

(i.e., heavier than they are at present). It is also striking that this fear of becoming fat typically intensifies as more weight is lost.

C. Disturbance in the way in which one's body weight or shape is experienced, undue influence of body weight on self-evaluation, or denial of the seriousness of the current low body weight.

Criterion C requires a serious disturbance in the individual's experience of his or her own shape and weight, and can be fulfilled in a number of ways. Individuals with anorexia nervosa often view themselves or, probably more frequently, parts of their bodies, as being too big. They may focus on their breasts, abdomen, buttocks, or thighs, and feel that even though they have lost weight, these parts of their bodies remain unsatisfactorily large. In most cases, this does not appear to be a primary perceptual disturbance. That is, individuals with anorexia nervosa usually *perceive* their size accurately. The problem is more often in the *judgment* that they make about the size that they see.

Individuals with anorexia nervosa also base much of their self-esteem on their weight and shape. If such individuals gain weight, they typically feel ashamed, frustrated, embarrassed, and frightened, whereas weight loss is accompanied by a feeling of deep accomplishment.

Particularly in anorexia nervosa patients with more chronic illness, the drive to lose weight and the satisfaction of being underweight may fade. These individuals continue to deny that their low body weight is worthy of serious concern or of medical or psychiatric intervention. They may, for example, grudgingly acknowledge that they may need to gain weight, but are unwilling to take consistent steps to achieve this goal.

D. In postmenarcheal females, amenorrhea, i.e., the absence of at least three consecutive menstrual cycles.

Criterion D requires that women with anorexia nervosa do not menstruate. Most women with anorexia nervosa have progressed normally through pubertal development and have begun to menstruate before the onset of their eating disorder. Therefore, the amenorrhea represent a loss of the physiological function that has developed normally. However, some girls develop anorexia nervosa before the onset of menstruation. Ovarian steroids, such as birth control pills, are capable of inducing menstrual periods in some individuals with anorexia nervosa who do not menstruate spontaneously. Thus, a woman who menstruates only while taking birth control pills is still viewed as fulfilling this criterion.

Although Criterion D does not apply to men, it should be noted that the male reproductive axis undergoes similar alterations in anorexia nervosa. Just as women with anorexia nervosa produce little estrogen, men with anorexia nervosa produce little testosterone. The ICD-10 criteria require that men exhibit a loss of sexual interest and potency.

It is likely that both physical and psychological factors play a role in the development of the menstrual disturbances of anorexia nervosa. Sufficient weight loss in any woman will eventually produce amenorrhea, but a significant percentage of women with anorexia nervosa develop amenorrhea before substantial weight loss has occurred.

Once a diagnosis of anorexia nervosa has been made, the clinician is asked to classify the patient into one of two mutually exclusive types, the restricting type or the binge-eating/purging type, according to the following criteria:

Restricting Type: during the current episode of Anorexia Nervosa, the person has not regularly engaged in binge-eating or purging behavior (i.e., self-induced vomiting or the misuse of laxatives, diuretics, or enemas)

Binge-Eating/Purging Type: during the current episode of Anorexia Nervosa, the person has regularly engaged in binge-eating or purging behavior (i.e., self-induced vomiting or the misuse of laxatives, diuretics, or enemas)

This subtyping scheme was introduced in DSM-IV to reflect information that has accumulated in the last 10 to 20 years concerning contrasting characteristics of individuals with anorexia nervosa who binge and/or purge, compared to those whose weight loss is maintained purely through restricting their diets and/or through exercising. It is reasonably well established that individuals who binge and/or purge and have anorexia nervosa, when compared to individuals with the restricting type of this illness, are more likely to show other disturbances

of impulse control (e.g., substance use disorders). They also usually have had the illness longer and are somewhat heavier. Individuals with the restricting type of anorexia nervosa are likely to be more obsessional in style and more socially awkward and isolated than those with the binge-eating/purging type.

It should be noted that although this subtyping scheme appears a useful one, uncertainty surrounds a number of its details. For example, the frequency of binge eating and purging that should cause an individual to be classified as having the binge-eating/purging type is not clear, nor is the precise meaning of "binge eating" for an individual who is underweight with anorexia nervosa (Garner, Garner, & Rosen, 1993). In addition, it is not clear whether there are important distinctions between those individuals with anorexia nervosa who binge and do not purge and those individuals who purge but do not binge.

BULIMIA NERVOSA

A. Recurrent episodes of binge eating. An episode of binge eating is characterized by both of the following:

   (1) eating, in a discrete period of time (e.g., within any 2-hour period), an amount of food that is definitely larger than most people would eat during a similar period of time and under similar circumstances
   (2) a sense of lack of control over eating during the episode (e.g., a feeling that one cannot stop eating or control what or how much one is eating)

The salient behavioral characteristic of bulimia nervosa is the frequent occurrence of binge-eating episodes. As Criterion A indicates, in DSM-IV a binge is defined on the basis of two elements: consumption of a large amount of food, and sense of loss of control during the eating episode. Investigators and the authors of DSM-IV have struggled to define when an episode of eating is "large." Many individuals with eating problems describe eating binges that are *not* objectively large (Walsh, 1993). For example, individuals may eat a normal serving of dessert, but because they had intended *not* to eat dessert, they view this as a binge and induce vomiting afterwards. Although this is clearly a behavioral problem, it does not meet the DSM-IV definition of an episode of binge eating, because the amount of food eaten is not larger than most people would eat for dessert. Thus, in making the diagnosis of bulimia nervosa, it is incumbent on the clinician to obtain a description of the individual's typical binge-eating pattern and to make a judgment about the degree to which the eating episodes involve the consumption of what would be clearly regarded as a large amount of food (Walsh, 1993).

In defining episodes of binge eating, the clinician should also consider the context in which the eating occurred. What may be an unusually large amount of food if eaten at 11 P.M. after a full dinner might not be excessive if consumed at a dinner party. The criterion also suggests that the eating occur within a "discrete period of time," implying that continual snacking throughout the day should not be viewed as a binge-eating episode.

Individuals with bulimia nervosa intend to consume a variety of food during eating binges. Perhaps most typical is the consumption of dessert or snack foods, such as cookies, ice cream, and cake. Individuals also often consume large amounts of liquid while binge-eating, perhaps because it enables them to induce vomiting more easily.

    B. Recurrent inappropriate compensatory behavior in order to prevent weight gain, such as self-induced vomiting; misuse of laxatives, diuretics, enemas, or other medications; fasting; or excessive exercise.

A second critical characteristic of bulimia nervosa is that following the eating binges, individuals engage in inappropriate attempts to rid themselves to avoid weight gain. In clinical samples, the most frequent inappropriate behavior is self-induced vomiting. Vomiting is often difficult to induce when the illness begins, but becomes less difficult and more habitual over time. Many individuals with bulimia nervosa eventually induce vomiting not only following binge episodes, but following the consumption of virtually any meal, whether large or small. Many individuals with bulimia nervosa also utilize medications in an attempt to counteract the binges (see Mitchell, Specker, & Edmonson, Chapter 23, this volume). Commonly they take large amounts of over-the-counter laxatives to induce diarrhea. Although laxative abuse certainly induces an acute loss of weight, this is secondary to dehydration rather than the loss of calories; laxatives have most of their effect on the large bowel, whereas calorie absorption occurs primarily in the small intestine (see Mitchell, Pomeroy, & Adson, Chapter 21, this volume).

Occasionally individuals attempt to manipulate their weights through other means, such as diuretics, enemas, and thyroid medication. There are also a number of reports of diabetics who omit insulin after binge-eating episodes (see Powers, Chapter 24, this volume).

Some individuals with bulimia nervosa do not purge, but use other techniques after they have binged—for example, eating nothing of caloric value for 24 hours, or excessive exercising. Although most clinicians agree that these are clinically important compensatory methods, it has proven difficult to provide explicit criteria for the definition of fasting and excessive exercise. DSM-IV suggests that fasting implies the absence of caloric consumption for 24 hours, and that exercise is excessive when it interferes with important activities, occurs at inappropriate times or settings, or continues to occur despite medical problems.

    C. The binge eating and inappropriate compensatory behaviors both occur, on average, at least twice a week for 3 months.

Like DSM-III-R (APA, 1987), DSM-IV requires that binge eating occur on average twice a week for a duration of 3 months for the diagnosis of bulimia nervosa. DSM-IV has added the requirement that the inappropriate compensatory behaviors also occur at this frequency. Although these are clearly arbitrary standards, they serve the useful purpose of restricting the diagnosis to those individuals who have a relatively recurrent and persistent problem. The unfortunate consequence is that many individuals whose problems appear quite similar to those of bulimia nervosa (e.g., individuals who binge-eat and vomit once a week for years) do not meet the formal criteria for bulimia nervosa, and must be classified at present as having an EDNOS.

    D. Self-evaluation is unduly influenced by body shape and weight.

Like patients with anorexia nervosa, individuals with bulimia nervosa are overconcerned with their body shape and weight, and their self-esteem is regulated in the extreme by these aspects of their appearance. They feel under intense pressure to diet and to avoid weight gain. When they do gain weight, they often report feeling extremely distressed.

> E. The disturbance does not occur exclusively during episodes of Anorexia Nervosa.

The purpose of Criterion E, which was introduced in DSM-IV, is to permit anorexia nervosa to "trump" bulimia nervosa. That is, an individual who meets criteria for both disorders (i.e., an underweight individual who binge-eats and vomits twice a week) is given the exclusive diagnosis of anorexia nervosa, binge-eating/purging type, and not a diagnosis of bulimia nervosa. This criterion serves to emphasize that this individual has one eating disorder, not two; it also emphasizes the seriousness of the low body weight, which is inherent to the diagnosis of anorexia nervosa. The introduction of Criterion E was a change from DSM-III-R, in which individuals who met criteria for both anorexia nervosa and bulimia nervosa were given both diagnoses.

This change introduces an apparent problem, in that it is unclear where the boundary lies between anorexia nervosa in partial recovery and bulimia nervosa. For example, a woman with anorexia nervosa, binge-eating/purging type, might regain weight and begin to menstruate, but continue to binge-eat and purge. She might be fairly viewed either as having partially recovered from her anorexia nervosa or as having the diagnosis of bulimia nervosa. However, it is important for the clinician to understand that the distinctions between these two eating disorders are really arbitrary, in the sense that the lines of demarcation have been simply defined by the diagnostic criteria themselves. They do not define conditions that are clinically distinct.

Having made the diagnosis of bulimia nervosa, the clinician is asked to specify the type:

Purging Type: during the current episode of Bulimia Nervosa, the person has regularly engaged in self-induced vomiting or the misuse of laxatives, diuretics, or enemas
Nonpurging Type: during the current episode of Bulimia Nervosa, the person has used other compensatory inappropriate behaviors, such as fasting or excessive exercise, but has not regularly engaged in self-induced vomiting or the misuse of laxatives, diuretics, or enemas

This subtyping scheme was introduced in DSM-IV for several reasons. First, it appears that individuals with the purging type of bulimia nervosa usually have lower body weights, more symptoms of depression, and greater concern with body shape and weight than do individuals with the nonpurging type (Willmuth, Leitenberg, Rosen, & Cado, 1988). In addition, they are much more likely to exhibit fluid and electrolyte disturbances. Finally, almost all the studies conducted on the efficacy of psychological and pharmacological treatment for bulimia have focused primarily on individuals with the purging subtype, and it is not clear to what degree the findings can be confidently extended to those with the nonpurging subtype.

EATING DISORDERS NOT OTHERWISE SPECIFIED

EDNOS diagnoses are reserved for a heterogeneous group of individuals who have eating disorders, but who do not meet the diagnostic criteria for the two main eating disorders, anorexia nervosa and bulimia nervosa. As indicated earlier, the term "not otherwise specified" could be misinterpreted as connoting eating problems of minor clinical significance. However, the clinical picture for individuals with EDNOS can be quite serious and can require prompt clinical attention. Therefore, the examples of EDNOS given in DSM-IV are briefly reviewed here. Although binge-eating disorder is actually sixth in DSM-IV's list of examples, we discuss it first.

Binge-Eating Disorder

For decades, it has been recognized that some individuals engage in uncontrollable episodes of binge eating, but do not engage regularly in the inappropriate compensatory behaviors (e.g., self-induced vomiting) characteristic of bulimia nervosa. Research criteria for binge-eating disorder are provided in Appendix B of DSM-IV to describe this syndrome. Binge-eating disorder is conceptually similar to bulimia nervosa, with the important absence of the inappropriate compensatory behaviors (Spitzer et al., 1992). The research criteria provided in DSM-IV are as follows:

A. Recurrent episodes of binge eating. An episode of binge eating is characterized by both of the following:

(1) eating, in a discrete period of time (e.g., within any 2-hour period), an amount of food that is definitely larger than most people would eat during a similar period of time under similar circumstances

(2) a sense of lack of control over eating during the episode (e.g., a feeling that one cannot stop eating or control what or how much one is eating)

It is suggested that the criteria for evaluating a binge in binge-eating disorder are identical to those used for individuals with bulimia nervosa. Pragmatically, however, this decision is more difficult, since the end of a binge-eating episode can be more difficult to establish in the absence of a discrete event such as vomiting. It also appears that many individuals who complain of binge eating also have episodes of overeating that are harder to distinguish from the eating of normal individuals.

B. The binge-eating episodes are associated with three (or more) of the following:

(1) eating much more rapidly than normal

(2) eating until feeling uncomfortably full

(3) eating large amounts of food when not feeling physically hungry

(4) eating alone because of being embarrassed by how much one is eating

(5) feeling disgusted with oneself, depressed, or very guilty after overeating

These characteristics were introduced, in part, to provide behavioral markers of episodes of binge eating among individuals who do not use inappropriate compensatory behaviors.

C. Marked distress regarding binge eating is present.

Individuals with binge-eating disorder are greatly troubled by what they view as a clear behavioral disturbance, because of both the loss of control and the implications of the binge eating for their weight and consequent medical health.

D. The binge eating occurs, on average, at least 2 days a week for 6 months.

Criterion D differs in some important details from the parallel one for bulimia nervosa. First, the criterion refers to the number of days per week on which eating binges occur. To a significant degree, this reflects the difficulty of defining the end of eating binges when such binges are not terminated by inappropriate compensatory behaviors. Thus, it is easier to enumerate days on which binges occur than the number of discrete episodes. Second, the binge eating is required to have occurred at this frequency for at least 6 months, in contrast to the 3 months required for bulimia nervosa. This higher degree of severity was introduced in order to set a higher threshold for this newly defined disorder.

E. The binge eating is not associated with the regular use of inappropriate compensatory behaviors (e.g., purging, fasting, excessive exercise) and does not occur exclusively during the course of Anorexia Nervosa or Bulimia Nervosa.

Criterion E explicitly distinguishes binge-eating disorder from anorexia nervosa and bulimia nervosa. As stated above, the critical distinction is the absence of the regular use of inappropriate compensatory behaviors. However, the specific definition of "regular use" is not clear. Some research studies have equated "regular" with a twice-a-week frequency of bulimia nervosa, and therefore have considered individuals who engage in these behaviors less then twice a week as eligible for the diagnosis of binge-eating disorder (e.g., Spitzer, et al., 1993). Other studies have required a virtual absence of these inappropriate compensatory behaviors (Brody, Walsh, & Devlin, 1994). Further research is needed to determine what is the most satisfactory level. An issue that this leaves unresolved is the demarcation between the nonpurging subtype of bulimia nervosa and binge-eating disorder. It appears that a number of individuals with the nonpurging subtype of bulimia nervosa are, like many patients with binge-eating disorder, overweight. Precisely at what point someone would be better classified as having bulimia nervosa versus binge-eating disorder is unclear at this time.

Other Examples of EDNOS

1. For females, all of the criteria for Anorexia Nervosa are met except that the individual has regular menses.

Individuals who meet all of the diagnostic criteria for anorexia nervosa, but who have regular menses, form a small but important subgroup. These individuals may present with a chronic eating disorder in which they have maintained a low body weight for many years. Since body fat levels in anorexia nervosa are typically below that thought critical for normal menstrual functioning, it is not known why some eating disorder patients menstruate at a low body weight. It is possible that there is biological adaptation to the low weight that allows resumption of menses in the presence of chronic starvation. This is consistent with reproductive patterns in countries in which famine is endemic. The view that amenorrhea is secondary to starvation has led some to argue that this should not be a diagnostic criterion for anorexia nervosa (Fairburn & Garner, 1986). The clinical management of this subgroup of patients is the same as for those with anorexia nervosa. However, according to both DSM-IV and the ICD-10, women who menstruate should not be given a diagnosis of anorexia nervosa, even if underweight.

2. All of the criteria for Anorexia Nervosa are met except that, despite significant weight loss, the individual's current weight is in the normal range.

This example is particularly relevant to the subgroup of obese individuals who lose a significant amount of body weight and maintain this loss only by extreme and sustained caloric restriction. They exhibit a level of preoccupation with eating and body weight that is as marked as that seen in anorexia nervosa. These individuals often pose a troublesome clinical predicament, since they may see themselves, and also may be seen by others, as being "recovered" from a serious disorder (i.e., obesity). These individuals will point to the medical and psychosocial improvements in their life that have accompanied weight loss. Thus, they are extremely reluctant to relax their pattern of rigid dietary restriction and other symptoms, because this pattern is seen as necessary to prevent weight regain. It is important for individuals with this variant of EDNOS to be helped to fully appreciate the degree of psychosocial and physical impairment created by their eating disorder symptoms. They require extraordinary support while gradually relaxing their rigid eating patterns, particularly if this relaxation results in weight gain.

3. All of the criteria for Bulimia Nervosa are met except that the binge eating or inappropriate compensatory mechanisms occur at a frequency of less than twice a week or for a duration of less than 3 months.

This example of EDNOS highlights the importance of the binge-eating threshold required for a diagnosis of bulimia nervosa. As mentioned earlier, the rationale for specifying the binge-eating frequency threshold is that it restricts the diagnosis of bulimia nervosa to those who have a recurrent and persistent problem. In this regard, it is important to note that the binge-eating threshold for bulimia nervosa applies to binge eating *and* inappropriate compensatory behaviors (rather than compensatory behaviors alone). For example, the EDNOS diagnosis would apply to an individual who binges less than twice a week on average, but who has vomited many times a day and abused laxatives for years. This apparent incongruity may be moot, since most individuals who frequently vomit usually meet the frequency criterion for binge eating. Nevertheless, problems in classification could result from precise enforcement of the definition of "binge eating," since research has shown that it is difficult to determine exactly how much patients have eaten prior to vomiting. Although there is a high correlation between recalled and actual food intake, bulimia nervosa patients' recall of the size of binge meals may be greater than the actual size of the binge meals (Hadigan, LaChaussee, Walsh, & Kissileff, 1992). Again, little is known about the extent to which persistent vomiting occurs in individuals who fail to meet the threshold for binge eating required for a diagnosis of bulimia nervosa. However, it is important for the clinician to be aware that metabolic disturbances and serious health risks are more closely tied to vomiting and laxative abuse than to binge eating (see Mitchell et al., Chapter 21, this volume). Thus, the clinical management of this particular variant of EDNOS would not differ from that of bulimia nervosa.

4. The regular use of inappropriate compensatory behavior by an individual of normal body weight after eating small amounts of food (e.g., self-induced vomiting after the consumption of two cookies).

This example of EDNOS overlaps with the one just described. However, in this case, the individual could fail to meet more than one of the criteria required for a diagnosis of bulimia nervosa as long as they regularly engaged in inappropriate compensatory behavior. Self-induced vomiting following the ingestion of small amounts of food may occur among individuals who are so terrified of eating that they cannot tolerate any food in their stomachs. Such individuals may label eating a tiny amount of food as "a binge." Again, because serious health risks are primarily associated with vomiting and laxative abuse rather than with binge eating per se, individuals who conform to this EDNOS example present clinical concerns similar to those of patients who receive a diagnosis of bulimia nervosa. In some cases, they may be particularly resistant to treatment, because their vomiting is ego-syntonic and is not offset by the distress that most bulimia nervosa patients experience with their recurrent binge eating.

5. Repeatedly chewing and spitting out, but not swallowing, large amounts of food.

This example applies to a small minority of individuals and illustrates that in order for an abnormal eating episode to qualify as binge eating, the food must be ingested during the episode. Applying this definition to anorexia nervosa would mean that individuals who repeatedly chew and spit out large amounts of food, and do not engage in purging behavior, would be classified as having the "restricting type" of the disorder.

RELATIONSHIP BETWEEN DIAGNOSTIC SUBGROUPS

The DSM-IV diagnostic criteria highlight the distinctions between subgroups of eating disorders; however, it is extremely important to recognize that these nominal designations should be viewed against the backdrop both of the key similarities *across* diagnostic categories and of the marked heterogeneity *within* each subgroup (Garner et al., 1993). Regardless of diagnostic subclassification, most individuals with eating disorders are extremely concerned about their weight and/or shape. Self-evaluation is unduly influenced by body weight for bulimia nervosa by definition. It applies equally to anorexia nervosa, and is a feature common for most of those receiving a diagnosis of EDNOS. Most individuals with eating disorders engage in periods of severe calorie restriction (dieting), or

compensatory behaviors, in order to lose weight or to avoid weight gain. These features can remain relatively stable over time, even though the diagnostic classification for an individual may change (e.g., an individual with anorexia nervosa, restricting type may begin with binge eating and/or purging). Even significant weight loss, which most obviously applies to anorexia nervosa, also occurs with many individuals with bulimia nervosa. In fact, many bulimia nervosa patients have lost as much weight as those with anorexia nervosa, the difference being that the bulimia nervosa patients simply began losing weight from higher initial levels. Key variables in determining which DSM-IV diagnostic category applies are: 1) body weight, 2) the presence or absence of binge eating, and 3) the presence or absence of compensatory behaviors such as vomiting and laxative abuse. Figure 1 is a simplified schematic illustrating the intersection of these traits. While most individuals with eating disorders try to restrict their food intake to lose weight or avoid weight gain, a subset binge-eat, an overlapping subset purge, and another subset do neither. Again, Figure 1 illustrates that these behaviors occur at a statistically "normal" body weight, for some, and well below (anorexia nervosa) or well above the norms for body weight for others. In sum, the DSM-IV criteria are intended to provide clinically meaningful diagnostic distinctions; however, accentuating the similarities may help in overcoming the temptation to view the different eating disorder diagnoses as completely separate clinical entities.

A second caveat relates to the recognition of the extraordinary variability *within* each of the diagnostic subgroups on a wide range of demographic, clinical, and psychological dimensions (Welch, Hall, & Renner, 1990). Individuals with the same diagnosis differ markedly in terms of symptom severity and type, psychopathology, family background and functioning, and responsiveness to treatment.

SUMMARY

This chapter has reviewed the DSM-IV diagnostic criteria for eating disorders, as well as the rationale for certain diagnostic distinctions according to DSM-IV. Examples of EDNOS have been reviewed, indicating that individuals can have a clinically significant eating disorder without meeting the DSM-IV diagnostic criteria for either anorexia nervosa or bulimia nervosa. It cannot be overemphasized that a diagnosis of EDNOS should not be used to exclude an individual from adequate evaluation and treatment. Even though there are limitations to the DSM-IV diagnostic system, it represents a major advancement over its predecessors. It offers a guidepost for clearer communication among clinicians, and it can facilitate research. Let us hope that the increased precision offered by this system will lead to improved understanding and treatment of the eating disorders.

ACKNOWLEDGMENT

The diagnostic criteria and examples of EDNOS presented and discussed in this chapter are reprinted with permission from the *Diagnostic and Statistical Manual of Mental Disorders,* Fourth Edition (pp. 544–545, 549–550, 731). Copyright 1994 by the American Psychiatric Association.

REFERENCES

American Psychiatric Association (APA). (1987). *Diagnostic and statistical manual of mental disorders* (3rd ed., rev.). Washington, DC: Author.

American Psychiatric Association (APA). (1994). *Diagnostic and statistical manual of mental disorders* (4th ed.). Washington, DC: Author.

Brody, M. L., Walsh, B. T., & Devlin, M. J. (1994). Binge-eating disorder: Reliability and validity of a new diagnostic category. *Journal of Consulting and Clinical Psychology, 62,* 381–386.

Fairburn, C. G., & Garner, D. M. (1986). The diagnosis of bulimia nervosa. *International Journal of Eating Disorders, 5,* 403–419.

Garner, D. M., Garner, M. V., & Rosen, L. W. (1993). Anorexia nervosa "restrictors" who purge: Implications for subtyping anorexia nervosa. *International Journal of Eating Disorders, 13,* 171–185.

Hadigan, C. M., LaChaussee, J. L., Walsh, B. T., & Kissileff, H. R. (1992). 24-hour dietary recall in patients with bulimia nervosa. *International Journal of Eating Disorders, 22,* 107–111.

Russell, G. F. M. (1988). The diagnostic formulation in bulimia nervosa. In D. M. Garner & P. E. Garfinkel (Eds.), *Diagnostic issues in anorexia nervosa and bulimia nervosa* (pp. 3–25). New York: Brunner/Mazel.

Spitzer, R. L., Devlin, M., Walsh, B. T., Hasin, D., Wing, R., Marcus, M., Stunkard, A., Wadden, T., Yanovski, S., Agras, S., Mitchell, J., & Nonas, C. (1992). Binge-eating disorder: A multisite field trial of the diagnostic criteria. *International Journal of Eating Disorders, 11,* 191–203.

Spitzer, R. L., Yanovski, S., Wadden, T., Wing, R., Marcus, M. D., Stunkard, A., Devlin, M., Mitchell, J., Hasin, D., & Horne, R. L. (1993). Binge-eating disorder: Its further validation in a multisite study. *International Journal of Eating Disorders, 13,* 137–153.

Walsh, B. T. (1993). Binge eating in bulimia nervosa. In C. G. Fairburn & G. T. Wilson (Eds.), *Binge eating: Nature, assessment, and treatment* (pp. 37–49). New York: Guilford Press.

Welch, G., Hall, A., & Renner, R. (1990). Patient subgrouping in anorexia nervosa using psychologically-based classification. *International Journal of Eating Disorders, 9,* 311–322.

Willmuth, M. E., Leitenberg, H., Rosen, J. C., & Cado, S. (1988). A comparison of purging and nonpurging normal weight bulimics. *International Journal of Eating Disorders, 7,* 825–835.

World Health Organization (WHO). (1992). *The ICD-10 classification of mental and behavioral disorders: Clinical descriptions and diagnostic guidelines.* Geneva: Author.

CHAPTER 4

Assessment

JANIS H. CROWTHER
NANCY E. SHERWOOD

Eating disorders are multifaceted behavior problems that require comprehensive, multidimensional assessment. Not surprisingly, the literature devoted to the assessment of eating disorders has expanded dramatically in recent years. In addition to the proliferation of new self-report measures and the revision of several well-established instruments—for example, the Bulimia Test—Revised (BULIT-R; Thelen, Farmer, Wonderlich, & Smith, 1991) and the Eating Disorder Inventory—2 (EDI-2; Garner, 1991)—structured clinical interviews have become more widely accepted, particularly in clinical and epidemiological research. Furthermore, increased attention has been paid to evaluating the psychometric strength of these assessment tools, ensuring that they possess adequate reliability and validity.

Before focusing specifically on the methods that may be used to assess eating-related symptomatology, we would like to emphasize some general information that may have relevance for the assessment of individuals with eating disorders. First, it may be helpful for the clinician working with such individuals to conceptualize assessment as a *process* that occurs over several sessions (Maloney & Ward, 1976). Second, within this context assessment is likely to serve several purposes, including (but not limited to) establishing a diagnosis and obtaining information relevant to treatment planning. Third, given the heterogeneity in eating-related symptomatology and comorbid psychopathology characterizing the eating disorders (e.g., Crowther & Mizes, 1992; Tobin, Johnson, Steinberg,

Staats, & Dennis, 1991), an assessment of the severity of eating-related and associated symptomatology may be essential for effective treatment planning. Finally, a thorough assessment of eating-related psychopathology is likely to be multimodal in nature, integrating information from interviews, a carefully selected battery of self-report questionnaires, and self-monitoring data.

The major goal of this chapter is to review the methods of assessment available to clinicians working with eating-disordered individuals, including the interview, self-report questionnaires, and self-monitoring. The interview is necessary for establishing a diagnosis; self-report questionnaires offer more detailed information regarding various dimensions of eating-related symptomatology and more general psychopathology; and self-monitoring provides relevant information about eating behavior in the naturalistic setting. Although we realize that this categorization may be somewhat simplistic, since all three methods contribute information that is important for diagnosis and treatment planning, it is our intent that it serve as an organizational framework to guide the assessment process (e.g., Rosen & Srebnik, 1990).

THE INTERVIEW: MAKING THE DIAGNOSIS

Anorexia nervosa and bulimia nervosa are the two principal eating disorders appearing in the fourth edition of the *Diagnostic and Statistical*

Manual of Mental Disorders (DSM-IV; American Psychiatric Association [APA], 1994; see Walsh & Garner, Chapter 3, this volume).[1] The distinguishing clinical feature of anorexia nervosa is extreme restriction of food intake, resulting in extensive weight loss (or a failure to gain expected weight during growth periods). In contrast, bulimia nervosa is characterized by recurring episodes of binge eating accompanied by inappropriate behaviors to compensate for the eating and prevent weight gain. Interestingly, some anorexics also engage in episodes of bingeing and purging (e.g., Bemis, 1978; Casper, Eckert, Halmi, Goldberg, & Davis, 1980; Garner, 1993). Research suggesting important differences between individuals with eating disorders who restrict their food intake and individuals with eating disorders who purge (e.g., Mitchell, 1992; Wilson & Walsh, 1991) led to the introduction of the restricting and binge-eating/purging subtypes of anorexia nervosa and the nonpurging and purging subtypes of bulimia nervosa in DSM-IV (APA, 1994; see Walsh & Garner, Chapter 3, this volume). Clinicians must familiarize themselves with the diagnostic criteria for anorexia nervosa and bulimia nervosa in order to thoroughly assess the body image disturbance, abnormal eating behaviors, and extreme weight control measures characterizing these disorders.

Weight and Body Image

Body image disturbance plays a prominent role in the psychopathology of eating disorders. Historically, either the perceptual or the cognitive–affective components of body image disturbance (i.e., body image distortion or body image dissatisfaction) have been incorporated into the diagnostic criteria for both anorexia nervosa (APA, 1980, 1987, 1994; Russell, 1970) and bulimia nervosa (APA, 1987, 1994; Russell, 1979). In DSM-IV (APA, 1994), the applicable diagnostic criteria have been modified slightly to focus on the influence of body shape and weight on self-evaluation.

During the interview, the clinician should obtain information regarding the woman's current weight and height and her weight history.[2] Of particular interest are her highest and lowest weights since she attained her current height, and the frequency with which she has experienced significant weight fluctuations. The interviewer can probe gently about the relationships between significant life events and weight fluctuations. Weight fluctuations among women with eating disorders may be associated with life stressors, particularly interpersonal stressors (e.g., Abraham & Beumont, 1982; Hawkins & Clement, 1984). Although the interviewer and patient may see a pattern emerging between specific life events and weight fluctuations that may provide important information about the function of the eating-disordered symptomatology, a lack of insight on the part of the patient is not uncommon.

The interviewer can also ask about weight during childhood and early adolescence. Being overweight as children and/or experiencing critical incidents of teasing may have been salient experiences for these women (Fabian & Thompson, 1989; Grilo, Wilfley, Brownell, & Rodin, 1994; Warren, 1968). For example, compared to parents of women without eating disorders, parents of women with bulimia nervosa reported making more negative comments about their daughters' bodies and encouraging them to diet (Moreno & Thelen, 1990). Since women's retrospective recall of their weight during childhood may be unreliable (e.g., Johnson, 1985), it may be more productive to ask about a woman's perceptions of her weight during this time, focusing on whether she felt overweight as a child, received negative feedback from family members about her weight and physical appearance, or was teased about her weight by her peers.

After obtaining information about the woman's current weight and height and her weight history, the interviewer should ask about the woman's ideal weight, since provision of information about an acceptable weight range and subsequent acceptance of that weight range are important goals in many treatments. Typically, women with eating disorders will report an unrealistically low ideal weight. Moreover, as Fairburn (1985) has noted, they will often report a rather arbitrary weight that falls under a given threshold figure (e.g., under 110 or 120 pounds in the United States, or under 7 or 8 stone in Great Britain).

With the weight history completed, the interviewer can further explore the body image disturbance that characterizes anorexia nervosa and bulimia nervosa. Traditionally, body image disturbance has not been regarded as a unitary concept (Garner & Garfinkel, 1981; Rosen, 1992; Rosen & Srebnik, 1990). In their review, Garner and Garfinkel (1981) stated that body image disturbance can be manifested in two ways: as a disturbance in perception (i.e., body image distortion), in which the woman views selected body parts as unrealistically large; and as a disturbance in cognition and affect (i.e., body image dissatisfaction), in which the woman evaluates her physical appearance negatively. Rosen and his colleagues (Rosen, 1992; Rosen, Srebnik, Saltzberg, & Wendt, 1991) have added a third component to this multidimensional conceptualization of body image disturbance: a disturbance in behavior (i.e., body image avoidance), in which the woman engages in repetitive "body-checking" behavior and avoids situations that provoke anxiety about her body.

During the interview, the clinician needs to be sensitive to the presence and severity of these manifestations of body image disturbance, and to their impact on the woman's self-esteem and life adjustment. Assessing the degree of body image distortion may be important (e.g., Johnson, 1985; Rosen, 1992); although degree of overestimation appears restricted to self-estimates, it has been predictive of severity of clinical presentation and treatment outcome, particularly in anorexia nervosa (e.g., Freeman, Thomas, Solyom, & Koopman, 1985; Garfinkel, Moldofsky, & Garner, 1977; Garner & Bemis, 1982). Underlying the body image dissatisfaction in anorexia nervosa and bulimia nervosa is the faulty assumption that weight, shape, or thinness is the primary source of self-worth and value (Garner & Bemis, 1982; Fairburn, 1985). Women with eating disorders will often spontaneously admit to "feeling fat," being fearful of gaining weight, or being dissatisfied with their weight or specific body parts (most notably their waists, hips, and thighs) (Fisher, 1986). Cooper and Fairburn (1987) believe that responses to questions about "feeling fat" or "being afraid of gaining weight" may not be sufficient to determine whether a woman has the overvalued concern about physical appearance characteristic of eating disorders. Thus, in addition to questioning the woman about her perceptions and feelings about her weight and shape, the interviewer should assess the meaning attached to attaining (or maintaining) her ideal weight; the impact that weight gain (or weight loss) has on her thoughts and feelings about herself; others' perceptions of her weight and shape; and the degree to which she avoids or restricts her involvement in activities that involve some bodily exposure (e.g., swimming, physical activity, physical intimacy, etc.).

Abnormal Eating Behaviors

Binge eating has two major characteristics: (1) eating an amount of food in a specified time period that is larger than that which most individuals would consume during a similar time period and in similar circumstances, and (2) feeling a lack of control over eating during the binge (APA, 1994). Since binge eating is a necessary symptom of bulimia nervosa and occurs among some anorexics as well (e.g., Bemis, 1978; Casper et al., 1980), the clinician must assess whether or not the woman is engaging in binge eating.

The definition of a binge episode has been a controversial issue. Historically, there has been considerable reluctance to specify a minimum caloric intake for a binge episode; it has only been required that the individual consume a large amount of food (APA, 1980, 1987). Continuing in this tradition, DSM-IV (APA, 1994) also provides no definition, but requires the clinician to take into consideration the *context* within which the eating occurs (e.g., Fairburn & Wilson, 1993; Wilson, 1993). Thus, the initial tasks for the clinician are to determine whether or not the binge involves the consumption of a quantity of food that is definitely larger than others would consume in similar circumstances, and whether or not the individual experiences a loss of control over her eating during the eating episode. Many women who binge report that they cannot stop bingeing once they start (i.e., the binge episode must "go its course") and/or cannot prevent a binge once the urge to binge has occurred.

If binge eating is present, the clinician should obtain information about the onset of binge eating, the frequency and severity of binges, and the woman's perception of control—that is, whether she can prevent the occurrence of a binge once the urge to binge is present or interrupt a binge once she has started (e.g., Fairburn & Cooper, 1993). Although self-monitoring (see below) will provide the most detailed information regarding daily eating patterns, including information about the food and caloric composition of a binge and its topographical characteristics, it is often informative to ask for a description of daily eating patterns, including a typical meal and a typical binge. The clinician can also gather information about the timing of binges during the day and common antecedents and consequences, including specific events or affective states that recurrently precipitate binge episodes and the affective states and somatic conditions that follow. Whereas information about the nature and frequency of binge episodes is diagnostically helpful, topographical information allows the clinician to formulate working hypotheses regarding the function of the binge episodes.

With respect to clinical presentation, the clinician is likely to note considerable variability in the frequency and duration of, and caloric consumption during, binge episodes. The literature suggests that bulimics binge, on the average, three to five times per week (Crowther, Lingswiler, & Stephens, 1984; Johnson & Larson, 1982; Lingswiler, Crowther, & Stephens, 1989), although some bulimics report bingeing daily or several times per day (e.g., Russell, 1979). Some bulimics report that their binges last "all day," but the average duration is 1–2 hours (e.g., Mitchell & Laine, 1985; Pyle, Mitchell, & Eckert, 1981). Although there have been examples of bulimics consuming up to 20,000 kilocalories during a binge (Russell, 1979), bulimics typically do not consume significantly more calories than normal controls during the day (Crowther et al., 1984); their more severe binges may average between 2,000 and 5,000 calories per binge (e.g., Kaye, Gwirtsman, George, Weiss, & Jimerson, 1986; Kissileff, Walsh, Kral, & Cassidy, 1986; Mitchell & Laine, 1985; Rosen, Leitenberg, Fisher, & Khazam, 1986; Rossiter & Agras, 1990), and a substantial minority of their binges may be under 600 calories (e.g., Kirkley, Burge, & Ammerman, 1988; Rosen et al., 1986; Rossiter & Agras, 1990).

Women with eating disorders also may adhere to a highly selective diet, often consuming only those foods perceived as "safe" or "good" and completely avoiding those foods considered "forbidden" or "bad." We have seen several young women with anorexia nervosa who severely limited their food choices: One patient would eat only tuna fish and lettuce, a second would allow herself no foods with fat, and a third would only consume foods listed in a commercially available diet plan. For women who binge, consumption of even a small amount of "forbidden" food may trigger bingeing and/or vomiting (e.g., Orleans & Barnett, 1984; Polivy & Herman, 1985; Rosen & Leitenberg, 1985). "Forbidden" foods are likely to be those high in calories, such as baked goods, salty snacks, candy, and other high-carbohydrate foods (e.g., Abraham & Beumont, 1982; Leon, Carroll, Chernyk, & Finn, 1985; Loro & Orleans, 1981);

however, the actual food items avoided may be idiosyncratic to the individual. Since treatment often involves increasing the variety of foods consumed, including the introduction of previously "forbidden" food items, the clinician should ask the patient to identify foods that cause distress and/or foods she enjoys but avoids eating.

Weight Control Measures

Women with eating disorders usually have an extensive history of dieting (e.g., Polivy & Herman, 1985). Typically, their attempts at chronically restricting their food intake are punctuated by episodes of bingeing (e.g., Fairburn, 1985; Heatherton & Polivy, 1992) and accompanied by the use of other extreme measures to control their weight. Frequent weighing (up to several times per day) is not uncommon. The clinician should question the patient about the initial onset, frequency, and preferred methods of dieting. Since some girls report dieting as early as the third grade (Thelen, Powell, Lawrence, & Kuhnert, 1992), the clinician should be aware that some women may have prolonged dieting histories. Moreover, since a period of severely restrictive dieting often precedes the onset of anorexia nervosa and bulimia nervosa (Polivy & Herman, 1985), the clinician should emphasize this most recent period of dieting; in particular, he or she should assess whether a relationship exists between any stressors and the onset of dieting, and how the woman is restricting her food intake. Anecdotally, we have been impressed with how frequently our patients report that an interpersonal stressor (e.g., the death of a family member or the ending of a romantic relationship) preceded the onset of their most recent dieting.

Central to the diagnosis of bulimia nervosa is the regular use of inappropriate compensatory methods to prevent weight gain. A substantial proportion of women with anorexia nervosa also engage in some form of purging, although purging is not required for this diagnosis (e.g., Garner, Garner, & Rosen, 1993). Furthermore, it is not uncommon for patients to use more than one compensatory method (Garner et al., 1993; Wolf & Crowther, 1992). In our experience, women with eating disorders may be relatively open about severely restrictive dieting, but they are less likely to spontaneously offer information about purging. Consequently, the clinician must ask the patient about her use of self-induced vomiting; laxatives, diuretics, enemas, appetite suppressants, or other medications (including syrup of ipecac); fasting; and excessive exercise. Although the clinician may introduce the issue with an open-ended question (e.g., "Tell me about the methods you use to control your weight"), he or she may need to probe more specifically about each method. Particularly in the case of exercise, it is important to ensure that the motivation for exercising is control of weight and shape. Questions about the onset, history, and frequency of use of these methods should follow.

Psychiatric History

It is not unusual for women with bulimia nervosa to have a history of anorexia nervosa (Johnson & Connors, 1987; Russell, 1979). Women with eating disorders may also experience other psychiatric disorders, including mood disorders (e.g., Hinz & Williamson, 1987; Hudson, Pope, Jonas, & Yurgelun-Todd, 1983), anxiety disorders (Piran, Kennedy, Garfinkel, & Owens, 1985), personality disorders (Vitousek & Manke, 1994; Wonderlich & Mitchell, 1988), and substance use disorders (e.g., Casper et al., 1980). The clinician needs to be sensitive to the presence of comorbid psychopathology, and to determine whether the onset of other symptoms precedes or follows the onset of the eating disorder. The presence of comorbid psychopathology may affect treatment recommendations. For example, treatment with antidepressant medication may be instituted for anorexics and bulimics with a coexisting major depressive disorder (Andersen, Morse, & Santmyer, 1985; Garfinkel, Garner, & Kennedy, 1985; Fairburn, 1985). Research has also indicated that bulimics who do not respond to standard cognitive-behavioral interventions are likely to meet the diagnostic criteria for borderline personality disorder (e.g., Dennis & Sansone, Chapter 25, this volume; Johnson, Tobin, & Enright, 1989; Rossiter, Agras, Telch, & Schneider, 1993; Wonderlich, Fullerton, Swift, & Klein, 1994). For these individuals, as well as those misusing alcohol or other drugs, more long-term, intensive treatments may need to be considered (e.g., Johnson, 1985; Lacey, 1985).

To complete the clinical interview, the clinician should gather information about the patient's family and social history, educational and occupational history, and motivation for treatment. Clinicians must be aware not only that women with anorexia nervosa experience amenorrhea (APA, 1994), but that women with bulimia nervosa also experience menstrual irregularities (Garner, Rockert, Olmsted, Johnson, & Coscina, 1985; Johnson, Stuckey, Lewis, & Schwartz, 1982). Since a goal weight above a woman's menstrual threshold is typically established at the onset of treatment (Garner & Bemis, 1985), and a return to regular menses is essential (particularly for anorexics), a menstrual history should be obtained. Furthermore, because anorexia nervosa and bulimia nervosa are not medically benign conditions (Mitchell, 1986a; 1986b; see Mitchell, Pomeroy, & Adson, Chapter 21, this volume), patients should be evaluated by a physician and followed during the course of treatment. Clinicians interviewing women with eating disorders should be sensitive to complaints about nausea, dizziness, weakness, lethargy, fatigue, and cardiac and gastrointestinal problems, and should refer patients with these symptoms for further medical evaluation.

Interview Issues

Women with eating disorders have been regarded as notoriously unreliable informants. Vitousek, Daly, and Heiser (1991) note that "the challenge of getting eating disorder clients to tell us what they think and feel—and the difficulty of trusting them when they do—have long figured prominently among the concerns of clinicians and researchers who work with this population" (p. 647). Clinical research suggests that denial of illness is quite common among individuals with eating disorders, although it is potentially more prominent among anorexics than among bulimics (e.g., Szmukler & Tantum, 1984; Vandereycken & Vanderlinden, 1983; Vitousek et al., 1991). However, the motivation for deliberate distortion may differ by diagnosis. Vitousek et al. (1991) suggest that the anorexic may be motivated to falsify her self-report for self-protective reasons, while the bulimic does so because of feelings of shame about her poor self-control.

Establishment of a strong therapeutic relationship characterized by genuineness, acceptance, honesty, and warmth is a prerequisite to eliciting accurate information from the patient. The clinician must also communicate awareness and an empathic understanding of the ambivalence women with eating disorders may experience about beginning treatment. Although these individuals are often anxious for recovery, anorexics are fearful about eating and the associated weight gain, while bulimics are fearful of potential increases in their weight and shape. Vitousek et al. (1991) argue that most women with eating disorders will provide basic information about their symptoms in response to gentle questioning by a knowledgeable clinician. These authors provide alternatives to confrontation that may be clinically useful for reducing denial, including gathering information about clinical status from collateral informants; asking hypothetical, inverse, and third-person questions; and asking patients to make choices between two alternatives.

A related issue involves the use of structured interviews. The past decade has seen the publication of several structured interviews, including the Clinical Eating Disorder Rating Instrument (CEDRI; Palmer, Christie, Cordle, Davies, & Kenrick, 1987), the Eating Disorder Examination (EDE; Cooper & Fairburn, 1987; Fairburn & Cooper, 1993), the Interview for Diagnosis of Eating Disorders (IDED; Williamson, 1990), and the Structured Interview for Anorexia and Bulimia Nervosa (SIAB; Fichter et al., 1991). Although all four structured interviews provide essential information about eating-related symptomatology, the EDE, IDED, and SIAB can be used to establish a diagnosis, while the CEDRI and SIAB provide information about general and/or familial psychopathology related to the eating disorders.

Of these structured interviews, the EDE has been the most extensively researched. The EDE yields four subscales measuring different dimensions of eating-related psychopathology (Restraint, Eating Concern, Shape Concern, and Weight Concern), as well as a global measure of overall severity (the mean of the four subscales). The 12th edition of the EDE also generates operationally defined eating disorder diagnoses (Fairburn & Cooper, 1993). The EDE has acceptable psychometric characteristics (for a review, see Fairburn & Cooper, 1993) and has proven to be sensitive to the effects of psychological treatment (e.g., Fairburn, Jones, Peveler, Hope, & O'Connor, 1993). Since unstructured interviews offer the clinician more flexibility with respect to rapport building and the exploration of the more unique aspects of the person, structured interviews are not widely adopted in clinical practice (Groth-Marnat, 1990). However, the EDE has several advantages, including a conceptual framework for

viewing different forms of overeating (Wilson, 1993), an organizational framework through which very detailed information about eating-related symptomatology can be gathered, and questioning procedures designed to facilitate accuracy (Wilson, 1993).

SELF-REPORT QUESTIONNAIRES: EXPANDING THE ASSESSMENT PROCESS

Self-report questionnaires have multiple uses in the assessment of eating-related and other symptomatology. First, although they cannot replace a clinical interview for diagnostic purposes, these measures can serve as screening instruments for the presence and/or severity of eating-related symptomatology and other concerns. Second, given the heterogeneity in symptom presentation, self-report measures can inform treatment planning by identifying and clarifying those issues requiring emphasis during the course of treatment. In a related vein, since women with eating disorders often experience other psychological difficulties, it may be useful to incorporate instruments that measure general psychological distress and other psychiatric symptomatology. Finally, these measures may also be useful in assessing progress, as they can be easily administered repeatedly during the course of treatment.[3]

Body Image Disturbance

As mentioned previously, multiple facets of body image disturbance have been identified, including body image distortion, body image dissatisfaction, and body image avoidance (Cash & Brown, 1987; Rosen, 1992). Although these three dimensions of body image disturbance are highly correlated, women with eating disorders are likely to differ in the extent to which each dimension is problematic (Cash & Brown, 1987). Self-report measures can be useful in delineating which component(s) of body image disturbance to target during treatment. Patients with more severe body size distortion may benefit most from treatment that focuses on correction of size and weight overestimation. When body image dissatisfaction is most prominent, modifying negative and distorted thoughts and working toward acceptance of one's body may be indicated. Finally, treatment incorporating exposure to situations that provoke anxiety-provoking thoughts about appearance will be beneficial for those patients who exhibit extreme avoidant behaviors.

Body size distortion has been commonly assessed by means of (1) techniques for estimating body part size, (2) distorting-image techniques, and (3) silhouettes. The "visual size estimation task" (Reitman & Cleveland, 1964; Slade & Russell, 1973), the Body Image Detection Device (Ruff & Barrios, 1986), and the "image-marking procedure" (Askevold, 1975), are body part size estimation procedures that have received attention in the research literature. Each of these procedures asks the individual to estimate the width of various body regions, and yields an index of perceptual accuracy based on her perceived versus her actual size. Among the frequently used distorting-image techniques are the "distorting-photograph technique" (Glucksman & Hirsch, 1969), and the "video distortion technique" (Allebeck, Hallberg, & Espmark, 1976). Distorting-image techniques generate an estimate of overall body size, as opposed to estimates of specific body parts. Finally, silhouettes have been used as a measure of perceptual distortion (e.g., the Body Image Assessment procedure; Williamson, 1990). Subjects are presented with a series of silhouettes of differing sizes, and are asked to select the silhouettes representing their current and ideal sizes.

Clinicians using body image distortion measures should be aware that although these measures have acceptable test–retest reliability, research on their abilities to discriminate women with eating disorders from non-eating-disordered controls has yielded discrepant findings (Cash & Brown, 1987; Rosen & Srebnik, 1990). Although overestimation of body size occurs among eating-disordered populations, women without eating disorders may also overestimate their body size (Cash & Brown, 1987). Some research suggests that patients with eating disorders may underestimate their body size as well (Slade, 1985). These discrepancies are partially a function of different measurement techniques. For example, distorting-image techniques are more likely to yield underestimation of body size than are body part size estimation techniques (Slade, 1985). Even so, assessing the discrepancy between perceived and ideal body size appears to be useful, given that eating-disordered women report significantly greater discrepancies than their non-eating-disordered counterparts (e.g., Lindholm & Wilson, 1988;

Williamson, 1990). Given equipment requirements, it may be impractical to use many of the body size distortion techniques in clinical practice; however, the image-marking or silhouette techniques can be easily included in an assessment battery.

Among the measures for assessing body image dissatisfaction are the Body Cathexis Scale (Secord & Jourard, 1953; Jourard & Secord, 1954), the Body Dissatisfaction subscale of the EDI-2 (Garner, 1991), and the Body Shape Questionnaire (Cooper, Taylor, Cooper, & Fairburn, 1987). One of the earliest instruments designed to measure body dissatisfaction, the Body Cathexis Scale measures the extent of satisfaction with a wide variety of body parts. The Body Dissatisfaction Scale subscale of the EDI-2 also measures the level of satisfaction with a wide variety of body parts; however, this measure focuses particularly on those areas that are of greatest concern to eating disorder patients, including the stomach, hips, thighs, and buttocks (Garner, 1991). The Body Shape Questionnaire measures concerns about body shape, self-deprecation because of physical appearance, and the experience of "feeling fat." The psychometric characteristics of the EDI-2 Body Dissatisfaction subscale and the Body Shape Questionnaire are quite promising (e.g., Cooper et al., 1987; Garner, 1991; Gross, Rosen, Leitenberg, & Willmuth, 1986). Rosen and Srebnik (1990) argue that the content of the Body Shape Questionnaire may have the greatest utility for patients with eating disorders.

Fewer instruments are available to assess the third component of body image disturbance—body image avoidance. Avoidance of situations that trigger anxiety about physical appearance is relatively common among women with eating disorders and may contribute to social and psychological impairment (Rosen & Leitenberg, 1988). Rosen et al. (1991) developed the Body Image Avoidance Questionnaire, a 19-item self-report measure, to assess this component of body image disturbance. Initial data suggest that this measure has adequate reliability and validity, and that it may serve as a useful adjunct to a battery of body image disturbance measures.

Maladaptive Eating Attitudes, Behaviors, and Cognitions

Given the prevailing sentiment that clinical interviews are necessary for diagnosis, self-report questionnaires assessing these domains may be most valuable when employed as screening measures, as quantitative indices of the severity of eating-related symptomatology, and as measures of treatment progress and outcome. Among the measures used for evaluating eating-related symptomatology are the Eating Attitudes Test (EAT) and its factor-analytically derived, abbreviated version, the EAT-26 (Garner & Garfinkel, 1979; Garner, Olmsted, Bohr, & Garfinkel, 1982); the EDI Symptom Checklist and the EDI-2 (Garner, 1991); the BULIT-R (Thelen et al., 1991); the Binge Scale (Hawkins & Clement, 1980); and the Binge Eating Scale (Gormally, Black, Daston, & Rardin, 1982). Each measure has been employed in both clinical and research contexts, and possesses adequate reliability and validity (for reviews, see Rosen & Srebnik, 1990; Williamson, 1990; Wilson, 1993).

The EAT was originally developed to assess attitudes and behaviors characteristic of anorexic patients. It not only discriminates anorexic samples from control samples, but also discriminates bulimic samples from controls (Gross et al., 1986). The EAT may be most appropriately used as an index of the severity of concerns typical among women with eating disorders, particularly drive for thinness, fear of weight gain, and restrictive eating (Williamson, 1990).

The EDI-2 provides a comprehensive assessment of the behavioral and psychological dimensions characteristic of eating disorders. Its major advantage is that it generates a psychological profile that can be used to target treatment goals. In addition to the Body Dissatisfaction subscale described above, the EDI-2 includes Drive for Thinness, Bulimia, Ineffectiveness, Interpersonal Distrust, Perfectionism, Interoceptive Awareness, and Maturity Fears subscales. The EDI-2 also has three scales that were not included in the original EDI: Asceticism, Impulse Regulation, and Social Insecurity. The EDI (and EDI-2) possesses good internal consistency (Crowther, Lilly, Crawford, & Shepherd, 1992; Garner, 1991), test–retest reliability (Wear & Pratz, 1987; Crowther et al., 1992), and validity (for a review, see Garner, 1991). Finally, the EDI is sensitive to changes as a result of psychological treatment (e.g., Mitchell et al., 1990; Wooley & Kearney-Cooke, 1986).

The EAT-26 and EDI-2 can also be used as screening measures for the presence of eating disorders. When used as the first stage of a two-stage screening process, the EAT-26 or EDI-2 can be accompanied by questions about other behaviors that confer risk for an eating disorder (Garner, 1995). For the EAT-26, a cutoff score of 20 is recommended; this score identifies a significant proportion of women with eating disorders or subclinical forms of these disorders that warrant further evaluation, and minimizes the false-negative rate (Garner, 1995; King, 1989, 1991). Although less widely used than the EAT-26, the EDI-2, particularly the Drive for Thinness subscale, has some utility as a screening instrument (see Garner, 1991). With the EDI-2, Garner (1991) argues that cutoff scores established in a two-stage screening process are not fixed or predetermined. Rather, clinicians may adjust the cutoff scores used, depending on the purpose of the screening and the base rate of eating problems in a given sample.

The BULIT was initially developed and validated in 1984 (Smith & Thelen, 1984), and the revised form, the BULIT-R, was developed in response to changes in the diagnostic criteria for bulimia nervosa (Thelen et al., 1991). The BULIT-R has good psychometric characteristics and discriminates individuals with bulimia nervosa from those with anorexia nervosa and those without eating disorders (Smith & Thelen, 1984; Thelen et al., 1991; Thelen, Mann, Pruitt, & Smith, 1987; Welch, Thompson, & Hall, 1993). Although the BULIT-R may be best utilized as a measure of the severity of bulimic symptomatology, Thelen et al. (1991) recommend a cutoff score of 104 to identify bulimic individuals. If the BULIT-R is being used for screening purposes, lower cutoff scores are recommended to minimize the number of false negatives (Thelen et al., 1991; Welch et al., 1993).

Other widely used measures of bingeing behavior include the Binge Scale, the Binge Eating Scale, and the Bulimia subscale of the EDI-2. The Binge Scale was originally designed to measure the attitudes and behaviors that accompany bulimia. The Binge Eating Scale was developed to assess the presence of binge eating in obese subjects and measures behaviors, feelings, and cognitions associated with binge eating (Gormally et al., 1982). This measure discriminates between patients with bulimia nervosa and normal controls, and between obese individuals with and without binge-eating problems (Marcus, 1993; Marcus, Wing, & Hopkins, 1988). The Bulimia subscale of the EDI-2 is a psychometrically sound measure that assesses the tendency to think about and engage in episodes of binge eating (Garner, 1991). Since these measures do not present patients with an objective definition of "binge eating" (Rosen & Srebnik, 1990), clinicians should consider providing patients with such a definition before they complete questionnaires assessing the presence of this symptom. There is some evidence that this may enhance the accuracy of self-report (Loeb, Pike, Walsh, & Wilson, 1994).

As mentioned previously, eating disorder patients have a tendency to dichotomize foods into "good" and "bad" foods and to avoid "bad" foods. Since one goal of treatment may be to decrease avoidance of these "forbidden" foods and facilitate a return to normal eating, clinicians may need to systematically assess the food choices of women with eating disorders. The Forbidden Food Survey (Ruggiero, Williamson, Davis, Schlundt, & Carey, 1988) is a self-report measure that assesses the degree of discomfort associated with 45 foods representative of the North American diet. This measure can be used to target the primary classes of foods feared and avoided by an eating disorder patient (Williamson, 1990).

Finally, although women with eating disorders hold irrational and maladaptive cognitions about eating, shape, and weight (Zotter & Crowther, 1991), and cognitive-behavioral interventions identify such cognitions for modification, measures of this domain have not been systematically incorporated into clinical practice. The Bulimic Thoughts Questionnaire (BTQ; Phelan, 1987), the Mizes Anorectic Cognitions (MAC) questionnaire (Mizes & Klesges, 1989), and the Bulimic Cognitive Distortions Scale (Schulman, Kinder, Powers, Prange, & Glenhorn, 1986) are psychometrically sound instruments useful in identifying maladaptive cognitions associated with eating disorders. Each questionnaire focuses on different domains. The BTQ is composed of three factors: self-schema regarding physical appearance; self-efficacy regarding ability to control weight; and characteristic beliefs about eating and loss of control of eating. The MAC questionnaire also assesses several cognitive domains related to anorexia and bulimia, including rigid weight regulation; self-control of eating and self-esteem; and appearance, weight, and approval. All three measures have good internal consistency and discriminate between individuals with bulimia nervosa and various control groups

(Bonifazi, Crowther, & Mizes, 1996; Phelan, 1987; Mizes, 1988, 1992; Schulman et al., 1986). Thus, clinicians can choose the measure that is most consistent with their perspective regarding the cognitive characteristics of eating disorders. Of particular importance is the sensitivity of the MAC questionnaire and the BTQ to cognitive changes associated with treatment.

Assessment of General Psychopathology

As mentioned previously, women with eating disorders may also receive comorbid Axis I and Axis II diagnoses (Casper et al., 1980; Cooper et al., 1988; Hudson et al., 1983; Vitousek & Manke, 1994). Even if women with eating disorders do not receive a comorbid diagnosis, they may experience other psychological difficulties, including depression, anxiety, obsessiveness, affective instability, poor impulse control, low self-esteem, passivity and lack of assertiveness, dependence and need for approval, and interpersonal difficulties (Bemis, 1978; Rosch, Crowther, & Graham, 1992). Self-report measures may be useful in the assessment of secondary psychopathology, since the presence of such pathology may affect the course of treatment (Williamson, 1990). If other psychological difficulties are present, the clinician will need to determine whether these difficulties must be addressed prior to or simultaneously with interventions for the eating disorder.

Supported by an extensive research history (Graham, 1993), the Minnesota Multiphasic Personality Inventory—2 (MMPI-2; Butcher, Dahlstrom, Graham, Tellegen, & Kaemmer, 1989) allows the clinician to thoroughly assess the personality characteristics and psychopathology of an individual. Initial research on the use of the original MMPI with eating-disordered populations focused on clinical scale elevations, with Scales 2, 4, 7, and 8 emerging as the most prominent elevations (Prather & Williamson, 1988; Rosch et al., 1991; Vitousek & Manke, 1994). Although no modal two-point code types for anorexic and bulimic populations have been identified (Root & Friedrich, 1989), research has suggested at least two groups of bulimics: a more severely disturbed, polysymptomatic group, often with characterological features, and a "neurotic depressive" group (Rosch et al., 1991; Rybicki, Lepkowsky, & Arndt, 1989). Clinicians should examine the pattern of clinical scale elevations to determine which personality descriptors and psychopathological features best characterize each patient. The clinician may also obtain useful information from selected MMPI-2 content scales, including Low Self-Esteem, Depression, Anxiety, Obsessiveness, Family Problems, and Negative Treatment Indicators. The MMPI-2 Addiction Potential and Addiction Acknowledgement scales may be particularly useful in screening for the presence of substance use disorders in eating-disordered populations.

Depending on a patient's initial presentation, the clinician can incorporate selected self-report instruments into a test battery, either to screen for or to assess further selected dimensions of psychopathology. Given the prevalence of Axis II disorders, particularly among women with bulimia nervosa (Vitousek & Manke, 1994; Wonderlich, Swift, Slotnick, & Goodman, 1990; Yates, Sieleni, Reich, & Brass, 1989), the clinician may wish to *screen* for personality disorders with a measure comparable to the Personality Diagnostic Questionnaire—Revised (PDQ-R; Hyler & Rieder, 1987). The PDQ adapts Axis II criteria to a self-report format and yields probable diagnoses consistent with the entire range of DSM-III-R personality disorders. The Symptom Checklist 90—Revised (Derogatis, 1977) is a psychometrically sound, multidimensional measure with three global indices of psychopathology and nine primary symptom dimensions: Somatization, Obsessive–Compulsive, Interpersonal Sensitivity, Depression, Anxiety, Hostility, Phobic Anxiety, Paranoid Ideation, and Psychoticism. In contrast, the clinician may select one or more scales that measure single symptoms or traits and are easy to administer and score—for example, the Beck Depression Inventory (Beck, 1972) or the Maudsley Obsessional–Compulsive Inventory (Hodgson & Rachman, 1977).

SELF-MONITORING: NATURALISTIC ASSESSMENT OF EATING BEHAVIOR

Finally, self-monitoring is a behavioral assessment procedure that can provide detailed information about the eating behavior of women with eating disorders. At the very minimum, self-monitoring provides an assessment of the frequency and timing of meals and snacks, the frequency and timing of binge episodes, the use of compensatory weight control methods, the types and quantities of food consumed, and the nutritional composition of the diet. Should the clinician desire more detailed information (particularly with respect to the more functional aspects of eating), information about location, persons present, and affect and thoughts associated with eating can be incorporated into an eating diary.

Self-monitoring as an assessment tool may serve several other functions during the course of treatment. Since self-monitoring is an important element of eating disorder treatments, particularly cognitive-behavioral treatments (e.g., Fairburn, 1985; Wilson, 1993), the eating diary can serve as a "focal point for interventions which are aimed at changing eating behavior" (Rosen & Srebnik, 1990, p. 238). For example, recording events that create distress for the patient may clarify the relationship between these events and binge episodes, whereas recording feelings of hunger and satiety may help the patient become more aware of these internal states and their relationship to eating (or the restriction of eating). Self-monitoring also provides information that can be used to examine treatment progress and outcome (Rosen & Srebnik, 1990; Williamson, 1990; Wilson, 1993).

Although self-monitoring is frequently used to assess the eating behavior of women with eating disorders, the reliability and validity of self-recorded food intake are salient issues. Research has yielded discrepant findings about the accuracy of self-recorded food intake among obese and normal-weight individuals, with some studies providing support (e.g., Krantzler et al., 1982; Stunkard & Waxman, 1981) and others raising substantial questions about accuracy (Bandini, Schoeller, Cyr, & Dietz, 1990; Lichtman et al., 1992). To assess the reliability of self-monitoring of binge eating, Crowther et al. (1984) had subjects self-monitor their food intake for 2 weeks. Family members or roommates were also asked to record subjects' food intake independently whenever they were with the subjects. The mean percentage of agreement between subjects and observers was 89.7% for types and quantities of food consumed during binges. There were also no significant differences in the types or amounts of food consumed during eating episodes matched for time of day and location in which an observer was present or absent. Although these results are encouraging, women with eating disorders may be more likely to record information about bingeing and purging without sufficient detail, or to deliberately omit some information. Even so, since bingeing and purging are relatively secretive behaviors and family members may be unable to serve as accurate informants, self-monitoring may be the most practical way to gather this information (e.g., Rosen & Srebnik, 1990).

Clinicians can either develop their own self-monitoring form or select one that has been published (e.g., Fairburn, 1985; Johnson & Connors, 1987; Williamson, 1990). With self-monitoring forms, clinicians should instruct their patients to complete one form for each day, recording the day and date; time of consumption, types and quantities of food and liquid consumed; location; whether the eating episode was a meal, snack, or binge; and whether or not the patients vomited or used laxatives, diuretics, or appetite suppressants. In a "Comments" column, patients may be asked to record other information (e.g., events or feelings associated with their eating). If clinicians are interested in collecting more detailed affective or cognitive information, a self-monitoring form completed for each eating episode may be more desirable than one completed for each day. When providing instructions about self-monitoring, clinicians must encourage the patients to fill out the form completely, recording *everything* they consumed. Since immediate recording yields more accurate information than records completed at the end of the day (e.g., Krantzler et al., 1982), clinicians must also emphasize the importance of completing the forms *immediately* after eating. Although training in the estimation of food servings using standard units of measurement may increase the accuracy of self-report (e.g., Rosen & Srebnik, 1990), patients should not be instructed to weigh and measure their foods or to count calories, since this may increase their preoccupation with food (Wilson, 1993).

Clinicians are likely to find that some women with eating disorders are reluctant to complete self-monitoring forms. It is not uncommon to find that some women only complete the self-monitoring forms on some days (often "good" days), that others complete them but "forget" to bring them to the office, and that still others fail to complete them at all. Williamson (1990) provides some suggestions for increasing compliance with self-monitoring; these include providing a thorough rationale for the use of self-monitoring, providing careful instructions, and explaining the relationship between the information yielded by self-monitoring and treatment recommendations. Fairburn (1985) suggests that therapists should "anticipate" women's reluctance to complete this task and assure them that self-monitoring is an initial step toward confronting their eating disorder. When we introduce self-monitoring, we often predict that a patient may have times when she may feel ashamed or embarrassed to record what she has eaten, and suggest that recording may provide the most important information at these very times. The clinician must be prepared to process the patient's feelings about self-monitoring and reassure her that she will not be evaluated on the basis of her eating.

One question that arises is how long self-monitoring should continue. Here, two factors must be considered. First, Wilson (1993) has suggested that self-monitoring may influence the nature and frequency of binge eating. Although research has found that the frequencies of binge episodes obtained from self-report are higher than those obtained from self-monitoring (e.g., Yates & Sambrailo, 1984), it is not clear whether these findings reflect the reactivity of self-monitoring or the inaccuracy of self-report. Second, of great concern among women with eating disorders is the chaotic nature of their eating patterns, with considerable fluctuations in the frequency of binge episodes. Although 1 week of diary data may be representative of the frequency of binge episodes and vomiting (e.g., Loeb et al., 1994), 2 weeks of self-monitoring prior to the onset of therapy are often recommended (e.g., Williamson, 1990). However, the clinician may choose to continue self-monitoring until he or she believes that representative information regarding eating patterns has been obtained.

SUMMARY

In summary, in order to establish a diagnosis and make effective treatment recommendations, the clinician will need to integrate information from the interview, a carefully selected battery of self-report questionnaires, and eating diaries. We have argued that a clinical interview is necessary to establish a diagnosis; that self-report measures offer more detailed information about the presence and severity of various dimensions of eating-related and secondary psychopathology; and that diary data provide important information about the functional aspects of eating. Although we have identified the areas that should be addressed in assessing women with eating disorders and have discussed representative measures of these dimensions in this chapter, clinicians may prefer to use other well-validated measures of the constructs we have outlined. Finally, we would like to promote the conceptualization of assessment as an ongoing process that continues across the course of treatment, with self-report measures and self-monitoring procedures assuming a greater role in the assessment of treatment progress and outcome.

NOTES

1. Although DSM-IV (APA, 1994) has also included binge-eating disorder as a diagnostic category for further study, we do not specifically address this diagnosis, although the assessment methods reviewed here are likely to be applicable to this disorder as well.

2. For the remainder of this chapter, we use feminine nouns and pronouns to refer to individuals with eating disorders. Although we recognize that a small percentage of individuals with eating disorders are male, the overwhelming majority are female.

3. The self-report measures discussed in this section have been chosen as representative measures; the section is not an exhaustive review of the measures available. For more extensive reviews, refer to Cash and Brown (1987), Rosen and Srebnik (1990), and Williamson (1990).

REFERENCES

Abraham, S. F., & Beumont, P. J. V. (1982). How patients describe bulimia or binge eating. *Psychological Medicine, 12,* 625–635.

Allebeck, P., Hallberg, D., & Espmark, S. (1976). Body image: An apparatus for measuring disturbances in estimation of size and shape. *Journal of Psychosomatic Research, 20,* 583–589.

American Psychiatric Association (APA). (1980). *Diagnostic and statistical manual of mental disorders* (3rd ed.). Washington, DC: Author.

American Psychiatric Association (APA). (1987). *Diagnostic and statistical manual of mental disorders* (3rd ed., rev.). Washington, DC: Author.

American Psychiatric Association (APA). (1994). *Diagnostic and statistical manual of mental disorders* (4th ed.). Washington, DC: Author.

Andersen, A. E., Morse, C., & Santmyer, K. (1985). Inpatient treatment for anorexia nervosa. In D. M. Garner & P. E. Garfinkel (Eds.), *Handbook of psychotherapy for anorexia nervosa and bulimia* (pp. 311–343). New York: Guilford Press.

Askevold, F. (1975). Measuring body image: Preliminary report on a new method. *Psychotherapy and Psychosomatics, 26,* 71–77.

Bandini, L. G., Schoeller, D. A., Cyr, H. N., & Dietz, W. H. (1990). Validity of reported energy intake in obese and nonobese adolescents. *American Journal of Clinical Nutrition, 52,* 421–425.

Beck, A. T. (1972). *Depression: Causes and treatment.* Philadelphia: University of Pennsylvania Press.

Bemis, K. M. (1978). Current approaches to the etiology and treatment of anorexia nervosa. *Psychological Bulletin, 85,* 593–617.

Bonifazi, D. Z., Crowther, J. H., & Mizes, J. S. (1996). *The validity of questionnaires for assessing cognitions in bulimia nervosa.* Manuscript submitted for publication.

Butcher, J. N., Dahlstrom, G. W., Graham, J. R., Tellegen, A., & Kaemmer, B. (1989). *MMPI-2: A guide to administration and scoring.* Minneapolis: University of Minnesota Press.

Cash, T. F., & Brown, T. A. (1987). Body image in anorexia nervosa and bulimia nervosa: A review of the literature. *Behavior Modification, 11,* 487–521.

Casper, R. C., Eckert, E. D., Halmi, K. A., Goldberg, S. C., & Davis, J. M. (1980). Bulimia: Its incidence and clinical importance in patients with anorexia nervosa. *Archives of General Psychiatry, 37,* 1030–1035.

Cooper, J. L., Morrison, T. L., Bigman, O. L., Abramowitz, S. I., Blunden, D., Nassi, A., & Krener, P. (1988). Bulimia and borderline personality disorder. *International Journal of Eating Disorders, 7,* 43–49.

Cooper, P. J., Taylor, M. J., Cooper, Z., & Fairburn, C. G. (1987). The development and validation of the Body Shape Questionnaire. *International Journal of Eating Disorders, 6,* 485–494.

Cooper, Z., & Fairburn, C. G. (1987). The Eating Disorder Examination: A semi-structured interview for the assessment of the specific psychopathology of eating disorders. *International Journal of Eating Disorders, 6,* 1–8.

Crowther, J. H., Lilly, R. S., Crawford, P. A., & Shepherd, K. L. (1992). The stability of the Eating Disorder Inventory. *International Journal of Eating Disorders, 12,* 97–101.

Crowther, J. H., Lingswiler, V. M., & Stephens, M. A. P. (1984). The topography of binge eating. *Addictive Behaviors, 9,* 299–303.

Crowther, J. H., & Mizes, J. S. (1992). Etiology of bulimia nervosa: Conceptual, research, and methodological issues. In J. H. Crowther, D. L. Tennenbaum, S. E. Hobfoll, & M. A. P. Stephens (Eds.), *The etiology of bulimia nervosa: The individual and familial context* (pp. 225–244). Washington, DC: Hemisphere.

Derogatis, L. (1977). *SCL-90-R: Administration, scoring, and procedures manual-I for the revised version.* Baltimore: Clinical Psychometric Research.

Fabian, L. J., & Thompson, J. K. (1989). Body image and eating disturbance in young females. *International Journal of Eating Disorders, 8,* 63–74.

Fairburn, C. G. (1985). Cognitive-behavioral treatment for bulimia. In D. M. Garner & P. E. Garfinkel (Eds.), *Handbook of psychotherapy for anorexia nervosa and bulimia* (pp. 160–192). New York: Guilford Press.

Fairburn, C. G., & Cooper, Z. (1993). The Eating Disorder Examination (12th edition). In C. G. Fairburn & G. T. Wilson (Eds.), *Binge eating: Nature, assessment, and treatment* (pp. 317–360). New York: Guilford Press.

Fairburn, C. G., Jones, R., Peveler, R. C., Hope, R., & O'-Connor, M. E. (1993). Psychotherapy and bulimia nervosa: The longer-term effects of interpersonal psychotherapy, behavior therapy, and cognitive behavior therapy. *Archives of General Psychiatry, 50,* 419–428.

Fairburn, C. G., & Wilson, G. T. (1993). Binge eating: Definition and classification. In C. G. Fairburn & G. T. Wilson (Eds.), *Binge eating: Nature, assessment, and treatment* (pp. 3–14). New York: Guilford Press.

Fichter, M. M., Elton, M., Engel, K., Meyer, A. E., Mall, H., & Poustka, F. (1991). Structured Interview for Anorexia and Bulimia Nervosa (SIAB): Development of a new instrument for the assessment of eating disorders. *International Journal of Eating Disorders, 10,* 571–592.

Fisher, S. (1986). *Development and structure of the body image* (Vol. 1). Hillsdale, NJ: Erlbaum.

Freeman, R. J., Thomas, C. D., Solyom, L., & Koopman, R. F. (1985). Clinical and personality correlates of body size overestimation in anorexia nervosa and bulimia nervosa. *International Journal of Eating Disorders, 4,* 439–456.

Garfinkel, P. E., Garner, D. M., & Kennedy, S. (1985). Special problems of inpatient management. In D. M. Garner & P. E. Garfinkel (Eds.), *Handbook of psychotherapy for anorexia nervosa and bulimia* (pp. 344–359). New York: Guilford Press.

Garfinkel, P. E., Moldofsky, H., & Garner, D. M. (1977). Prognosis in anorexia nervosa as influenced by clinical features, treatment, and self-perception. *Canadian Medical Journal, 177,* 1041–1045.

Garner, D. M. (1991). *Eating Disorders Inventory—2.* Odessa, FL: Psychological Assessment Resources.

Garner, D. M. (1993). Binge eating in anorexia nervosa. In C. G. Fairburn & G. T. Wilson (Eds.), *Binge eating: Nature, assessment, and treatment* (pp. 50–76). New York: Guilford Press.

Garner, D. M. (1995). *Proposed national eating disorders screening project: The Eating Attitudes Test.* Unpublished manuscript.

Garner, D. M., & Bemis, K. M. (1982). A cognitive-behavioral approach to anorexia nervosa. *Cognitive Therapy and Research, 6,* 123–150.

Garner, D. M., & Bemis, K. M. (1985). Cognitive therapy for anorexia nervosa. In D. M. Garner & P. E. Garfinkel (Eds.), *Handbook of psychotherapy for anorexia nervosa and bulimia* (pp. 107–146). New York: Guilford Press.

Garner, D. M., & Garfinkel, P. E. (1979). The Eating Attitudes Test: An index of the symptoms of anorexia nervosa. *Psychological Medicine, 9,* 273–279.

Garner, D. M., & Garfinkel, P. E. (1981). Body image in anorexia nervosa: Measurement, theory, and clinical implications. *International Journal of Psychiatry in Medicine, 11,* 263–284.

Garner, D. M., Garner, M. V., & Rosen, L. W. (1993). Anorexia nervosa "restrictors" who purge: Implications for subtyping anorexia nervosa. *International Journal of Eating Disorders, 13,* 171–185.

Garner, D. M., Olmsted, M. P., Bohr, Y., & Garfinkel, P. E. (1982). The Eating Attitudes Test: Psychometric features and clinical correlates. *Psychological Medicine, 12,* 871–878.

Garner, D. M., Rockert, W., Olmsted, M. P., Johnson, C. L., & Coscina, D. V. (1985). Psychoeducational principles in the treatment of bulimia and anorexia nervosa. In D. M. Garner & P. E. Garfinkel (Eds.), *Handbook of psychotherapy for anorexia nervosa and bulimia* (pp. 513–572). New York: Guilford Press.

Glucksman, M. L., & Hirsch, J. (1969). The response of obese patients to weight reduction: III. The perceptions of body size. *Psychosomatic Medicine, 31,* 1–7.

Gormally, J., Black, S., Daston, S., & Rardin, D. (1982). The assessment of binge eating severity among obese persons. *Addictive Behaviors, 7,* 47–55.

Graham, J. R. (1993). *MMPI-2: Assessing personality and psychopathology.* New York: Oxford University Press.

Grilo, C. M., Wilfley, D. E., Brownell, K. D., & Rodin, J. (1994). Teasing, body image, and self-esteem in a clinical sample of obese women. *Addictive Behaviors, 19*(4), 443–450.

Gross, J., Rosen, J. C., Leitenberg, H., & Willmuth, M. E. (1986). Validity of the Eating Attitudes Test and the Eating Disorder Inventory in bulimia nervosa. *Journal of Consulting and Clinical Psychology, 54,* 875–876.

Groth-Marnat, G. (1990). *Handbook of psychological assessment.* New York: Wiley.

Hawkins, R., & Clement, P. (1980). Development and construct validation of a self-report measure of binge eating tendencies. *Addictive Behaviors, 7,* 47–55.

Hawkins, R. C., & Clement, P. F. (1984). Binge eating: Measurement problems and a conceptual model. In R. C. Hawkins, W. J. Fremouw, & P. F. Clement (Eds.), *The binge–purge syndrome: Diagnosis, treatment, and research* (pp. 229–253). New York: Springer.

Heatherton, T. E., & Polivy, J. (1992). Chronic dieting and eating disorders: A spiral model. In J. H. Crowther, D. L. Tennenbaum, S. E. Hobfoll, & M. A. P. Stephens (Eds.), *The etiology of bulimia nervosa: The individual and familial context* (pp. 133–155). Washington, DC: Hemisphere.

Hinz, L. D., & Williamson, D. A. (1987). Bulimia and depression: A review of the affective variant hypothesis. *Psychological Bulletin, 102,* 150–158.

Hodgson, R. J., & Rachman, S. (1977). Obsessional–compulsive complaints. *Behaviour Research and Therapy, 15,* 389–395.

Hudson, J. I., Pope, H. G., Jonas, J. M., & Yurgelun-Todd, D. (1983). Family history study of anorexia and bulimia. *British Journal of Psychiatry, 142,* 133–138.

Hyler, S. E., & Rieder, R. O. (1987). *PDQ-R: Personality Diagnostic Questionnaire—Revised.* New York: New York State Psychiatric Institute.

Johnson, C. L. (1985). Initial consultation for patients with bulimia and anorexia nervosa. In D. M. Garner & P. E. Garfinkel (Eds.), *Handbook of psychotherapy for anorexia nervosa and bulimia* (pp. 19–51). New York: Guilford Press.

Johnson, C. L., & Connors, M. E. (1987). *The etiology and treatment of bulimia nervosa: A biopsychosocial perspective.* New York: Basic Books.

Johnson, C. L., & Larson, R. (1982). Bulimia: An analysis of moods and behavior. *Psychosomatic Medicine, 44,* 341–351.

Johnson, C. L., Stuckey, M., Lewis, L. D., & Schwartz, D. (1982). Bulimia: A descriptive study of 316 cases. *International Journal of Eating Disorders, 2,* 1–15.

Johnson, C. L., Tobin, D. L., & Enright, A. B. (1989). Prevalence and clinical characteristics of borderline patients in an eating disordered population. *Journal of Clinical Psychiatry, 50,* 9–15.

Jourard, S. M., & Secord, P. F. (1954). Body size and body cathexis. *Journal of Consulting Psychology, 18,* 184.

Kaye, W. H., Gwirtsman, H. E., George, D. T., Weiss, S. R., & Jimerson, D. C. (1986). Relationship of mood alterations to bingeing behavior in bulimia. *British Journal of Psychiatry, 149,* 479–485.

King, M. B. (1989). Eating disorders in a general practice population: Prevalence, characteristics, and follow-up at 12 to 18 months. *Psychological Medicine, 19*(Monograph Suppl. 14), 1–34.

King, M. B. (1991). The natural history of eating pathology in attenders to primary medical care. *International Journal of Eating Disorders, 10,* 379–387.

Kirkley, B. G., Burge, J. C., & Ammerman, A. (1988). Dietary restraint, binge eating and dietary behavior patterns. *International Journal of Eating Disorders, 7,* 771–778.

Kissileff, H. R., Walsh, B. T., Kral, J. G., & Cassidy, S. M. (1986). Laboratory studies of eating behavior in women with bulimia. *Physiology and Behavior, 38,* 563–570.

Krantzler, N. J., Mullen, B. J., Schutz, H. G., Grivetti, L. E., Holden, C. A., & Meiselman, H. L. (1982). Validity of telephoned diet recalls and records for assessment of food intake. *American Journal of Clinical Nutrition, 36,* 1234–1242.

Lacey, J. H. (1985). Time-limited individual and group treatment for bulimia. In D. M. Garner & P. E. Garfinkel (Eds.), *Handbook of psychotherapy for anorexia nervosa and bulimia* (pp. 431–457). New York: Guilford Press.

Leon, G. R., Carroll, K., Chernyk, B., & Finn, S. (1985). The bulimia–purging syndrome and associated habit patterns with college student and clinically identified populations. *International Journal of Eating Disorders, 4,* 43–57.

Lichtman, S. W., Pisarska, K., Berman, E. R., Pestone, M., Dowling, H., Offenbacher, E., Weisel, H., Heshka, S., Matthews, D. E., & Heymsfield, S. B. (1992). Discrepancy between self-reported and actual caloric intake and exercise in obese subjects. *New England Journal of Medicine, 327,* 1893–1898.

Lindholm, L., & Wilson, G. T. (1988). Body image assessment in patients with bulimia nervosa and normal controls. *International Journal of Eating Disorders, 7,* 527–539.

Lingswiler, V. M., Crowther, J. H., & Stephens, M. A. P. (1989). Affective and cognitive antecedents to eating episodes in bulimia and binge eating. *International Journal of Eating Disorders, 8,* 533–539.

Loeb, K. L., Pike, K. M., Walsh, B. T., & Wilson, G. T. (1994). Assessment of diagnostic features of bulimia nervosa: Interview versus self-report format. *International Journal of Eating Disorders, 16,* 75–81.

Loro, A. D., Jr., & Orleans, C. S. (1981). Binge eating in obesity: Preliminary findings and guidelines for behavioral analyses and treatment. *Addictive Behaviors, 6,* 155–166.

Maloney, M. P., & Ward, M. P. (1976). *Psychological assessment: A conceptual approach.* New York: Oxford University Press.

Marcus, M. D. (1993). Binge eating in obesity. In C. G. Fairburn & G. T. Wilson (Eds.), *Binge eating: Nature, assessment, and treatment* (pp. 77–96). New York: Guilford Press.

Marcus, M. D., Wing, R. R., & Hopkins, J. (1988). Obese binge eaters: Affect, cognitions, and response to behavioral weight control. *Journal of Consulting and Clinical Psychology, 56,* 433–439.

Mitchell, J. E. (1986a). Anorexia nervosa: Medical and physiological aspects. In K. D. Brownell & J. P. Foreyt (Eds.), *Handbook of eating disorders: Physiology, psychology, and treatment of obesity, anorexia, and bulimia* (pp. 266–282). New York: Basic Books.

Mitchell, J. E. (1986b). Bulimia: Medical and physiological aspects. In K. D. Brownell & J. P. Foreyt (Eds.), *Handbook of eating disorders: Physiology, psychology, and treatment of obesity, anorexia, and bulimia* (pp. 379–388). New York: Basic Books.

Mitchell, J. E. (1992). Subtyping of bulimia nervosa. *International Journal of Eating Disorders, 11,* 327–332.

Mitchell, J. E., & Laine, D. C. (1985). Monitored binge eating behavior in patients with bulimia nervosa. *International Journal of Eating Disorders, 4,* 177–183.

Mitchell, J. E., Pyle, R. L., Eckert, E. D., Hatsukami, D., Pomeroy, C., & Zimmerman, R. (1990). A comparison study of antidepressants and structured intensive group psychotherapy in the treatment of bulimia nervosa. *Archives of General Psychiatry, 47,* 149–157.

Mizes, J. S. (1988). Personality characteristics of bulimic and non-eating disordered female controls: A cognitive behavioral perspective. *International Journal of Eating Disorders, 7,* 541–550.

Mizes, J. S. (1992). Validity of the Mizes Anorectic Cognitions scale: A comparison between anorectics, bulimics, and psychiatric controls. *Addictive Behaviors, 17,* 283–289.

Mizes, J. S., & Klesges, R. C. (1989). Validity, reliability, and factor structure of the Anorectic Cognitions questionnaire. *Addictive Behaviors, 14,* 589–594.

Moreno, A., & Thelen, M. H. (1990, August). *Familial factors related to bulimia nervosa.* Paper presented at the annual meeting of the American Psychological Association, Boston.

Orleans, C. T., & Barnett, L. R. (1984). Bulimarexia: Guidelines for behavioral assessment and treatment. In R. C. Hawkins, W. J. Fremouw, & P. F. Clement (Eds.), *The binge–purge syndrome: Diagnosis, treatment, and research* (pp. 144–182). New York: Springer.

Palmer, R., Christie, M., Cordle, C., Davies, D., & Kenrick, J. (1987). The Clinical Eating Disorder Rating Instrument (CEDRI): A preliminary description. *International Journal of Eating Disorders, 6,* 9–16.

Phelan, P. W. (1987). Cognitive correlates of bulimia: The Bulimic Thoughts Questionnaire. *International Journal of Eating Disorders, 6,* 593–607.

Piran, N., Kennedy, S., Garfinkel, P. E., & Owens, M. (1985). Affective disturbance in eating disorders. *Journal of Nervous and Mental Disease, 173,* 395–400.

Polivy, J., & Herman, C. P. (1985). Dieting and bingeing: A causal analysis. *American Psychologist, 40,* 193–201.

Prather, R. C., & Williamson, D. A. (1988). Psychopathology associated with bulimia, binge eating, and obesity. *International Journal of Eating Disorders, 7,* 177–184.

Pyle, R. L., Mitchell, J. E., & Eckert, E. (1981). Bulimia: A report of 34 cases. *Journal of Clinical Psychiatry, 42,* 60–64.

Reitman, E. E., & Cleveland, S. E. (1964). Changes in body image following sensory deprivation in schizophrenic and control groups. *Journal of Abnormal and Social Psychology, 68,* 168–176.

Root, M. P. P., & Friedrich, W. N. (1989). MMPI code types and heterogeneity in a bulimic sample. *Psychotherapy in Private Practice, 7,* 97–113.

Rosch, D. S., Crowther, J. H., & Graham, J. R. (1992). MMPI-derived personality description and personality subtypes in bulimia. *Psychology of Addictive Behaviors, 5,* 15–22.

Rosen, J. C. (1992). Body-image disorder: Definition, development, and contribution to eating disorders. In J. H. Crowther, D. L. Tennenbaum, S. E. Hobfoll, & M. A. P.

Stephens (Eds.), *The etiology of bulimia nervosa: The individual and familial context* (pp. 157–177). Washington, DC: Hemisphere.

Rosen, J. C., & Leitenberg, H. (1985). Exposure plus response prevention treatment of bulimia. In D. M. Garner & P. E. Garfinkel (Eds.), *Handbook of psychotherapy for anorexia nervosa and bulimia* (pp. 193–209). New York: Guilford Press.

Rosen, J. C., & Leitenberg, H. (1988). Eating behavior in bulimia nervosa. In B. T. Walsh (Ed.), *Eating behavior in eating disorders* (pp. 161–174). Washington, DC: American Psychiatric Press.

Rosen, J. C., Leitenberg, H., Fisher, C., & Khazam, C. (1986). Binge-eating episodes in bulimia nervosa: The amount and type of food consumed. *International Journal of Eating Disorders, 5,* 255–257.

Rosen, J. C., & Srebnik, D. (1990). Assessment of eating disorders. In P. McReynolds, J. C. Rosen, & G. J. Chelune (Eds.), *Advances in psychological assessment* (Vol. 7, pp. 229–260). New York: Plenum Press.

Rosen, J. C., Srebnik, D., Saltzberg, E., & Wendt, S. (1991). Development of a body image avoidance questionnaire. *Psychological Assessment: A Journal of Consulting and Clinical Psychology, 3,* 32–37.

Rossiter, E. M., & Agras, W. S. (1990). An empirical test of the DSM-III-R definition of binge. *International Journal of Eating Disorders, 9,* 513–518.

Rossiter, E. M., Agras, W. S., Telch, C. F., & Schneider, J. A. (1993). Cluster B personality disorder characteristics predict outcome in the treatment of bulimia nervosa. *International Journal of Eating Disorders, 13,* 349–357.

Ruff, G. A., & Barrios, B. A. (1986). Realistic assessment of body image. *Behavioral Assessment, 8,* 237–251.

Ruggiero, L., Williamson, D. A., Davis, C. J., Schlundt, D. G., & Carey, M. P. (1988). Forbidden Food Survey: Measure of bulimics' anticipated emotional reactions to specific foods. *Addictive Behaviors, 13,* 267–274.

Russell, G. F. M. (1970). Anorexia nervosa: Its identity as an illness and its treatment. In J. H. Price (Ed.), *Modern trends in psychological medicine* (Vol. 2, pp. 131–164). London: Butterworths.

Russell, G. F. M. (1979). Bulimia nervosa: An ominous variant of anorexia nervosa. *Psychological Medicine, 9,* 429–448.

Rybicki, D. J., Lepkowsky, C. M., & Arndt, S. (1989). An empirical assessment of bulimic patients using multiple measures. *Addictive Behaviors, 14,* 249–260.

Schulman, R. G., Kinder, B. N., Powers, P. S., Prange, M., & Glenhorn, A. (1986). The development of a scale to measure cognitive distortions in bulimia. *Journal of Personality Assessment, 50,* 630–639.

Secord, P. F., & Jourard, S. M. (1953). The appraisal of body cathexis: Body-cathexis and the self. *Journal of Consulting Psychology, 17,* 245–252.

Slade, P. D. (1985). A review of body-image studies in anorexia nervosa and bulimia nervosa. *Journal of Psychiatric Research, 19,* 255–265.

Slade, P. D., & Russell, G. F. M. (1973). Awareness of body dimensions in anorexia nervosa: Cross-sectional and longitudinal studies. *Psychological Medicine, 3,* 188–199.

Smith, M. C., & Thelen, M. H. (1984). Development and validation of a test for bulimia. *Journal of Consulting and Clinical Psychology, 52,* 863–872.

Stunkard, A. J., & Waxman, M. (1981). Accuracy of self-reports of food intake. *Journal of the American Dietetic Association, 79,* 547–551.

Szmukler, G. I., & Tantam, D. (1984). Anorexia nervosa: Starvation dependence. *British Journal of Medical Psychology, 57,* 303–310.

Thelen, M. H., Farmer, J., Wonderlich, S., & Smith, M. (1991). A revision of the Bulimia Test: The BULIT-R. *Psychological Assessment: A Journal of Consulting and Clinical Psychology, 3,* 119–124.

Thelen, M. H., Mann, L. M., Pruitt, J., & Smith, M. (1987). Bulimia: Prevalence and component factors in college women. *Journal of Psychosomatic Research, 31,* 73–78.

Thelen, M. H., Powell, A. L., Lawrence, C., & Kuhnert, M. E. (1992). Eating and body image concerns among children. *Journal of Clinical Child Psychology, 21,* 41–47.

Tobin, D. L., Johnson, C. L., Steinberg, S., Staats, M., & Dennis, A. B. (1991). Multifactorial assessment of bulimia nervosa. *Journal of Abnormal Psychology, 100,* 14–21.

Vandereycken, W., & Vanderlinden, J. (1983). Denial of illness and the use of self-reporting measures in anorexia nervosa patients. *International Journal of Eating Disorders, 2,* 101–107.

Vitousek, K. B., Daly, J., & Heiser, C. (1991). Reconstructing the internal world of the eating-disordered individual: Overcoming denial and distortion in self-report. *International Journal of Eating Disorders, 10,* 647–666.

Vitousek, K. B., & Manke, F. (1994). Personality variables and disorders in anorexia nervosa and bulimia nervosa. *Journal of Abnormal Psychology, 103,* 137–147.

Warren, M. (1968). A study of anorexia nervosa in young girls. *Journal of Child Psychology and Psychiatry, 9,* 27–40.

Wear, R. W., & Pratz, O. (1987). Test–retest reliability for the Eating Disorder Inventory. *International Journal of Eating Disorders, 6,* 767–769.

Welch, G., Thompson, L., & Hall, A. (1993). The BULIT-R: Its reliability and clinical validity as a screening tool for DSM-III-R bulimia nervosa in a female tertiary education population. *International Journal of Eating Disorders, 14,* 95–105.

Williamson, D. A. (1990). *Assessment of eating disorders: Obesity, anorexia, and bulimia nervosa.* Elmsford, NY: Pergamon Press.

Wilson, G. T. (1993). Assessment of binge eating. In C. G. Fairburn & G. T. Wilson (Eds.), *Binge eating: Nature, assessment, and treatment* (pp. 227–249). New York: Guilford Press.

Wilson, G. T., & Walsh, B. T. (1991). Eating disorders in the DSM-IV. *Journal of Abnormal Psychology, 100,* 362–365.

Wolf, E. M., & Crowther, J. H. (1992). An evaluation of behavioral and cognitive-behavioral group interventions for the treatment of bulimia nervosa in women. *International Journal of Eating Disorders, 11,* 3–15.

Wooley, S. C., & Kearney-Cooke, A. (1986). Intensive treatment of bulimia and body image disturbance. In K. D. Brownell & J. P. Foreyt (Eds.), *Handbook of eating disorders: Physiology, psychology, and treatment of obesity, anorexia, and bulimia* (pp. 476–502). New York: Basic Books.

Wonderlich, S. A., Fullerton, D., Swift, W. J., & Klein, M. H. (1994). Five year outcome from eating disorders: The relevance of personality disorders. *International Journal of Eating Disorders, 15,* 233–243.

Wonderlich, S. A., & Mitchell, J. E. (1988). Eating disorders and personality disorders. In J. Yager (Ed.), *Special problems in managing eating disorders* (pp. 51–86). Washington, DC: American Psychiatric Press.

Wonderlich, S. A., Swift, W. J., Slotnick, H. B., & Goodman, S. (1990). DSM-III-R personality disorders in eating-disorder subtypes. *International Journal of Eating Disorders, 9,* 607–616.

Yates, W. R., & Sambrailo, F. (1984). Bulimia nervosa: A descriptive and therapeutic study. *Behaviour Research and Therapy, 22,* 502–518.

Yates, W. R., Sieleni, B., Reich, J., & Brass, C. (1989). Comorbidity of bulimia nervosa and personality disorder. *Journal of Clinical Psychiatry, 50,* 57–59.

Zotter, D. L., & Crowther, J. H. (1991). The role of cognitions in bulimia nervosa. *Cognitive Therapy and Research, 15,* 413–426.

CHAPTER 5

Sequencing and Integration of Treatments

DAVID M. GARNER
LAWRENCE D. NEEDLEMAN

The number of psychotherapeutic options available in treating eating disorders has expanded remarkably in the past decade. The major approaches to psychotherapy have been well articulated, along with a growing list of alternative forms of treatment. The trend has been for clinical formulations to reflect a particular orientation to treatment of eating disorders; indeed, the main chapters in this volume are organized accordingly. At the same time, there has been a seemingly opposite movement in the general field of psychotherapy toward eclecticism and integration of different therapeutic approaches (Garfield, 1994; Garfield & Bergin, 1994). It is not clear why the integration of different treatments for eating disorders has not been more popular. However, the wisdom of considering integration of different psychotherapeutic procedures is increasingly evident with the demonstrated effectiveness of different forms of treatment.

The impressive advancement in the technology of treatment for eating disorders has largely derived from carefully controlled studies using detailed treatment manuals. However, results from these treatment studies do not always generalize to the clinical situations actually faced by the practitioner. This is because the aim of treatment research is clearly different from that of the clinician. The objective in treatment research is to study the effects of delivering a standard or "pure" form of treatment on a precisely defined patient sample. The clinician, in con-

trast, sees a wide range of patients, many of whom would not meet entry criteria for a study. Moreover, the clinician must decide how to alter the approach for patients who fail to respond to treatment or who relapse. Thus, controlled treatment research may leave the clinician with a number of questions: To what degree are treatments used in research studies generalizable to patients when they do not meet research inclusion criteria? What factors should be considered in choosing various treatment options? What viable alternative treatments are available? What treatments should be considered when patients do not respond favorably to the "standard" clinical approach? What treatments should be considered if patients relapse? Thus, the practitioner is vitally interested in the logic behind matching treatments to individuals, as well as in the conditions under which treatments should be altered, integrated, or changed.

The notion of applying different treatments to different eating disorder patients is not new and has formed the basis for multidimensional approaches to psychotherapy (see Garner, Garfinkel, & Bemis, 1982). However, there has been more recent interest in stepped care, decision-tree, or integration models, which rely on set rules for the delivery of the various treatment options (Agras, 1993; Fairburn & Peveler, 1990; Fairburn, Agras, & Wilson, 1992; Garner, Garfinkel, & Irvine, 1986; Tiller, Schmidt, & Treasure, 1993). These overlapping concepts of treatment delivery share the value system of nonallegiance to a single theoretical orientation, but they have somewhat different points of emphasis.

The "stepped-care" approach involves sequencing empirically or logically-derived interventions into graded levels or "steps," based on level of intensity, cost and probability of success. Typically, all patients follow the same sequence. Initially, a patient is provided with the lowest-step intervention—the one that is least intrusive, dangerous, and costly, even if it does not have the highest probability of success. If the first level intervention fails, then the second step on the treatment hierarchy is initiated. The sequencing of treatments is followed until the patient responds favorably.

The "decision-tree" model provides numerous choice points resulting in different paths for treatment, depending on the clinical features of the patient as well as the response to each treatment delivered. Thus, the treatment decision at each juncture may depend on answers to key questions. For instance, the clinician may ask, "Is the patient in acute medical danger?" If the answer is "yes," the patient is referred to an inpatient program. If the answer is "no," the clinician asks, "Is the patient 18 years old or younger and living at home?" If the answer is "yes," the patient is referred to family therapy. If the answer is "no," the patient is referred to individual therapy, and so on. The decision-tree approach follows the clinical application of treatments more closely.

The "integration" concept has played an increasingly important role in the field of psychotherapy in recent years. It has been used in different ways to denote the combination of two or more forms of psychotherapy (Garfield, 1994). The term "integration" overlaps with "eclecticism." However, there appears to be general agreement that "integration" tends to signify the combination of two or more theoretical orientations, whereas "eclecticism" connotes the selection of techniques and procedures regardless of their theoretical origin (Garfield, 1994).

At this time, proposals for integrating and sequencing different forms of treatment have not been empirically tested in the area of eating disorders. This is partly because of the formidable practical and theoretical impediments to a research protocol required to test complex stepped-care, decision-tree, and integration models. Nevertheless, existing treatment research combined with current clinical knowledge provides a foundation for rational recommendations regarding the selection of treatments in the management of eating disorders. The literature on the application of stepped-care, decision-tree, and integration approaches to eating disorders is reviewed below, followed by the proposal of a general model for making decisions about treatment.

LITERATURE REVIEW AND A GENERAL DECISION-MAKING MODEL

Giles, Young, and Young (1985) introduced a stepped-care procedure in an early uncontrolled study of cognitive-behavioral therapy for bulimia nervosa. They found that brief cognitive-behavioral therapy was beneficial for the majority of patients, but that a subgroup of recalcitrant patients might benefit from being exposed to a succession of procedures over a longer duration. Those patients who failed to improve were moved to the next stage of treatment. The graded steps included (1) training a significant other to supervise *in vivo* exposure between sessions; (2) having an experienced therapist supervise two cafeteria meals a week; (3) introducing tricyclic antidepressants; and (4) recommending hospitalization. One of the six recalcitrant patients responded well and three showed moderate improvement with this regimen.

Garner et al. (1986) proposed a model for integrating and sequencing different forms of treatment of eating disorder patients. In this model, treatments were graded from the less complicated and intrusive approaches to those that are more disruptive, costly, or carry greater risks. At each step, specific decisions were guided by considerations such as (1) age of the patient; (2) current living arrangements; (3) duration of the disorder; (4) current symptomatology (presence of bingeing, vomiting, or purgative abuse; stable or unstable weight; deteriorating symptom picture); (5) previous treatments; (6) premorbid functioning, with particular reference to depression, problems with impulse control, and personality disorders; and (7) medical condition, including (but not limited to) degree of weight loss and electrolyte disturbances. The authors recommended an educational approach as the initial intervention for the least disturbed bulimia nervosa patients and as an adjunct to other forms of treatment for other eating disorder patients, including those with anorexia nervosa. They recommended family therapy as the primary treatment modality if a patient was young and living at home. They considered pharmacotherapy as an option in bulimia nervosa (but not anorexia nervosa) when patients failed to respond to psychosocial treatments. For patients with serious medical complications or a need to gain substantial body weight, the authors recommended inpatient treatment as the initial intervention. Finally, they recommended day treatment for patients who did not require hospitalization but did need a high level of treatment intensity and meal supervision. Although this integration and sequencing model was a novel attempt to specify the decision-making process in delivering different forms of treatment for both of the main eating disorders, it lacked clear criteria for determining how patients would be allocated reliably to different treatment options.

Fairburn and Peveler (1990) outlined a more modest five-level stepped-care approach limited to bulimia nervosa patients. The steps were (1) self-help or written materials; (2) dietary education and advice, perhaps in a group setting; (3) antidepressant drug treatment (desipramine or fluoxetine) in combination with advice and support; (4) outpatient cognitive-behavioral treatment; and (5) day or inpatient care with subsequent outpatient treatment. Fairburn et al. (1992) proposed a similar model for managing bulimia nervosa that did not include antidepressant drugs "because their position in the scheme is debatable" (p. 334). The model by Fairburn and colleagues was novel because it formally introduced the use of supervised self-help, which is potentially more economical than other treatment options.

Agras (1993) described a more detailed decision-tree model for the treatment of binge eating that was more precise than earlier recommendations. In cases of severe binge eating, he advised assigning patients to either cognitive-behavioral therapy or interpersonal psychotherapy, depending on whether dietary or interpersonal problems were predominant. When binge eating was less severe, he recommended psychoeducational treatment. This model had and still has intuitive appeal, despite the fact that there is no empirical evidence that cognitive-behavioral therapy and interpersonal psychotherapy are differentially effective based on these clinical features. Finally, Agras proposed that obese patients who became abstinent from binge eating should go on to weight loss treatment—a point that remains controversial (Garner & Wooley, 1991).

Tiller et al. (1993) outlined a stepped-care program that was similar in some ways to those presented earlier. They divided the decision-making process into five phases, adding additional treatments if patients failed to respond or if they showed only partial improvement. The steps involved (1) minimal interventions such as psychoeducation, bibliotherapy, or referral to self-help groups; (2) standard cognitive-behavioral therapy for bulimia nervosa; (3) antidepressant medication; (4) cognitive analytical therapy (Ryle, 1990) or interpersonal psychotherapy (Klerman, Weissman, Rounsaville, & Chevron, 1984); and (5) inpatient or day treatment. Inpatient or day treatment was recommended for those who failed to respond to earlier interventions or who presented with a medical or psychiatric crisis. Thus, the model presented by Tiller et al. combined elements of earlier stepped-care and the decision-tree models.

These models continue to have clinical appeal, but they offer only limited criteria for decision making and only a narrow range of treatment options that would be considered by most knowledgeable clinicians. Figure 5.1 is a diagrammatic representation of a further development of the decision-making process for sequencing and integration of treatments for people with eating disorders. At first blush, Figure 5.1 may seem a bit onerous in its complexity, but it is actually quite a simple set of questions (represented by boxes with rounded corners, mostly on the left side of the figure) and treatment options (represented by boxes with sharp corners, mostly in the middle of the figure). Beginning in the upper left corner with the question "Is pt [patient] in serious physical danger?", it is possible to work gradually through the flow chart. Figure 5.1 does not include all possible treatment alternatives, but concentrates on those for which there is good clinical or empirical support. With this in mind, we briefly discuss these treatments, as well as the clinical criteria for their integration and sequencing.

MAJOR TREATMENT OPTIONS

Inpatient Hospitalization and Partial Care

During the 1980s, there was a convergence of extraordinary economic incentives for inpatient

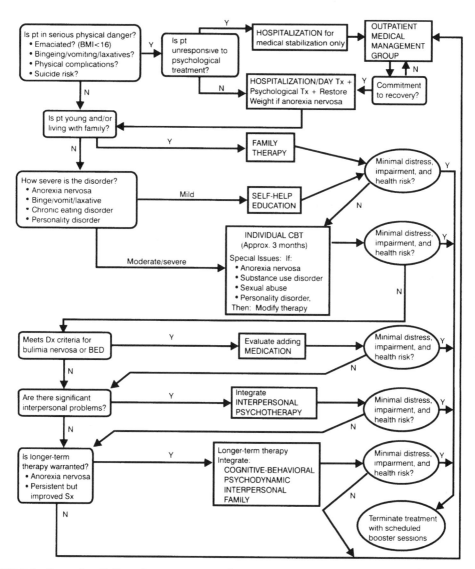

FIGURE 5.1. General guidelines for integration and sequencing major treatment options for eating disorder patients. Begin in the upper left corner with the question "Is pt in serious physical danger?" Further criteria for decision making, including symptom areas, patient characteristics, and response to previous treatments, are indicated by boxes with rounded corners (mostly on the left side of the figure). The treatment options are represented by boxes with sharp corners (hospitalization, family therapy, self-help/education, individual therapy, etc.). The figure does not delineate all treatment alternatives or all considerations for decision making. However, it does include the main interventions for which there is good clinical and/or empirical support, and key variables to consider in determining the most appropriate type and intensity of treatment. Abbreviations: pt, patient; BMI, body mass index; 5×/wk, five times a week; Dx, diagnostic; BED, binge-eating disorder; Tx, treatment; CBT, cognitive-behavioral therapy.

care, surging demands for clinical services, and widespread misinformation regarding optimal treatment; this convergence led to the unnecessary hospitalization of many eating disorder patients who could have been easily managed on an outpatient basis. The abuse of inpatient treatment has been followed by a backlash, resulting in inappropriate denial of hospital coverage or absurd limitations of coverage for eating disorder patients, which have put many such patients at unnecessary risk for chronic illness or death. Part of the problem has been a failure to clearly articulate two different sets of objectives for hospitalization, requiring different treatment protocols. Hospitalization either can be a strategic step aimed at recovery from an eating disorder or can be aimed solely at medical stabilization. When aimed at treating physical complications, hospitalization is a medical priority not requiring a commitment by the patient to recover from the eating disorder. This contrasts with hospitalization intended as a critical step in the recovery process (see Anderson, Bowers, & Evans, Chapter 17, this volume). As part of recovery, hospitalization is aimed at addressing both the physical and the psychological aspects of the disorder. Considerable effort is required to enlist the patient's genuine commitment to participate in every stage of the treatment process.

Hospitalization is required under certain circumstances. These are (1) to achieve weight restoration or interrupt steady weight loss in patients who are emaciated and in medical danger; (2) to interrupt bingeing, vomiting, and/or laxative abuse that poses medical risks or complications; (3) to evaluate and treat other potentially serious physical complications; and (4) to manage associated conditions, such as severe depression, risk of self-harm, or substance use disorders. Failure to offer hospitalization under these circumstances is perilous, considering the extremely high mortality rates associated with anorexia nervosa (Sullivan, 1995). On rare occasions, hospitalization may be required to "disengage" a patient from a social system that both contributes to the maintenance of the disorder and disrupts outpatient treatment. Thus, as indicated in Figure 5.1, the first major treatment consideration is whether or not an eating disorder patient is in sufficient medical danger to require hospitalization. If a careful evaluation of prior treatment and current motivation for treatment leads to the conclusion that the patient is clearly unresponsive to psychological treatment, then it is appropriate to consider hospitalization for medical stabilization only and referral to outpatient medical maintenance, discussed below.

More typically, there is reason for optimism about recovery from the eating disorder. In these cases the hospitalization can usually be brief, again aimed at medical stabilization, but with the addition of psychological counseling followed by referral to outpatient psychotherapy. Again, the most common exception to brief hospitalization is the emaciated anorexia ner-

vosa patient, for whom longer hospitalization is usually required to make steady headway in the renourishment process. It is generally pointless to negotiate with patients or insurance carriers in regard to the duration of hospitalization required for weight restoration, since the time needed is relatively straightforward and easy to calculate. At a minimum, it is the number of weeks or months required for the patient to reach at least 90% of expected weight, assuming a weight gain rate of about 2 to 3 pounds a week and optimal compliance with the treatment program. Even though weight restoration can be a time-consuming and expensive process, premature discharge is not cost-effective: It leads to high rates of rehospitalization and entrenchment of symptoms, compared to allowing patients to achieve a normal weight before discharge (Baran, Weltzin, & Kaye, 1995). A chronic eating disorder inflicts a heavy price, in both monetary and emotional terms. At the same time, it is legitimate to question the validity or timing of a lengthy hospitalization aimed at renutrition if steady weight gain does not occur.

Another situation in which hospitalization may be necessary is a patient's failure to improve in protracted outpatient therapy. Such a patient may simply be unable to make improvement without the structure and containment offered by the inpatient environment. Indefinite outpatient treatment may be fruitless or even deleterious, in the sense that it inadvertently colludes with the patient's ambivalence about recovery. It is like years of insight-oriented psychotherapy with an elevator phobic without ever requiring a ride on an elevator. Without some exposure, the therapist cannot ever assist the patient in confronting fears associated with weight restoration. The patient may perceive the recommendation for hospitalization as a threat or as abandonment, but should be reassured that it is a humane alternative to the tremendous emotional and financial expense of prolonged and unproductive outpatient therapy. Psychotherapy can achieve only modest goals, given the limits imposed by dietary chaos or chronic starvation.

Day treatment or partial hospitalization is the preferred alternative to inpatient care for most eating disorder patients. These programs provide structure around mealtimes, plus the possibility for intensive therapy, without requiring a patient to become totally disengaged from the supports and the therapeutic challenges outside the hospital. Partial-care programs offer the distinct advantage of being more economical than full hospitalization. They can also provide a useful bridge between inpatient and outpatient care. There are various models for day treatment programs, which generally share many features with inpatient programs (see Kaplan & Olmsted, Chapter 18, this volume). The major difference is that patients receive the therapeutic services without staying overnight.

Outpatient Medical Management for Chronic Patients

Concluding that a patient is unresponsive to psychological treatment, and then referring the patient to outpatient medical management (see Figure 5.1), require careful analysis and considerable reflection. However, some chronic or recalcitrant patients have participated in various forms of competently delivered treatment over the course of many years and reach the point at which they, in consultation with their clinicians, believe that further psychotherapy at this time has a very low probability of success. In these cases, further psychotherapy *aimed at recovery* can be highly frustrating for both therapists and patients, often leading to their termination from therapy with inadequate follow-up plans. These patients are reluctant to seek further assistance if and when their medical or psychological condition deteriorates. The key issue in evaluating these patients is determining whether there really has been sufficient exposure to truly adequate treatment, since patients can have had extensive exposure to poor treatment or to therapists who are not knowledgeable about eating disorders.

If careful evaluation leads to the conclusion that such a patient has had an adequate course of psychotherapy, then termination from psychotherapy may be very appropriate as long as it is made conditional on the patient's agreeing to weekly medical management (Figure 5.1), conducted in an individual or a group format and with concrete emergency backup. A goal of the medical management group should be to insure that body weight, electrolytes, and vital signs are checked at appropriate intervals, with appropriate referral to medical specialists as needed. These groups afford patients the added benefits of group support and sharing with similarly afflicted patients. In some cases, medical management groups set the stage for renewed efforts to pursue psychological treatment. In

sum, the goal of medical management is very different from that of psychotherapy: Rather than focusing on "overcoming the eating disorder," it is aimed at maintaining medical and psychological stability. The criteria for medical management are (1) repeated failures to respond to appropriate psychological or nutritional treatments; (2) no logical basis for pursuing another form of treatment; (3) no immediate psychological or medical crises; and (4) sufficient symptoms to suggest ongoing medical risk.

Education-Based Interventions and Self-Help

Psychoeducation and Nutritional Management

Figure 5.1 indicates that psychoeducation or some other sort of educational intervention should be considered for bulimia nervosa patients with milder symptoms (see Garner, Chapter 8, this volume). In the past decade, education has played an important role in the treatment of eating disorders. It was integrated into early descriptions of cognitive-behavioral treatment for eating disorders, based on the premise that certain faulty assumptions evinced by patients were maintained at least in part by misinformation (e.g., Fairburn, 1985; Garner & Bemis, 1982). There was considerable variation in the content of early treatments identified as "educational"; they stressed dietary management, social skills, assertiveness, relaxation training, or some combination of these approaches (Beumont, O'Connor, Touyz, & Williams, 1987; Connors, Johnson, & Stuckey, 1984; Garner, Rockert, Olmsted, Johnson & Coscina, 1985; Wolchik, Weiss, & Katzman, 1986). An early psychoeducational primer (Garner et al., 1985) emphasized several key issues: (1) the conflict between Western cultural pressures on women to diet (since most patients with eating disorders are female) and biological compensatory mechanisms that tend to defend a set point for body weight; (2) recommendations for establishing regular eating patterns; (3) self-monitoring or meal planning, (4) gradual incorporation of forbidden foods; and (5) specific methods for interrupting bingeing and purging. A study comparing the presentation of this educational material in a group classroom format (five 90-minute sessions during a 1-month period) with individual cognitive-behavioral therapy indicated, for the least symptomatic 25–45% of patients, that both treatments were equally effective on important measures of outcome (Olmsted et al., 1991).

Nutritional counseling or nutritional management (Beumont, Beumont, Touyz, & Williams, Chapter 9, this volume; Beumont et al., 1987; Hsu, Holben, & West, 1992) overlaps with the psychoeducational approach described above. Laessle et al. (1991) compared nutritional management with stress management and found that both treatments led to marked improvement in eating disorder symptoms and general psychopathology at the end of treatment and at a 12-month follow-up. However, nutritional management produced a significantly more rapid reduction in binge eating, greater abstinence rates, and greater improvements on some measures of psychopathology.

Self-Help and Guided Self-Help

Some eating disorder patients with relatively mild symptoms may experience marked improvement or complete recovery with self-help or education-based interventions. Self-help organizations for eating disorders have been very popular for almost 20 years (Baker Enright, Butterfield, & Berkowitz, 1985). In the last decade, there has been a remarkable increase in the number of self-help books available for eating disorder patients and their families (Santrock, Minnett, & Campbell, 1994). Interest in testing the efficacy of self-help has been slower to develop, but there are now a number of studies indicating that some forms of self-help or guided self-help may be quite effective with some eating disorders (see Fairburn & Carter, Chapter 30, this volume). Again, and as indicated in Figure 5.1, self-help is recommended for patients with less severe eating disorder symptoms.

Huon (1985) was the first to test the effectiveness of a structured self-help program. Binge-eating subjects were recruited from a woman's magazine article, and the 32% who followed a self-help manual were found to be symptom-free at a 6-month follow-up, compared to only 7% of a comparison group. Two later studies indicated short-term benefits of following a self-help manual, but neither presented follow-up data (Schmidt, Tiller, & Treasure, 1993; Treasure et al., 1994). In contrast to "pure" self-help, Cooper, Coker, and Fleming (1994, 1996) have reported that self-help supervised by a professional can be effective for some patients. Cooper et al. (1996) followed up 82 patients after 4 to 6 months and found that 16 (20%) had dropped out of the program, but that 22 (33%) of those remaining had not binged or vomited over the past month. Thus, although self-help is not sufficient for most patients, a significant subgroup can benefit from this economical intervention.

In sum, there is general agreement that some sort of educational treatment, in the form of either self-help manuals, accurate educational readings, or educational groups, can be a valuable adjunct to most forms of treatment. Education is not a necessary ingredient, since interpersonal psychotherapy, with no educational component, is an effective treatment for bulimia nervosa (Fairburn, Chapter 14, this volume). It is not known whether the integration of educational material and interpersonal psychotherapy would accelerate improvement. For people with mild eating disorder symptoms (Figure 5.1), clinicians should consider educational groups or guided self-help before proceeding to more costly interventions.

Family Therapy

Family therapy (Figure 5.1) is the initial treatment choice for anorexia nervosa patients who are 18 years old or younger and living at home (Russell, Szmukler, Dare, & Eisler, 1987; Dare & Eisler, Chapter 16, this volume). Family therapy (or strategically employed family sessions) may also be a desirable adjunct to individual therapy with older patients, particularly when family conflicts predominate. Even when family therapy is not the primary mode of treatment, a comprehensive family assessment can be critical in order to fully understand and then address specific therapeutic issues (Andersen, 1985; Crisp, 1970; Garner et al., 1982; Vandereycken, Kog, & Vanderlinden, 1989; Wooley & Lewis, 1989).

Family therapists have argued convincingly that an eating disorder may reflect certain dysfunctional roles, alliances, conflicts, or interactional patterns within a family (Minuchin, Rosman, & Baker, 1978; Selvini Palazzoli, 1974). This can be manifested in many ways. An eating disorder can deflect members of the family away from potentially threatening developmental expectations emergent in a child's transition to puberty. It can function as a maladaptive solution to the adolescent's struggle to achieve autonomy in a family in which any move toward independence is perceived as a threat to family unity. It can also become a powerful diversion, enabling the parents and the child to avoid major sources of conflict.

For young patients, there are practical as well as theoretical reasons for recommending family therapy. From a strictly practical point of view, parents or guardians are legally responsible for a minor patient's well-being. Moreover, parents have the potential to provide powerful directives in support of therapeutic goals. Regardless of theoretical orientation of treatment, family members need assistance in dealing with a young eating-disordered patient. Often the family is so terrified by an anorexic patient's increasingly skeletal appearance that members vacillate between desperate attempts at overcontrol and failure to set appropriate limits when confronted with bizarre dietary rituals. As indicated in Figure 5.1, it may be appropriate to integrate family therapy into the longer-term treatment plan. It can be a valuable adjunct to individual therapy in addressing trauma (e.g., sexual abuse) within a family (Wooley & Lewis, 1989).

Cognitive-Behavioral Therapy

Cognitive-behavioral therapy has become the standard treatment for bulimia nervosa and forms the theoretical base for much of the treatment of anorexia nervosa. As indicated in Figure 5.1, cognitive-behavioral therapy is the treatment of choice for patients whose age does not mandate family therapy, and whose symptoms are moderate to severe.

The cognitive-behavioral therapy developed by Fairburn and colleagues for bulimia nervosa (Fairburn, 1985; Fairburn, Marcus, & Wilson, 1993; Wilson, Fairburn, & Agras, Chapter 6, this volume) has the following major points of emphasis: (1) self-monitoring of food intake and of bingeing and purging episodes, as well as the thoughts and feelings that trigger these episodes; (2) regular weighing; (3) specific recommendations (e.g., introducing avoided foods and meal planning) designed to normalize eating behavior and curb restrictive dieting; (4) cognitive restructuring directed at habitual reasoning errors and underlying assumptions that are relevant to the development and maintenance of the eating disorder; and (5) preventing relapse.

Cognitive-behavioral therapy is also effective in stabilizing the eating patterns of obese individuals who experience recurrent episodes of binge eating (Agras et al., 1992; Telch, Agras, Rossiter, Wilfley, & Kenardy, 1990; Wilfley et al., 1993). The results of cognitive-behavioral therapy with binge-eating disorder patients are promising; however, its long-term effectiveness with this group remains unclear.

In the case of anorexia nervosa, cognitive-behavioral therapy has been recommended largely on clinical grounds (Garner, 1986, 1988; Garner & Bemis, 1982, 1985; Garner & Rosen, 1990; Garner, Vitousek, & Pike, Chapter 7, this volume; Pike, Loeb, & Vitousek, 1996). Case studies and preliminary research provide some grounds for optimism (Cooper & Fairburn, 1984; Channon, DeSilva, Helmsley, & Perkins, 1989); however, current data are insufficient to permit meaningful conclusions regarding effectiveness to be drawn.

There are many areas of overlap between the versions of cognitive-behavioral therapy offered for anorexia nervosa and bulimia nervosa, as well as some significant differences (see Garner et al., Chapter 7, this volume). A major focus for both disorders is the patient's underlying assumption that "weight, shape, or thinness can serve as the sole or predominant referent for inferring personal value or self-worth" (Garner & Bemis, 1982, p. 142). Fear of body weight gain is a central theme for both anorexia nervosa and bulimia nervosa; however, most bulimia nervosa patients can be reassured that treatment will probably result in little weight gain (Fairburn, Marcus, & Wilson, 1993). In contrast, therapeutic strategies for anorexia nervosa must specifically target weight gain, despite the patients' implacable resistance to change. Anorexia nervosa patients are typically less motivated for change, since many of their symptoms are ego-syntonic. Cognitive-behavioral therapy for anorexia nervosa is usually longer in duration than the 3 months recommended for bulimia nervosa. Moreover, the content domain is focused beyond that typically described for bulimia nervosa. It includes integrating methods for addressing interpersonal and family problems (see Garner et al., Chapter 7, this volume). In the subset of anorexia nervosa patients who do not engage in binge eating, and those who show no obvious serious physical complications, there may be extraordinary resistance to complying with the therapeutic objectives of weight gain. As long as there is gradual improvement in symptoms (Figure 5.1), outpatient cognitive-behavioral therapy is recommended; however, if the patient's physical condition deteriorates, hospitalization must be considered.

Interpersonal Psychotherapy

For the past decade, the prevailing view has been that cognitive-behavioral therapy's effectiveness with eating disorder patients is fundamentally related to its focus on attitudes about weight and shape that cause severely restrictive dieting and extreme weight-controlling behaviors. However, a recent series of studies using interpersonal psychotherapy adapted to bulimia nervosa has prompted a reexamination of these assumptions, because this form of therapy does not focus directly on eating problems (Fairburn et al., 1991; Fairburn, Jones, Peveler, Hope, & O'Connor, 1993; Fairburn et al., 1995). Interpersonal psychotherapy was originally formulated by Klerman et al. (1984) as a short-term treatment for depression. Interpersonal psychotherapy for eating disorders is divided into three stages (Fairburn, Chapter 14, this volume). The first stage involves identifying the interpersonal problems that have led to the development and maintenance of the eating problems. The second stage consists of a therapeutic contract for working on these interpersonal problems. The final stage addresses issues related to termination. Fairburn et al. (1991) found interpersonal psychotherapy somewhat less effective than cognitive-behavioral therapy at the end of treatment; however, patients who received interpersonal psychotherapy gradually improved during the follow-up period, so that after 1 year both treatments were equally effective (Fairburn, Jones, et al., 1993). These findings were maintained over the longer term, with patients receiving either cognitive-behavioral therapy or interpersonal psychotherapy doing significantly better than those receiving behavior therapy (Fairburn et al., 1995). This pattern of improvement during follow-up was not found with a very different form of interpersonally oriented therapy, supportive–expressive therapy (Garner, Rockert, Garner, Davis, & Olmsted, 1993). These findings suggest that the interpersonal therapies offered in the Oxford trials contain specific therapeutic ingredients that facilitate change. Further support for the effectiveness of interpersonal psychotherapy comes from Wilfley et al. (1993) in a study of nonpurging bulimic patients, many of whom

presented with obesity. They found cognitive-behavioral therapy and interpersonal psychotherapy to be equally effective in reducing binge eating, assessed both at the end of treatment and at a 1-year follow-up.

The evidence that certain interpersonal therapies are as effective as cognitive-behavioral therapy with binge eating has implications for the decision process illustrated in Figure 5.1. It could be argued that either interpersonal psychotherapy or cognitive-behavioral therapy could be the initial treatment of choice for bulimia nervosa, because both treatments are equally effective in the long term. Certainly a therapist well trained in one of the interpersonal therapies described by Fairburn and colleagues should not be encouraged to abandon this form of treatment in favor of cognitive-behavioral therapy. However, we are still inclined to recommend cognitive-behavioral therapy as the preferred initial treatment, because it has been shown to have a more rapid effect on symptoms. Moreover, the efficacy of interpersonal psychotherapy for bulimia nervosa has been demonstrated in just one center, whereas many studies have supported the effectiveness of cognitive-behavioral therapy. If the findings from the Oxford trials are replicated in other centers, then interpersonal psychotherapy may become another "standard" initial treatment for bulimia nervosa. At this time, there is no empirical basis for suggesting that interpersonal psychotherapy should be applied differentially to patients on the basis of premorbid features such as interpersonal conflicts. However, integrating interpersonal psychotherapy into treatment should be considered for bulimia nervosa patients who fail to respond favorably to an initial course of cognitive-behavioral therapy when interpersonal conflicts predominate, according to Figure 5.1. In the treatment of anorexia nervosa, many of the elements of interpersonal psychotherapy are already integrated into the longer-term cognitive-behavioral therapy (see Garner et al., Chapter 7, this volume).

Psychodynamic Therapy

There have been no controlled comparisons between long-term psychodynamic psychotherapy and other forms of treatment; however, dynamically oriented treatments have been well articulated for eating disorders and may be recommended on clinical grounds when other short-term treatments are ineffective (Figure 5.1). Psychodynamic treatment for eating disorders may be roughly divided into two schools of thought. The first presumes that eating disorders do not require fundamental modifications to orthodox dynamic interventions, because neither the symptoms nor the disorders represent a unique underlying process. The second conceptualization implies that eating disorders are distinctive, in that they require major modifications to traditional dynamic therapy to meet the patients' special psychological and physical needs. There has been considerable movement among dynamically oriented writers toward integrating psychodynamic therapy with active symptom management principles in treating eating disorders (Crisp, 1980 and Chapter 13, this volume; Bruch, 1973; Casper, 1982; Goodsitt, 1985 and Chapter 11, this volume; Stern, 1986; Strober, Chapter 12, this volume; Strober & Yager, 1985). However, there are still some who espouse a traditional interpretive framework (Lerner, 1991; Sugarman, 1991; Sands, 1991). We recommend the modified forms of dynamic therapy as a viable alternative to long-term cognitive-behavioral therapy for eating disorder patients who do not show progress with less expensive approaches.

Feminist Therapies

A new generation of feminist therapists is deviating from the traditional views by incorporating the growing literature on the psychology of women into dynamic formulations regarding the etiology and treatment of eating disorders (Fallon, Katzman, & Wooley, 1994; Fallon & Wonderlich, Chapter 22, this volume; Katzman, 1994; Perlick & Silverstein, 1994; Steiner-Adair, 1994; Striegel-Moore, 1994; Wooley, 1994; Wooley & Kearney-Cooke, 1986). These theorists emphasize sociopolitical themes that should be considered (Perlick & Silverstein, 1994; Steiner-Adair, 1994), as well as therapist gender and treatment (Katzman, 1994; Wooley, 1994) and the need to realign mainstream psychology to include the feminist perspective (Striegel-Moore, 1994). They have highlighted the importance of addressing such issues as role conflicts, identity confusion, sexual abuse, and other forms of victimization in the development, maintenance, and treatment of eating disorders. Treatments are described in interactive terms, emphasizing the importance of

women's interpersonal relationships. Although controlled studies are still lacking on the efficacy of feminist therapies, this is true for many other treatment approaches to eating disorders. Recent advances in articulating feminist therapeutic principles as they relate to eating disorders (Fallon et al., 1994; Fallon & Wonderlich, Chapter 22, this volume) set the stage for evaluative studies using methods and measures that better address feminist views on treatment. At this time, a therapist's orientation, rather than the special needs of a patient, probably determines the decision to apply feminist therapy to eating disorders. However, many of the views articulated by feminist therapists have influenced the applications of other forms of therapy. Feminist therapy offers specific treatment principles designed to assist patients who have a history of physical or sexual abuse (Fallon & Wonderlich, Chapter 22, this volume). Other approaches to therapy should integrate these methods when abuse issues emerge during the course of treatment (Figure 5.1).

Pharmacotherapy

The issue of pharmacotherapy for eating disorders is complex, and the present discussion cannot be anything other than cursory. However, a number of basic principles can be derived from major reviews of the literature (Garfinkel & Garner, 1987; Garfinkel & Walsh, Chapter 20, this volume; Mitchell, Raymond, & Specker, 1993). First, medication should rarely be the primary method of treatment for bulimia nervosa, and when it is used, it should be as a supplement to education, nutritional rehabilitation, and psychotherapy. Second, cognitive-behavioral therapy is generally superior to antidepressant medication alone with bulimia nervosa. Third, antidepressant medications may add to the effectiveness of psychotherapy for bulimia nervosa. Fourth, the role of medication for anorexia nervosa is very limited.

A multisite collaborative study (Fluoxetine Bulimia Nervosa Collaborative Study Group, 1992; Goldstein et al., 1995) indicated that fluoxetine hydrochloride (Prozac) is currently the first medication of choice in treating bulimia nervosa (daily dosages of 60 mg were generally superior to 20 mg), and probably should be used at least as an adjunct to psychotherapy in many cases not responding to a course of adequate psychological treatment (Figure 5.1). However, there are several reasons for not using medication alone in the treatment of bulimia nervosa, including (1) the overall effectiveness of well-established psychological interventions; (2) the high dropout rates reported in most medication trials; (3) the risks of drug side effects; and (4) data suggesting high relapse rates with drug discontinuation. However, extensive and well-controlled research comparing the effectiveness of antidepressant medications, psychotherapy, and their combination in the treatment of bulimia nervosa has yielded relatively consistent findings: The combination of treatments produces added benefits on important parameters of change (see Garfinkel & Walsh, Chapter 20, this volume). Tricyclic antidepressants may be an alternative to fluoxetine for some patients, but side effects, high dropout rates, and greater incidence of lethality with overdose may be sources of concern (Leitenberg et al., 1994; Mitchell et al., 1990; Walsh, Hadigan, Devlin, Gladis, & Roose, 1991). There are limited circumstances under which the clinician may want to consider integrating other medications in the treatment of bulimia nervosa (Garfinkel & Walsh, Chapter 20, this volume). Monoamine oxidase inhibitors may be useful in a small minority of patients who fail to respond to fluoxetine and tricyclics. There is some evidence that patients who fail to respond to one tricyclic may benefit from changing to an alternative medication (see Mitchell et al., 1993). However, the decision to avoid prescribing medication can be therapeutic in some cases (Raymond, Mitchell, Fallon, & Katzman, 1994).

There is little evidence for changing the early recommendation that pharmacotherapy has limited value with emaciated anorexia nervosa patients and should never be the sole treatment modality (Garfinkel & Garner, 1982). A few patients may benefit from medication to deal with overwhelming anxiety, severe depression, or intolerable gastric discomfort after meals, but this applies only to a small minority (Andersen, 1985; Garfinkel & Garner, 1982).

In sum, psychotropic medication is generally not necessary or useful in most cases of anorexia nervosa. There is a role for medication with bulimia nervosa, but probably not as the initial treatment of choice (see Figure 5.1). The high dropout and relapse rates in studies using medication alone suggest that the best use of medication at this time is as an adjunct to one of the psychosocial treatments with proven effectiveness.

CAVEATS REGARDING INTEGRATION AND SEQUENCING MODELS

Models of treatment relying on the integration and sequencing of approaches are predicated on the assumption that less intensive treatments should be applied initially because they are cost-effective and less intrusive. There is some information on costs and effectiveness of several treatments for eating disorders; however, proper cost-effectiveness analyses per se have not been conducted. In the absence of these studies, decision making should not be overly influenced by treatments just because they are economical. The failure of an economical treatment may have an iatrogenic effect by making the patient more resistant to subsequent interventions. This potential concern might dictate that all bulimia nervosa patients (with the exception of the small percentage requiring inpatient or partial care) should be exposed to an initial trial of cognitive-behavioral therapy, since at the present time it is the method with the best empirical support. This recommendation has the practical advantage of not requiring each clinical setting to train staff members to competently apply the broad range of treatments described in this chapter. However, months of individual cognitive-behavioral therapy may be more treatment than many patients require. Educational treatments are relatively easy to administer, and as long as a competent clinician is able to triage patients who require more intensive treatments, education alone is suitable for many patients.

One of the greatest pitfalls of the stepped-care, decision-tree, and integration models is that their complexity makes rigorous research on effectiveness exceedingly difficult. The ideal research protocol would allow the efficacy of each treatment to be tested separately and in combination. It would also allow examination of the effects of treatments presented in different sequences. Finally, it would provide complete information concerning the interactions between each treatment (and treatment combination) and key patient characteristics. Needless to say, the resulting hypothetical matrix of treatment combinations and patient features would be enormous and impractical. A more realistic approach is to conduct studies using larger sample sizes and comparing different treatment sequences that are particularly relevant from a clinical point of view. For example, it may be practical to assess the relative efficacy of the "best-shot" treatment, compared to a predetermined and limited decision-tree approach. For example, it would be feasible to compare standard cognitive-behavioral therapy for bulimia nervosa with an approach that systematically adds educational, cognitive-behavioral, interpersonal, and drug treatments.

Another potential problem with the integration and sequencing approach is that it could compromise the understanding and cogent application of different methods. It may be that the components are really not complementary or that integrating treatments dilutes overall efficacy. Trying to mix and match methods may weaken the training of therapists, undermine the decision-making process, and lead to a bewildering application of conflicting treatment principles. At its worst, "eclecticism" connotes a failure to distinguish meaningful theoretical constructs, which leads to the naive application of techniques. However, in the general field of psychotherapy, and in the treatment of eating disorders in particular, there is an increasing movement toward the systematic integration of different approaches in a seamless fashion (Garfield, 1994).

CONCLUSION

The aim of this chapter has been to refine and extend stepped-care, decision-tree, and integration models for treating eating disorders. All available treatment options have not been covered; however, the main treatments have been discussed on the basis of current knowledge of patient clinical features and response to treatment. We hope that this will provide a background for students and beginning clinicians in the decision-making process, and will enable them to consider the major treatment options knowledgeably. In the future, this process will be updated continually by empirical research that is informed by acute clinical insights. The result will be increasingly cost-effective interventions.

REFERENCES

Andersen, A. E. (1985). *Practical comprehensive treatment of anorexia nervosa and bulimia.* Baltimore: Johns Hopkins University Press.

Agras, W. S. (1993). Short-term psychological treatments for binge eating. In C. G. Fairburn & G. T. Wilson (Eds.), *Binge eating: Nature, assessment, and treatment* (pp. 50–76). New York: Guilford Press.

Agras, W. S., Rossiter, E. M., Arnow, B., Schneider, J. A., Telch, C. F., Raeburn, S. D., Bruce, B., Perl, M., & Koran, L. M. (1992). Pharmacologic and cognitive-behavioral treatment for bulimia nervosa: A controlled comparison. *American Journal of Psychiatry, 149,* 82–87.

Baker Enright, A., Butterfield, P., & Berkowitz, B. (1985). Self-help and support groups in the management of eating disorders. In D. M. Garner & P. E. Garfinkel (Eds.), *Handbook of psychotherapy for anorexia nervosa and bulimia* (pp. 491–512). New York: Guilford Press.

Baran, S. A., Weltzin, T. E., & Kaye, W. H. (1995). Low discharge weight and outcome in anorexia nervosa. *American Journal of Psychiatry, 152,* 1070–1072.

Beumont, P. J. V., O'Connor, M., Touyz, S. W., & Williams, H. (1987). Nutritional counseling in the treatment of anorexia and bulimia nervosa. In P. J. V. Beumont, G. D. Burrows, & R. C. Casper (Eds.), *Handbook of eating disorders: Part 1. Anorexia and bulimia nervosa* (pp. 349–359). New York: Elsevier.

Bruch, H. (1973). *Eating disorders: Obesity, anorexia nervosa and the person within.* New York: Basic Books.

Casper, R. C. (1982). Treatment principles in anorexia nervosa. *Adolescent Psychiatry, 10,* 86–100.

Channon, S., DeSilva, P., Hemsley, D., & Perkins, R. (1989). A controlled trial of cognitive-behavioural and behavioural treatment of anorexia nervosa. *Behaviour Research and Therapy, 27,* 529–535.

Connors, M. E., Johnson, C. L., & Stuckey, M. K. (1984). Treatment of bulimia with brief psychoeducational group therapy. *American Journal of Psychiatry, 141,* 1512–1516.

Cooper, P. J., Coker, S., & Fleming, C. (1994). Self-help for bulimia nervosa: A preliminary report. *International Journal of Eating Disorders, 16,* 401–404.

Cooper, P. J., Coker, S., & Fleming, C. (1996). An evaluation of the efficacy of cognitive behavioral self-help for bulimia nervosa. *Journal of Psychosomatic Research, 40,* 281–287.

Cooper, P. J., & Fairburn, C. G. (1984). Cognitive behavioral treatment for anorexia nervosa: Some preliminary findings. *Journal of Psychosomatic Research, 28,* 493–499.

Crisp, A. H. (1970). Anorexia nervosa: 'Feeding disorder', nervous malnutrition or weight phobia? *World Review of Nutrition, 12,* 452–504.

Crisp, A. H. (1980). *Anorexia nervosa: Let me be.* New York: Grune & Stratton.

Fairburn, C. G. (1985). Cognitive-behavioral treatment for bulimia. In D. M. Garner & P. E. Garfinkel (Eds.), *Handbook of psychotherapy for anorexia nervosa and bulimia* (pp. 160–192). New York: Guilford Press.

Fairburn, C. G., Agras, W. S., & Wilson, G. T. (1992). The research on the treatment of bulimia nervosa: Practical and theoretical implications. In G. H. Anderson & S. H. Kennedy (Eds.), *Biology of feast and famine* (pp. 317–340). San Diego: Academic Press.

Fairburn, C. G., Jones, R., Peveler, R. C., Carr, S. J., Solomon, R. A., O'Connor, M. E., Burton, J., & Hope, R. A. (1991). Three psychological treatments for bulimia nervosa: A comparative trial. *Archives of General Psychiatry, 48,* 463–469.

Fairburn, C. G., Jones, R., Peveler, R. C., Hope, R. A., & O'Connor, M. E. (1993). Psychotherapy and bulimia nervosa: The longer-term effects of interpersonal psychotherapy, behavior therapy and cognitive behavior therapy. *Archives of General Psychiatry, 50,* 419–428.

Fairburn, C. G., Marcus, M. D., & Wilson, G. T. (1993). Cognitive-behavioral therapy for binge eating and bulimia nervosa: A comprehensive treatment manual. In C. G. Fairburn & G. T. Wilson (Eds.), *Binge eating: Nature, assessment, and treatment* (pp. 361–404). New York: Guilford Press.

Fairburn, C. G., Norman, P. A., Welch, S. L., O'Connor, M. E., Doll, H. A., & Peveler, R. C. (1995). A prospective study of outcome in bulimia nervosa and the long-term effects of three psychological treatments. *Archives of General Psychiatry, 52,* 304–312.

Fairburn, C. G., & Peveler, R. C. (1990). Bulimia nervosa and a stepped care approach to management. *Gut, 31,* 1220–1222.

Fallon, P., Katzman, M. A., & Wooley, S. C. (Eds.). (1994). *Feminist perspectives on eating disorders.* New York: Guilford Press.

Fluoxetine Bulimia Nervosa Collaborative Study Group. (1992). Fluoxetine in the treatment of bulimia nervosa. *Archives of General Psychiatry, 49,* 139–147.

Garfield, S. L. (1994). Eclecticism and integration in psychotherapy: Developments and issues. *Clinical Psychology: Science and Practice, 1,* 123–137.

Garfield, S. L., & Bergin, A. E. (1994). Introduction and historical overview. In A. E. Bergin & S. L. Garfield (Eds.), *Handbook of psychotherapy and behavior change* (4th ed., pp. 3–18). New York: Wiley.

Garfinkel, P. E., & Garner, D. M. (1982). *Anorexia nervosa: A multidimensional perspective.* New York: Brunner/Mazel.

Garfinkel, P. E., & Garner, D. M. (Eds.). (1987). *Psychotropic drug therapies for eating disorders* [Monograph]. New York: Brunner/Mazel.

Garner, D. M. (1986). Cognitive therapy for anorexia nervosa. In K. D. Brownell & J. P. Foreyt (Eds.), *Handbook of eating disorders: Physiology, psychology, and treatment of obesity, anorexia, and bulimia* (pp. 301–327). New York: Basic Books.

Garner, D. M. (1988). Anorexia nervosa. In M. Hersen & C. G. Last (Eds.), *Child behavior therapy casebook* (pp. 263–276). New York: Plenum Press.

Garner, D. M., & Bemis, K. M. (1982). A cognitive-behavioral approach to anorexia nervosa. *Cognitive Therapy and Research, 6,* 123–150.

Garner, D. M., & Bemis, K. M. (1985). Cognitive therapy for anorexia nervosa. In D. M. Garner & P. E. Garfinkel (Eds.), *Handbook of psychotherapy for anorexia nervosa and bulimia* (pp. 107–146). New York: Guilford Press.

Garner, D. M., Garfinkel, P. E., & Bemis, K. M. (1982). A multidimensional psychotherapy for anorexia nervosa. *International Journal of Eating Disorders, 1,* 3–46.

Garner, D. M., Garfinkel, P. E., & Irvine, M. J. (1986). Integration and sequencing of treatment approaches for eating disorders. *Psychotherapy and Psychosomatics, 46,* 67–75.

Garner, D. M., Rockert, W., Garner, M. V., Davis, R., Olmsted, M. P., & Eagle, M. (1993). Comparison of cognitive-behavioral and supportive-expressive therapy for bulimia nervosa. *American Journal of Psychiatry, 150,* 37–46.

Garner, D. M., Rockert, W., Olmsted, M. P., Johnson, C. L., & Coscina, D. V. (1985). Psychoeducational principles in the treatment of bulimia and anorexia nervosa. In D. M. Garner & P. E. Garfinkel (Eds.), *Handbook of psychotherapy for anorexia nervosa and bulimia* (pp. 513–572). New York: Guilford Press.

Garner, D. M., & Rosen, L. W. (1990). Anorexia nervosa and bulimia nervosa. In A. S. Bellack, M. Hersen, & A. E. Kazdin (Eds.), *International handbook of behavior modification and therapy* (2nd ed., pp. 805–817). New York: Plenum Press.

Garner, D. M., & Wooley, S. C. (1991). Confronting the failure of behavioral and dietary treatments for obesity. *Clinical Psychology Review, 11,* 729–780.

Giles, T. R., Young, R. R., & Young, D. E. (1985). Case studies and clinical replication series: Behavioral treatment of severe bulimia. *Behavior Therapy, 16,* 393–405.

Goldstein, D. J., Wilson, M. G., Thompson, V. L., Potvin, J. H., Rampey, A. H., & the Fluoxetine Bulimia Nervosa Research Group. (1995). Long-term fluoxetine treatment of bulimia nervosa. *British Journal of Psychiatry, 166,* 660–666.

Goodsitt, A. (1985). Self psychology and the treatment of anorexia nervosa. In D. M. Garner & P. E. Garfinkel (Eds.), *Handbook of psychotherapy for anorexia nervosa and bulimia* (pp. 55–84). New York: Guilford Press.

Huon, G. F. (1985). An initial validation of a self-help program for bulimia. *International Journal of Eating Disorders, 4,* 573–588.

Hsu, L. K. G., Holben, B., & West, S. (1992). Nutritional counseling in bulimia nervosa. *International Journal of Eating Disorders, 11,* 55–62.

Katzman, M. A. (1994). When reproductive and productive worlds meet: Collusion or growth? In P. Fallon, M. A. Katzman, & S. C. Wooley (Eds.), *Feminist perspectives on eating disorders* (pp. 132–151). New York: Guilford Press.

Klerman, G. L., Weissman, M. M., Rounsaville, B. J., & Chevron, E. S. (1984). *Interpersonal psychotherapy of depression.* New York: Basic Books.

Laessle, R. G., Beumont, P. J. V., Butow, P., Lennerts, W., O'Connor, M., Pirke, K. M., Touyz, S. W., & Waadi, S. (1991). A comparison of nutritional management and stress management in the treatment of bulimia nervosa. *British Journal of Psychiatry, 159,* 250–261.

Leitenberg, H., Rosen, J. C., Wolf, J., Vara, L. S., Detzer, M. J., & Srebnik, D. (1994). Comparison of cognitive-behavior therapy and desipramine in the treatment of bulimia nervosa. *Behavior Research and Therapy, 32,* 37–45.

Lerner, H. D. (1991). Masochism in subclinical eating disorders. In C. Johnson (Ed.), *Psychodynamic treatment of anorexia nervosa and bulimia* (pp. 109–127). New York: Guilford Press.

Minuchin, S., Rosman, B. L., & Baker, L. (1978). *Psychosomatic families: Anorexia nervosa in context.* Cambridge, MA: Harvard University Press.

Mitchell, J. E., Pyle, R. L., Eckert, E. D., Hatsukami, D., Pomeroy, C., & Zimmerman, R. (1990). A comparison study of antidepressants and structured intensive group psychotherapy in the treatment of bulimia nervosa. *Archives of General Psychiatry, 47,* 149–157.

Mitchell, J. E., Raymond, N., & Specker, S. (1993). A review of the controlled trials of pharmacotherapy and psychotherapy in the treatment of bulimia nervosa. *International Journal of Eating Disorders, 14,* 229–247.

Olmsted, M. P., Davis, R., Garner, D. M., Rockert, W., Irvine, M. J., & Eagle, M. (1991). Efficacy of a brief group psychoeducational intervention for bulimia nervosa. *Behavior Research and Therapy, 29,* 71–83.

Perlick, D., & Silverstein, B. (1994). Faces of female discontent: Depression, disordered eating, and changing gender roles. In P. Fallon, M. A. Katzman, & S. C. Wooley (Eds.), *Feminist perspectives on eating disorders* (pp. 77–93). New York: Guilford Press.

Pike, K. M., Loeb, K., & Vitousek, K. (1996). Cognitive-behavioral therapy for anorexia nervosa and bulimia nervosa. In J. K. Thompson (Ed.), *Body image: Eating disorders and obesity* (pp. 253–302). Washington, DC: American Psychological Association.

Raymond, N. C., Mitchell, J. E., Fallon, P., & Katzman, M. A. (1994). A collaborative approach to the use of medication. In P. Fallon, M. A. Katzman, & S. C. Wooley (Eds.), *Feminist perspectives on eating disorders* (pp. 231–250). New York: Guilford Press.

Russell, G. F. M., Szmukler, G. I., Dare, C., & Eisler, I. (1987). An evaluation of family therapy in anorexia nervosa and bulimia nervosa. *Archives of General Psychiatry, 44,* 1047–1056.

Ryle, A. (1990). *Cognitive analytic therapy: Active participation in change.* Chichester, England: Wiley.

Sands, S. (1991). Bulimia, dissociation, and empathy: A self-psychological view. In C. Johnson (Ed.), *Psychodynamic treatment of anorexia nervosa and bulimia* (pp. 34–50). New York: Guilford Press.

Santrock, J. W., Minnett, A. M., & Campbell, B. D. (1994). *The authoritative guide to self-help books.* New York: Guilford Press.

Schmidt, U., Tiller, J., & Treasure, J. (1993). Self-treatment of bulimia nervosa: A pilot study. *International Journal of Eating Disorders, 13,* 273–277.

Selvini Palazzoli, M. P. (1974). *Self-starvation.* London: Chaucer.

Steiner-Adair, C. (1994). The politics of prevention. In P. Fallon, M. A. Katzman, & S. C. Wooley (Eds.), *Feminist perspectives on eating disorders* (pp. 381–394). New York: Guilford Press.

Stern, S. (1986). The dynamics of clinical management in the treatment of anorexia nervosa and bulimia: An organizing theory. *International Journal of Eating Disorders, 5,* 233–254.

Striegel-Moore, R. H. (1994). A feminist agenda for psychological research on eating disorders. In P. Fallon, M. A. Katzman, & S. C. Wooley (Eds.), *Feminist perspectives on eating disorders* (pp. 438–454). New York: Guilford Press.

Strober, M., & Yager, J. (1985). A developmental perspective on the treatment of anorexia nervosa in adolescents. In D. M. Garner & P. E. Garfinkel (Eds.), *Handbook of psychotherapy for anorexia nervosa and bulimia* (pp. 363–390). New York: Guilford Press.

Sugarman, A. (1991). Bulimia: A displacement from psychological self to body self. In C. Johnson (Ed.), *Psychodynamic treatment of anorexia nervosa and bulimia* (pp. 3–33). New York: Guilford Press.

Sullivan, P. F. (1995). Mortality in anorexia nervosa. *American Journal of Psychiatry, 152,* 1073–1074.

Telch, C. F., Agras, W. S., Rossiter, E. M., Wilfley, D., & Kenardy, J. (1990). Group cognitive-behavioral treatment for the non-purging bulimic: An initial evaluation. *Journal of Consulting and Clinical Psychology, 58,* 629–635.

Tiller, J., Schmidt, U., & Treasure, J. (1993). Treatment of bulimia nervosa. *International Review of Psychiatry, 5,* 75–86.

Treasure, J., Schmidt, U., Troop, N., Tiller, J., Todd, G., Keilen, M., & Dodge, E. (1994). First step in managing bulimia nervosa: Controlled trial of therapeutic manual. *British Medical Journal, 308,* 686–689.

Vandereycken, W., Kog, E., & Vanderlinden, J. (1989). *The family approach to eating disorders.* New York: PMA.

Walsh, B. T., Hadigan, C. M., Devlin, M. J., Gladis, M., & Roose, S. P. (1991). Long-term outcome of antidepressant treatment for bulimia nervosa. *American Journal of Psychiatry, 148,* 1206–1212.

Wilfley, D. E., Agras, W. S., Telch, C. F., Rossiter, E. M., Schneider, J. A., Cole, A. G., Sifford, L., & Raeburn, S. D. (1993). Group cognitive-behavioral and group interpersonal psychotherapy for the nonpurging bulimic individual: A controlled comparison. *Journal of Consulting and Clinical Psychology, 61,* 296–305.

Wolchik, S. A., Weiss, L., & Katzman, M. A. (1986). An empirically validated, short-term psychoeducational group treatment program for bulimia. *International Journal of Eating Disorders, 5*(1), 21–34.

Wooley, S. C. (1994). Sexual abuse and eating disorders: The concealed debate. In P. Fallon, M. A. Katzman, & S. C. Wooley (Eds.), *Feminist perspectives on eating disorders* (pp. 171–211). New York: Guilford Press.

Wooley, S. C., & Kearney-Cooke, A. (1986). Intensive treatment of bulimia and body-image disturbance. In K. D. Brownell & J. P. Foreyt (Eds.), *Handbook of eating disorders: Physiology, psychology, and treatment of obesity, anorexia, and bulimia* (pp. 476–502). New York: Basic Books.

Wooley, S. C., & Lewis, K. G. (1989). The missing woman: Intensive family-oriented treatment of bulimia. *Journal of Feminist Family Therapy, 1,* 61–83.

II

COGNITIVE-BEHAVIORAL AND EDUCATIONAL APPROACHES

CHAPTER 6

Cognitive-Behavioral Therapy for Bulimia Nervosa

G. TERENCE WILSON
CHRISTOPHER G. FAIRBURN
W. STEWART AGRAS

The use of cognitive-behavioral therapy (CBT) for bulimia nervosa in North America, Great Britain, Europe, and Australia/New Zealand derives directly from Fairburn's first formulation of this approach in Oxford in a treatment manual in the early 1980s (Fairburn, 1981). The publication of that detailed treatment manual greatly facilitated the dissemination of CBT and research on its effectiveness (Fairburn, 1985; Fairburn & Cooper, 1989). A somewhat expanded version of this manual was published in 1993 (Fairburn, Marcus, & Wilson, 1993).

Although there are differences in the ways in which CBT has been implemented across different clinical and research settings, the current Oxford manual is increasingly being adopted in major clinical research centers. For example, we are presently engaged in two major multisite treatment outcome studies in the United States. The participating research centers include Columbia University and the New York Psychiatric Institute, Cornell Medical School, Rutgers University, University of Minnesota Medical School, and Stanford University School of Medicine. All have adopted the Oxford manual as the standard form of CBT for bulimia nervosa.

The present chapter should be seen as a supplement to the Oxford CBT manual (Fairburn, Marcus, & Wilson, 1993). We summarize the manual, elaborate on how it should be imple-

mented, and discuss common problems and issues in the clinical treatment of bulimia nervosa. Many of the issues we discuss in regard to the clinical use of this treatment approach come from our collective experience in training therapists in the use of this manual-based treatment, and in monitoring their implementation of the principles and procedures of this approach. Before we address these issues, however, it is important to review what we know about the effectiveness of CBT in general and the Oxford manual in particular. It is because manual-based CBT has been shown to be an effective treatment in well-controlled clinical studies that a detailed analysis of its clinical application is warranted.

EFFECTIVENESS OF COGNITIVE-BEHAVIORAL THERAPY

In the opening of his chapter on the treatment of bulimia nervosa in the Garner and Garfinkel (1985) anthology, Fairburn noted: "Several different psychological and pharmacological approaches have been advocated [for the treatment of bulimia nervosa], but there have been no satisfactory treatment studies, and it is not known whether any intervention influences the long-term outcome" (1985, p. 160). Over a decade later, the situation is quite different. Different groups of investigators in different countries have completed a number of randomized controlled trials. These studies have demonstrated the specific clinical effectiveness of CBT as a treatment for bulimia nervosa.

The effectiveness of CBT can be gauged in different ways. One method is simply to compile an average—a box score estimate—of the overall outcome of all available studies. For example, Craighead and Agras's (1991) summary of 10 studies yielded a mean reduction in purging of 79%, with a 57% remission figure. The results for binge eating were similar. However, simple averages such as these are compiled from studies varying widely in procedures, measurement, and methodological rigor; as a result, they can be misleading (Kazdin & Wilson, 1978).

An alternative strategy is to select what we judge to be the most recent and best-controlled studies (Fairburn, Agras, & Wilson, 1992). These show a mean percentage reduction in binge eating ranging from 93% to 73%; the comparable figures for purging range from 94% to 77%. Mean remission rates for binge eating range from 51% to 71%, and for purging from 36% to 56% (Agras, Schneider, Arnow, Raeburn, & Telch, 1989; Agras et al., 1992; Fairburn et al., 1991; Garner et al., 1993). Aside from clinically significant reductions in binge eating and purging, studies have consistently shown that dietary restraint is reduced (Fairburn et al., 1991; Garner et al., 1993; Wilson, Eldredge, Smith, & Niles, 1991), with an increase in the amount of food eaten between bulimic episodes (Rossiter, Agras, Losch, & Telch, 1988). Attitudes to shape and weight—which constitute a key psychopathological feature, and one that is central to the cognitive-behavioral view of the disorder—also improve (Fairburn et al., 1991; Garner et al., 1993; Wilson et al., 1991).[1]

Other reliable findings have been the broad effects of CBT on associated psychopathology. Most studies have shown striking improvements in measures of depression, self-esteem, social functioning, and personality disorder (e.g., Fairburn, Kirk, O'Connor, & Cooper, 1986; Fairburn et al., 1992; Garner et al., 1993).

As a whole, studies of CBT have shown reasonably good maintenance of change at both 6-month and 1-year follow-ups (Agras et al., 1994; Fairburn, Jones, Peveler, Hope, & O'Connor, 1993; Wilson et al., 1991). The longest follow-up has been reported by the Oxford group, which conducted a rigorous evaluation of treatment outcome an average of 5.8 years following therapy. The results showed that at posttreatment the effects of CBT were maintained (an abstinence rate of 48%) (Fairburn et al., 1995). The good maintenance at 1 year, combined with Fairburn et al.'s (1995) long-term findings, stands in marked contrast to Keller, Herzog, Lavori, Bradburn, and Mahoney's (1992, p. 7) characterization of "extraordinarily high" rates of chronicity, relapse and recurrence in patients with bulimia nervosa. None of Keller et al.'s (1992) sample of patients was treated with CBT.

CBT versus Antidepressant Drug Treatment

Aside from CBT, the most intensively researched treatment for bulimia nervosa has been antidepressant medication. Both tricyclics and fluoxetine have been shown to be significantly more effective than a pill placebo (Mitchell & deZwaan, 1993). Consequently, antidepressant medication provides a stringent standard of comparison for the effects of CBT or any other psychological treatment.

Five studies have directly evaluated the relative and combined effectiveness of CBT and antidepressant drug treatment in controlled studies (Agras et al., 1992; Fichter et al., 1991; Leitenberg et al., 1994; Mitchell et al., 1990;[2] Walsh et al., in press). The different designs of these studies provide more than one way of assessing the comparative effectiveness of CBT.

One comparison is CBT versus medication only. The two studies that permitted this comparison both showed that CBT was significantly superior to the tricyclic desipramine (Agras et al., 1992; Leitenberg et al., 1994). A second comparison is CBT plus medication versus medication only. The four studies that make this analysis possible all showed the superiority of the combined treatment (Agras et al., 1992; Leitenberg et al., 1994; Mitchell et al., 1990; Walsh et al., in press). A third comparison is CBT plus medication versus CBT alone. The two studies that included this comparison both indicated that no advantage was attached to the combined treatment in terms of reducing binge eating and purging (Agras et al., 1992; Leitenberg et al., 1994). The final comparison is CBT plus medication versus CBT plus a pill placebo. Two of the three studies including this comparison showed no difference (Fichter et al., 1991; Mitchell et al., 1990). In the third study, although the difference was not statistically significant, the drug-plus-CBT condition had a higher remission rate for binge eating and vomiting (50%) than placebo plus CBT (24%).

Taken as a whole, these five studies indicate that CBT is superior to medication alone; that combining CBT with medication is significantly more effective than medication alone; and that combining the two produces what, at best, are modest incremental benefits over CBT alone. Also favoring CBT are the findings that it is more acceptable to patients and results in fewer dropouts during treatment (Wilson & Fairburn, in press). Perhaps the most important finding is that in contrast to the data on CBT, there is virtually no evidence of the long-term effect of pharmacological treatment. The single exception to this dearth of evidence on the durability of drug treatment is the Agras et al. (1994) study, showing that 6 months of treatment with desipramine produced lasting improvement even after the medication was withdrawn.

CBT versus Alternative Psychological Therapies

CBT has proved to be significantly more effective than, or at least as effective as, any psychological treatment with which it has been compared in a controlled study. The following studies illustrate this general pattern.

At Stanford, Agras et al. (1989) showed that CBT was more effective than supportive psychotherapy at the end of treatment and at a 6-month follow-up. In Toronto, Garner et al. (1993) compared CBT with supportive–expressive therapy (SET). The two treatments were equally effective in reducing binge eating, but CBT was significantly superior to SET in decreasing purging, lessening dietary restraint, and modifying dysfunctional attitudes to shape and weight. Significantly, CBT produced greater improvement in depression, self-esteem, and general psychological distress.

In Oxford, Fairburn et al. (1991) compared CBT with two alternative treatments. One was behavior therapy (BT), consisting of the CBT treatment minus cognitive restructuring, and behavioral and cognitive methods for modifying abnormal attitudes about weight and shape. The second was interpersonal psychotherapy (IPT), which was adapted from Klerman, Weissman, Rounsaville, and Chevron's (1984) interpersonal treatment of depression. At posttreatment, the three therapies were equally effective in reducing binge eating. CBT, however, was significantly more effective than IPT in reducing purging, dietary restraint, and attitudes to shape and weight, and superior to BT on the latter two variables despite equivalent ratings of suitability of treatment and expectations of outcome. This pattern of results shows that CBT has specific effects on different measures of outcome, consistent with its theoretical rationale.

The closed 1-year follow-up of this study revealed a different picture (Fairburn, Jones, et al., 1993). Fully 48% of the BT group dropped out or were withdrawn from the study because of lack of improvement. The dropout rate was 20% for CBT, which maintained its improvement throughout follow-up. IPT showed continuing improvement, to the point where it was as successful as CBT on all measures at 8- and 12-month evaluations. Forty-four percent of IPT patients had ceased all binge eating and purging at the 1-year follow-up. The 5.8-year follow-up of this study showed the same pattern of results. Forty-eight percent of patients treated with CBT, and 52% of those treated with IPT, were abstinent; the comparable figure for BT was 18%. These data rebut the argument that all treatments are equally effective. BT was clearly inferior to CBT and IPT. Similarly, the striking differences in the temporal pattern of results between CBT and IPT suggests that each treatment has specific effects, probably via different mechanisms.

How Broadly Applicable Is Manual-Based CBT?

Patients with bulimia nervosa show a wide range of associated psychopathology (Fairburn & Cooper, 1984; Laessle, Wittchen, Fichter, & Pirke, 1989; Schwalberg, Barlow, Alger, & Howard, 1992). Nonetheless, there are few circumstances in which manual-based CBT cannot be recommended as the preferred treatment. Contraindications include psychotic states, severe depression or the risk of suicide, and substance use disorders that effectively prevent patients from fully engaging in the treatment for their eating disorder.

Predictors of treatment success in bulimia nervosa remain to be firmly established for any form of therapy. Available evidence suggests that low self-esteem predicts lack of improvement (Fairburn, Jones, et al., 1993). In addition, comorbid personality disorders—namely, the cluster B disorders—have been associated with a poorer response to CBT (Coker, Vize, Wade, & Cooper, 1993; Fahy & Russell, 1993; Fairburn, Jones, et al., 1993; Rossiter et al., 1988). However, as Fairburn, Marcus, and Wilson (1993), p. 362) have pointed out, this is no reason not to use CBT. Contrary to the speculations of some clinicians (Johnson, Tobin, & Dennis, 1990), there is no evidence that alternative psychological treatments are any more helpful for bulimia nervosa patients with comorbid personality disorders. The contention that psychodynamic therapy is better suited than CBT for the treatment of borderline personality disorder has no empirical support in the case of either eating disorders or other psychiatric disorders (Wilson, 1995).

SUMMARY DESCRIPTION OF THE TREATMENT MANUAL

CBT for bulimia nervosa, as described in the current version of the Oxford manual (Fairburn, Marcus, & Wilson, 1993), is based on a model that emphasizes the critical role of both cognitive and behavioral factors in the maintenance of the disorder. Figure 6.1 summarizes this model. Of primary importance is the value attached to an idealized body weight and shape. This leads women[3] to restrict their food intake in rigid and unrealistic ways—a process that

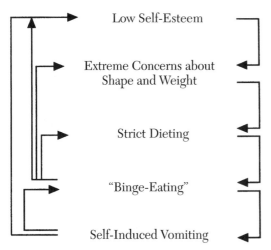

FIGURE 6.1. The cognitive-behavioral model of the maintenance of bulimia nervosa. From Fairburn, Marcus, and Wilson (1993, p. 369). Copyright 1993 by The Guilford Press. Reprinted by permission.

leaves them physiologically and psychologically susceptible to periodic loss of control over eating (i.e., binge eating). Purging and other extreme forms of weight control are the patients' attempts to compensate for the effects of binge eating. Purging helps maintain binge eating by reducing the patients' anxiety about potential weight gain and disrupting learned satiety that regulates food intake. In turn, binge eating and purging cause distress and lower self-esteem, thereby reciprocally fostering the conditions that will inevitably lead to more dietary restraint and binge eating.

It follows from this model that treatment must address more than the presenting behaviors of binge eating and purging. In addition, dietary restraint must be replaced with more normal eating patterns, and dysfunctional thoughts and feelings about the personal significance of body weight and shape must be altered.

In this manual-based treatment program, CBT consists of 19 sessions of individual treatment spanning roughly 20 weeks. Exemplifying the practice of CBT in general, treatment is problem-oriented and focused primarily on the present and future. As is also true of all forms of CBT, a good therapist–patient relationship is essential. The therapist must earn the patient's trust and respect. The success of CBT depends in large part on the willingness of the patient to play an active role in treatment and follow through on homework assignments that can prove very threatening. Patients with eating disorders often feel ashamed about their behavior, and are very sensitive to cues of disapproval and rejection. Accordingly, a therapist must convey acceptance of a patient and understanding of her problem.

The treatment has three stages.

Stage 1

The aims of the first stage, which is focused mainly on behavior change and spans the first eight sessions, are as follows:

To establish a sound therapeutic relationship.
To educate the patient about the cognitive view of the maintenance of bulimia nervosa, and to explain the need for both behavior and cognitive change.
To establish regular weekly weighing.
To educate the patient about body weight regulation; the adverse effects of dieting; and the physical consequences of binge

eating, self-induced vomiting, and laxative abuse.

To reduce the frequency of overeating by introducing a pattern of regular eating and the use of alternative behavior.

The cognitive-behavioral model of the maintenance and modification of the disorder is explained, and its relevance to the patient's current problems is made clear. It is important to emphasize that therapy involves change in all facets of the eating disorder, as described in the model (see Figure 6.1). The structure and goals of treatment, as well as the likely possible outcome, are discussed.

Self-Monitoring

In the first session, the therapist introduces self-monitoring. Patients are instructed to record everything they eat on monitoring sheets. They record the time of day; what was consumed; where; whether it was a meal, snack, or binge; whether it led to purging; and associated thoughts and feelings. Calorie counting should be discouraged. Patients are urged to record intake shortly after it occurs, and not wait until the end of the day. The importance of self-monitoring cannot be overemphasized; it is the basis on which the rest of treatment is built. Accordingly, the therapist must explain the twofold importance of self-monitoring: (1) It provides the therapist with a detailed assessment of the eating problem and the circumstances under which it occurs; and (2) by increasing a patient's awareness of what she eats and how this is related to specific triggering events, it helps her regain control.

Weekly Weighing

Patients are instructed to weigh themselves once a week. As a result of their overconcern with weight and shape, these patients typically weigh themselves too often (e.g., several times a day) or not at all. Both groups may have difficulty with this intervention. The therapist, however, can point out how this behavioral intervention begins to address patients' excessive concern with weight and shape. Moreover, as patients make changes in their eating patterns, it is important for them to have feedback on what each change does—or does not do—to their weight. It is made clear to patients that the focus of treatment is on eliminating binge eating and restoring regular eating patterns. Only then can the issue of weight be usefully examined. Patients are educated about normal variability in weight and urged to accept a weight range (e.g., 6 pounds) rather than a specific number.

Educating the Patient about Weight and Eating

Information about weight regulation, the negative effects of rigid dieting and binge eating, and the adverse physical consequences of vomiting and laxative abuse is presented in some detail. In regard to purging, it is explained that laxatives are completely ineffective as a means of controlling weight. Self-induced vomiting is only partially effective; its negative reinforcing quality derives largely from the subjective sense of immediate relief that it affords. Throughout treatment the therapist remains active in offering information, advice, and encouragement. We now recommend that all patients read the recent Fairburn (1995) book in eating disorders characterized by binge eating. This book provides a "user-friendly" source of education about the nature of binge eating and bulimia nervosa.

Prescription of Regular Eating Patterns

Most patients with bulimia nervosa skip meals as part of highly restrictive dieting. As early as the third session, patients are asked to begin eating three meals a day plus two planned snacks. This is a critical behavioral intervention and one that often meets with resistance from patients, who fear they will gain weight. Patients can be reassured that the majority of those who cease binge eating and purging in CBT do not gain weight. Among the reasons is the simple fact that the adoption of more regular eating patterns reduces the number of binges and hence the overall amount of calories they consume.

To help overcome patients' resistance, they are allowed to eat for their meals even small amounts of what they regard as "safe" foods. The focus here is on *when* they eat rather than *what* they eat. Even so, many patients will experience significant discomfort and anxiety over eating more regular meals. Patients commonly complain about feeling full, and often attribute the feeling to having eaten too large a quantity of food. This reaction provides therapists with another opportunity to flag the importance of patients' subjective appraisal of their eating, and to relate it to the cognitive-behavioral model of the maintenance of bulimia nervosa. It is explained to patients that the subjective feeling of fullness is likely to be a function of the unfamiliar sensations of more regular eating. Moreover, fear of gaining weight results in patients' being overly sensitive to sensations of fullness. (These interventions lay the groundwork for the more systematic cognitive restructuring that is part of Stage 2.) Patients are strongly encouraged to "wait out" the aversive feelings of fullness or anxiety. In the field of substance use disorders, this is known as "urge surfing." (See Marlatt & Gordon, 1985, pp. 237–244, for a useful account of how patients can learn to resist urges that lead to loss of control.) It is helpful to draw a graph illustrating patients' perceptions that the negative feelings will continue to increase uncontrollably, as opposed to the reality that they will rapidly peak and then more slowly, but surely, decrease in intensity (see Figure 6.2). Engaging in distracting activities immediately after eating is useful in this regard, but patients need to learn to tolerate negative affect and to realize that it will gradually diminish.

Although the emphasis during this early stage tends to be on behavioral change, the therapist uses this change to influence patients' thoughts and feelings. For example, it is often possible to show patients, using their own weight histories, that their weight increases rather than decreases when they restrict intake and thereby trigger the binge–purge cycle. Moreover, patients often confuse regaining control over their eating behavior with weight control, as illustrated in the following case:

> Approximately 2 months into therapy, Janet, very distressed, complained that she had "lost control." She had weighed herself that morning and found that she had gained 3 pounds. Her clothes were tighter, and she felt fat and hated her body. Her first thought had been to binge and then purge to "get rid of" the hated fat. The therapist then reviewed with the patient her progress over the previous 2 months. It showed that she had significantly reduced her binge–purge frequency; she was less preoccupied with thoughts of food; and her actual eating patterns were more normal and not the source of constant conflict and anxiety they had once been. This helped Janet see that she had in fact significantly increased her control over her eating and bulimic behavior. She was more "in control" than she had been for years. Unfortunately, at the time, her weight had not decreased as she had hoped. The therapist explained that weight control was not under her direct control. What she could realistically take responsibility for—namely, her actual eating behavior, she had. Although Janet was still unhappy with her weight, she felt much better about herself, and her mood improved considerably. As a result, she did not binge-eat or purge that day or that week.

Self-Control Strategies

The therapist can draw on several self-control techniques to help patients refrain from binge eating. One strategy is the planned use of behaviors that are incompatible with binge eating. Patients are asked to identify high-risk situations for binge eating; they are then asked to generate a list of alternative activities that are both pleasurable and feasible. Examples include taking a walk, listening to music, talking to a friend on the phone, or taking a bath. The therapist can draw on Marlatt's model of a balanced lifestyle—in this connection, a balance between "shoulds" and "wants" (Marlatt & Gordon, 1985). A patient is encouraged to be "good to herself" in ways that are not self-defeating but are healthier. Patients with bulimia nervosa are typically characterized by very high, rigid standards, and are prone to be self-critical and evaluative. Restoring a better balance between

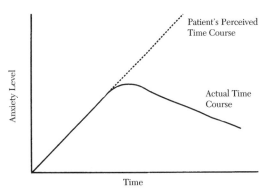

FIGURE 6.2. Schematic representation of the time course of an urge to purge.

"shoulds" and "wants" helps to address both of these dysfunctional cognitions.

Stimulus control is another useful strategy for restructuring healthy eating patterns. Particularly in the early stages of treatment, patients should limit the availability of "binge" foods in the house. Patients should avoid shopping for food, or engaging in other obvious exposure to food, when they feel that their self-control is shaky. Eating should be confined to particular places at regular times. For example, patients should avoid eating while driving or otherwise "on the run."

Stage 2

In the second stage (sessions 9 through 16), the techniques from Stage 1 are supplemented with a variety of procedures for reducing dietary restraint and developing cognitive and behavioral coping skills for resisting binge eating. It has an increasingly cognitive focus.

Eliminating Dieting

By this stage, patients will have an understanding of how rigid dieting predisposes them to binge eating. Having made changes in their patterns of eating, patients are now helped to alter what and how much they eat. Patients are asked to generate a list of roughly 40 "forbidden foods"—namely, those that they have been avoiding. They rank them in terms of the degree to which they find them threatening, and are then instructed to include them progressively in their meals, beginning with the least threatening. Each forbidden food must not be a substitute for a meal, but should be incorporated into what patients would normally eat. The goal is to experiment systematically with consuming modest amounts of these foods as part of regular meals or snacks, until patients are no longer anxious about losing control. In short, this is another way of implementing the principle of exposure to disconfirm dysfunctional expectations and increase self-efficacy. Finally, once patients are flexibly incorporating a range of different foods into their diet, the emphasis switches to ensuring that they eat a sufficient amount of food.

Patients should also be encouraged to eat under a wide range of different circumstances they would previously have avoided. For example, they are asked to eat in restaurants and oth-er people's houses, where they do not have complete control over what food is served or how it is prepared. These assignments provide important sources of exposure to previously avoided situations. Patients need to learn to cope with uncertainty.

Teaching Problem-Solving Skills

Binge eating is triggered by a variety of events, including specific thoughts, negative emotions, and interpersonal stressors. CBT is designed to allow patients to develop the cognitive and behavioral skills for coping with these situations without resorting to such maladaptive behaviors as binge eating or purging. One of the strategies involves improving patients' problem-solving skills.

There are several specific steps to be followed: (1) identifying and specifying the problem; (2) generating different ways of coping with the problem; (3) evaluating the feasibility and likely effectiveness of each possible solution; (4) choosing the best alternative and specifying how it is to be implemented; (5) carrying out the alternative; and (6) evaluating the outcome and overall effectiveness of the process. Patients should record their attempts at problem solving so that they can review the process in detail with the therapist. These principles are illustrated in the following vignette.

> Susan, a college sophomore, had experienced a lot of loneliness during her first year away from home and was currently in therapy for bulimia nervosa. In her second year as a student, she had become friendly with a small group of students whose companionship she greatly valued. At least once a week this group would make a late-night visit to a popular local hangout, where they would eat pizza and drink beer. Susan described how the past Friday night she had declined to accompany her friends because she would not allow herself to eat pizza—one of her many forbidden foods. Alone in the dormitory on a Friday night when everyone else was out having fun, Susan felt lonely and unhappy. She was also hungry, having eaten very little for dinner that night. This combination of energy and emotional deprivation resulted in her going to a local convenience store, buying food, and returning to her room, where she binged and purged.

The therapist asked Susan to problem-solve this situation in retrospect. What alternatives had there been? After considering several options, she decided that it would have been best to go with her friends and avoid the feeling of being left out. But what about eating "binge food," as she put it, when she was there? She somewhat grudgingly agreed that she probably could have eaten one piece of pizza and drunk some beer without necessarily going on to binge, especially since she would have been feeling happy to be part of the group. The calories she would have consumed there were far fewer than those involved in the binge that had occurred. The joint analysis of this event proved to be an eye-opener for Susan. She readily took to using these problem-solving principles in a variety of life situations, and reported that actively considering alternatives to problematic situations gave her a sense of "empowerment."

The therapist was also able to use this event to make two additional therapeutic interventions. First, it provided a cogent illustration of how Susan had setup the conditions that left her vulnerable to binge eating: She had eaten too little for dinner and made no provision for a planned snack (which gave the therapist an opportunity to reinforce the dangers of dieting); and she had exposed herself to the old feelings of loneliness. And second, the therapist was able to reinforce the importance of a balanced lifestyle, and to show how extreme or dysfunctional thinking led to binge eating.

Cognitive Restructuring

Patients with eating disorders typically present with a number of problematic thoughts and attitudes about their eating and body weight. Examples include dichotomous ("all-or-nothing") thinking, such as food's being either "good" or "bad," or the patients' being completely "in control" or totally "out of control"; and dysfunctional attitudes, such as "To be thin is to be attractive, successful, and happy, whereas to be fat is to be unattractive, unsuccessful and unhappy." These commonplace themes are made pathological by the intensity and rigidity with which they are held. Some of these dysfunctional cognitions will have been addressed by this point in the therapy. For example, the common assumption that eating a previously forbidden food inevitably results in total loss of control over eating and consequent weight gain will have been disconfirmed. The focus now shifts to more formal treatment of problematic thoughts and attitudes, using cognitive restructuring.

Cognitive restructuring is adapted from Beck's cognitive therapy for depression (Beck, Rush, Shaw, & Emery, 1979). The first step is to help the patient identify and specify a problematic thought and the context in which it occurred. The second and third steps require the patient to dispute the validity of the problematic thought; the patient is asked to evaluate the evidence for and against her thought. The fourth and final step consists of the patient's coming to "a reasoned conclusion" (a shift in her thinking) as a result of challenging the problematic thought. This should lead to a change in her behavior. The process is illustrated in the following example:

Joan was a college student who had asked her boyfriend to visit her for the weekend. He had said that he could not make it—an event that triggered a series of problematic thoughts. In the first step of cognitive restructuring she was able to specify these thoughts: "I have been rejected," and "It is because I'm fat and unattractive." It followed, therefore, that she would have to lose weight in order to be more attractive. That evening she vomited after a modest dinner because of her concern about losing weight. In the second and third steps, the therapist helped Joan to challenge these problematic thoughts. On weighing the available evidence, Joan agreed that she was not fat and unattractive, even though she would still like to lose some weight. Her boyfriend often told her that he liked her body, and she had received compliments from other friends. On considering alternative views of the situation, she concluded that her boyfriend had not visited because he had already made other plans. She remembered that she had left it until the last minute to invite him. In the fourth step she resolved to invite him again with adequate preparation, and to resist the urge to resume dieting in order to lose weight. She was also able to appreciate that the feeling of being "fat" was influenced by her sense of rejection—a transitory emotional state—and that having this feeling did not mean that she was actually overweight.

Cognitive restructuring can be implemented in different ways (e.g., Garner & Bemis, 1985; Wilson & Pike, 1993). In the program based on the Oxford CBT manual, patients are instructed to record their efforts at cognitive restructuring on the back of their self-monitoring sheets. What is important is that patients actively write down their problematic thoughts and how they try to challenge them, and that they bring their notes to the next session so that they can review them with the therapist.

Abnormal attitudes about body shape and weight are more generalized and less well-articulated cognitions that are not as easy to identify as problematic thoughts (Fairburn, Marcus, & Wilson, 1993, pp. 388–89). They may have to be inferred from a patient's behavior rather than elicited by direct questioning. The same principles of cognitive restructuring for modifying specific thoughts can be used to alter these abnormal attitudes.

For example, one patient believed that "I must be thin to be attractive and successful. If I gain any weight, I will be fat and ugly; no one will want me." Not surprisingly, she greatly restricted her food intake and frequently induced vomiting even after eating modest amounts of food at meals. This attitude had resulted in her resisting the therapist's attempt to have her adopt more normal eating patterns. Cognitive restructuring was aimed at addressing this problem according to the principles summarized above. However, in addition to evaluating the evidence for and against the attitude, the therapist challenged the patient with the following questions: "What is the effect of clinging to this attitude? How does it affect the way you feel and what you do? What are its advantages and disadvantages? Is there an alternative way of viewing things that would be more helpful to you?"

Such questions are designed to prompt attitudinal change. The patient in question here readily conceded that her attitude made her feel miserable. She was constantly preoccupied with concerns about eating and weight. Moreover, this preoccupation had begun to interfere with her work and had led to her withdrawing from social activities she once enjoyed. (When pushed, many if not most patients will acknowledge that they are unlikely to be satisfied even if they lost weight.) And, of course, it had led directly to the dieting that she now accepted was linked to binge eating and purging, which further eroded her self-esteem. The therapist prompted her to draw the conclusion that her attitude about shape and weight was highly dysfunctional. Compared with this "no-win" situation, the alternative of making changes, albeit scary, seemed more reasonable than ever before. By loosening her rigid dietary restraint she would overcome her binge-eating problem, even though some weight gain was a possibility. Either way, she would feel more in control. Moreover, she would no longer be so preoccupied with concerns about eating and its putative effects on weight. This would free her to get on with her life, to become more socially active, and to function more efficiently at work.

Other Strategies for Addressing Shape and Weight Concerns

The cognitive methods for overcoming extreme concern with body weight and shape are complemented by behavioral techniques. These involve the flexible implementation of the principle of exposure to a feared or avoided stimulus. Some patients actively avoid allowing others to see their bodies. For example, they may typically wear "fat clothes"—loose-fitting, shapeless garments that conceal their shape. Just as patients are asked to eat avoided foods, so they are instructed to reveal more of their bodies. Typical assignments include wearing tighter and more revealing clothes; going swimming; and deliberately looking at their bodies in the mirror.

In contrast to these patients, others scrutinize their body parts (e.g., their stomachs, hips, and thighs) constantly, either by examining themselves in the mirror or by using certain clothes (e.g., a pair of jeans) of known tightness. As in the case of too frequent weighing, these patients are asked to limit this behavior. Finally, patients can be encouraged to compare their shape and weight with those of other women who are regarded as attractive. The goal is to have them realize that these attractive women have imperfections too. Using exposure in this way invariably provokes problematic thoughts about shape and weight that can be addressed by means of using cognitive restructuring.

Stage 3

In the third stage, the focus moves to the use of relapse prevention strategies to ensure the maintenance of change following treatment. Sessions are typically held every 2 weeks. This provides an extended opportunity for the patient to review what has worked for her, to consolidate the improvement she has made, and to continue addressing any remaining problem areas.

The major goal is for a patient to anticipate future difficulties and prepare ways of coping with them. Forewarned is forearmed! Patients are told that even if they have completely ceased binge eating and purging, they will probably always be vulnerable to the recurrence of eating problems, particularly if they encounter unusually stressful circumstances. In other words, they should expect the occasional setback. Nevertheless, they can learn to cope with sporadic setbacks without allowing these lapses to precipitate a full-blown relapse.

It is important to anticipate specific circumstances that might pose a problem, and to rehearse effective strategies for coping with these. A typical example might be the following: Imagine that therapy is concluding successfully at the end of January. Using imagery, the patient is asked to "fast-forward" to June. The weather is warm and sunny, and she has been invited to the shore. She immediately thinks about how she will look in a bikini. She feels uncomfortable, and thinks that she would look much more attractive if she were to lose "a few pounds." Her mind automatically reverts to contemplating dieting.

This is a high-risk situation for relapse. The patient is advised to recall immediately how she responded to such circumstances during treatment. Also, what had happened in the past when she reverted to dieting? Was it not a set-up for continued restriction and subsequent binge eating? In addition, the patient is encouraged to examine her overly self-critical thinking about her appearance, and to find a swimsuit that is attractive at her current weight. Other predictable triggers for renewed dieting should be anticipated (e.g., weight gain following childbirth).

Each patient is asked to prepare a written "maintenance plan" she can follow after therapy ends. The therapist reviews this plan with the patient to ensure that it is realistic. It should include the following points:

1. If eating problems recur, the first step is for the patient to be aware of what is happening.

2. The patient reinstitutes self-monitoring of all eating and the circumstances under which it occurs. This will allow her to uncover life events that are associated with the reemergence of the eating problem.
3. The patient makes a concerted effort to follow what worked before, such as eating three meals a day plus planned snacks.
4. The patient uses problem-solving strategies to cope with difficult life circumstances.
5. The patient reinstitutes cognitive restructuring aimed at reducing concern with weight and shape, or coping with other stressors.
6. The patient sets short-term, realistic goals, taking one day at a time. She tries to keep in mind that one or more episodes of binge eating or even purging do not mean that she has relapsed and lost all the improvement she made during therapy. Setbacks are to be expected, and can be overcome with the strategies learned during therapy.

CLINICAL ISSUES IN IMPLEMENTING THE MANUAL-BASED TREATMENT

We now have extensive collective experience in training a variety of therapists to use the CBT manual. These therapists have ranged from novice graduate students to experienced clinical psychologists and psychiatrists, and from those whose training and theoretical background are psychodynamic to those steeped in the theory and practice of CBT. In the course of this training, we have noted important procedural points that need to be made more explicit in the manual. We have also identified interventions that not infrequently pose problems for therapists mastering the manual, and result in less than optimal treatment. Our purpose in this section of the chapter is to highlight these components of manual-based CBT and to elaborate on their implementation.

Treatment Structure

Manual-based CBT for bulimia nervosa is a highly structured treatment. The structure is important for several reasons: It ensures a highly focused and systematic approach to the eating disorder, and it knits together the many different therapeutic elements of the CBT program in a planned fashion. CBT is not a miscellany of procedurally disconnected or conceptually disembodied techniques.

Patients with bulimia nervosa exhibit disturbed and often chaotic eating patterns. Many of them also report highly disorganized lifestyles; this disorganization tends to fuel their sense of being out of control. The focused and structured approach that CBT entails can contribute importantly to restoring some measure of orderliness and purpose in the lives of patients. In this way, its structure is well suited to combating patients' sense of "demoralization" and expediting the process of "remoralization" (Ilardi & Craighead, 1994). We believe that this structure also enhances adherence to the specific therapeutic interventions that define CBT.

We can distinguish between two forms of structure. One is the overall structure across therapy sessions; the other is the degree of structure with each session.

Structure across Treatment

It cannot be emphasized too much that manual-based CBT is a coordinated course of treatment. Therapists must ensure that patients understand this point. The manual distinguishes among three stages of treatment. In general, the early emphasis on behavior change blends into a more explicit focus on cognitive change. Interventions are cumulative, and therapists should routinely check to ensure that patients are adhering to earlier strategies as they introduce additional techniques later in the course of therapy.

A useful way of illustrating the integrative nature of the therapy is for the therapist to return frequently to the treatment model. Using a copy of the model (see Figure 6.1), the therapist can show patients where they are still experiencing problems. The therapist can also point out how the different behavioral and cognitive interventions complement one another in addressing each part of the model.

Therapists should follow the sequence of interventions described in the manual, although the pace at which the different elements are introduced may vary according to each patient's needs. For example, some patients respond rapidly and cease binge eating and purging before the end of the eight sessions of Stage 1. In these cases it makes sense to accelerate the introduction of cognitive restructuring to address abnormal attitudes about body weight and shape, which typically take longer to change than eating behavior.

Alternatively, it may make sense to accelerate the introduction of cognitive restructuring if a patient shows little sign of change. For example, a patient may cut down on binge eating but continue to vomit even after normal meals or small amounts of food. The patient may contend that she purges to get rid of the "excessive" amount of food she has consumed, when in fact she has eaten only a light meal. She may also justify vomiting in order to reduce the size of what she characterizes as her "huge stomach." These problematic thoughts and attitudes will need to be addressed directly, using both behavioral and cognitive techniques.

The shift from a primarily behavioral to a more cognitive focus from Stage 1 to Stage 2 is seamless. The transition from Stage 2 to Stage 3, however, is more marked. In Stage 3, the explicit emphasis on relapse prevention means that therapy focuses on the future rather than the present. The goal is to help patients disengage from the day-to-day details of treatment and think ahead. If patients have improved markedly, the objective is to help them plan how they will cope with possible setbacks in the months ahead. If they have shown little or no improvement, the objective is to motivate them to continue trying to implement the treatment strategies.

Structure within Sessions

Treatment sessions are divided into four parts: (1) a review of the patient's self-monitoring forms; (2) setting and implementing the agenda for the session; (3) a wrap-up of what was covered during the session; and (4) the assignment of specific homework tasks.

After the introduction of self-monitoring in Session 1, each subsequent session begins with a review of the patient's monitoring sheets. As the manual indicates, these sheets should be discussed in great detail in the first few sessions (Fairburn, Marcus, & Wilson, 1993, pp. 371–372). The purpose is twofold. One goal is to develop a complete picture of the patient's eating habits. A second goal is to encourage and reinforce the patient's active compliance with a seminal homework assignment. Systematic self-monitoring is crucial to the success of CBT, and a patient's cooperation in this regard is related in large part to the attention the therapist pays it. Establishing the value of detailed self-monitoring lays the foundation for compliance with the remainder of the CBT program.

After the first few sessions, when the patient is complying successfully with these instructions, the review of monitoring sheets becomes briefer (ranging from 5 to 15 minutes, depending on the particular patient and circumstances). The goals of this review are as follows: (1) to check and reinforce continuing compliance with monitoring and other homework assignments; (2) to monitor progress and problems, with a view to determining what the agenda for that particular session should be; and (3) to identify and reinforce specific improvements the patient has made. The emphasis on improvements sets a positive tone for the session, and reflects the general emphasis in CBT on patients' strengths and assets rather than weaknesses and deficits.

Some therapists learning to use the manual get waylaid in reviewing the first problem detected on a monitoring sheet. They can also become bogged down in unnecessary detail by doggedly going through each meal of each day. This is unsatisfactory, since it prevents the therapist from prioritizing the treatment agenda, starts off the session on a negative footing, and usually takes too much valuable time. With practice, therapists can learn to review the monitoring sheets quickly to identify the major themes that require attention. For example, it is very apparent if a patient has been restricting her food intake on most of the days during the preceding week. This indicates that the therapist needs to address the general issue of dieting as part of the agenda for the session. When addressing the dieting problem later in the session, the therapist need only use one or two good examples of how restriction of food intake led to problems during the week, without covering every meal. Similarly, a patient may have recorded a number of episodes of binge eating on her monitoring sheets. The review is not the time to explore each of these episodes or to begin to intervene with a view to eliminating them. Rather, the therapist notes the need to address these occurrences later in the session, at which point one or two selected examples, which illustrate the overall problem with binge eating, should be the focus of analysis.

Once the review is completed, the therapist decides on an agenda for the remainder of the session. The specific agenda is driven by the joint considerations of the stage of treatment on the one hand, and the review of monitoring sheets on the other. The therapist sets the agenda, but explains the choice to the patient and invites her input with questions such as "Does this make sense to you?" and "Is there anything else you would like to add?" Here as elsewhere, it is important to foster the active collaboration between therapist and patient in understanding and modifying the eating disorder.

Covering the agenda that is set then occupies most of the session. Therapists need to remain aware of the time, and plan to leave enough time (5 to 10 minutes) to wrap up the session and assign homework. The wrap-up is a summary of what issues were covered and what was agreed upon during the preceding agenda. The purpose of the wrap-up is to organize and underscore information and experience from the session; it leads naturally to spelling out homework assignments prior to the next session.

Departing from the Treatment Agenda

Time-limited, manual-based therapy demands strict adherence to the overall structure of treatment and the agenda of individual sessions. This requires that the therapist be disciplined and well prepared. Nevertheless, there are times when it is necessary to depart from a set agenda.

Sometimes a patient will enter a therapy session intent on talking about an experience that has little if any direct relevance to the goals for that session. Usually the patient is emotionally distressed. The causes are virtually limitless, ranging from an unexpectedly stressful situation at work to the death of a family member. In this type of situation, the therapist allows the patient to vent her feelings and explain her distress for the first 5 to 10 minutes of the session. In responding to such situations, the therapist must keep in mind the necessity of developing and maintaining a good therapeutic relationship. The patient's immediate needs must be addressed. After active listening and appropriate expressions of support and understanding, the therapist must decide whether or not to refocus the patient on the specific agenda for that session. In most cases, this presents little difficulty. In a few cases, however, the therapist may decide to postpone the session; the patient may be too upset and distracted to derive any benefit from the manual-based agenda.

Commitment to Treatment

Again, we should underscore the point that manual-based CBT is a coordinated course of treatment. This must be made clear to prospective patients. Accordingly, it is unwise to begin treatment unless patients are able to commit to attending therapy sessions on a regular basis for the next 4 to 6 months. Participation in therapy is a priority. Significant life events that would necessarily interfere with making it a priority are grounds for postponing therapy (e.g., imminent business or holiday travel for an extended period of time).

Some patients enter treatment committed to overcoming their eating disorder. Within the framework of the Prochaska and DiClemente (1986) model of stages of psychological change, they are either in the "determination" or "action" stages. They are ready to change and readily amenable to working on the manual-based program. Other patients, who are less committed to change, may be characterized as in the "contemplation" stage of change. They are ambivalent. Part of them wants to stop binge eating and purging, but another part is less sure. The ambivalence derives mainly from uncertainty about the consequences of change, and from the fear that this uncertainty breeds. It is the task of the cognitive-behavioral therapist to reduce this ambivalence and strengthen these patients' motivation to change. Developing commitment to change is a continuing task. Motivation waxes and wanes over the course of treatment, and it may require continual attention.

The cognitive-behavioral approach to developing commitment and motivation to change differs sharply from that of alternative therapeutic systems. CBT does not embrace the psychodynamic emphasis on resistance motivated by unconscious psychological processes. CBT also rejects the seminal assumption of treatments based on the Twelve-Step philosophy of Alcoholics Anonymous—that patients who are ambivalent about change are necessarily "in denial," and therefore must be openly confronted. Readers interested in a fuller discussion of the differences between CBT and these alternative treatments regarding commitment to change are referred to Lazarus and Fay (1982), Marlatt and Gordon (1985), Miller and Rollnick (1991), and O'Leary and Wilson (1987). (Miller & Rollnick's [1991] text on *Motivational Interviewing,* although based on the treatment of alcohol abuse and dependence, is a particularly useful source of practical suggestions for fostering motivation to change that is also applicable to patients with bulimia nervosa.) The following is a summary of some of the strategies therapists should adopt in promoting commitment to the treatment program.

Expectations of Outcome

An important element of Session 1 of the CBT program is orienting patients to treatment (Fairburn, Marcus, & Wilson, 1993, p. 367). Patients can be assured that the likely outcome will be positive; treatment works for the majority of patients. This message may bear repeating in later sessions. Some patients may become discouraged over their apparent lack of progress. Some will read popular or professional articles that misleadingly describe bulimia nervosa as "intractable," or they may read accounts of the much less positive outcome of treatment for anorexia nervosa and confuse anorexia with their own problem. Patients with a long history of bulimia nervosa often feel that they are less likely to succeed; they can be reassured that duration of the eating disorder does not predict a poor outcome.

Patients should not expect "overnight success." The orientation should make clear that the eating disorder is unlikely to disappear within a few weeks. Similarly, it is unrealistic to anticipate smooth and steady progress; uneven progress marked by occasional setbacks is more common. The setbacks need to be framed as learning opportunities for identifying and overcoming remaining obstacles to change.

It is not uncommon for patients who are struggling early in treatment to feel pessimistic about change. It can be helpful to point out that it would be premature to conclude that treatment is ineffective until they go through the full program. The therapist can also emphasize that the treatment program includes many different treatment strategies, which are differentially helpful with some patients.

It is the rare patient who does not encounter difficulties in implementing treatment strategies. Patients should be constantly encouraged to persevere, despite difficulty in following the therapist's instructions and despite limited or little improvement. Some patients who are still symptomatic at the end of CBT nonetheless cease binge eating and purging over the course of the following year (Agras et al., 1994; Fairburn et al., 1995).

Analysis of the Advantages and Disadvantages of Change

Patients' ambivalence can be overcome by amplifying the personal costs of maintaining the status quo and clarifying the short- and long-term benefits of change. The therapist can help patients spell out the costs of severe dieting with its attendant binge eating and purging. These include potential medical complications; psychological sequelae (e.g., guilt, self-hatred, and the tyranny of constant preoccupation with eating and body weight/shape); interpersonal problems (e.g., secrecy); and school- and job-related difficulties (e.g., impaired concentration). It can be made clear that these problems will not spontaneously disappear. They are likely to be chronic; if anything, their severity may worsen. The purpose here is to highlight the personal costs to a patient of hanging on to the thoughts and actions that constitute the eating disorder.

For many patients, the fear of potential weight gain outweighs the disadvantages of their disordered eating. Here the therapist can emphasize the consistent research findings indicating that the majority of patients who overcome bulimia nervosa and return to more normal eating patterns do not gain weight, even at long-term follow-up (Fairburn et al., 1995). It is often possible to show patients, on the basis of their own self-monitoring records (or their weight histories), that their weight is more likely to increase than to decrease during periods of binge eating and purging.

In seeking to develop what Miller and Rollnick (1991) describe as the discrepancy between a patient's present maladaptive state and the more adaptive alternative, a therapist should be careful to remain Socratic and not directly pressure or coerce the patient. Direct confrontation is likely to be perceived as a personal attack and to elicit defensiveness (Garner & Bemis, 1985). Therapists must resist the temptation to spell out the maladaptive nature of eating disorder symptoms as they see them. Instead, therapists should prompt patients to spell out the positive and negative consequences that the patients themselves have experienced.

Patients must genuinely believe the analysis

of the personal costs and benefits of change. The early sessions on education and advice regarding eating lend themselves well to developing this discrepancy. Subsequently, cognitive restructuring provides a particularly useful means of challenging reservations patients may have about making changes and engaging in therapy (Fennell, 1989; see Fairburn, Marcus, & Wilson, 1993, p. 388).

Compliance with Homework Assignments

For CBT to be effective, patients must comply with treatment instructions and complete homework assignments. Accordingly, therapists must be alert to problems with compliance from the outset. A guiding principle of CBT is that lack of compliance is a behavioral problem to be solved. It is not viewed as a trait-like characteristic that patients either have or do not have; as a manifestation of "denial" or as an expression of some unconscious, intrapsychic resistance. Hence the various cognitive and behavioral strategies described in the CBT manual can be used to overcome problems with compliance.

As an illustration, imagine that a patient comes to Session 11 without having completed homework assignments for the previous week. She explains that she is thinking of terminating because therapy is making the problem worse. She objects particularly to planning daily meals and snacks and to monitoring food intake, because this makes her anxious and preoccupied with her eating problems. In CBT, therapists hypothesize that problematic thoughts are responsible, at least in part, for this lack of engagement in treatment. The thoughts have to be identified and challenged by means of cognitive restructuring, just as other negative thinking regarding dieting or body weight has to be addressed. For example, the therapist can target the thought "Therapy is making me worse." What is the patient's evidence "for" and "against" this notion? Have her pretreatment frequencies of binge eating and purging changed? Is her weight different? How can this objective information lead to different conclusions about therapeutic progress or lack thereof?

In the hypothetical case in point, the patient's binge eating and purging are slightly improved, and her weight is unchanged. But she reports anxiety and displeasure about focusing on planning and eating three meals a day. The therapist should make this distinction clear, and, while expressing empathy and understanding, should urge the patient to persevere. It can be explained that the anxiety is likely to be a temporary state and should pass as the patient's new eating habits become established. This may also be a good time to draw out the consequences of returning to dieting and unplanned eating in the hope that the problem will go away.

The CBT manual is designed to promote compliance. The structure of the treatment program provides clear and concretely defined interventions that follow a logical and systematic course, and that are linked to an explicit model of the maintenance of the disorder. These qualities are known to facilitate compliance (Meichenbaum & Turk, 1988). The manual is not only structured but also graded. For example, the early focus is on making the least difficult behavioral changes—namely, restoring a pattern of regular eating. Patients are allowed to restrict intake and eat "safe" foods, provided that they eat three meals a day plus planned snacks. The typically more threatening tasks of increasing the amount of food consumed, and including previously avoided foods in meals, are tackled in Stage 2. Graduating behavior change assignments maximizes the likelihood of early progress and positive reinforcement. Assigning manageable tasks, in which patients can succeed counters feelings of hopelessness and rapidly, results in the important "remoralization" process of therapy. It is probably this process that accounts for the rapid improvement in the first few weeks of therapy (Jones, Peveler, Hope, & Fairburn, 1993). It is no coincidence that CBT produces rapid change not only in bulimia nervosa, but also in depression (Ilardi & Craighead, 1994) and anxiety disorders (Clark et al., 1994).

The style of treatment, which can be characterized as "collaborative empiricism," similarly promotes compliance. Cognitive-behavioral therapists seek to develop an open, trusting relationship with patients, in which they cooperate in identifying and solving problems. Each patient is an active collaborator in her therapy. Feedback on the therapist's approach and behavior is encouraged; the traditional role of the (medical) patient as a relatively passive recipient of an authoritative doctor's orders is deliberately avoided. The emphasis is not on "control" but on patient choice.

Referring to this therapeutic style, Guidano and Liotti (1983) made the following observation:

> This policy [of active cooperation and collaboration] prevents many hidden competitive and resentful feelings and many artful tactics of the patient to check the therapist's "omniscience" and "omnipotence." It is probably for this reason that the "resistance" phenomenon is so remarkably uncommon in cognitive therapy [we would add also behavior therapy] as compared to psychodynamic therapies. If a cooperative relationship exists, the patient does not feel the need to "countercontrol," and the therapist can plainly consider any disagreement, noncompliance, or irritation on the patient's part not as a form of "resistance," but as a source of information in the patient's way of perceiving or construing the therapist's feelings and behavior. (p. 123)

The commitment to active collaboration between therapist and patient is also consistent with the view that therapy is analogous to scientific reasoning. Particularly in CBT, patients are encouraged to view their cognitions as hypotheses that need to be continually tested and evaluated, in the manner that scientists presumably carry out their investigations. A major goal of this therapy is for patients to adopt a new conceptualization of their problems; to this end, they are prompted to be open to "anomalous data" and to reconsider key beliefs that may be responsible for their difficulties.

The CBT manual consistently calls for this process of collaborative empiricism. In setting the agenda for each session, the therapist specifically invites patient input. In developing homework assignments, therapists ask patients for feedback and for possible suggestions. It is helpful to have patients think through the obstacles they are likely to encounter in completing the homework assignment, and how they might overcome them. Therapists are most likely to invite noncompliance if they unilaterally tell their patients what to do. Specific techniques such as problem solving and cognitive restructuring are based on collaborative empiricism.

The therapeutic relationship is crucial to obtaining good compliance. Unless patients trust their therapists, feel understood by them, and find them competent and credible, compliance will suffer. As a general rule, successfully implementing the CBT manual calls for a judicious blend of empathy and firmness.

Empathy is important because patients with eating disorders are extremely sensitive to disapproval, as we have noted earlier in this chapter. Some may be disclosing the details of their eating problems for the first time. They are also very apprehensive about abandoning extreme (albeit maladaptive) methods of weight control for fear of gaining weight.

Firmness is demanded by the content of the manual. Among other requirements of the manual, patients must keep food records. Some patients are initially uncomfortable with self-monitoring, claiming that it merely increases their preoccupation with food. (This is more common and more problematic in patients with anorexia nervosa than in those with bulimia nervosa, however.) The therapist takes a sympathetic but unyielding stance in pointing out the necessity of self-monitoring. Patients can be prompted to think about their recent history and to realize that their preoccupation with eating and body weight and shape was extreme prior to therapy. They can be reassured that this is likely to be a temporary reaction that will pass as they begin to move through the treatment program. The manual suggests that therapists respond to failure to self-monitor with surprise or puzzlement, since it effectively undermines treatment (Fairburn, Marcus, & Wilson, 1993, pp. 371–372).

(Readers unfamiliar with the cognitive-behavioral conceptualization of compliance and resistance are referred to the more general literature on this topic—e.g., Fennell, 1989; Lazarus & Fay, 1982; Meichenbaum & Turk, 1988; and O'Leary & Wilson, 1987.)

Therapist Training

We have underscored the importance of a good therapeutic relationship in the treatment of bulimia nervosa. The effective implementation of manual-based treatment requires well-trained, competent therapists. It takes therapeutic skill to keep patients focused on the treatment. Although the treatment is standardized, therapists still make judgments about when to introduce different components of the therapy and which elements they emphasize. The more patients trust and believe in their therapists, the more likely they are to comply with treatment prescriptions. Manual-based therapy should not be confused with mechanistic or rote administration of preset techniques.

In the controlled clinical studies summarized in an earlier section of this chapter, CBT was carried out by therapists explicitly trained in its

use. How effective manual-based CBT is when administered by therapists with different degrees of training and expertise remains to be determined (Wilson, 1995). However, our experience in training a variety of therapists with different theoretical backgrounds and levels of clinical experience suggests that the manual-based therapy is broadly exportable.

We are often asked whether the gender of the therapist is important. Our answer is that it does not appear to be so. The critical variables are how well trained therapists are and how well they communicate their understanding of bulimia nervosa to patients, not whether the therapists are male or female.

Problems with Implementing Cognitive Restructuring

Of all the CBT techniques, cognitive restructuring is probably the most difficult to do well and requires the most technical skill. In our experience, it is the technique that is most commonly misapplied in the treatment of bulimia nervosa.

Conceptual Issues

The CBT manual prescribes a basic version of cognitive restructuring. A more elaborate version of fundamentally the same intervention is described by Fennell (1989) and Clark (1989) for the treatment of depression and anxiety disorders, respectively. These sources provide invaluable background reading on the clinical practice of cognitive restructuring. In addition, Garner and Bemis (1985) have described cognitive restructuring for the treatment of patients with anorexia nervosa; their description is closer to the original Beck et al. (1979) treatment approach.

In their evaluation of the effectiveness of the Oxford CBT manual, Hollon and Beck (1994) had the following to say:

> Despite the apparent success of [this approach], it is still not clear that cognitive change procedures have been operationalized in the most powerful manner possible . . . for example, the manual used by Fairburn and colleagues in their recently published trial makes no reference to teaching patients to chart beliefs or to distinguish among specific lines of inquiry (e.g., evidence, alternatives, and implications) when evaluating their accuracy. . . . Moreover, attention has often been restricted to specific beliefs regarding weight and food, rather

than being extended to more generic concerns about one's self-worth and the nature of interpersonal relationships. (p. 444)

We agree that the manual offers a less expansive and probably a less intensive focus on cognitive restructuring than is possible. Nevertheless, we continue to recommend that therapists follow the technique described in the manual, for a number of reasons. Our experience in training a wide range of different therapists in the use of the manual has taught us that cognitive restructuring can be difficult to master; adopting a still more complex and elaborate form of the technique would be an even more formidable task. We are concerned about how "exportable" cognitive restructuring is. We also have serious reservations about therapists' using this technique without systematic training in CBT in general, and CBT for eating disorders in particular.

A more elaborate form of cognitive restructuring, even if administered by a suitably trained therapist, would almost certainly involve more time than is available in the 19-session program described by Fairburn, Marcus, and Wilson (1993). The trade off of additional therapy sessions versus the putative benefits of using the expanded technique requires careful consideration. Hollon and Beck (1994) speculate that the added focus on cognitive restructuring might enhance the effectiveness of CBT. Of course, this is an empirical question. In the meantime, there are no data from other disorders showing that a heavier cognitive focus produces better results. For example, in the treatment of panic disorder, Barlow's panic control treatment (Craske & Barlow, 1993) includes a form of cognitive restructuring that is less elaborate than the one used by Clark et al. (1994). Although there has been no direct comparison, the results to date do not indicate the superiority of the latter. We can envisage situations in which it might be important to pursue the sort of in-depth cognitive restructuring Hollon and Beck (1994) have in mind. One would be patients' failure to respond to manual-based CBT. The other would be the case of the more difficult-to-treat eating disorder of anorexia nervosa (Garner & Bemis, 1985).

Procedural Details

The most common problem with the clinical use of cognitive restructuring is that therapists become too didactic and begin to lecture patients. Consider this hypothetical example: A patient says that she is "disgustingly fat," and claims that her "butt is getting bigger by the day." The therapist may have the inclination to jump in to point out that the patient's body mass index (BMI) is low-normal; that neither her friends nor her boyfriend regards her as "fat" or "disgusting"; and that it is normal for women in Western society to be especially concerned about the size of their hips and stomachs. Of course the therapist is correct in these assertions. The information is accurate, but it is unlikely to have much impact. This type of intervention is really a form of verbal persuasion, which is known to be largely ineffective as a means of changing cognitions or behavior (Bandura, 1986). Beliefs do not change as a result of simple self-statements; therapy would be a simple matter if this were the case. Changing emotionally laden beliefs and attitudes requires much more.

Another problem with the sort of didactic intervention summarized above is that invites opposition and counterargument from the patient. In this example, the patient may insist that her butt really is big—or at least bigger than those of her friends, and certainly bigger than what she desires. She may also insist that she is "fat" regardless of what a BMI chart says. It is common for therapists inexperienced in the use of cognitive restructuring to find themselves arguing with patients over who is "right" about the patients' statements. As a rule of thumb, a therapist who feels that he or she is arguing with a patient should stop and refocus the session.

Cognitive restructuring, as opposed to verbal persuasion, demands that a therapist adopt a Socratic style. Patients must be guided to arrive at their own reevaluation of problematic thoughts and attitudes; this is an example of the collaborative empiricism noted above.

For example, one patient, who was having great difficulty breaking away from severely restrictive dieting, declared that immediately after eating she could feel her "fat cells expanding." It would have been easy (and very likely futile) to point out authoritatively that this is not biologically possible—that food is not processed that quickly, that fat cell expansion cannot be directly sensed, and so on.

Once a problematic thought such as this has been identified, the CBT manual requires that the patient explore the evidence "for" and "against" the thought. In support of the thought, the patient responded that she felt tingling, especially in her thighs where "I always put on weight." Initially, she could not come up with evidence to the contrary. Upset and adamant, she claimed it was obviously true. At this point, a direct cross-examination of the patient's logic would have been counterproductive. Instead, the therapist patiently validated the patient's distress, and then gently but firmly reminded her that feelings, real and important as they may be, are not evidence. The therapist helped the patient review her self-monitoring sheets, which showed that only after eating certain cookies (a forbidden food) one day after lunch (violating one of the patient's rigidly held dietary rules) had she felt her fat cells expanding. There were many other days when she had eaten more food than on the occasion in question, but when she had not experienced her fat cells expanding. The therapist asked that patient to make sense of these different pieces of evidence. The therapist also asked the patient how else she could explain the tingling sensations in her thighs. What about her sensitivity and her focus of attention on her thighs? Here the therapist suggested possible alternative interpretations of the feelings (although it is always preferable for the patient to try to generate alternative explanations).

As a result of this carefully directed questioning, the patient tearfully agreed that it was her sensitivity to eating sugar cookies that had led to a terror of gaining weight and the feelings she had experienced. The reasoned conclusion she was able to draw from this analysis was that she could eat food without gaining weight, and that she needed to work on coming to terms with her fear about eating cookies and other forbidden foods. She was encouraged to make the prediction, which could be tested by the behavioral experiment of eating more normally, that eating a less restrictive range of foods would not necessarily lead to weight gain.

It should be stressed that it is not necessary for patients to believe fully an alternative view of their problematic thought or attitude. As the manual makes clear, what is important is that the cognitive work, especially the reasoned conclusion that is reached, leads to action. The resulting behavioral change will reinforce changes in thoughts and attitudes. The focus of cognitive restructuring is tailored to the individual patient's problems.

Overweight or obese patients with bulimia nervosa are relatively rare. Nevertheless, they require adjustments in using cognitive restructuring. For example, the objective reality is that they are "fat." Cognitive restructuring can only be effective to the extent that it is authentic and credible to patients. In these cases the cognitive challenging that makes up the second and third steps of restructuring can be targeted at the implications of being overweight or obese. The course of action that this condition leads to is what can be usefully challenged. The question therefore becomes this: What is the evidence for the value of rigid dieting or purging as an attempt to lose weight? What has happened when the patient has done this in the distant and recent past? The evidence against such a course of action is usually unambiguous. First, it triggers binge eating and its maladaptive sequelae—purging, emotional distress, and self-recrimination. Second, it is almost always futile; it does not work as a lasting weight reduction strategy. Again, although the treatment literature on weight loss allows the therapist to make a confident statement about the ineffectiveness of rigid dieting in controlling weight, the patient must reach this verdict on the basis of her own experience. Finally, the reasoned conclusion is that rigid dieting is an unsatisfactory response. (Additional information on the use of cognitive restructuring in obese patients is provided in Fairburn, Marcus, & Wilson, 1993, pp. 398–399.)

The primary goal of the treatment program is to have patients learn and then use cognitive restructuring as a skill. It is useful for therapists to work through one or more specific examples of using the technique during sessions, but patients then need to implement it consistently between sessions as a means of resisting or coping with binge–purge episodes. It is vital that patients write out their attempts to use cognitive restructuring. Identifying and then challenging problematic thoughts in writing make this cognitive work more focused and systematic than it would otherwise be. If not, the cognitive work is often reduced to the perfunctory recitation of homilies that patients have heard, unavailingly, many times before (e.g., "I'm not perfect").

Finally, it is commonplace for patients to label themselves in harshly critical terms (e.g., "I'm a fat pig"). Patients should be urged to desist from this practice. Therapists can help patients see that this negative labeling does not lead to any useful or constructive action. Moreover, it undermines their already battered self-image. Therapists can refer to the model (Figure 6.1) to emphasize the self-perpetuating downward spiral that a reduction in self-esteem entails.

SUPPLEMENTARY OR ADDITIONAL TREATMENT

As we have noted above, it is commonplace for bulimia nervosa patients to report a range of associated psychopathology. It is important to reiterate that the effectiveness of the CBT manual has been demonstrated in patients with significant psychiatric comorbidity (Wilson & Fairburn, in press). The myth that CBT is appropriate only for so-called "discrete" cases of bulimia nervosa dies hard. Patients with additional problems should be encouraged to complete the treatment for bulimia nervosa before seeking supplementary or additional therapy. The exceptions, as we have noted above, include severe depression and suicidal states, and serious substance use problems. Patients can be told that the chances are favorable that successful treatment of their eating disorder will result in improvement in other psychological problems. Measures of anxiety, depression, interpersonal functioning, self-esteem, and personality disorder have all shown improvement following successful CBT (e.g., Fairburn et al., 1986; Garner et al., 1993).

Circumstances may arise during the course of treatment that interfere with the effective implementation of manual-based CBT. In these relatively rare cases, it may be necessary to postpone treatment of the eating disorder and to address the more salient problem. A strategic switch in tactics is illustrated in the following case:

Jenny was a 23-year-old woman who sought treatment for bulimia nervosa. In addition to her eating disorder, Jenny reported depressive symptoms and periodic alcohol abuse. The latter often preceded her cutting herself on the arm. Despite these problems, Jenny initially responded well to manual-based CBT, with significant decreases in binge eating, purging, and depressive symptoms. At Session 11, however, she appeared tearful and depressed; she was unusually unresponsive to the therapist's attempt to address her eating problems.

The therapist's inquiry into reasons for Jenny's despondent state revealed that her relationship with her boyfriend had deteriorated to such an extent that he had become physically abusive during the previous week. Jenny confided that she was thinking about dropping out of treatment because she was "a failure" as far as the eating problem was concerned. At the following session, the therapist proposed a strategic postponement of addressing the eating disorder in favor of work on the patient's relationship with her boyfriend. Jenny expressed relief and gratitude, disclosing further that she had been contemplating seeking some form of alternative therapy for the problem. The therapist was also careful to frame the switch in tactics in a way that challenged Jenny's perception that she had "failed" CBT for bulimia nervosa. Following six sessions focused on disengaging from the abusive boyfriend, CBT for bulimia nervosa was resumed.

Similarly, a patient who becomes seriously depressed or develops some other clinical disorder will require treatment for the more pressing problem. In the case of depression, it may be possible to combine concurrent antidepressant drug therapy with CBT, depending on the patient's ability to engage in the manual-based CBT.

Many patients will still be somewhat symptomatic at the end of the 19-session manual-based treatment. In our clinical experience, patients in the United States, with its ready availability of different forms of psychological therapy and a tradition of largely open-ended treatment,[4] will often wish to seek additional therapy at the end of the 19 sessions of CBT. We reiterate the caveat issued by Fairburn, Marcus, and Wilson (1993, pp. 364–365) about the inadvisability of a rush into further therapy. Patients should be encouraged to follow through on their maintenance plans and to "be their own therapists'" as CBT has emphasized. If after a period of some months their problems have not improved, or possibly deteriorated, they can then seek additional treatment.

NONRESPONDERS TO MANUAL-BASED TREATMENT: OTHER TREATMENT OPTIONS

CBT is an effective treatment, but this cannot obscure the reality that no more than about 50% of patients cease binge eating and purging. Of the remainder, many show partial improvement, whereas a small number derive no benefit at all. The question is how best to treat these nonresponders.

Expanding the Scope of CBT

Although the CBT manual that has been evaluated in controlled trials allows the therapist considerable flexibility in using a variety of behavioral and cognitive techniques, it remains a truncated version of the unrestricted clinical practice of CBT in general. By carrying out a more idiographic assessment of individual patients' particular problems, and by drawing upon the wider range of cognitive and behavioral strategies, practitioners should, in principle, be able to tailor therapy to the patients' particular needs.

Exposure Treatments

Expanding CBT for bulimia nervosa can take several forms (Wilson, 1996b). The most obvious prospects are variations of the exposure component of treatment (Carter & Bulik, 1993; Wilson, 1988). The most thoroughly studied variation has been the exposure plus response prevention (ERP) method for preventing self-induced vomiting (Rosen & Leitenberg, 1985). The manual suggests the use of this therapist-assisted, in-session exposure treatment in cases where patients cannot comply with instructions to eat forbidden foods or where even small meals lead to purging (Fairburn, Marcus, & Wilson, 1993, p. 383). In this technique, patients are instructed to eat their typical "binge" foods to the point at which they would ordinarily induce vomiting. Under the guidance of the therapist, patients are helped to resist vomiting and to cope with the anxiety that they experience (see Rosen & Leitenberg, 1985, for details of this procedure). Although the original application of this technique was viewed as a means of extinguishing the association between eating-induced anxiety and vomiting (Leitenberg, Rosen, Gross, Nudelman, & Vara, 1988), other investigators have conceptualized it in cognitive terms as a means of enhancing self-efficacy for coping with triggers for vomiting (Wilson, 1988).

Another variation of exposure treatment focuses on the cues that trigger binge eating rather than vomiting. In this method, the patient eats a small amount of a forbidden food, which would typically lead to uncontrolled overeating; she is then guided by the therapist in preventing a subsequent binge (Jansen, Broekmate, & Heymans, 1992).

It is still unclear whether ERP enhances the effectiveness of the generic CBT program. One study showed no incremental benefit of adding in-session ERP to individual CBT (Wilson et al., 1991). Another indicated that the addition of ERP actually detracted from the effectiveness of CBT (Agras et al., 1989). Leitenberg (1994), however, has argued that neither study provided an adequate test of ERP. In the Agras et al. (1989) study, for example, therapy sessions were only 50 to 60 minutes in duration, whereas Leitenberg et al. (1988) have used sessions lasting 2 hours. The effective use of ERP is likely to require longer sessions. Leitenberg (1994) suggests that trying to fit ERP into the normal course of 50- to 60-minute sessions not only provided an inadequate test of ERP, but also may have compromised the basic CBT program. Similarly, Leitenberg (1994) faults the Wilson et al. (1991) study for including too few sessions of ERP to make a significant difference. Some of the methodological difficulties in testing the incremental benefits of combining ERP with the now-standard CBT program are discussed by Carter and Bulik (1993).

Another variation of exposure treatment that is adaptable to the treatment of bulimia nervosa is known as "worry exposure" (Craske, Barlow, & O'Leary, 1992). In this procedure, patients are asked to concentrate on anxiety-provoking thoughts about body weight or shape (e.g., "I ate too much and now my stomach is huge"). They are instructed to conjure up a detailed and vivid image of this feared outcome, and then to stay with the thought/image for at least 25 to 30 minutes, despite the discomfort it causes. It is important that patients experience the emotional upset that this exposure entails, and that they not attenuate the exposure through any form of cognitive avoidance. At the end of this period of exposure, patients use cognitive restructuring to challenge the problematic thoughts and attitudes the exposure scene has brought to the fore. As in all forms of exposure treatment, these trials should be repeated in a systematic and planned fashion. The goal of worry exposure is habituation to unrealistic anxiety-eliciting thoughts and feelings. The rationale derives from the learning theory principle of extinction. As such, it differs from what has been called "pure" or "focused" cognitive restructuring, in that the latter is designed to provide corrective information aimed strictly at cognitive change (Hollon & Beck, 1994).

Interpersonally Oriented CBT

Another clinical expansion of CBT is an increased focus on interpersonal issues. The treatment manual addresses interpersonal issues only insofar as they constitute proximal triggers for specific episodes of binge eating or purging (Fairburn, Marcus, & Wilson, 1993). Imposing this boundary has allowed researchers to compare CBT with IPT without the methodological problem of procedural overlap between the two treatments (Fairburn et al., 1991). However, this has entailed excluding commonly used cognitive-behavioral strategies. The clinical practice of CBT in general often focuses on interpersonal anxieties, conflicts, and deficits, using a number of different treatment techniques (O'Leary & Wilson, 1987). IPT has been shown to be an effective treatment for bulimia nervosa (Fairburn et al., 1995). What is unknown is whether its effectiveness is attributable to the focus on the interpersonal domain of functioning, or to the structure and style of the IPT itself. It is possible that a focus on interpersonal issues from a CBT perspective might produce similar results.

Day Program and Inpatient CBT

CBT as described in the manual is outpatient treatment. An insufficiently explored option is a day hospital program, or full hospitalization, for more direct and intensive treatment of the patient's disordered eating habits. Food intake can be better regulated, and binge eating and purging prevented, in such a structured setting. Day hospital treatment is preferred because it is less expensive and does not completely remove the patient from the psychosocial situations associated with binge eating and purging.

Tuschen and Bent (1995) describe a promising example of intensive inpatient CBT. Treatment lasts 10 to 14 days, with direct therapist contact for as much as 10 to 12 hours a day. From the beginning, patients are exposed to a daily routine of regular eating consisting of 2,000 calories. In the course of this eating plan, they are systematically exposed to eating previously forbidden food and foods that have triggered binge eating. For example, in eating forbidden food, patients are asked to "verbalize its taste, smell, appearance and consistency. In order to

obtain habituation, any avoidance behavior is prevented. A primary goal of these exposure sessions is to reduce anxiety and to enhance self-control over regular eating and the consumption of moderate portions of high caloric food" (Tuschen & Bent, 1995, p. 356). Exposure to body shape is provided by having patients use a mirror that furnishes a full view of the body, as well as by videotaping patients' bodies.

An important feature of this German program is that the therapists attempt to introduce real-life stressors (e.g., negative mood states) during the inpatient stay, in order to capture naturalistic triggers of binge eating more faithfully. Treatment of the anxiety disorders has shown that exposure is most effective if all relevant stimulus cues are included in the session (Butler, 1989). There is evidence that combining affective and interpersonal cues with food-specific cues produces increased physiological reactivity and craving in bulimia nervosa patients (Carter & Bulik, 1993; Laberg, Wilson, Eldredge, & Nordby, 1991). These findings point to the importance of incorporating relevant affective cues in exposure treatment (Wilson, 1988).

This inpatient program is the logical extension of the rationale and theoretical principles of the Oxford manual. The structure and intensive supervision ensure implementation of procedures, in a way that is not possible in outpatient therapy. Given the sound theoretical grounding and obvious clinical appeal of this innovative program, we look forward to the systematic evaluation of its results.

Alternative Therapies

When CBT fails, instead of modifying it, therapists can switch to a different approach. IPT is currently the logical choice as far as psychotherapy is concerned. It has been shown to be effective in the treatment of depression (Klerman & Weissman, 1993) and of bulimia nervosa (Fairburn, 1993). Note that this switching of treatment tactics is not a form of therapeutic integration, in which therapists incorporate a treatment into their own conceptual framework and possibly make changes in how it is implemented. By switching to IPT, the therapist abandons both the style and content of CBT. IPT is a nondirective (albeit focused) approach that is procedurally and conceptually immiscible with CBT (see Fairburn, Chapter 14, this volume). The two treatments can be sequenced but not integrated.

Should CBT fail, it may also be useful to try a

course of antidepressant medication. Tricyclics, and more recently fluoxetine, have been shown to produce significant short-term improvement in eating disorder symptoms and associated depression (Mitchell & deZwaan, 1993). Whether or not patients who fare badly with CBT will respond to antidepressant medication is currently unknown, although the issue is under clinical investigation.

Exploring alternative treatment interventions for patients who do not respond well to manual-based CBT is a priority. Nevertheless, this search should be tempered by the realization that some patients will not respond, regardless of the type of treatment they receive. Bulimia nervosa patients who do not respond to CBT may prove intractable. For example, Fairburn et al. (1995) reported that of those patients who were diagnosed with an eating disorder at the 5.8-year follow-up, two-thirds had received additional psychiatric treatment to no avail.

A Cautionary Note about "Nonresponders"

We caution against dichotomizing treatment outcome into simple "responder" and "nonresponder" categories. There are degrees of treatment response that range along a continuum.

Ideally, a bulimia nervosa patient will have ceased all binge eating and purging, will have abandoned rigid and unhealthy dieting, and will attach less importance to body shape and weight in self-evaluation by the end of treatment. A rigorous way of assessing such a composite outcome might be to use the global score on the Eating Disorder Examination (EDE; Fairburn & Cooper, 1993). The EDE, a semi-structured clinical interview with established validity, provides the most comprehensive assessment of specific eating disorder psychopathology (Wilson, 1993). Fairburn et al. (1995) used a cutoff of one standard deviation within the mean for young women as a way of defining overall treatment outcome.

The reality, however, is that patients respond to treatment with varying degrees of improvement. For example, some patients cease binge eating and purging, but they continue to restrict their food intake because of excessive concerns about body shape and weight, which have remained unchanged. Other patients resume normal eating and change their abnormal attitudes about shape and weight, but continue sporadic binge eating, which may or may not be accom-

panied by self-induced vomiting. In these cases, as emphasized above, we recommend that patients first try to "be their own therapists" in overcoming remaining problems before seeking additional therapy. Consider the following case:

Norma, by Session 8 of manual-based treatment, had stopped binge eating and purging, although she continued to restrict her eating because she had slowly gained weight. She reported frequent urges to binge, but she was able to fight these off. At Session 18, however, she described a major setback: She had binged and purged several times each day for most of the preceding week and a half. Frustrated with the weight gain and "sick of dealing with my eating disorder," she described how she had "gone on strike," abandoning the various CBT strategies she had been using. The therapist helped her to accept once more that the alternative to adhering to the treatment program was a life of disordered eating and purging. Two weeks later, in her final therapy session, Norma reported regaining partial control of her eating and had succeeded in resisting binge eating and purging on most of the intervening days. Following the manual, the therapist encouraged Norma to continue using the strategies she had learned, reminding her how successful she had been when she had complied with the program.

We believe that it would have been inadvisable for Norma to seek additional therapy at that point. What was needed was a commitment on her part to tackling her eating problem on a day-to-day basis. She had the necessary tools to cope with the eating disorder. Entering into more therapy could well have undermined her opportunity to exercise the self-control that seemed called for. As we have noted earlier in this chapter, some patients who are still symptomatic following manual-based CBT show significant improvement at a 1-year follow-up (Agras et al., 1994; Fairburn et al., 1995; Maddocks, Kaplan, Woodside, Langdon, & Piran, 1992).

A STEPPED-CARE MODEL OF TREATMENT

If individual, manual-based CBT is not always sufficient to overcome bulimia nervosa, neither is it always necessary. Another priority in the field is the development of the most cost-effective and easily disseminable form of the treatment.

Many of the early applications of CBT to bulimia nervosa involved group treatment (e.g., Kirkley, Schneider, Agras, & Bachman, 1985; Mitchell et al., 1990). The CBT manual lends itself readily to group application, and it remains a plausible means of more efficient treatment. Whether the greater efficiency is offset by any loss in effectiveness has yet to be tested. There has been no well-controlled comparison of manual-based individual and group CBT (Agras, 1993).

An alternative means of efficiently implementing the principles and procedures of manual-based CBT would be psychoeducational group therapy. Using a program of five 90-minute group sessions, Olmsted et al. (1991) have reported encouraging results. This brief intervention was roughly comparable in effectiveness to 19 sessions of individual CBT for patients with less severe binge-eating problems.

Another promising development is the supervised use of a self-help version of the CBT manual. Cooper, Coker, and Fleming (1994) have treated bulimia nervosa patients with a self-help manual entitled *Bulimia Nervosa: A Guide to Recovery* (Cooper, 1993), which is based on the Oxford manual. In an initial study, Cooper et al. (1994) provided patients with their self-help guide, in conjunction with 6 to 12 brief (20- to 30-minute) sessions with a social worker who focused on implementing the self-help manual. The data suggest that more than half the patients reported marked clinical improvement. No follow-up data were reported, however. (The possibilities of using a self-help program are discussed by Fairburn and Carter in Chapter 30 of the present volume.) At this point, there is little doubt that many bulimia nervosa patients may need no more than the self-help manual, with or without guided assistance, or psychoeducational therapy. Identifying predictors of which patients are appropriate for these interventions would represent an important clinical advance.

MANUAL-BASED THERAPY: PROS AND CONS

The manual-based CBT used in controlled clinical trials may differ from the more flexible and expansive application of CBT in unrestricted clinical practice. Whether or not this difference influences treatment outcome is ultimately an empirical question.

On the face of it, the greater range and flexibility of an idiographic implementation of CBT are clinically appealing. Nonetheless, there are reasons to question whether a more idiographically based intervention would improve upon the CBT manual (Fairburn, Marcus, & Wilson, 1993, p. 364). First, the CBT manual has been repeatedly shown to be effective. Second, the manual makes CBT more disseminable; it is easier for therapists to acquire skill in using this approach. Third, the highly structured and time-limited nature of this treatment focuses the attention of both therapist and patient in working hard to make well-defined changes. This feature is especially attractive, given the reality of managed care and the corresponding need for treatment to be cost-effective. Finally, adding additional elements to the treatment would require either replacing some aspects or making it longer. Both options have disadvantages. It is unclear whether extending treatment has any advantages. Patients are being helped to be their own therapists so that they can continue to make progress following the termination of formal treatment.

Beyond these considerations, there is a more fundamental issue—namely, that of clinical judgment versus actuarial prediction. It is well established that when it comes to predicting behavior, highly trained clinical experts who assess all available information, and integrate it into their own understanding of the niceties of the individual case, do no better and possible worse than actuarial prediction (Dawes, Faust, & Meehl, 1989). The explanation is well known: Human judgment is not as effective as systematic research in selecting robust predictors of behavioral outcomes. Is this finding about predicting behavior similar to the therapist's task of idiographically assessing an individual patient, with a view to selecting from an array of often competing and incompatible treatment techniques?

Some therapists are likely to object to manual-based treatment that precludes the opportunity to improvise—to modify or even disregard the protocol—based on their clinical experience and expert assessment of the patient. The hallmark of behavioral assessment and therapy has been the functional analysis of the individual case (O'Leary & Wilson, 1987). It goes against the grain to ignore this dictum and fit a standardized treatment to a particular diagnosis. Clinical psychologists are especially likely to object to this practice, on the grounds that it does not provide a psychological analysis of the presenting problem. Bulimia nervosa, like most clinical disorders, is heterogeneous in nature. The specific variables that maintain the problem probably vary from case to case.

Nevertheless, it can be argued that the value of idiographic assessment has been overrated in CBT and in psychotherapy in general (Wilson, 1996a). In conducting an idiographic clinical assessment, therapists will be guided by their personal experience. Research has shown that such cognitive processes as the availability heuristic and confirmatory bias undermine the utility of personal experience (Garb, 1994). O'Donohue and Szymanski (1994) point out that "Clinicians tend to find relationships between variables based on their prior expectations of what relationships they expect should exist rather than what relationships actually exist" (p. 32). Weighting the findings of clinical research more heavily by using a validated treatment manual should reduce the potential influence of such biases.

The fine-grained analysis of the individual case will yield more information, but does this increase effectiveness in selecting and implementing effective techniques? More information often increases judges' confidence in their decisions, but it does not increase their accuracy (O'Donohue & Szymanski, 1994). Therapists would be better advised to follow the empirically derived guideline that the preferred treatment for someone meeting diagnostic criteria for bulimia nervosa is manual-based CBT. If this does not work, they can then move to the next empirically validated method, or the approach that is most consistent with what is known about effective treatment.

CONCLUDING REMARKS

The present chapter must be read as a supplement to the CBT manual described by Fairburn, Marcus, and Wilson (1993). This manual-based treatment has been rigorously evaluated in controlled clinical trials by different groups of clinical investigators in different countries, and these trials have shown it to be effective. It is acceptable and broadly applicable to patients with bulimia nervosa.

On the basis of these and other considerations, manual-based CBT is likely to become the standard of treatment for bulimia nervosa. This development should have distinct advantages. In our own therapist training and supervision, as part of our collaborative clinical research, the adoption of a uniform approach has helped us detect differences in our respective treatment and training programs, has led to fruitful discussions about clinical practice, and has produced refinements in how we have used manual-based CBT. We anticipate a still wider range of feedback from other clinical centers as they adopt this manual-based treatment.

The use of a standardized treatment method in different clinical studies will remove one of the most formidable obstacles to comparing outcome results across studies. The application of a standardized treatment to different patient samples across widely varying settings by different therapists should provide invaluable information about largely unexplored issues, such as the disseminability of the treatment and the moderating influence of different patient characteristics.

Finally, it is important to note that this development does not herald the premature standardization of treatment of bulimia nervosa. Nor does it curtail clinical innovation in any manner. On the contrary, we believe that common clinical experience in implementing manual-based CBT will spur clinical innovation by encouraging a more focused dialogue among clinicians. It will also provide an impetus to a new generation of clinical studies focusing on the treatment of patients who do not respond to an established treatment.

ACKNOWLEDGMENTS

Preparation of this chapter was made possible in part by support from the McKnight Foundation and Grant No. MH 49886 from the National Institute of Mental Health.

NOTES

1. The Fairburn et al. (1991) study used the manual summarized in the present chapter. The Garner et al. (1993) study "generally followed the manual described by Fairburn and Cooper (1989), supplemented by our own adaptation of cognitive-behavioral principles for eating disorders" (Garner et al., 1993, p. 40). The Stanford manual employed by Agras and his colleagues was originally derived from

the Oxford manual (Agras et al., 1989, 1992), as was the manual used by Wilson et al. (1991).

2. The Mitchell et al. (1990) study evaluated an intensive group psychotherapy condition that differed in important ways from CBT as discussed in this chapter. We include it in this analysis because it contained many of the core components of what is now recognized as the standard CBT approach.

3. Because the vast majority of patients with bulimia nervosa are female, we use feminine nouns and pronouns throughout the chapter to refer to such patients.

4. The changes in health care, especially the growth of managed care, are beginning to alter this long-standing practice. If this continues, empirically validated, manual-based treatments such as CBT for bulimia nervosa will be increasingly adopted (Barlow, 1994; Wilson, 1995).

REFERENCES

Agras, W. S. (1993). Short-term psychological treatments for binge eating. In C. G. Fairburn & G. T. Wilson (Eds.), *Binge eating: Nature, assessment and treatment* (pp. 270–286). New York: Guilford Press.

Agras, W. S., Rossiter, E. M., Arnow, B., Schneider, J. A., Telch, C. F., Raeburn, S. D., Bruce, B., Perl, M., & Koran, L. M. (1992). Pharmacologic and cognitive-behavioral treatment for bulimia nervosa: A controlled comparison. *American Journal of Psychiatry, 149*, 82–87.

Agras, W. S., Rossiter, E. M., Arnow, B., Telch, C. F., Raeburn, S. D., Bruce, B., & Koran, L. (1994). One-year follow-up of psychosocial and pharmacologic treatments for bulimia nervosa. *Journal of Clinical Psychiatry, 55*, 179–183.

Agras, W. S., Schneider, J. A., Arnow, B., Raeburn, S. D., & Telch, C. F. (1989). Cognitive-behavioral treatment with and without exposure plus response prevention in the treatment of bulimia nervosa: A reply to Leitenberg and Rosen. *Journal of Consulting and Clinical Psychology, 57*, 778–779.

Bandura, A. (1986). *Social foundations of thought and action: Social cognitive theory.* Englewood Cliffs, NJ: Prentice-Hall.

Barlow, D. H. (1994). Psychological interventions in the era of managed competition. *Clinical Psychology, 1*, 109–122.

Beck, A. T., Rush, A. J., Shaw, B. F., & Emery, G. (1979). *Cognitive therapy of depression.* New York: Guilford Press.

Butler, G. (1989). Phobic disorders. In K. Hawton, P. M. Salkovskis, J. Kirk, & D. M. Clark (Eds.), *Cognitive behavior therapy for psychiatric problems* (pp. 97–128). New York: Oxford University Press.

Carter, F. A., & Bulik, C. M. (1993). Exposure treatments for bulimia nervosa: Procedure, efficacy, and mechanisms. *Advances in Behaviour Research and Therapy, 15*, 1001–1053.

Clark, D. M. (1989). Anxiety states: Panic and generalized anxiety. In K. Hawton, P. M. Salkovskis, J. Kirk, & D. M. Clark (Eds.), *Cognitive behavior therapy for psychiatric*

problems (pp. 52–96). New York: Oxford University Press.

Clark, D. M., Salkovskis, P. M. Hackman, A., Middleton, H., Anastisiades, P., & Gelder, M. (1994). A comparison of cognitive therapy, applied relaxation and imipramine in the treatment of panic disorder. *British Journal of Psychiatry, 6*, 759–769.

Coker, S., Vize, C., Wade, T., & Cooper, P. J. (1993). Patients with bulimia nervosa who fail to engage in cognitive behavior therapy. *International Journal of Eating Disorders, 13*, 35–40.

Cooper, P. J. (1993). *Bulimia nervosa: A guide to recovery.* London: Robinson.

Cooper, P. J., Coker, S., & Fleming, C. (1994). Self-help for bulimia nervosa: A preliminary report. *International Journal of Eating Disorders, 16*, 401–404.

Craighead, L. W., & Agras, W. S. (1991). Mechanisms of action in cognitive-behavioral and pharmacological interventions for obesity and bulimia nervosa. *Journal of Consulting and Clinical Psychology, 59*, 115–125.

Craske, M. G., & Barlow, D. H. (1993). Panic disorder and agoraphobia. In D. H. Barlow (Ed.), *Clinical handbook of psychological disorders* (2nd ed., pp. 1–47). New York: Guilford Press.

Craske, M. G., Barlow, D. H., & O'Leary, T. (1992). *Mastery of your anxiety and worry.* New York: Graywind.

Dawes, R. M., Faust, D., & Meehl, P. E. (1989). Clinical versus actuarial judgment. *Science, 243*, 1668–1674.

Fahy, T. A., & Russell, G. F. M. (1993). Outcome and prognostic variables in bulimia nervosa. *International Journal of Eating Disorders, 14*, 135–146.

Fairburn, C. G. (1981). A cognitive behavioural approach to the management of bulimia. *Psychological Medicine, 11*, 707–711.

Fairburn, C. G. (1985). Cognitive-behavioral treatment for bulimia. In D. M. Garner & P. E. Garfinkel (Eds.), *Handbook of psychotherapy for anorexia nervosa and bulimia* (pp. 160–192). New York: Guilford Press.

Fairburn, C. G. (1993). Interpersonal psychotherapy for bulimia nervosa. In G. R. Klerman & M. M. Weissman (Eds.), *New applications of interpersonal psychotherapy* (pp. 353–378). Washington, DC: American Psychiatric Press.

Fairburn, C. G. (1995). *Overcoming binge eating.* New York: Guilford Press.

Fairburn, C. G., Agras, W. S., & Wilson, G. T. (1992). The research on the treatment of bulimia nervosa: Practical and theoretical implications. In G. H. Anderson & S. H. Kennedy (Eds.), *The biology of feast and famine: Relevance to eating disorders* (pp. 318–340). New York: Academic Press.

Fairburn, C. G., & Cooper, P. J. (1984). The clinical features of bulimia nervosa. *British Journal of Psychiatry, 144*, 238–246.

Fairburn, C. G., & Cooper, P. (1989). Eating disorders. In K. Hawton, P. M. Salkovskis, J. Kirk, & D. M. Clark (Eds.), *Cognitive behavior therapy for psychiatric problems* (pp. 277–314). New York: Oxford University Press.

Fairburn, C. G., & Cooper, Z. (1993). The Eating Disorder Examination. In C. G. Fairburn & G. T. Wilson (Eds.), *Binge eating: Nature, assessment, and treatment* (pp. 317–360). New York: Guilford Press.

Fairburn, C. G., Jones, R., Peveler, R. C., Carr, S. J., Solomon, R. A., O'Connor, M. E., Burton, J., & Hope, R. A. (1991). Three psychological treatments for bulimia nervosa. *Archives of General Psychiatry, 48*, 463–469.

Fairburn, C. G., Jones, R., Peveler, R. C., Hope, R. A., & O'Connor, M. (1993). Psychotherapy and bulimia nervosa: The longer-term effects of interpersonal psychotherapy, behavior therapy and cognitive behavior therapy. *Archives of General Psychiatry, 50,* 419–428.

Fairburn, C. G., Kirk, J., O'Connor, M., & Cooper, P. J. (1986). A comparison of two psychological treatments for bulimia nervosa. *Behaviour Research and Therapy, 24,* 629–643.

Fairburn, C. G., Marcus, M. D., & Wilson, G. T. (1993). Cognitive-behavioral therapy for binge eating and bulimia nervosa: A comprehensive treatment manual. In C. G. Fairburn & G. T. Wilson (Eds.), *Binge eating: Nature, assessment, and treatment* (pp. 361–404). New York: Guilford Press.

Fairburn, C. G., Norman, P. A., Welch, S. L., O'Connor, M. E., Doll, H. A., & Peveler, R. C. (1995). A prospective study of outcome in bulimia nervosa and the long-term effects of three psychological treatments. *Archives of General Psychiatry, 52,* 304–312.

Fennell, M. (1989). Depression. In K. Hawton, P. M. Salkovskis, J. Kirk, & D. M. Clark (Eds.), *Cognitive behaviour therapy for psychitric problems* (pp. 169–234). New York: Oxford University Press.

Fichter, M. M., Leibl, K., Rief, W., Brunner, E., Schmidt-Auberger, S., & Engel, R. R. (1991). Fluoxetine versus placebo: A double-blind study with bulimic inpatients undergoing intensive psychotherapy. *Pharmacopsychiatry, 24,* 1–7.

Garb, H. N. (1994). Judgment research: Implications for clinical practice and testimony in court. *Applied and Preventive Psychology, 3,* 173–184.

Garner, D. M., & Bemis, K. M. (1985). Cognitive therapy for anorexia nervosa. In D. M. Garner & P. E. Garfinkel (Eds.), *Handbook of psychotherapy for anorexia nervosa and bulimia* (pp. 107–146). New York: Guilford Press.

Garner, D. M., & Garfinkel, P. E. (Eds.). (1985). *Handbook of psychotherapy for anorexia nervosa and bulimia.* New York: Guilford Press.

Garner, D. M., Rockert, W., Davis, R., Garner, M. V., Olmsted, M. P., & Eagle, M. (1993). Comparison between cognitive-behavioral and supportive–expressive therapy for bulimia nervosa. *American Journal of Psychiatry, 150,* 37–46.

Guidano, V. F., & Liotti, G. (1983). *Cognitive processes and emotional disorders.* New York: Guilford Press.

Hollon, S. D., & Beck, A. T. (1994). Cognitive and cognitive-behavioral therapies. In S. L. Garfield & A. E. Bergin (Eds.), *Handbook of psychotherapy and behavior change: An empirical analysis* (4th ed., pp. 428–466). New York: Wiley.

Ilardi, S. S., & Craighead, W. E. (1994). The role of nonspecific factors in cognitive-behavior therapy for depression. *Clinical Psychology, 1,* 138–156).

Jansen, A., Broekmate, J., & Heymans, M. (1992). Cue-exposure vs self-control in the treatment of binge eating: A pilot study. *Behaviour Research and Therapy, 30,* 235–241.

Johnson, C., Tobin, D. L., & Dennis, A. (1990). Differences in treatment outcome between borderline and nonborderline bulimics at one-year follow-up. *International Journal of Eating Disorders, 9,* 617–627.

Jones, R., Peveler, R. C., Hope, R. A., & Fairburn, C. G. (1993). Changes during treatment for bulimia nervosa: A comparison of three psychological treatments. *Behaviour Research and Therapy, 31,* 479–485.

Kazdin, A. E., & Wilson, G. T. (1978). *Evaluation of behavior therapy: Issues, evidence, and research strategies.* Cambridge, MA: Ballinger.

Keller, M. B., Herzog, D. B., Lavori, P. W., Bradburn, I. S., & Mahoney, E. M. (1992). The naturalistic history of bulimia nervosa: Extraordinarily high rates of chronicity, relapse, recurrence, and psychosocial morbidity. *International Journal of Eating Disorders, 12,* 1–10.

Kirkley, B. G., Schneider, J. A., Agras, W. S., & Bachman, J. A. (1985). Comparison of two group treatments for bulimia. *Journal of Consulting and Clinical Psychology, 53,* 43–48.

Klerman, G. L., & Weissman, M. M. (Eds.). (1993). *New applications for interpersonal psychotherapy.* Washington, DC: American Psychiatric Press.

Klerman, G. L., Weissman, M. M., Rounsaville, B. J., & Chevron, E. S. (1984). *Interpersonal psychotherapy of depression.* New York: Basic Books.

Laberg, J., Wilson, G. T., Eldredge, K., & Nordby, H. (1991). Effect of mood on heart rate reactivity in bulimia nervosa. *International Journal of Eating Disorders, 10,* 169–178.

Laessle, R. G., Wittchen, H. U., Fichter, M. M., & Pirke, K. M. (1989). The significance of subgroups of bulimia and anorexia nervosa: Lifetime frequency of psychiatric disorders. *International Journal of Eating Disorders, 8,* 569–574.

Lazarus, A. A., & Fay, A. (1982). Resistance or rationalization? A cognitive-behavioral perspective. In P. I. Wachtel (Ed.), *Resistance: Psychodynamic and behavioral approaches.* New York: Plenum Press.

Leitenberg, H. (1994, July). *Cognitive-behavioral treatment of bulimia nervosa.* Keynote address presented at the 17th National Australian Behaviour Modification Conference, Fremantle, Western Australia.

Leitenberg, H., Rosen, J., Gross, J., Nudelman, S., & Vara, L. (1988). Exposure plus response-prevention treatment of bulimia nervosa. *Journal of Consulting and Clinical Psychology, 56,* 535–541.

Leitenberg, H., Rosen, J. C., Wolf, J., Vara, L. S., Detzer, M. J., & Srebnik, D. (1994). Comparison of cognitive-behaviour therapy and desipramine in the treatment of bulimia nervosa. *Behaviour Research and Therapy, 32,* 37–46.

Maddocks, S. E., Kaplan, A. S., Woodside, D. B., Langdon, L., & Piran, N. (1992). Two year follow-up of bulimia nervosa: The importance of abstinence as the criterion of outcome. *International Journal of Eating Disorders, 12,* 133–142.

Marlatt, G. A., & Gordon, J. (Eds.). (1985). *Relapse prevention.* New York: Guilford Press.

Meichenbaum, D. H., & Turk, D. (1988). *Facilitating treatment adherence.* New York: Plenum Press.

Miller, W. R., & Rollnick, S. (1991). *Motivational interviewing.* New York: Guilford Press.

Mitchell, J. E., & deZwaan, M. (1993). Pharmacological treatments of binge eating. In C. G. Fairburn & G. T. Wilson (Eds.), *Binge eating: Nature, assessment, and treatment* (pp. 250–269). New York: Guilford Press.

Mitchell, J. E., Pyle, R. L., Eckert, E. D., Hatsukami, D., Pomeroy, C., & Zimmerman, R. (1990). A comparison study of antidepressants and structured intensive group psychotherapy in the treatment of bulimia nervosa. *Archives of General Psychiatry, 47,* 149–157.

O'Donahue, W., & Szymanski, J. (1994). How to win friends and not influence clients: Popular but problematic ideas that impair treatment decisions. *The Behavior Therapist, 17,* 30–33.

O'Leary, K. D., & Wilson, G. T. (1987). *Behavior therapy: Application and outcome* (2nd ed.). Englewood Cliffs, NJ: Prentice-Hall.

Olmsted, M. P., Davis, R., Garner, D. M., Rockert, W., Irvine, M. J., & Eagle, M. (1991). Efficacy of a brief group psychoeducational intervention for bulimia nervosa. *Behaviour Research and Therapy, 29,* 71–83.

Prochaska, J. O., & DiClemente, C. C. (1986). Toward a comprehensive model of change. In W. R. Miller & N. Heather (Eds.), *Treating addictive behaviors: Processes of change* (pp. 3–27). New York: Plenum Press.

Rosen, J. C., & Leitenberg, H. (1985). Exposure plus response prevention treatment of bulimia. In D. M. Garner & P. E. Garfinkel (Eds.), *Handbook of psychotherapy for anorexia nervosa and bulimia* (pp. 193–209). New York: Guilford Press.

Rossiter, E. M., Agras, W. S., Losch, M., & Telch, C. F. (1988). Dietary restraint of bulimic subjects following cognitive-behavioral or pharmacological treatment. *Behaviour Research and Therapy, 26,* 495–498.

Schwalberg, M. D., Barlow, D. H., Alger, S. A., & Howard, L. J. (1992). A comparison of bulimics, obese binge eaters, social phobics, and individuals with panic disorder on comorbidity across DSM-III-R anxiety disorders. *Journal of Abnormal Psychology, 101,* 675–681.

Tuschen, B., & Bent, H. (1995). Intensive brief inpatient treatment of bulimia nervosa. In K. D. Brownell & C. G. Fairburn (Eds.), *Eating disorders and obesity: A comprehensive handbook* (pp. 354–360). New York: Guilford Press.

Walsh, B. T., Wilson, G. T., Loeb, K. L., Devlin, M. J., Pike, K. M., Roose, S. P., Fleiss, J., & Waternaux, C. (in press). *Medication and psychotherapy in the treatment of bulimia nervosa. American Journal of Psychiatry.*

Wilson, G. T. (1988). Cognitive-behavioral treatment of bulimia nervosa: The role of exposure. In K. M. Pirke, W. Vandereycken, & D. Ploog (Eds.), *The psychobiology of bulimia nervosa* (pp. 137–145). Berlin: Springer-Verlag.

Wilson, G. T. (1993). Assessment of binge eating. In C. G. Fairburn & G. T. Wilson (Eds.), *Binge eating: Nature, assessment, and treatment* (pp. 227–249). New York: Guilford Press.

Wilson, G. T. (1995). Empirically validated treatments as a basis for clinical practice: Problems and prospects. In S. C. Hayes, V. M. Follette, R. M. Dawes, & K. E. Grady (Eds.), *Scientific standards of psychological practice: Issues and recommendations* (pp. 163–196). Reno, NV: Context Press.

Wilson, G. T. (1996a). Manual-based treatments: The clinical application of research findings. *Behaviour Research and Therapy, 34,* 295–315.

Wilson, G. T. (1996b). Treatment of bulimia nervosa: When CBT fails. *Behaviour Research and Therapy, 34,* 197–212.

Wilson, G. T., Eldredge, K. L., Smith, D., & Niles, B. (1991). Cognitive-behavioural treatment with and without response prevention for bulimia. *Behaviour Research and Therapy, 29,* 575–583.

Wilson, G. T., & Fairburn, C. G. (in press). Treatment of eating disorders. In P. E. Nathan & J. M. Gorman (Eds.), *Psychotherapies and drugs that work: A review of the outcome studies.* New York: Oxford University Press.

Wilson, G. T., & Pike, K. M. (1993). Eating disorders. In D. H. Barlow (Ed.), *Clinical handbook of psychological disorders* (2nd ed., pp. 278–317). New York: Guilford Press.

CHAPTER 7

Cognitive-Behavioral Therapy for Anorexia Nervosa

DAVID M. GARNER
KELLY M. VITOUSEK
KATHLEEN M. PIKE

Cognitive-behavioral therapy has established an impressive empirical track record during the past decade in the treatment of bulimia nervosa, and is now considered the treatment of choice for this eating disorder. In contrast, research on the effectiveness of cognitive-behavioral therapy for anorexia nervosa has been conspicuous by its absence. There have been more than 60 follow-up studies of anorexia nervosa published since 1953 (Steinhausen & Glanville, 1983; Steinhausen, Rauss-Mason, & Seidel, 1991), but there are few controlled trials comparing different treatment approaches. This relates in part to practical obstacles in treatment research for this eating disorder. Compared to bulimia nervosa, anorexia nervosa has a lower incidence (Hoek, 1993) and requires a longer duration of treatment; in addition, treatment design is complicated by the need for hospitalization for some patients. Although other reasons for the lack of comparative treatment research are not obvious, they may relate to the widespread view that emaciated anorexic patients often require not only intensive inpatient treatment, but years of complicated outpatient psychotherapy.

There have been several case reports indicating that cognitive-behavioral therapy is effective (Cooper & Fairburn, 1984; Channon, DeSilva, Hemsley, & Perkins, 1989). However, the dearth of controlled treatment research on anorexia nervosa means that support for this approach rests largely on clinical evidence (American Psychiatric Association, 1993; Garner, 1986, 1988, 1992; Garner & Bemis, 1982, 1985; Garner & Friedman, 1994; Garner, Garfinkel, & Bemis, 1982; Garner & Friedman, 1994; Garner & Rosen, 1990, 1994; Hollon & Beck, 1994; Orimoto & Vitousek, 1992; Pike, Loeb, & Vitousek, 1996; Vitousek & Hollon, 1990; Vitousek & Ewald, 1993; Vitousek & Orimoto, 1993). Early conceptualizations of anorexia nervosa from a cognitive perspective were based on clinical literature indicating that abnormal attitudes toward food and weight are common and persistent features in anorexia nervosa, greatly interfering with full recovery from the disorder (Bruch, 1973, 1978; Dally & Gomez, 1979; Gladstone, 1974; Ushakov, 1971). Dally and Gomez (1979) observed that these attitudes "are the most distressing and long lasting features of anorexia nervosa . . . and are likely to continue or to recur in situations of crisis for many years" (pp. 134–135). Theander (1970) reported that virtually none of the patients in his follow-up study were free from "neurotic fixations" on body weight. Our experience is consistent with these earlier observations and led to our original proposal of a cognitive-behavioral therapy for anorexia nervosa (Garner & Bemis, 1982; Garner et al., 1982).

The current chapter is a further refinement of methods previously described. The cognitive procedures we recommend are largely adaptations of those described by Beck and his colleagues (Beck, 1976; Beck, Freeman, & Associates, 1990; Beck, Rush, Shaw, & Emery, 1979); however, other cognitive theorists have also influenced our approach (Ellis, 1962; Goldfried, 1971, 1980; Guidano & Liotti, 1983; Liotti, 1993; Mahoney, 1974; Meichenbaum, 1974; Safran & Segal, 1990; Teasdale & Barnard, 1993). A manual format is adopted in the current chapter to facilitate teaching, clinical training, and controlled research. It divides cognitive-behavioral procedures for anorexia nervosa into three treatment phases, outlining specific interventions at each stage. Specification of the content and structure of interventions has obvious advantages; however, cautions are also in order. Patient and therapist factors may make rigid adherence to the manual unrealistic in many clinical situations. Also, this manual has not been empirically validated, so its utility remains open to question. It is intended to provide a framework within which methods can be tested, adapted, and further developed.

COGNITIVE THERAPY FOR ANOREXIA NERVOSA VERSUS BULIMIA NERVOSA

Anorexia nervosa and bulimia nervosa have many features in common (Garner, Garner, & Rosen, 1993), so it is not surprising that cognitive approaches to therapy for the two disorders overlap to a significant degree. Similar cognitive restructuring approaches are recommended for both disorders to address characteristic attitudes about weight and shape. Education about regular eating patterns, body weight regulation, starvation symptoms, vomiting, and laxative abuse is a strategic element in the treatment of both disorders. Finally, similar behavioral methods are also required, particularly for the binge-eating/purging subgroup of anorexia nervosa patients. Comparing early reports advancing cognitive therapy for anorexia nervosa (Garner & Bemis, 1982; Garner et al., 1982) and for bulimia nervosa (Fairburn, 1981) with later publications indicates a reassuring convergence of cognitive principles for both eating disorders over the last 15 years. Nevertheless, there are differences in the treatment recommendations made for these two eating disorders. As noted by Vitousek (1995), this may partially reflect differences in the personalities, background, and training of the main contributors to the cognitive-behavioral literature for these two eating disorders. However, key distinctions can also be made between these disorders in terms of motivation for treatment and weight gain as a target symptom; both of these require variations in the style, pace, and content of cognitive-behavioral therapy. These contrasts are highlighted below and elaborated further in later sections.

Motivation for Treatment

Enlisting motivation for treatment can be difficult with eating disorder patients with any diagnosis. However, those with anorexia nervosa are particularly reluctant to commit to the main goal of treatment—namely, weight gain. Thus, a key ingredient in the initial phase of treatment for anorexia nervosa is cultivating and sustaining motivation for change. In contrast, bulimia nervosa patients usually accept elimination of binge eating as the primary goal of treatment.

Addressing Weight and Weight Gain in Treatment

The topic of body weight is approached from entirely different perspectives for anorexia nervosa and bulimia nervosa. Fairburn, Marcus, and Wilson (1993) recommend that bulimia nervosa patients "should be told that in most cases treatment has little or no effect on body weight, either during treatment itself or afterwards" (p. 376). Patients who are reluctant to eat meals or snacks due to fear of weight gain, "should be reassured that this rarely occurs . . . [and that they] will discover that they can eat much more than they thought without gaining weight" (p. 378). In anorexia nervosa, this reassurance is not available, since weight gain *is* a major aim of treatment. The significance of this contrast cannot be overemphasized. As noted above, it affects motivation to initiate and then to continue treatment; it also determines the content of sessions early in treatment. Although patients with both of these eating disorders experience a morbid fear of becoming "fat," in the case of anorexia nervosa, this fear must be addressed while the patient is actually becoming "fatter."

In the treatment of bulimia nervosa, weekly weighing is left up to the patient, "in part because sessions can become dominated by the subject of weight at the expense of other more important issues" (Fairburn et al., 1993, p.

372–374). In contrast, with anorexia nervosa, weight and weight gain cannot be sidestepped but must be directly confronted. Weight must be regularly checked by the therapist or another reliable source. As described in later sections on treatment, changes in body weight dramatically affect the interpretation of session content.

Introducing Self-Monitoring

For bulimia nervosa, Fairburn et al. (1993) recommend that self-monitoring be introduced "toward the end of the first session" (p. 370), with the rationale that it is "the cornerstone of treatment and is essential for progress to be made" (p. 371). In anorexia nervosa, the patient may begin treatment with minimal or no interest in "progress," particularly if it means gaining weight. The subgroup of anorexia nervosa patients who engage in binge eating may be less resistant to self-monitoring, but compliance is still affected by the implications for weight change. Fairburn et al. (1993) recommend for bulimia nervosa that it is appropriate for the therapist to react to failure to self-monitor "with some surprise, since not monitoring will effectively sabotage treatment" (p. 372). In contrast, with anorexia nervosa, the therapist should react with shock and surprise if the patient *fails* to sabotage treatment! Anorexia nervosa patients may require the more gradual introduction of self-monitoring as motivation increases. Many patients require "meal planning" because it provides even greater structure around mealtimes (Garner et al., 1982; Garner, Rockert, Olmsted, Johnson, & Coscina, 1985).

Discussing the Cognitive Model

Fairburn et al. (1993) recommend that the first session should include discussion of the rationale underlying the cognitive-behavioral approach to treatment, using a diagram showing the following causal sequence: (1) low self-esteem, (2) extreme concerns about shape and weight, (3) strict dieting, (4) binge eating, and (5) self-induced vomiting. Thus, the self-perpetuating cycle of bingeing and dieting is emphasized with bulimia nervosa patients. It is obvious that this paradigm must be changed for anorexia nervosa patients who do not binge-eat. Moreover, anorexia nervosa patients often report that their "self-esteem" has improved significantly since they have lost weight. The for-

mal discussion of the cognitive model presupposes agreement regarding the targets of treatment—a process that usually evolves more gradually in anorexia nervosa.

Interpersonal Focus in Treatment

Cognitive-behavioral therapy and interpersonal psychotherapy have been developed as distinct forms of treatment for bulimia nervosa; however, both appear to be equally effective for this disorder (Fairburn et al., 1995). Involvement of significant others is recommended for bulimia nervosa; however, few details have been provided regarding the integration of these others into treatment (Fairburn, 1985; Fairburn et al., 1993). The marked social deficits observed in anorexia nervosa, the need to involve the family in many cases, and the longer duration of therapy have formed the basis for the explicit integration of interpersonal themes in early descriptions of cognitive-behavioral therapy for anorexia nervosa (Garner, 1988; Garner & Bemis, 1982, 1985; Garner et al., 1982; Guidano & Liotti, 1983). The rationale for addressing interpersonal processes in cognitive therapy has been well developed in recent years (Beck et al., 1990; Linehan, 1993; Liotti, 1993; Safran & Segal, 1990), and it is our view that this emphasis is particularly relevant to the treatment of anorexia nervosa.

Integration of Family Therapy

Particularly with young anorexia nervosa patients, who require the involvement of the family for practical as well as theoretical reasons, cognitive-behavioral principles must be adapted to include a family therapy format (Garner, 1988; Garner et al., 1982). Many principles articulated by family systems theorists can be understood in cognitive terms and therefore integrated without compromising fidelity to cognitive theory.

Other Content Differences

There are other differences in the content of interventions for anorexia nervosa and bulimia nervosa. With anorexia nervosa, there is a greater need for awareness of the potential medical risks and criteria for hospitalization or partial care. Detailed discussion of the psychobiology of starvation is another point of departure. Setting a session agenda is equally appropriate for both eating disorders; however, the therapist may need to take a more directive role in anorexia nervosa, since patients commonly deflect attention away from ego-syntonic symptoms.

DURATION AND STRUCTURE OF THERAPY

Treatment for anorexia nervosa typically lasts from 1 to 2 years—much longer than the 19 sessions over 20 weeks recommended for bulimia nervosa (Fairburn, 1985; Fairburn et al., 1993). The longer duration of treatment is required in most cases of anorexia nervosa because of the time required to overcome motivational obstacles, achieve appropriate weight gain, and occasionally implement inpatient or partial hospitalization. Therapy for anorexia nervosa is divided into three "phases": (I) building trust and setting treatment parameters; (II) changing beliefs related to food and weight, then broadening the scope of therapy; and (III) preventing relapse and preparing for termination. Sessions are normally scheduled twice a week during Phase I (the first month), weekly during Phase II (1 year), and every other week to monthly during Phase III (6 months). It is often desirable to plan the initial meeting to last from 2 to 3 hours, to allow sufficient time to cover the relevant content and motivational issues.

The structure of individual therapy sessions is similar to that described for bulimia nervosa (Fairburn et al., 1993), but is modified to take into consideration the special needs of the anorexia nervosa patient. For example, as we describe later, the age of the patient and the clinical circumstances determine whether the format of meetings is individual, family, or a mix of family and individual meetings. The session structure can be summarized as follows:

1. The patient's weight is checked and discussed within the context of goals.
2. Potential physical complications are reviewed.
3. The agenda is set within the context of weight and potential complications.
4. Meal planning and self-monitoring are reviewed or modified.
5. Dysfunctional behaviors and schemas are identified and changed.
6. The session is summarized.
7. Homework assignments are specified.

If weight goals are met, then personal and interpersonal issues identified by the patient take priority. If weight goals are *not* met, practical implications are reviewed, motivation is reelicited, and problem solving aimed at meeting weight and eating goals is instituted. Identifying and changing behaviors and schemas occupy the main part of the session. Checking weight and reviewing physical complications becomes unnecessary as the patient's physical condition improves.

The essential content areas for each phase of treatment are summarized in Table 7.1. Although many of these are introduced in Phase I of treatment, in actual practice these issues are revisited periodically throughout the course of therapy.

PHASE I: BUILDING TRUST AND SETTING TREATMENT PARAMETERS

Phase I, which occupies the first month of treatment, consists of eight sessions (two sessions a week). A glance ahead in this manual reveals the disproportionate amount of space devoted to Phase I. Those preferring symmetry might raise questions such as "How can all of this material be covered in a month?" and "why is so much space devoted to this phase?" First, it is crucial to establish the foundations of therapy in Phase I, in order to maximize the probability of even reaching Phase II. A substantial amount of specific information is transmitted in the initial phase of therapy, laying the groundwork for the content and process of therapy. Second, as noted above, therapy is additive: Most of the issues covered in Phase I resurface periodically during the course of treatment. Third, the fact that the course of treatment for anorexia nervosa is typically lengthy, with manifold pathways of change, defies precise delineation of later "stage-specific" techniques along with their timing and variations. Moreover, as therapy progresses, cognitive techniques described for other disorders (e.g., depression and anxiety) become more relevant to the eating disorder patient. These need not be repeated here.

Building a Positive Therapeutic Alliance

Historically, behavioral therapies minimized the specific role of the therapeutic relationship in the process of change; however, cognitive-be-

TABLE 7.1. Major Content Areas for Cognitive Therapy

Phase I

Building a positive therapeutic alliance

Assessing key features of the eating disorder

Providing education about starvation symptoms and other selected topics

Evaluating and treating medical complications

Explaining the multiple functions of anorexic symptomatology

Differentiating the "two tracks" of treatment

Presenting the cognitive rationale for treatment

Giving rationale and advice for restoring normal nutrition and weight

Implementing self-monitoring and meal planning

Prescribing normalized eating patterns

Interrupting bingeing and vomiting

Implementing initial cognitive interventions

Increasing motivation for change

Challenging cultural values regarding weight and shape

Determining optimal level of family involvement

Phase II

Continuing the emphasis on weight gain and normalized eating

Reframing relapses

Identifying dysfunctional thoughts, schemas, and thinking patterns

Developing cognitive restructuring skills

Modifying self-concept

Developing an interpersonal focus in therapy

Involving the family in therapy

Phase III

Summarizing progress

Reviewing fundamentals of continued progress

Summarizing areas of continued vulnerability

Reviewing the warning signs of relapse

Clarifying when to return to treatment

---

havioral therapy has long maintained the need for therapist warmth, accurate empathy, genuineness, trust, and a collaborative relationship (Beck et al., 1979; Goldfried, 1982). Beck et al. (1979, 1990) have focused on the importance of a collaborative approach to therapy, emphasizing the patient's active role in setting treatment goals, establishing session priorities, homework assignments, and gathering data to examine the validity or functionality of beliefs. Nevertheless, critics of early cognitive formulations argued that they lacked a systematic theoretical framework for integrating the therapeutic relationship and technical aspects of treatment (Wachtel, 1982). This has been countered in recent years with refinement of the conceptual framework for considering the patient–therapist rela-tionship in cognitive-behavioral psychotherapy (Jacobson, 1989; Linehan, 1993; Liotti, 1993; Safran & Segal, 1990). Adaptations of cognitive-behavioral therapy to anorexia nervosa have underscored the need for a strong therapeutic alliance as a prerequisite for effective psychotherapy (Garner, 1986, 1988; Garner & Bemis, 1982, 1985; Garner et al., 1982; Guidano & Liotti, 1983). The relevance of the therapeutic relationship is ubiquitous; however, several aspects deserve special emphasis in the treatment of anorexia nervosa.

The Decision to Initiate Treatment

The circumstances surrounding the initiation of treatment for an anorexia nervosa patient differ from those of the more typical psychiatric patient, who readily admits to psychological discomfort. It is not uncommon for an anorexia nervosa patient to seek therapy at the insistence of parents, a spouse, or other mediators, often after months of bitter struggle. The patient arrives for the consultation poised to resist, anticipating the same pressures for change from the therapist. If this is the case, the therapist needs to disaffiliate from the motives of others and redefine the purpose of therapy as the exploration and resolution of issues that are truly relevant to the patient. Therapy is doomed if it is perceived by the patient as simply carrying out the objectives of others for weight gain or the elimination of weight control behaviors. Since cognitive, affective, and behavioral material is largely dependent on self-report data, a strong therapeutic alliance is required to gather the information necessary for treatment.

Overall Quality of the Therapeutic Bond

Surveying the entire psychotherapy literature, Orlinsky, Grawe, and Parks (1994) found the overall quality of the therapeutic bond to be a strong predictor of outcome, and these findings were even more robust when viewed from the patient's perspective. Data in the eating disorder literature on this issue have been scarce, but there is little reason to assume that the association would be different. In a study of bulimia nervosa, Garner, Rockert, et al. (1993) found that patient satisfaction with treatment was positively associated with outcome. Particularly in light of the anorexia nervosa patient's ambivalence about the goals of treatment, it is vital that the therapist be cognizant of the patient's ongoing appraisal of the quality of the relationship. The therapist must strive to convey qualities of appropriate warmth, sensitivity, compassion, genuineness, honesty, flexibility, engagement, acceptance, and positive regard; he or she must also be acutely attuned to how the patient is feeling about treatment progress, and about the therapist's role in this process. The patient's confidence in the therapist's emotional fortitude and technical skills is pivotal in establishing a therapeutic connection.

Instilling Hope

Anorexia nervosa is often a chronic disorder (Theander, 1985) and has the highest mortality rate of any psychiatric disorder (Sullivan, 1995).

Patients may have failed to respond to treatment before, and although it is important for the therapist to provide a realistic appraisal of potential outcome, it is also crucial to convey an honest sense of hope for recovery. Many patients who recover do so after multiple earlier treatment failures. Thus, the premise that change is possible should be presented at the initial assessment and emphasized throughout the course of treatment. Those who are unable to commit to treatment at this time can be assisted in coping with symptoms while remaining optimistic about the prospects for future change.

In-Session Samples of Interpersonal Schemas

Cognitive theorists have been reluctant to acknowledge the idea that a patient's way of construing the therapeutic relationship may be linked to present and past relationships in a way that can be used in cognitive therapy, possibly because this sounds perilously close to the psychodynamic construct of "transference." However, early behavior therapy innovators argued that the patient's behavior in therapy provides useful samples of enduring interpersonal problems (e.g., Goldfried & Davison, 1976). The patient's reaction to the therapist can be regarded as providing important clues about problematic interpersonal styles or schemas. In recent years, cognitive theory has evolved to integrate interpersonal processes into therapy in a way that maintains complete fidelity to the cognitive approach (Beck et al., 1990; Guidano & Liotti, 1983; Jacobson, 1989; Liotti, 1993; Safran & Segal, 1990). In regard to anorexia nervosa, Garner and Bemis (1985) have maintained that "the relationship provides a conduit for examining distortions and misperceptions that the patient applies to her interpersonal world. When the patient's reactions to the therapist are viewed within the context of other current or past relationships, they provide data that may illuminate beliefs, assumptions, and attitudes that are salient for the patient" (p. 111).[1]

Resistance to Change

The concept of "resistance" has been ignored or even rejected by many cognitive-behavioral theorists, with notable exceptions (Beck et al., 1979, 1990; Goldfried, 1982; Guidano & Liotti, 1983; Liotti, 1987; Safran & Segal, 1990; Wachtel, 1982). Clearly, the concept of resistance is germane to the discussion of anorexia nervosa. These patients have been labeled as resistant, stubborn, defiant, and intractable. They can generate "strong feelings of aggression in the therapist" (Selvini Palazzoli, 1978, p. 128) and "intense emotional reactions . . . perhaps the most intense encountered in a therapeutic relationship" (Cohler, 1977, p. 353). Perhaps these reactions have been responsible for the malevolent and punitive forms of treatment occasionally reported (see Garner, 1985, and Goldner, Birmingham, & Smye, Chapter 26, this volume, for reviews). As we have indicated earlier, reluctance to participate in psychotherapy may also be a reflection of more general mistrust in relationships. It is not unusual for patients to have felt inferior, incompetent, and vulnerable to influence in earlier relationships, even though they have responded with compliance and passivity.

It is a common but false assumption that all anorexic patients are distrustful of the therapeutic relationship and unmotivated to change. Most approach the initial consultation aware of their fragile physical and emotional state, as well as the fact that their disorder has deprived them of a "normal" existence. Except for the minority truly paralyzed by prolonged malnutrition, patients are aware of their need for help, but fear that parting with their ego-syntonic symptoms will throw them into an even deeper state of distress and confusion. The decision to commit to treatment often hinges on the patient's evaluation of the therapist's ability to fathom the personal unhappiness signified by the disorder, and to command the resources to traverse the frightening road ahead. As we describe later, establishing a strong therapeutic alliance is a key to motivating patients to confront dreaded eating patterns and weight gain, as well as unnerving emotional and interpersonal predicaments.

The Therapist as Role Model

The impact of the therapist as a role model for problem solving has been long recognized by cognitive therapists (Goldfried, 1971; Mahoney, 1974). Safran and Segal (1990) state that "the basic values and philosophical perspective one has as a therapist are ultimately transmitted to the patient regardless of how much or how little one talks about them in therapy" (p. 224). This concept is supported by a series of critical reviews of research indicating that "clients tend to adopt the personal values of their therapists

during the course of successful psychotherapy" (Beutler, Machado, & Neufeldt, 1994, p. 241). In the treatment of anorexia nervosa, the therapist's beliefs and values regarding such key concepts as perfectionism, competence, competitiveness, self-control, affective expression, and self-acceptance, as well as the specific topics of dieting, obesity, fitness, and physical attractiveness, are of the utmost importance. Obviously, the patient's wholesale adoption of values held by the therapist would be countertherapeutic; however, recognition of the inevitable process of integration needs to be acknowledged in the process of fostering the patient's own identity (Safran & Segal, 1990).

Assessing Key Features of the Eating Disorder

Assessment is certainly not exclusive to the initial sessions; it should be considered integral to the ongoing treatment process. Details of a comprehensive assessment plan have been presented elsewhere (Crowther & Sherwood, Chapter 4, this volume; Garner, 1991, 1995; Garner & Parker, 1993; Vitousek & Hollon, 1990; Williamson, Anderson, & Gleaves, 1996). However, as summarized in Table 7.2, several points need to be underscored in the initial sessions in the treatment of anorexia nervosa.

Ruling Out the Need for Hospitalization or Urgent Care

The topic of hospitalization may need to be addressed at different points throughout treatment. There are several possible reasons for hospitalization: (1) to achieve weight restoration or interrupt steady weight loss in patients who are emaciated and in medical danger; (2) to interrupt bingeing, vomiting, and/or laxative abuse if any of these poses medical risks; (3) to evaluate and treat other potentially serious physical complications; and (4) to manage associated conditions such as severe depression, risk of self-harm, or substance use disorders (see Garner & Needleman, Chapter 5, this volume). It is difficult to determine a precise weight requiring admission, since all of the factors above must be considered. Clearly, a weight corresponding to a body weight 75% of that expected for age and height, or a body mass index (BMI) of 13 or below, is extreme (Fichter, 1995). If hospitalization is required, then reducing resistance to inpatient care is a prime focus in the

TABLE 7.2. Clinical Interview Checklist

1. Demographic features; treatment history; circumstances surrounding the initiation of treatment and the decision to involve the family

2. Current body weight and weight history
   a. Current weight and height
   b. Weight range at current height
      • Highest and lowest weight
      • Highest stable weight prior to disorder onset
      • Chronology of weight changes year by year

3. Weight-controlling behavior (frequency, intensity, duration)
   a. Dieting, fasting
   b. Vomiting
   c. Spitting food
   d. Exercise
   e. Substance misuse to control weight
      • Laxatives
      • Diuretics
      • Emetics
      • Amphetamines
      • Cocaine
      • Alcohol

4. Binge eating and eating behavior
   a. Frequency of binge eating over past 3 months (note fluctuations and longest period of abstinence)
   b. "Binge foods" (foods eaten and those that trigger episodes)
   c. Typical times and settings for binge eating
   d. Mood before, during, and after episodes
   e. Experience of loss of control?
   f. Description of eating
      • Intake when adhering to restrictive dieting
      • Intake when violating restrictive pattern
      • Estimated caloric intake when adhering to restrictive pattern
      • Specific dietary "rules"

5. Attitudes toward weight and shape
   a. Level of disparagement (whole body and specific regions)
   b. Misperceptions of shape
   c. Hypothetical question: "If gaining 5 pounds would eliminate all symptoms, could you tolerate the gain?" What effect would the gain have on mood and self-esteem?
   d. Frequency of weighings, weight preoccupations, intrusive thoughts about weight, response to weighing
   e. Perception of others' attitudes about patient's weight

6. Physical symptoms (see Mitchell, Pomeroy, & Adson, Chapter 21, this volume, for details)

7. Psychological, interpersonal, and familial data
   Cover all standard assessment areas, with particular emphasis on depression, substance use disorders, impulse control, sexual abuse, vocational capacity, and quality of interpersonal and family relationships.

initial sessions. When hospitalization is not medically necessary, it still may be desirable to promote weight gain. On rare occasion, involuntary hospitalization may be required; however, the potentially iatrogenic effects of this scenario must be carefully considered, along with associated moral and ethical dilemmas, which we describe toward the end of this chapter.

Current Body Weight and Weight History

A thorough weight history provides important information regarding the nature and temporal sequence of events in the development of the eating disorder. It is also a relatively nonthreatening area for discussion that allows for the development of rapport. In most cases, it is preferable for the weight history to be elicited in an individual interview, since details related to weight may have highly personal significance to the patient. With a younger patient, it may be desirable to obtain this information in an interview involving both the parents and the patient. Within this context, it is important to be mindful of the fact that weight has probably become an emotionally charged topic within the family.

*Binge Eating, Vomiting, Laxative Abuse, and
Other Weight-Controlling Behaviors*

The observation that binge eating occurs in
about half of all anorexia nervosa patients presenting for treatment led to the original subclassification of a "bulimic subtype" of the disorder (Casper, Eckert, Halmi, Goldberg, &
Davis, 1980; Garfinkel, Moldofsky, & Garner,
1980). Despite the important historical role of
binge eating in describing variants of anorexia
nervosa, it is noteworthy that very little is actually known about the nature, frequency, and significance of this behavior (Garner, 1993; Garner, Garner, & Rosen, 1993). Early reports defined binge eating as recurrent and involving
large amounts of food, as well as the experience
of loss of control (Garfinkel et al., 1980). However, it is important to stress that patients may
purge even after eating a small amount of food
(i.e., an amount that does not meet the technical definition of "a binge"), and these patients
have a presentation similar to that of patients
who engage in binge eating (Favaro & Santonastaso, 1996; Garner, Garner, & Rosen,
1993). Since medical risks, chronicity, emotional disturbance, impulsivity, suicidal risk, and
poor outcome are more closely tied to vomiting
and laxative abuse than to the amount of food
eaten, it has been argued that diagnostic formulations should be based on these potentially
dangerous compensatory behaviors, not on
binge eating (Garner, 1993). Nevertheless,
binge eating is very distressing to patients and
should be one of the targets of cognitive-behavioral interventions.

Thus, assessment should include careful
questioning regarding the duration and frequency of binge eating, vomiting, and laxative
abuse. It should also cover other weight controlling behaviors such as other drug or alcohol
use to control appetite, chewing and spitting
food out before swallowing, prolonged fasting,
and vigorous exercise for the purpose of controlling body weight. Diabetic patients may manipulate insulin levels to control weight and patients taking thyroid replacement may alter
their dosage to control their weight (Garfinkel
& Garner, 1982).

Attitudes toward Weight and Shape

The psychopathology related to weight or shape
has been described in various ways over the
years, including a drive for thinness, fear of fatness, shape and weight dissatisfaction, body size
misperception, body image disturbance, and
fears associated with physical maturity (Garner
& Garfinkel, 1981; Thompson, 1996). Dissatisfaction with overall body shape and disparagement directed toward specific bodily regions are
common in eating disorders and should be a focus of assessment. Some patients may actually
overestimate their body size. Although research
has shown that overestimation is not unique to
eating disorder patients, it may have clinical importance, particularly for emaciated patients. A
crucial psychopathological feature in anorexia
and bulimia nervosa is that patients must be
more than merely dissatisfied with their body;
they rely on weight or shape as the predominant
or even the sole criterion for judging their self-
worth (Garner & Bemis, 1982). It is the magnitude of the overconcern about weight and shape
and the lengths that the individual is willing to go
in the interests of weight control that distinguish
the individual who is merely dissatisfied with
weight and shape from those who meet the criteria for a clinical eating disorder. This information can be obtained from standardized self-report measures as well as structured interview
methods (Williamson et al., 1996).

Personality and Premorbid Functioning

Marked personality changes mimicking primary
personality disorders may actually stem from
prolonged undernutrition. Therefore, the assessment should include a careful evaluation of
premorbid personality features. Patients may
recall being more sociable and confident prior
to the onset of the disorder. As the disorder has
progressed, they may have become more sullen
and isolated from others. Other patients describe a passive, compliant, and reserved premorbid personality style (Rastam, Gilberg, &
Gilberg, 1995).

Premorbid personality disorders, including
affective disorders and Cluster C personality
disorders of the *Diagnostic and Statistical Manual of Mental Disorders*, third edition, revised
(APA, 1987 i.e., avoidant, dependent, obsessive–compulsive, and passive–aggressive) have
been identified as common in anorexia nervosa
(Braun, Sunday, & Halmi, 1994; Halmi et al.,
1991; Toner, Garfinkel, & Garner, 1988). Moreover, certain personality traits have been shown
to persist long after recovery from the eating
disorder. Casper (1990) found that even after
8–10 years of recovery, traits such as risk avoid-

ance, restraint in emotional expression and initiative, and conformity to authority were common. Srinivasagam et al. (1995) reported that perfectionism as well as an obsessive need for symmetry and exactness persisted after long-term recovery from anorexia nervosa.

Formal personality testing may be useful in some cases; however, the confounding of primary and secondary symptoms is a concern (see Crowther & Sherwood, Chapter 4, this volume). When primary personality disturbance is identified, it usually means a longer duration of therapy with a more difficult course. Adaptations are required for patients whose disorder is complicated by substance use problems, physical abuse, or sexual abuse.

Providing Education about Starvation Symptoms and Other Selected Topics

Starvation Symptoms

Eating disorder patients typically fail to interpret their food preoccupations, urges to binge-eat, emotional distress, cognitive impairment, and social withdrawal as secondary to their severe attempts to reduce or control their weight. These symptoms are commonly thought of as specific to eating disorders; however, it is useful for the therapist to reattribute them to dieting or starvation (Garner & Bemis, 1982). The therapist needs to carefully review the array of starvation symptoms identified in a well-known study of the effects of semistarvation on normal volunteers (Keys, Brozek, Henschel, Mickelsen, & Taylor, 1950; Pirke & Ploog, 1987; see Garner, Chapter 8, this volume and Table 7.3). The description of the "starvation state" as normal physiological consequences of weight suppression can mitigate guilt or defensiveness about what may have been perceived as "primary psychopathology." It also introduces the notion that the current starved state seriously impedes the assessment of personality. This implies that biological equilibrium must be restored if fundamental emotional problems are to be changed. Trying to make meaningful psychological changes with an anorexic patient in this starved state is analogous to trying to address underlying issues with an alcoholic patient who is intoxicated. This concept must be presented sensitively, to avoid minimizing the patient's current experiences or suggesting that the distortions imposed by starvation are the only symptoms warranting treatment.

TABLE 7.3. Effects of Starvation

Attitudes and behavior toward food
    Food preoccupation
    Collection of recipes, cookbooks, and menus
    Unusual eating habits
    Increased consumption of coffee, tea, and spices
    Gum chewing
    Binge eating

Emotional and social changes
    Depression
    Anxiety
    Irritability, anger
    Lability
    "Psychotic" episodes
    Personality changes on psychological tests
    Decreased self-esteem
    Social withdrawal

Cognitive changes
    Decreased concentration
    Poor judgment
    Apathy

Physical changes
    Sleep disturbances
    Weakness
    Gastrointestinal disturbances
    Hypersensitivity to noise and light
    Edema (water retention, particularly in ankles)
    Hypothermia and feeling cold
    Paresthesia
    Decreased metabolic rate
    Decreased sexual interest
    Dry skin
    Hair loss
    Lanugo (fine, soft hair on face and elsewhere)

Note. Symptoms are from Keys, Brozek, Henschel, Mickelsen, and Taylor (1950).

Effects of Dieting on Binge Eating

Patients should also be educated about the effects of dieting on the tendency to engage in binge eating (Polivy & Herman, 1985; Garner et al., 1985; see Garner, Chapter 8, this volume). If this symptom is not part of the clinical presentation, the rationale for pursuing treatment should be bolstered by the fact that this ego-dystonic symptom develops in a significant minority of "pure restricting" patients. Hsu (1988) indicated that restricting anorexics develop bulimia about twice as often as bulimic anorexics move to a restricting subtype. Kreipe, Churchill, and Strauss (1989) reported that although only 6 of 49 adolescent anorexia nervosa patients (13%) had a history of binge eating before hospitalization, 22 (45%) initiated the symptom during the mean 6.5-year follow-up period. Diminishing the probability of binge eating developing is one aim of treatment.

Ineffectiveness of Dieting

Long-term follow-up studies of obesity treatment consistently indicate that 90–95% of those who lose weight will regain it within several years (see Garner & Wooley, 1991). It is no longer a mystery why diets have such a poor long-term record of success. The failure of traditional dietary treatments is rooted in biology: Body weight tends to be "defended," in that weight loss leads to metabolic adaptations designed to return body weight to the level normally maintained (Keesey, 1993). This pattern of findings led Brownell (1982) to conclude that if "cure from obesity is defined as reduction to ideal weight and maintenance of that weight for 5 years, a person is more likely to recover from most forms of cancer than from obesity" (p. 820). The relevance of these studies for anorexia nervosa is that "set point" for body weight is a relentless adversary in the battle to lose weight. Patients cannot expect to relax their guard permanently and ever really adjust to a lower weight. Overriding the set-point mechanism can only be done at great personal sacrifice, in the face of constant biological pressure to return to higher body weight levels.

The Self-Perpetuating Cycle of Binge Eating and Vomiting

Self-induced vomiting and laxative abuse usually begin as methods of preventing weight gain by "undoing" the caloric effects of normal eating or binge eating. It becomes self-perpetuating because it allows the patient to acquiesce to the urge to eat, but eliminates the feedback loop that would stem underlying hunger and food cravings. This is a paradox, since the strategy that begins as a means of establishing or regaining "control" typically escalates into chaotic eating patterns, with the patient experiencing a complete breakdown of control. For some patients, vomiting occurs after eating even small amounts of food and is not associated with loss of control over eating (Garner, Garner, & Rosen, 1993).

Laxative Abuse

Laxative abuse is dangerous because it contributes to electrolyte imbalance and other physical complications. Perhaps the most compelling argument for discontinuing the use of laxatives is that they are an ineffective method of trying to prevent the absorption of calories. Laxatives primarily affect the emptying of the large intestine, which occurs after calories have already been absorbed in the small bowel (BoLynn, Santa-Ana, Morawski, & Fordtran, 1983). Once patients learn that laxatives cause wide swings in weight because of changes in water balance, but do not cause malabsorption, they usually agree to immediate or gradual discontinuation (Garner, Chapter 8, this volume; Garner et al., 1985).

Anorexia Nervosa as a Disorder

Finally, attention should be given to clarifying myths resulting from inaccurate or conflicting reports regarding the etiology and complications of the disorder. Patients should be aware of the likely time and course of treatment; the high mortality rates (Sullivan, 1995; Theander, 1985); the poor long-term outcome associated with minimal treatment (Theander, 1985); the common residual psychosocial symptoms (Casper, 1990; Stonehill & Crisp, 1977), starvation symptoms (Garner, Chapter 8, this volume), and medical complications, (Mitchell, Pomeroy, & Adson, Chapter 21, this volume; Sharp & Freeman, 1993); and the more optimistic prospects associated with adequate treatment (Crisp, Callender, Halek, & Hsu, 1992; Hsu, Crisp, & Callender, 1992; Steinhausen et al., 1991). Some patients find it useful to review the "evidence" in the form of written educational material as an adjunct to therapy (Garner, Chapter 8, this volume). If the patient has not previously received a formal diagnosis, giving the disorder a name may be useful. Confirming the presence of such a serious disorder sets the stage for formal agreement to treatment.

Evaluating and Treating Medical Complications

Anorexia nervosa patients should have a medical evaluation to determine overall physical status and to identify or rule out physical complications associated with starvation and certain extreme weight loss behaviors (Comerci, 1990; Mitchell, 1986; Mitchell et al., Chapter 21, this volume; Sharp & Freeman, 1993). Occasionally, a medical evaluation will reveal that weight loss has been precipitated by an underlying physical disorder (Comerci, 1990). As stressed above, patients should be made aware of the serious physical complications associated with starvation, self-induced vomiting, and purgative abuse. These include electrolyte disturbances, general fatigue, muscle weakness, cramping, edema, constipation, cardiac arrhythmias, paresthesia, kidney disturbances, swollen salivary glands, dental deterioration, finger clubbing, dehydration, bone demineralization, and cerebral atrophy (Mitchell et al., Chapter 21, this volume). Strategic review of these complications, with an emphasis on their being inherent to the eating disorder, can be helpful in enlisting motivation for change. In all cases, arrangements should be made for a medical consultation with a physician who is knowledgeable about the medical risks and complications associated with anorexia nervosa.

Explaining the Multiple Functions of Symptomatology

After the careful gathering of background data, it is often useful to present the patient with a conceptual framework of the multilevel adaptive functions served by anorexia nervosa. This begins with a functional analysis of specific positive and negative reinforcement contingencies that probably play a role in maintaining the eating disorder.

Negative Reinforcement

The principle of negative reinforcement, through not cast in explicitly behavioral terms, has been a central explanatory principle in one of the most influential theories of the etiology of anorexia nervosa (Crisp, 1970, 1980; see Crisp, Chapter 13, this volume). According to Crisp and colleagues, anorexia nervosa is best viewed as a "weight phobia" or "fat phobia," because its development and maintenance conform to an avoidance- or escape-learning paradigm. Dieting and weight loss are maintained by negative reinforcement (i.e., the offset of aversive stimuli) by allowing the avoidance (or reversal) of a prepubertal shape—the harbinger

of overwhelming psychosexual challenges and conflicts. Other theories evoke an avoidance paradigm in accounting for anorexia nervosa as a retreat from fears associated with sexuality, high performance expectations, separation from the family, and family conflicts, though again this paradigm is not framed in behavioral terms.

Once avoidance learning is acquired, its durability hinges on the fact that behavioral patterns are established that insulate against recognizing when aversive contingencies are no longer operative. Cognitive variables may contribute to this process. Beck (1976) has observed that avoidance behavior may be perpetuated by "hyperactive" cognitive sets, which eventually operate in an autonomous fashion. An idiosyncratic belief system develops, propelled by internal avoidance contingencies, acting as a Procrustean mold that incoming information is shaped to fit. Over time, anticipated exposure to feared stimuli, such as certain foods or a higher weight on the scale, creates such anxiety that rigid rules are adopted to guard against encountering the feared consequences. The dread leads to rules or biases erring in the direction of safety, involving gradual exclusion of feared foods and setting of lower weight limits.

An aspect of the anorexic's avoidance behavior that appears to be unique to the disorder is that the patient cannot really place much distance between herself and the "phobic object," since the feared stimulus is *herself* at higher weight levels (Garner & Bemis, 1982). Since total escape from the aversive stimulus is impossible, it may be controlled only through constant vigilance. Unlike patients with other disorders in which avoidance plays a major role, the anorexia nervosa patient may not want to be relieved of anxiety about food and weight gain. These aversive experiences are functional, in that they assist the patient in the difficult task of oral self-restraint, despite voracious hunger (Garner & Bemis, 1982).

Positive Reinforcement

In addition to being motivated by a "phobic fear of fatness," anorexia nervosa patients are driven by positive reinforcement—that is, the sense of triumph, mastery, self-control, and superiority they feel at successful weight loss (Garner & Bemis, 1982). Bemis (1983) noted this feature as widespread in early clinical accounts of patients as "exhilarated," "elated," "delighted," "triumphant," "powerful," and "proud"; weight loss is viewed as an "accomplishment," "achievement," "virtue," "source of positive pleasure," and "sensuous delight." Selvini Palazzoli's (1978) description captures the allure of self-reinforcement derived from the success in resisting corporal needs: "every victory over the flesh is a sign of greater control over one's biological impulses . . . [and a] magic key to power . . . [in the search for] freedom, beauty, intelligence and morality" (pp. 72–74). The fact that most patients extol the virtues of their pathological state, actively pursuing ego-syntonic symptoms, distinguishes anorexia nervosa from a simple "weight phobia." A claustrophobic patient typically panics in closed spaces, but does not typically report euphoria or a sense of power in a open field.

In the early stages of the disorder, there also may be considerable social reinforcement for initial weight loss and the self-control required in adherence to a diet. It is not difficult to understand why an adolescent female, struggling with extreme feelings of ineffectiveness, might embrace the idea that a thinner shape could enhance her value. As indicated earlier, the resounding media message is that ultra-thinness is a sign of beauty, success, self-control, and social competence. The weight loss industry and the folk culture surrounding dieting provide the remedies. Positive social reinforcement may take other forms. Initial weight loss may win parental concern or attention. It is not uncommon for patients to strive for and then cling to an "anorexic identity" because of its associations with celebrity status and socially desirable traits. However, social reinforcement fails to account adequately for the development of anorexia nervosa, since the emaciated state achieved by most patients is beyond the societal standards for shape. Once the disorder is initiated, it is the cognitive self-reinforcement that becomes a key factor in regulating it.

The Adaptive Functions of Anorexia Nervosa

It is often useful to provide the patient with a tentative and more abstract formulation of the personal "meaning" of the disorder, making it clear that it is usually much more than dieting that has spiraled out of control. If the patient describes specific premorbid fears and conflicts at this point, then these can be integrated into

the tentative understanding of the functions of symptoms. If specific fears are denied, then it is possible to present a "generic" and "hypothetical" scenario, with the suggestion that the functional nature of the disorder often becomes clearer during the course of recovery. This approach avoids direct confrontation and resulting defensiveness, but at the same time informs the patient of the therapist's commitment to addressing fears exposed during the process of recovery. Our approach has been to illustrate the multilevel adaptive functions of symptoms with an adaptation of Crisp's (1980) well-known diagram (Garner & Bemis, 1985). Figure 7.1 can be used (1) to underscore the concurrent physiological and psychological adaptation occurring with weight loss; (2) to illustrate the range of potential adaptive functions; (3) to explain how and why the adaptation may lead to resistance to change at particular points in the recovery process, highlighting the rationale for the therapist's commitment to helping the patient deal with the psychological distress that may follow weight restoration; and (4) to imply that recovery and maintenance of a suboptimal (submenstrual) weight are mutually exclusive events. Thus, weight gain and changed eating behaviors are placed within the context of achieving other personal goals, such as contentment, happiness, competence, and interpersonal skills. The following therapist monologue illustrates the key points:

This is a diagram illustrating your weight history and the way that anorexia nervosa can change life to resolve certain problems, but, unfortunately, at great personal cost. The problems solved aren't the same for everyone, and later we will want to understand the details of this process as it has applied to you. This is the natural process of weight gain into adolescence (*the therapist points to A on the diagram*). In addition to the obvious physical changes that occur as a girl enters into puberty, research has shown that there are important changes in thinking and overall experience that occur with menarche (*pointing to B*) and puberty. Entering adolescence can produce new challenges and problems. It is not uncommon for young women to feel insecure or distressed during this time (*pointing to C*) and to decide that dieting and weight loss might be a solution. Weight loss of the magnitude seen in anorexia nervosa causes changes in physical appearance, hormonal function-

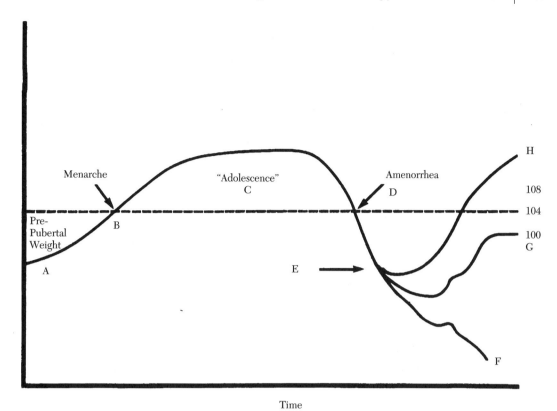

FIGURE 7.1. The weight course in anorexia nervosa. The dotted line represents the "menstrual weight threshold," which is approximately 47 kg (104 pounds) for a woman 163 cm (5′4″) tall (Frisch, 1983). A represents the natural process of weight gain into adolescence; B indicates the menarche; C represents normal adolescence; D indicates the menstrual weight threshold; E represents further weight loss; F indicates still further weight loss and possible death; G represents a pseudorecovery; and H represents full recovery. The two arrows at E and D represent weights at which anorexic patients typically express panic: at the initiation of weight gain and when they approach the "menstrual threshold." Adapted from Crisp (1980, p. 143). Copyright 1980 by Grune & Stratton. Adapted by permission.

ing, and general experience that turn back the developmental clock in some ways. Discomfort and conflicts associated with the move to adulthood no longer seem relevant and are replaced by feelings of control and confidence. [The therapist then elaborates on the specific positive and negative reinforcement contingencies that seem at this point to be relevant to this particular patient.] Amenorrhea develops (*pointing to D*), and this is a biological watershed—it means that you are now becoming more like you were back at A, in terms of shape, hormones, and perhaps even thinking, than you were at C. Thus, achieving a subpubertal weight and shape appear to "resolve" a host of potential developmental concerns. Further weight loss (*pointing to E*) becomes

like "money in the bank," keeping you at a distance from the shape and the experiences that have had negative associations, and maybe even allaying certain unexpressed fears in parents (*pointing to C*). From this point on, the course of the disorder becomes variable: Some do poorly (*pointing to F*); others try to walk the biological tightrope (*pointing to G*), never really resuming biological and psychological maturity [here the therapist elaborates on the biological significance of normal menstrual functioning, if necessary]; and others recover (*pointing to H*). Recovery does not mean simply gaining weight. It requires addressing the issues at C that may have made weight loss, with its "biopsychosocial regression" to A, attractive. If you were to become involved in therapy, these issues at C, if they indeed exist [since some patients deny problems at this juncture], will become an important focus of treatment. Thus, you can see why weight gain is necessary, but clearly not the only concern. You will need guidance to address other important issues that may be uncovered along the way.

Many patients readily appreciate this interpretation of their disorder as having psychological and developmental meaning. Although the foregoing monologue is based on Crisp's (1970) "phobic" response to perceived demands of adulthood and its consequent reversal of the normal hormonal substrate, it is remarkably similar to the observations of others arguing from very different theoretical perspectives.[2] Some patients are immediately able to recognize that there is a particular weight they fear most, and that this translates into a weight threshold for the return of the menses and associated normalization of hypothalamic–pituitary functioning. They sometimes seize this opportunity to elaborate upon fears of "growing up"; however, it must be cautioned that this theme is only relevant to a subset of patients and disregards the powerful influence of positively reinforcing aspects of anorexic symptomatology, described earlier.

At this point, the patient needs to acknowledge in general terms that "recovery" from the eating disorder is the goal. Typically the devil is in the details, but it is essential to establish that "recovery" is the theoretically desired outcome, even though any decision is tentative and experimental at this point. The "goal" of treatment is defined in general and nonthreatening terms at this juncture, with the understanding that it will be revisited in greater detail once there has been some change in body weight, eating behavior, and other symptoms. The following dialogue illustrates the first step in this process:

THERAPIST. Let's talk about some specific goals for treatment. At this point, what kind of problems, other than eating and weight, do you think are at the heart of the problem?

PATIENT. I feel disgusted about feeling fat.

THERAPIST. Tell me more. What does being fat mean to you?

PATIENT. It means I am a slob. I don't feel confident. I do not like myself very much.

THERAPIST. So you don't feel confident except when you are in control of your weight?

PATIENT. Yes.

THERAPIST. If treatment is to make any sense, priority must be given to help you find other ways to feel confident, other than weight control. This is important—let me write this goal down. What about other goals? What about relationships with your family?

PATIENT. My family is fine. The problem is me.

THERAPIST. OK, but if we should find later that you have concerns about your family, or if there are other issues that we need to address, we will add them to the list then.

The therapist purposely stops at this general goal, rather than pressing for a clearer operational definition of the patient's negative feelings. Clarification will be pursued in subsequent meetings; the purpose here is to establish that this non-weight-related subject domain will be a priority in therapy, and that other similar issues, including emergent family concerns, can be added later.

Differentiating the "Two Tracks" of Treatment

The content of therapy may be divided into "two tracks" (Garner, 1986). The first track pertains to issues related to weight, bingeing, vomiting, strenuous dieting, and other behaviors aimed at weight control. The second relates to psychological themes such as self-esteem, self-concept, self-control, perfectionism, impulse regulation, affective expression, family conflicts, and interpersonal functioning. Both tracks are characterized by reasoning errors, dysfunctional thinking, and distorted underlying assumptions. In practice, there is considerable switching back and forth between these content areas in therapy. Greater emphasis is placed on the first track early in therapy, emphasizing the interdependence between mental and physical function. Treatment gradually shifts to second-track issues as progress is made in the areas of eating behavior and weight. However, patients typically begin therapy more motivated to address second-track issues (at least in abstract terms) while avoiding symptoms related to eating and weight. The patient needs to be provided with the rationale that starvation symptoms and chaotic eating have such a great impact on psychological functioning that a certain amount of progress must be made on the first track in order even to understand, let alone make progress on, the second. With some patients, progress on the first track is driven by an implicit contingency system: Attention to the second track is contingent on the first.

Presenting the Cognitive Rationale for Treatment

The main principles of cognitive therapy govern the conduct and content of therapy from the beginning: (1) primary reliance on conscious experience rather than unconscious motivation; (2) explicit emphasis on beliefs, assumptions, schematic processing, and meaning systems as mediating variables accounting for maladaptive behaviors and emotions; (3) use of questioning as a major therapeutic device; (4) active and directive involvement on the part of the therapist; and (5) emphasis on work outside of the session as a means for exploring beliefs and patterns of thinking (Beck, 1976; Beck et al., 1979).

Discussion of the cognitive-behavioral model of treatment in anorexia nervosa must be tailored to fit the current motivation of the patient. In contrast to bulimia nervosa (where symptoms are usually more distressing to the patient), at this stage in the treatment of anorexia nervosa it is advisable to resist "teaching" the cognitive model or prematurely introducing techniques for identifying and correcting "dysfunctional beliefs." Patients are reticent to accept a model for belief change if they prefer their ego-syntonic symptoms and are not committed to treatment. It is advisable for cognitive-behavioral principles to unfold gradually in the initial phase of treatment. Education is the first "cognitive" procedure, since it is explicitly aimed at changing beliefs through new or corrective information. Another way to present the cognitive model early in therapy is by example. The therapist can use the language of cognitive therapy by emphasizing the importance of beliefs and assumptions in determining behavior. However, at this stage (as described in the earlier section on the multiple functions of anorexic symptomatology), the focus is on identifying the wider schematic context for the disorder, including its personal meaning for the individual. The initial rather oblique presentation of cognitive principles becomes more focused later, when automatic thoughts and cognitive restructuring are discussed. As we describe later, it is also guided by procedures aimed at cognitive change at the higher-order or generic schematic level (Teasdale & Barnard, 1993), intended to produce "downstream" changes in subsidiary beliefs and attitudes.

Giving a Rationale and Advice for Restoring Normal Nutrition and Body Weight

The formulation of goals related to body weight, eating behavior, and symptomatic control is dependent on the patient's current level of motivation. If delineating concrete weight goals is beyond the patient's level of commitment or tolerance for change, then attention needs to shift to increasing motivation for change, as described later. In the absence of a formal agreement to change the eating disorder symptoms, it is still possible to proceed with "experiments" aimed at stabilizing body weight; normalizing eating; and controlling bingeing, vomiting, and laxative abuse.

Explaining the Need to Assess Body Weight

A patient may arrive for the first interview determined to resist having her weight checked. At some point, once rapport has been established, it is desirable to obtain the patient's current weight in normal street clothing. This should be done in a sensitive but straightforward manner. If the patient resists stepping on the scale, it should be emphasized that there are several reasons why it is countertherapeutic, if not irresponsible, to ignore monitoring body weight in anorexia nervosa. First, monitoring weight emphasizes the interdependence between psychological and physical issues. Second, in the same way that it is inappropriate to ignore a suicidal patient's self-harm, it is inadvisable to disregard weight in anorexia nervosa. Third, even if a patient's weight is not dangerously low, weight changes are critical in evaluating cognitive processes. For example, the meaning and the approach taken in a particular session may be entirely different for the patient who reports improved mood and successful completion of all homework assignments, but has lost 2 pounds in the past week, in contrast to the same report within the context of gaining 2 pounds. Fourth, the therapist's assumption of responsibility for regularly monitoring weight may interrupt a patient's inappropriate patterns of self-assessment. Some patients obsessively weigh themselves many times throughout the day, while others avoid the scales altogether. Patients who protest that they do not want to know their weight may choose initially to stand backward on the scale. A matter-of-fact explanation in the initial session of the need to monitor weight carefully is usually sufficient to overcome resistance to subsequent regular weighing. Some clinicians prefer having the patient's weight checked by a family doctor, nurse, or other medical practitioner. However, not weighing the patient represents a missed opportunity, since the act of being weighed often generates valuable in-session cognitive, affective, and behavioral data. Body weight should be taken at each session as described earlier in the section on assessment, and it should be recorded on a body weight graph.

Determining Minimal Body Weight Threshold

Patients need to be told that *outpatient treatment can only proceed if their weight does not fall below a certain minimum* (Garner et al., 1982). If a patient is near this minimum at the initial meetings, then this weight needs to be clearly stipulated. However, there are no absolute rules regarding this minimum, since it depends on a patient's overall health, the presence of complications, and the patient's ability to make progress in outpatient treatment. If the patient's weight falls below the established minimum, other, more structured alternatives (e.g., partial or inpatient hospitalization) must be available, and the focus of therapy shifts to convincing the patient that these options are necessary. The point here is that the "minimum weight" should not become the subject of weekly renegotiation, with the therapist retreating to progressively lower standards. If weight has been stable, with no other indications for immediate hospitalization, then it is usually not necessary to specify a *specific* minimum weight for the patient at this time, since there is a risk that stipulating such a weight may be misinterpreted as an invitation to gravitate toward this new "safe weight threshold."

Setting a Target Body Weight Range

Setting a target weight range as a goal in the initial meeting(s) is dependent on the patient's current level of motivation and commitment to treatment. If the patient has no intention of gaining weight, establishing an explicit weight goal may be counterproductive. Nevertheless, the patient needs to understand the enormous biological significance of reaching a certain minimal body weight threshold (D on Figure 7.1), and to realize that the achievement of this weight status is essential to recovery. There are individual differences in this threshold; however, it generally corresponds to approximately 90% of expected weight for postmenarcheal women and elicits resumption of normal hormonal functioning and menstruation (Figure 7.1). The minimal weight necessary for a particular height for the restoration of menstrual cycles was proposed by Frisch and McArthur (1974) to be equivalent to about 22% body fat, or about 102 pounds (46.3 kg) for a 20-year-old woman who is 5'3" (160 cm) tall. Renutrition and normalization of body weight tend to result in return of normal menstrual function in anorexia nervosa (Katz, Boyar, Roffwarg, Hellman, & Weiner, 1977; Treasure, Wheeler, King, Gordon, & Russell, 1988). This argument for assuming a "normal" body weight may not be persuasive for some patients. However, the link among undernutrition, amenorrhea, and bone demineralization in anorexia nervosa patients (Bachrach, Guido, Katzman, Litt, & Marcus, 1990; Biller et al., 1989; Siemers, Chakmakjian, & Gench, 1996) and athletes (Ramos & Warren, 1995), as well as certain other biological sequelae (e.g., cerebral atrophy on computed tomography scan), generally elicit greater concern (Garner, Chapter 8, this volume).

A weight "range" of 3–5 pounds above this threshold has been recommended, because it accounts for normal weight fluctuations (Garner et al., 1982). It should be explained that this weight is a bit too high for some women and too low for others, but is a good initial estimate. Return to premorbid weight, rather than to a population average "normal" weight based on a normal BMI, has been found to be a better predictor of return of normal reproductive function in anorexia nervosa (Treasure et al., 1988) and bulimia nervosa (Devlin et al., 1989; Weltzin, Cameron, Berga, & Kaye, 1994). This concept is alarming for patients with a higher premorbid body weight. In these cases, the point should not be pressed at this stage of treatment, since it is theoretical and may not apply to an individual case.

Because body weight is influenced at least in part by constitutional factors, it is as much of an abuse of aggregate statistics to infer individual expected weight from weight norms as it would be to derive expected height from tables of norms for height. Timing and sensitivity are essential in relating this information to patients: Prematurely recommending a higher weight that is terrifying may drive a patient from treatment, whereas avoiding the topic entirely fails to address a primary treatment issue and is likely to lead to a therapeutic impasse.

Introducing the Experimental Model of Change

The therapist should emphasize that therapy will adhere to an "experimental" model, with each step carefully planned to gather and evaluate evidence before the therapist and patient decide to proceed to the next step. Reluctance to participate in therapy can be fueled by the mistaken assumption that the decision to gain even minimal weight will lead to an almost magical and irreversible commitment to recovery (Garner & Bemis, 1982). This belief is tied to the notion that the current system is precarious and that relaxing controls will lead to a complete breakdown of control.

Gaining a small amount of weight is proposed as part of an "experiment" rather than as a commitment to recovery. It will provide an opportunity to test the implications of beliefs about the impact of weight gain on experience, and the patient can, at least hypothetically, return to the lower weight if dissatisfied with the outcome of the experiment (Garner et al., 1982). Some patients indicate that they might consider a more structured hospital or partial program for renutrition, except that they feel they really do not require this type of intervention, since they believe that they can gradually gain weight on their own as outpatients. This may be true in some cases, but it is unrealistic in others. It may be useful to propose an "experiment" whereby these patients agree to gain 1–2 pounds a week for the next 2 weeks, to determine whether they are really "in control" of their weight. Typically, patients are unable to force their weight up even as a temporary measure to avoid hospitalization, and this serves as a poignant illustration of the fact that they are really "out of control" and require the added structure of partial or full hospitalization as the next step on the road to recovery.

Implementing Meal Planning

Patients who require more structure in complying with advice about normalizing their eating patterns may benefit from meal planning in contrast to self-monitoring, which is typically described for bulimia nervosa (Garner et al., 1982, 1985). Meal planning involves specifying the details of eating in advance. As described below, it includes prescribing the precise foods to be consumed and their amounts, as well as the eating context, such as place and time. It is highly recommended that the task of meal planning occur as part of therapy, rather than being necessarily relegated to a dietitian or nutritionist. Meal planning and elements of prescribing normalized eating are not only aimed at renutrition, but also at probing motivation and illuminating beliefs, which then become targets for cognitive interventions. The beginning of each session is devoted to evaluating the patient's ability to conform to the meal plan, as well as beliefs interfering with compliance. Some patients require an even more gradual approach to changing eating behavior and underlying beliefs. In these cases, meal planning can be conducted without written records, yet can still provide sufficient detail to allow meticulous exploration of beliefs and attitudes (Garner et al., 1982). The structure imposed by meal planning allows most patients to depart from their rigid rules about food with the security that they will not be allowed to go too far in the direction of overeating or undereating. This structure may also facilitate the identification of recurrent situations or emotions that lead to disturbed eating patterns.

Prescribing Eating Patterns

Again, securing agreement on goals related to changing eating patterns relates to motivation. Some patients will be unable to agree to making changes at the initial meetings; most will express willingness in principle, but will need encouragement, corrective feedback, and education for many months. Other patients will be ready to take action immediately.

Eating Mechanically

Eating should be done "mechanically" according to set times and a predetermined plan. In most cases, this involves completing a detailed written meal plan in the treatment session, specifying the precise foods to be consumed, their amounts, and the context, which should include when and where food is eaten. Figure 7.2 is an example of a completed meal plan form for 1 day. It includes the approximate caloric value for foods, which may be useful in allaying fears of overeating expressed by some patients, but may be unnecessary or even counterproductive for others.

Food should be thought of as "medication" prescribed to "inoculate" the patient against future extreme food cravings and the tendency to engage in binge eating (Garner et al., 1982). Temporarily taking the decision making out of eating is necessary early in treatment, when pa-

tients are particularly susceptible to becoming overwhelmed by anxiety and guilt in problematic eating situations. Deviations from the eating plan, whether undereating or overeating, should be discouraged equally. Mechanical eating minimizes the sense of virtue for not eating and guilt for giving in to the urge to eat. Patients need to accept that, at least for the present, they cannot permit their eating behavior to be determined by urges and transient shifts in thinking. New, "nonanorexic" rules for dietary intake need to be followed until regulation of eating can be more naturally determined by internal signals. Promoting mechanical eating appears to conflict with the therapeutic goal

Self-Monitoring & Meal Planning Form

Name: _____ Date: _____

Time/ Place	Food and Liquid Consumed	B	V	Thinking, Feeling and Interpersonal Context
9:00 Home	1 bagel (160) 1 oz. cream cheese (100) 1 banana (100) 1 cup plain tea (0)			
12:00 Work	1 tuna salad sandwich (400) [½ cup tuna (175) 2 slices wheat bread (130) 1 tbsp. mayo (100)]			
6:00 Home	Pasta (1 cup spaghetti with tomato sauce and cheese) (260) Salad (100) 1 tbsp. Ranch dressing (85) 1 hard roll (150) 1 tbsp. margarine (35)			
8:00 Home	2 small cookies (130) 1 glass (8oz) lowfat 1% milk (100)			
	Total = 2025			

FIGURE 7.2. Example of a completed self-monitoring and meal-planning form.

of fostering trust in internal sensations; however, it takes months and sometimes years for normal appetite to return. It is often helpful to use the analogy that mechanical eating is like a splint for a broken bone: Rigid structure is needed temporarily during the healing process.

Spacing Eating

Most eating disorder patients try to "save" calories for later in the day or hope that they may be able to avoid eating altogether. However, mounting hunger during the day can lead to binge eating in the evening. This oscillation between starving and overconsumption can ultimately lead to patients' establishing a higher body weight than they would without any dieting whatsoever. It is important for meals to be spaced throughout the day (Garner et al., 1985). Breakfast should never be omitted, and it is ideal for there to be three meals and one or two snacks spread throughout the day. It is also best to confine eating to set times on the clock, rather than relying on internal sensations in determining when to eat (Figure 7.2). The rationale for this type of plan is that it will minimize food cravings, urges to overeat or undereat, and loss of control.

Increasing the Quantity of Foodstuffs Consumed

The number of calories that a patient needs to consume daily depends on the individual's current weight, metabolic condition, eating patterns, and tolerance for change (Garner et al., 1985). Some emaciated patients have maintained their weight on as few as 600–900 calories per day (Russell, 1970). Gradually increasing caloric intake to achieve a 1- to 2-pound weight gain per week is ideal. For inpatients, the number of calories should be adjusted to achieve a 2- to 3-pound weight gain per week. The prescribed diet for inpatients should never be set below 1,500 calories per day and is usually increased to 1,800–2,400 calories within the first week. All meals need to be completed, so that a patient can gain confidence that calories prescribed can be assimilated according to the plan for weight gain or weight stabilization. As patients shift from a hypometabolic to a hypermetabolic state, daily consumption may need to be increased to as high as 3,500–4,000 calories. Patients with a personal or family history of obesity will usually need fewer calories to ac-

complish the desired rate of weight gain. For outpatients, the speed of weight gain is not as important as is moving steadily in the direction of gradual weight gain.

Broadening the Range of Foodstuffs Consumed

Most patients begin treatment with considerable confusion about what constitutes "normal" eating. Patients tend to divide food into "good" and "bad" categories, often on the basis of nutritional myths such as "Calories from dietary fat accumulate as body fat, in contrast to calories from protein and carbohydrate, which get burned off." Some of these ideas are extreme interpretations of sensible dietary guidelines. Rather than minimizing the intake of red meat, patients exclude it altogether. Dietary fat and sugar are eliminated rather than reduced. Only foods considered "calorie-sparing" are permitted. The result is usually an unappealing dietary regimen, but one that makes a patient feel "safe."

One goal of treatment is for a patient to feel more relaxed eating a wide range of foods. A weekly meal plan should gradually incorporate small amounts of previously avoided or forbidden foods. In most cases, patients who eat according to a vegetarian diet should be encouraged to abandon this diet during the process of recovery. Food preferences prior to the onset of the eating disorder should serve as a guideline for legitimate food choices. Patients should be encouraged to challenge the tendency to divide food into "good" and "bad" categories by recognizing that the calories of those foods previously considered "bad" really have no greater impact on weight than calorie-sparing food items. Patients who engage in binge eating should consume small amounts of the foodstuffs typically reserved for episodes of binge eating. Again, these foods should be redefined as "medication" that will help "inoculate" against binge eating by reducing psychological cravings as well as by establishing new responses to foods that previously represented "blowing" a diet. Even after considerable effort has been devoted to dispelling nutritional myths, patients often report overwhelming anxiety when confronted with certain food choices. This is why eating needs to be planned in advance, with the times and amounts of food predetermined. It can be useful to construct a hierarchy of feared foods, and to have patients gradually move up this scale over time. The amounts of these feared foods can be small, but they should be part of every meal.

Challenging specific irrational beliefs about food may require specialized nutritional knowledge, and clinicians need to develop the necessary informational background in this area to help patients combat food myths. Finally, persistent patterns of distorted thinking about food may reflect a more basic tendency toward faulty reasoning. Resistance to experimenting with different types of foods may require the application of more formal cognitive-behavioral therapy methods, as described later in this chapter.

Implementing Self-Monitoring

Self-monitoring has been consistently recommended in cognitive behavioral research studies with bulimia nervosa (see Wilson, Fairburn, & Agras, Chapter 6, this volume). Self-monitoring can be helpful in establishing a regular eating routine as well as gaining control over symptoms such as binge eating, vomiting, or laxative abuse. Self-monitoring involves keeping a daily written record of all food and liquid consumed as well as of incidents of binge eating, vomiting, laxative abuse, and other extreme weight-controlling behaviors. Patients are sometimes reluctant to complete self-monitoring forms, because they feel ashamed of their behavior or they feel that self-monitoring will only increase their preoccupation with food. These concerns need to be set aside, and the knowledge that self-monitoring is an extremely effective tool in obtaining control over eating disorder symptoms should be encouraged. Although there is general agreement on the value of self-monitoring, recommendations related to timing and flexibility in implementing this procedure in the treatment of anorexia nervosa vary. Some patients resist self-monitoring early in treatment, even when presented with the rationale that this is an important tool for recovery. Resistance to self-monitoring can be related to a patient's overall low motivation to change or to commit to the goals of treatment. With such patients, discussing failure to comply with self-monitoring forms or reviewing inaccurate forms may be pointless. It may be necessary to adopt a more gradual and flexible approach that focuses on basic motivational issues.

Patients who are able to comply with self-monitoring should be given written instructions (Fairburn, 1985) and should be encouraged to record all food and liquid ingested on a self-monitoring form (Figure 7.2) as soon after consumption as possible. Episodes of bingeing, vomiting, laxative abuse, and other weight-losing behaviors, as well as feelings and thoughts surrounding eating, should also be included. The self-monitoring forms should then be reviewed in depth during each meeting, with the aim of identifying problematic eating behavior and dysfunctional thoughts. Patients who are initially unable to benefit from self-monitoring may become more able to comply and profit from the procedure with time. In general, patients will tend toward greater detail or fine-grained analysis of beliefs during the course of treatment; however, it is our experience that the timing and type of self-monitoring must be tailored to meet the needs of the individual patient.

Interrupting the Binge-Eating and Vomiting Cycle

Anorexia nervosa patients who engage in vomiting in connection with binge eating, or even with the consumption of smaller amounts of food, require special treatment strategies. Self-monitoring, as described earlier, focuses attention on the binge–purge process and can lead to an overall reduction in symptoms. The detailed prescription of eating patterns as described above can be helpful in changing the connotation of certain foods, thus giving patients "permission" to eat them without interpreting their behavior as "a loss of control" or a "blown diet." Patients who regularly engage in episodes of vomiting and binge eating must become convinced that regular eating patterns and gradual weight gain offer the best protection against the continuation of this vicious cycle. However, most patients require additional practical strategies to resist the urge to purge.

Delaying

One strategy is to have the patient agree to delay binge eating or purging for a specific period of time (e.g., 30 minutes). This is useful because the urge to engage in these behaviors often subsides with time. A useful delay tactic is to have patients take 10 minutes to compose a "script" or detailed account of what would occur if they were either to proceed with or to avoid the episode (Orimoto & Vitousek, 1992). Patients are instructed to make detailed notes regarding what they would be thinking and feeling during and after a complete episode, or, alternatively, if they avoided the episode. The script-writing technique imposes a delay between the impulse to engage in the episode and the actual initiation of the behavior. It also underscores the adverse effects of the completed cycle (Orimoto & Vitousek, 1992).

Distracting

There are circumstances when patients are unable to employ sophisticated cognitive techniques to challenge assumptions underlying symptomatic behavior. It is common for patients to feel overwhelmed by anxiety after eating or when confronted by problematic interpersonal situations. The therapist can encourage a patient to plan for these times by developing strategies to distract her attention away from troublesome thoughts. This involves forcefully "changing the cognitive channel" rather than identifying and modifying dysfunctional thoughts (Garner & Bemis, 1985). The patient can develop a list of "coping phrases" with instructions to reread them in problematic situations such as after a meal when overwhelmed by the urge to binge or purge. Some sample phrases are as follows: "I must take my meal like medication," "Vomiting now will only increase the risk of bingeing later," "I can't trust my perceptions of my body now; I am like a color-blind person trying to pick out a tie." This same technique can be used to counter the urge to undereat: "Eating is protection," "I need food to keep me healthy," "Regardless of what I feel, I am at a thin normal weight." The purpose of using coping phrases is to interrupt the automatic cognitive sequence leading to symptomatic behavior.

Planning Alternative Behaviors

Another technique is to plan specific alternative behaviors that will break the cycle of binge eating and vomiting (Garner et al., 1985). These alternative behaviors need to be established in therapy sessions and ideally should be written down on paper or a 3 × 5″ card; the patient then needs to agree to execute the alternative behaviors before acting on the urge to binge and purge. The alternative behaviors should be practical yet salient enough to override anxiety and maladaptive thoughts that initiate the cycle. Alternative behaviors that can break the chain of events are, for example, abruptly leaving the house to go for a walk, making telephone calls to supportive friends, listening to loud music, or watching television. Obviously, the success of delay, distraction, and engaging in alternative behaviors depends on the patient's basic agreement regarding the desirability of interrupting the problematic behavior.

Implementing Initial Cognitive Interventions

Patients invariably encounter difficulties in implementing the behavioral prescriptions in Phase I, and this sets the stage for implementing initial cognitive interventions. Resistance to the specific prescriptions for normalizing eating and body weight stimulates discussion of underlying beliefs and assumptions. The therapist tends to take the lead in early cognitive interventions by probing the implications of the patient's specific behaviors and then gently countering them with data and pertinent arguments. This strategy quickly reveals the content and intensity of the patient's dysfunctional beliefs and thinking patterns. It also begins to reveal a wider set of coherent meaning systems or schemas that drive maladaptive behaviors.

Particular care must be taken to avoid allowing interventions to deteriorate into an inquisition or argument over points of logic. There is a delicate balance between being persuasive on the one hand and avoiding any hint of personal attack on the other. Probes and suggestions must occur in an atmosphere of acceptance. In the process of eliciting personal history, providing education, and prescribing more normal eating patterns, distorted and dysfunctional thinking patterns begin to emerge. Following are several examples of common dysfunctional beliefs, as well as initial therapist responses.

The Anorexic Wish

PATIENT. I must first resolve underlying conflicts before I can tackle eating symptoms. I can recover without giving up dieting or weight suppression techniques. I do not really need to gain weight or change my eating now; I want to focus on my emotional problems.

THERAPIST. It is not uncommon for patients to

express the wish to recover from their disorder without gaining weight. This is the "anorexic wish" and reflects the desire for two mutually exclusive events. It is like an elevator phobic's trying to overcome the fear of elevators by discussing theoretical issues in the office but without ever riding an elevator. Your situation is complicated by the fact that it is next to impossible to understand, let alone solve, your real psychological difficulties as long as your experiences are clouded by starvation, dieting, and chronic electrolyte disturbances. *If you choose to overcome your eating disorder, then at some point, you must normalize your eating and gradually gain weight.* Again, recovery is not mandatory; anorexia nervosa is not illegal. However, anorexia nervosa and normal functioning are mutually exclusive conditions. If you were to choose to pursue recovery, then you need reassurance that (1) treatment will provide explicit advice on how to accomplish this task; and (2) since the real aim of therapy is to help you feel truly better about yourself, restoration of normal eating and weight will not be the only emphasis in therapy. Therapy will continue as long as it is needed to address emotional or interpersonal issues that remain after eating symptoms are corrected.

The aim of this type of intervention is to increase cognitive dissonance and to begin to alter the schema the patient has about the disorder. Instead of its being a vehicle for self-expression, or a way to achieve competence, control, and mastery, the disorder is characterized as incompatible with achieving higher-order goals.

Fear of Losing Control

PATIENT. If I begin eating foods that I don't eat now, I am afraid that I will lose complete control and get fat. I just can't take that chance.

THERAPIST. I understand your feelings—this is a fear that most patients express. However, you are arguing from the standpoint of being starved. During the process of weight gain, you may experience periods of intense hunger, but once you have reached a healthy weight and have sustained it for some time, you will simply not have the urge to eat uncontrollably. The only way that you will learn that your fear won't materialize is to eat these foods in prearranged amounts and see that they do not lead to uncontrollable weight gain. Nevertheless, you deserve more than my word on this—you deserve protection. If you do find yourself losing control, every attempt will be made to interrupt it. If necessary, you can be hospitalized to protect you from uncontrollable overeating.

PATIENT. I do not want to give up the sense of control that I feel when I diet.

THERAPIST. I understand that losing weight and adhering to your current eating regimen give you a feeling of control, but I wonder if you are really "in control"? Is your rigid control around eating giving you the control you really want? Doesn't control imply choice? Shouldn't control lead to more rather than fewer options in your life? Aren't you like a person driving a car but only being able to turn the steering wheel one way?

PATIENT. Once I get into the habit of eating "nondietetic" foods, I am afraid I will lose control and not be able to stop. I will develop, or go back to, "unhealthy habits" that I will be unable to change. I will become a slob. I must not break from my routine of eating the same "safe" foods every day.

THERAPIST. In the same way that your current eating is not looking after your biological needs, it is hypothetically possible that your could eat in an "unhealthy" way that would be inconsistent with good health. Perhaps we need to agree now that the goal of therapy is not just to gain weight, but rather to make sure that your eating is consistent with your real health needs, and this is just as important in the future when others are no longer concerned about your weight as they are right now. We will stick with this process to make sure you have a truly healthy lifestyle after you have accomplished your eating and weight goals.

Fear of Shape Change

PATIENT. I cannot gain weight because it will all go to my stomach or thighs.

THERAPIST. Eating more may temporarily make your stomach bloated, and it is true that weight gain tends to come on as body fat [the therapist provides supportive evidence from starvation studies; see Garner, Chapter 8, this volume]. But the weight will redistribute itself automatically without any effort on your part. If your stomach were a bit bigger than you would like, what would it mean?

Beliefs about Food

PATIENT. I always eat "fat-free" foods because dietary fat gets converted into body fat. I never eat carbohydrate with fat because mixing the two [macronutrients] makes you fatter. I try to eat protein because it converts to muscle. I always exercise after I eat so that the calories will be burned up. I never eat before I go to sleep, because then the food will turn to fat.

THERAPIST. [For each of these] This is a common belief; let's review the accuracy of this notion. [The therapist provides correct nutritional information and relates it back to the unlikely event that any of these "tricks" could be expected to override the biological processes underlying "set point"; see Garner, Chapter 8, this volume.]

In each of the examples above, the therapist provides information and reassurance aimed at shifting beliefs and assessing resistance to change. Early in therapy, the therapist takes a more active and directive role, shifting to greater reliance on the Socratic method later in therapy. The rationale for this is that anorexia nervosa patients usually experience many of their symptoms as ego-syntonic. A patient's response to the therapist's advice allows the therapist to determine the nature and intensity of the patient's beliefs.

Increasing Motivation for Change

Safran and Segal (1990) note that "although cognitive-behavioral theory consistently eschews motivational concepts, there is little written in the cognitive-behavioral literature that explicitly clarifies the reasons for this omission" (p. 49). The cognitive model applied to anorexia nervosa has deviated from cognitive approaches to other disorders in emphasizing motivational

or functional features of beliefs and behavior (Garner, 1986; Garner & Bemis, 1982, 1985; Vitousek & Ewald, 1993; Vitousek & Hollon, 1990). Discussion of motivation is also relevant in addressing the resistance to change so commonly observed in anorexia nervosa.

Stages of Motivation

As indicated earlier, an initial focus of cognitive procedures is on increasing motivation for change. The model proposed by Prochaska, DiClemente, and colleagues for understanding changes in addictive behavior is applicable to anorexia nervosa (Prochaska & DiClemente, 1983; Prochaska, DiClemente & Norcross, 1992). The five stages of motivation to change, as described by Prochaska et al. (1992), can be summarized as follows:

1. Precontemplation (no intention to change).
2. Contemplation (aware of problem, thinking about problem, but no commitment to change).
3. Preparation (intending to take action, but not having done so in last year).
4. Action (modifying behavior, experiences, or environment to overcome problem).
5. Maintenance (relapse prevention and consolidation of gains).

Anorexia nervosa patients typically neither are troubled by their disorder nor have any intention to change at the beginning of the initial interview. Treatment often begins at the precontemplation stage, and unless medical risks dictate otherwise, the premature insistence that patients take action will result in their declining any further help. Thus, the initial aim for such patients is to heighten awareness of the disadvantages of the eating disorder, in order to facilitate movement to the contemplation stage. Those at the contemplation stage need to have their awareness of the problem fortified, and the intent is to have them commit themselves to action. Some patients begin treatment at the preparation stage and are willing to take action; however, this may reverse with further clarification of the behavioral goals of treatment. Those at the action stage are equally vulnerable to motivational decay, but at least at this point there has been agreement regarding the objectives and mechanics of recovery. It is not uncommon for patients to experience increasing cognitive dissonance, ambivalence, and distress with the presentation of educational material described in the earlier sections. Used properly, this can boost motivation for change.

Recognizing the "Spiral Pattern" of Change

The process of motivation for change is not linear. It is referred to as the "spiral pattern of change," because motivation fluctuates between stages (Prochaska et al., 1992). Motivational shifts, oscillation, vacillation, indecision, and ambivalence are common attributes in anorexia nervosa. These phenomena are closely tied to the perceived goals of treatment. A mismatch between the patient's current stage of motivation and the goals of treatment is as inappropriate for eating disorders as it has been found to be for addictions (Prochaska et al., 1992). Thus, in formulating goals, it is vital for the clinician to be aware of the patient's current motivational stage, as well as the shifting nature of motivation. At each stage, the spiral pattern of motivation for change is typical. Understanding this process can protect the patient and therapist against unnecessary discouragement.

Accepting the Patient's Beliefs as Currently Genuine

As mentioned earlier, regardless of the array of possible causal and maintaining factors, anorexia nervosa patients share the basic premise that "weight, shape, or thinness can serve as the sole or predominant referent for inferring personal value or self-worth" (Garner & Bemis, 1982, p. 142). It is ineffective to dispute the validity or rationality of this or related beliefs. This not only heightens shame, but can also trigger a retreat into what appears to be indifference but is really a tenacious resolve to maintain the status quo. Rather, the therapist needs to explicitly convey the understanding that these beliefs are currently genuine and functional for the patient (Garner & Bemis, 1982).

Analyzing the Pros and Cons of Maintaining the Disorder

The next step is assisting the patient in developing a detailed list of the pros and cons of maintaining the disorder at this time. In order to minimize defensiveness, the enumeration and analysis of advantages and disadvantages must emphasize the *adaptive* nature of symptoms. The exercise should not deteriorate into demanding that the patient defend the correctness of her behavioral patterns and beliefs. The aim is to identify functional higher-order goals related to effectiveness, mastery, autonomy, and interpersonal competence, and then to begin to introduce doubt about the practicality and utility of anorexia nervosa as the means for meeting these broader goals (Garner & Bemis, 1982).

The lines of inquiry illustrated in this therapist monologue may be helpful:

Let's try to come up with a list of some of the ways that weight control and thinness have made your life better. I can see the intended purpose of anorexia nervosa, but how well is it working now to accomplish your goals? What have you gotten and what have you had to give up as a result of your present state? What goals and values are really important to you? If you believe that there should be a connection between losing weight and attaining your other goals, how does it seem to be working out in practice? How are relationships different, compared to the way they were before the disorder? How is the quality of your life different? In a practical sense, is thinness achieving these goals now?

Vitousek and Orimoto (1993) have stressed the utility of employing the pros and cons technique early in therapy, and have suggested that it serves several specific purposes. First, the clinician's suggesting that there are advantages to anorexic symptomatology can have a disarming effect on patients who have been used to hearing only of the dangers of their disorder. Second, the list of pros and cons can provide an entry into psychoeducation about various aspects of the disorder. Third, the exercise allows assessment of the individual patient's motivational system and experience of the disorder. Finally, the technique allows the therapist to begin to introduce cognitive change strategies. For example, the claimed advantages and disadvantages can be cast as hypotheses that can be examined by prospective data gathering (Vitousek & Orimoto, 1993). Table 7.4 lists perceived advantages and disadvantages of anorexia nervosa.

Projecting into the Future

Early in therapy, motivation can be enhanced by encouraging patients to project the functionality of their current system of weight-control-

TABLE 7.4. Perceived Advantages and
Disadvantages of Anorexia Nervosa Symptoms

Advantages

I just like the way I feel when I am thin.

I get more respect and more compliments.

What everyone else tries to do, I am showing I can
do better.

I like the attention.

I like the clothes I can wear.

I look better this way.

Having fat on my body is really disgusting—now I do
not have to put up with it.

My family and my doctor worry about me.

I can keep people at a distance.

I don't have to have menstrual periods.

I feel like I am in touch with the suffering of the
world.

I feel healthier and more energetic when I'm low in
weight.

I feel more confident and capable when I am thin.

I like the feeling of self-control.

I feel more powerful when I don't eat.

When I am thin, I feel everything more keenly.

I feel special, pure, virtuous.

Disadvantages

Being thin takes up so much time and energy.

I think it is superficial to worry so much about how I
look.

People hassle me a lot about it.

I can't eat a lot of things I like.

I am so tired of being hungry.

I hate thinking about food all of the time.

There is too much pressure in social situations where
eating is expected.

I can't go on vacations because it is too hard to plan
eating.

My mood is negative and unstable.

Sometimes I have a hard time concentrating.

I don't like being cold all of the time.

My hair is falling out.

I hate binge eating.

I worry about being able to have children.

I worry about my future.

I hate being a cliché.

Note. Adapted from Vitousek and Orimoto (1993, p. 209).
Copyright 1993 by Academic Press. Adapted by permission.

ling behaviors from the present into the future
("decentering"). Often there is an unarticulated
belief that the disorder can be simply "switched
off" at some point in the future. Patients need
to comprehend that it is not uncommon for the
disorder to take a chronic course, and that those
who have followed that course probably once
shared the conviction that it could be easily reversed. The therapist might ask:

> Can you see a way that you will be able to re-
> ally fulfill your long-range goals and values on
> the course you are on? What role will your
> present concerns about weight play in your
> life 5 years from now? Ten years? Do you
> think that you will be able to keep up this
> struggle until you are 40? Can you see your-
> self being in greater control and more confi-
> dent in 10 years? If so, how will this happen?

*Using a Drug and Alcohol Analogy
(Reframing Ego-Syntonic Symptoms)*

Patients who insist that there is little reason to
change because their beliefs and behaviors are
so gratifying may respond with a spark of motivation when provided with the rationale that
their current system is functional for them in
the same way that alcohol and drugs are functional for addicts. The drug and alcohol analogy
is potentially problematic because it has so often been misapplied with eating disorders (Wilson, 1993); however, the parallel can be useful
in reframing ego-syntonic symptoms. Discontinuing the use of alcohol, cocaine, heroin, am-
phetamines, or other mood-enhancing substances requires addicts to forgo immediate
"pleasure" because of the recognition that their
addiction is inconsistent with future goals.
Though there is little evidence that anorexic
symptoms are truly "addicting," their potency
as positive reinforcers may be eroded as patients begin to realize that the immediate pleasure and safety they provide are incompatible
with their own higher-order goals. Like those of
some addictive substances, the initial effects of
anorexic symptoms are feelings of control, self-
confidence, and competence, but these fade
over time; the patients actually have little control and are slaves to their symptoms. Although
the pursuit of weight control may be pleasurable, patients are able to recognize that their
lives are consumed by this idea (just as addicts'
lives are), and that there are disadvantages to
permitting a single idea to dictate the conduct

of one's life or the contents of one's thoughts. Eating disorder symptoms can function like drugs and alcohol in another way, by distracting or deflecting individuals away from negative experience. Again, the symptoms are functional in the short term, but do not resolve the long-term issues of concern.

Challenging Cultural Values Regarding Weight and Shape

A recurrent theme throughout cognitive therapy with anorexia nervosa patients is examination of the personal effects of exposure to the intense cultural pressure on women to diet and to engage in "weight control" in order to meet the prevailing standards for thinness. The role models for shape have little to do with the actual shape of most women in Western society (Garner, Garfinkel, Schwartz, & Thompson, 1980). As indicated earlier, the disconcerting result is a norm in which women report being dissatisfied with their shape and feel guilty about eating even reasonable amounts of food (Heatherton, Nichols, Mahamedi, & Keel, 1995). Treatment for anorexia nervosa involves swimming against this cultural stream. Male therapists must develop a sincere appreciation of the unique subculture in which women live, and female therapists must develop sufficient distance from these values that they do not present conflicting messages to patients. Throughout the struggle to recover from their eating disorder, patients are bombarded by media messages glorifying the virtues of dieting and thinness. In some cases, these pressures are further amplified by family values or participation in sports subcultures in which thinness is emphasized. A central component of cognitive therapy is helping each patient identify and synthesize the personal implications of adopting the prevailing cultural standards related to weight and shape. How has the culture shaped and reinforced the patient's personal assumptions and self-definition? During this process, the therapist must remain acutely aware of the degree to which these values have been incorporated by the patient, and must not allow cultural rebukes to be translated into personal disparagement.

It can be useful for the therapist to prescribe homework assignments to underscore the cultural pressures on women to diet. Patients are encouraged to gather examples from magazine advertisements promoting unrealistic shapes or equating female worth with physical attractiveness in general and thinness in particular. Some patients eventually develop a healthy sense of indignation at the harsh and delimiting definitions of feminine attractiveness. This leads them to reframe the etiology of their disorder, at least in part, in cultural terms. However, most patients remain conflicted about cultural messages about weight and shape, and require ongoing support in challenging the social norms.

Determining the Optimal Level of Family Involvement

Regardless of the therapist's theoretical orientation, it is advisable for all members of a patient's family to participate in the evaluation when the patient is living at home, is in frequent contact with the family, or is financially dependent on the family (Garner et al., 1982). From a strictly practical point of view, parents or guardians are legally responsible for a minor patient's well-being. Moreover, parents have the potential to provide powerful directives in support of therapeutic goals. From a theoretical perspective, the interaction between the patient's thinking, feeling, and behavior and those of family members is usually so salient that it compels family involvement. For older patients, the psychological themes may be similar but the legal and ethical implications differ, since the patient must choose to participate in treatment as well as whether or not to involve family members. Nevertheless, family therapy or strategically employed family sessions may be a desirable adjunct to individual therapy with older patients, particularly when family conflicts predominate. With older patients living independently, it is preferable to see the individual alone for all or at least part of the initial assessment. This privacy denotes respect for the patient's autonomy (even though significant family problems may exist) and allows the clinician to gather information regarding eating symptoms that the patient may be reluctant to share in the presence of others. This format also underscores the primacy of the patient's personal goals as a focus of therapy.

As we elaborate later, theoretical principles guiding the cognitive approach to treatment must accommodate the undeniable need to involve the family when clinically indicated. It is possible to remain firmly anchored in cognitive theory, while taking advantage of the family therapy format. In each specific case, deciding whether to perform the assessment and subsequent treatment with the individual alone or whether to involve other family members depends on clinical issues that may vary during the course of therapy.

It is useful for parents to understand that family interactional patterns may indeed contribute to the maintenance of symptoms; however, extraordinary guilt and shame can stem from the view that the eating disorder is caused by poor parenting or family psychopathology. Parents need to be reassured that there is little empirical support for this notion. However, it should be expected that having an eating disorder in the family will create incredible stress within even the most "normal family."

PHASE II: CHANGING BELIEFS RELATED TO FOOD AND WEIGHT, THEN BROADENING THE SCOPE OF THERAPY

Phase II of treatment consists of weekly meetings that build on the motivational and educational foundations established earlier. Time is set aside in each session to review progress related to eating patterns, body weight gain, and the interruption of compensatory behaviors. Ongoing advice is given about the biological factors regulating body weight, nutritional myths, sociocultural influences, and the effects of starvation. Although the patient has been exposed to cognitive principles during Phase I, more formal cognitive methods, such as cognitive restructuring, are introduced as the commitment to therapy increases. During Phase II, the content of therapy is gradually broadened from food and weight to the personal meaning that thinness has acquired for the individual (see Table 7.1). The major aims of Phase II of treatment are identifying the particular meanings and functions of symptoms for the individual patient, and helping the patient to find more adaptive means of achieving constructive goals.

Continuing the Emphasis on Weight Gain and Normalized Eating

Particularly in the early stage of Phase II, the rationale for achieving a target weight range that allows normal biological functioning will need to be reiterated. Similarly, each session is structured to review self-monitored eating, adherence to meal planning, and episodes of overeating or undereating, as described in Phase I. Themes related to food and weight are visited and revisited from different angles during the course of therapy. Patients will continue to require help in breaking eating down into the components described earlier (spacing, quantity, and quality), and then in examining beliefs that interfere with adherence to prescribed patterns.

Reframing Relapses

The therapist needs to prepare patients in the binge-eating/purging subgroup for vulnerability to relapses in bingeing and vomiting, particularly during stressful times. After an episode of binge eating, patients chastise themselves with conclusions like these: "I have blown it; it doesn't matter any more," "Since I binged this morning, the rest of the day is ruined and I might as well continue bingeing," "All of my efforts are spoiled—now I must start over from square one," "Bingeing is evidence that I will never recover." These beliefs can lead to a vicious cycle, in which hopelessness and despair precipitate further symptomatic behavior. As suggested earlier, progress is rarely linear in nature; more commonly, it follows a variable pattern in which ultimate success can only be measured amidst intermittent setbacks. Patients need to be encouraged to refrain from applying dichotomous and perfectionistic thinking to relapses. They need to reframe relapses by stepping back and evaluating the episodes in light of the "big picture." On the other hand, episodes of binge eating and vomiting should not be taken casually. Concern and thoughtful exploration of the factors that led to a "slip" form the adaptive response. A common reaction to relapse is trying to compensate by skipping the next meal or undereating; this usually leads to increased food cravings and an escalation in binge eating. The therapist should encourage the patient to practice the "four R's" in reframing relapses:

1. *Reframe* the episode as a "slip," not as "blown recovery."
2. *Renew* the commitment to long-term recovery.
3. *Return* to the plan of regular eating without engaging in compensatory behaviors.
4. *Reinstitute* behavioral controls to interrupt future episodes.

If the tendency to binge-eat continues, the therapist and patient need to review the eating plan to ensure that the quantity of food it calls for is sufficient to quell food cravings. In addition to the amount eaten, it is important to review the quality of foods and the spacing of meals. Changes in the patient's weight may reveal a conscious or unintentional drift in the direction of undereating. The patient may rationalize the undereating as providing "money in the bank" that can be used later if she really feels hungry. However, the mounting caloric deficit increases the biological basis for food cravings, making the patient more vulnerable to binge episodes. The patient becomes a "walking time bomb with a hair-trigger on eating." In this case, it is helpful for the therapist to review the biological basis for binge eating and stress the need to make appropriate adjustments to food intake to correct the state of undernutrition. With practice, patients usually improve their ability to interrupt a vicious downward spiral by monitoring and challenging self-defeating beliefs.

Identifying Dysfunctional Thoughts, Schemas, and Thinking Patterns

The concept of dysfunctional thoughts or beliefs is developed more fully in Phase II, usually within the context of addressing resistance to making behavioral changes in the areas of eating, weight, and purging. The process typically begins by highlighting the predicament posed by noncompliance on the one hand, and most patients' assertions by this point in treatment that they really do want to recover on the other. Again, symptoms are often intended to further the attainment of laudable goals, whereas on another level they represent adaptive failure. The therapist needs to reassure a patient that her behavior is not motivated by defiance or self-sabotage; rather, it stems from beliefs and assumptions that can be identified, examined, and either affirmed or changed. At this point it is useful for the therapist to begin to describe some of the other properties of cognitive functioning, since these are useful in beginning to identify dysfunctional thoughts and cognitive processing errors. The therapist needs to acquaint the patient with the following concepts, to facilitate the development of the language for identifying and changing thinking patterns that maintain symptomatic behavior.

Automatic Thoughts

Beck et al. (1979) define "cognitions" as automatic, habitual, and believable thoughts or visual images that generally operate outside of the individual's immediate awareness, but that can be identified. The automatic operation of thinking is described as a normal and valuable process that is essential to everyday functioning. When a traffic light turns green, a person generally does not have to think consciously "Now I can cross the street"; however, it is clear that this belief is directing the person's behavior. To take another example, toothbrushing is based on automatic thoughts guiding the immediate behavior, as well as more abstract assumptions related to oral hygiene. Engaging in law-abiding behavior is dictated by certain assumptions, just as is lawlessness; the same can be said for political and religious beliefs. The way an individual interprets and responds to complex information in interpersonal situations is also determined by the relatively automatic operation of beliefs and assumptions. The therapist should select an automatic dysfunctional thought relevant to the patient to illustrate this concept. By examining what goes through the patient's head when she sees a thin person or when she looks at a food that has a "nondietetic" caloric connotation, it underscores the fact that behavior "makes sense" in light of this thought, and now can be examined to determine the ways in which it is adaptive and maladaptive.

Cognitive Schemas

Individuals tend to organize their social experiences and information about themselves into specific categories referred to as "self-schemata" or "schemas" (Markus, 1977, 1990; Markus, Crane, Bernstein, & Siladi, 1982; Rogers, Kuiper, & Kirker, 1977). Cognitive schemas are enduring cognitive structures or sets that function by processing, organizing, and integrating complex information. Jean Piaget described them as "mobile frames" automatically applied to various contents; the contents are adapted and molded to fit into the schema structure (Flavell, 1963). Beck et al. (1979) describe schemas as "relatively stable cognitive patterns [that] form the basis for the regularity of interpretations of a particular set of situations" (p. 12). Fiske and Taylor (1984) differentiate "person" schemas, "event" schemas and "procedural" schemas. Person and event schemas relate to content in these two domains, whereas procedural schemas are processing rules for linking information in a consistent fashion. The cognitive model attributes emotional disorders in part to an overreliance on certain rigid or extreme schemas, which lead to unrealistic, erroneous, or dysfunctional interpretations of experiences (Beck, 1976). In anorexia nervosa, experiences are organized according to weight-related self-schemas. Weight or shape becomes the frame of reference for self-evaluation. Weight is particularly appealing as a yardstick for self-rating, since it is objective, observable, and quantifiable.

The Enduring and Resistant Nature of Schemas

Because schemas are relatively stable organizing structures, they resist change. Whereas some beliefs change with the acquisition of new knowledge (e.g., laxatives do not work), schemas are more cohesive cognitive organizing structures that guide the processing of new data. Schemas are not immune to change; however, these mental frameworks or personal theories tend to organize, interpret, and assimilate new information or data to fit their mold.

The Motivation to Maintain Congruence among Schemas and Beliefs

Festinger (1957) hypothesized that "cognitive dissonance," or "the existence of nonfitting relations among cognitions, is a motivating factor in its own right" (p. 3). Accordingly, the person tries to reduce cognitive dissonance when it is present, and actively avoids situations and information that might increase dissonance. Similar concepts have reemerged in more recent cognitive models, again as motivational constructs (Teasdale & Barnard, 1993). Accordingly, the individual tries to reduce the discrepancy among current, past, and anticipated informational sources.

The Occurrence of Beliefs at Different Schematic Levels

Beliefs can occur at different levels. Patients may say, "I know intellectually that my worth is not related to my weight or shape, but I don't believe this emotionally." Beck et al. (1979) have suggested that this is simply a semantic problem: Since people cannot really believe something "emotionally," such patients are really expressing different "degrees of belief" (p. 302). However, Teasdale and Barnard (1993) have postulated a schematic cognitive model in which higher-level meaning ("implicational") may be qualitatively different from lower-level meaning ("propositional"). Implicational beliefs are really higher-order, affect-laden beliefs that are more fundamental. Also, according to this model, dissociation between beliefs on these two levels is to be expected. It follows that change at the higher, implicational level of meaning is the central goal of therapy. The lower-level, propositional beliefs may be markers of a "parent" schematic model from which they are derived, and thus can be useful targets for intervention. This bears some resemblance to Beck's (1976) "underlying assumptions," described as overarching or higher-order meanings or schemas from which automatic thoughts derive (Beck et al., 1979).

However, the Teasdale and Barnard (1993) model places much more emphasis on strategies that focus on the "schematic" level (i.e., the implicational meaning systems or the wider semantic context), in contrast to targeting the "truth value of specific propositional statements" (p. 242) or specific dysfunctional beliefs. This has implications for the conduct of therapy. Rather than the "search-and-destroy" strategy aimed at specific negative thoughts, the aim is to "create coherent, alternative, semantic 'packages'" (Teasdale & Barnard, 1993, p. 240). This multilevel concept of meaning systems is a useful guide in identifying dysfunctional thoughts held by the individual. It offers a framework for linking automatic thoughts such as "I am fat and disgusting" to the underlying assumption that "Being thin is directly related to my self-definition and self-worth." It also provides the heuristic framework for importing and integrating meaning systems that may be accessed more readily through interpersonal and family therapy. For example, metacommunication in interpersonal relationships is a reflection of multilevel meaning systems (Watzlawick, Beavin, & Jackson, 1967). Emphasis on the implicit and multilevel nature of cognition is consistent with the broader focus of cognitive therapy described as clinically useful for anorexia nervosa (Garner et al., 1982; Guidano & Liotti, 1983).

The Occurrence of Contradictory Beliefs

Even though there is a tendency toward consistency among beliefs, it is also true that beliefs can be contradictory. People can entertain two or more apparently mutually exclusive beliefs at the same time. A patient can hold such contradictory beliefs as "I want to induce vomiting" and "I do not want to induce vomiting." They both stem from separate "lines of logic" and may be activated with shifts in attention or in different situations. In part, this relates to cognitive limitations in recognizing contradictions or discrepancies between meaning systems when they occur on different information-processing levels. An individual may have a general schema "I am an honest person," but may do something that is dishonest. On one level, patients can believe that human worth cannot be measured in terms of simple traits; yet they may still infer their own value from weight or shape.

Reasoning or Information-Processing Errors

In trying to understand and change behavior, it is important to recognize that styles or patterns of thinking operate in a relatively automatic manner to influence the interpretation of experience. In most situations, with most people, these processes are highly adaptive. It is only in problematic situations that maladaptive thinking needs to be identified and corrected. Once certain schemas exist, then systematic information-processing errors can modify discrepant

---

TABLE 7.5. Common Reasoning Errors among Eating Disorder Patients

Selective abstraction, or basing a conclusion on isolated details while ignoring contradictory and more salient evidence.

Examples:

"I just can't control myself. Last night when I had dinner in a restaurant, I ate everything I was served, although I had decided ahead of time that I was going to be very careful. I am so weak."

"The only way that I can be in control is through eating."

"I am special if I am thin."

Overgeneralization, or extracting a rule on the basis of one event and applying it to other dissimilar situations.

Examples:

"When I used to eat carbohydrates, I was fat; therefore, I must avoid them now so I won't become obese."

"I used to be of normal weight, and I wasn't happy. So I *know* gaining weight isn't going to make me feel better."

Magnification, or overestimation of the significance of undesirable consequent events. Stimuli are embellished with surplus meaning not supported by an objective analysis.

Examples:

"Gaining five pounds would push me over the brink."

"If others comment on my weight gain, I won't be able to stand it."

"I've gained two pounds, so I can't wear shorts any more."

Dichotomous or all-or-none reasoning, or thinking in extreme and absolute terms. Events can be only black or white, right or wrong, good or bad.

Examples:

"If I'm not in complete control, I lose all control. If I can't master this area of my life, I'll lose everything."

"If I gain one pound, I'll go on and gain a hundred pounds."

"If I don't establish a daily routine, everything will be chaotic and I won't accomplish anything."

Personalization and self-reference, or egocentric interpretations of impersonal events or overinterpretations of events relating to the self.

Examples:

"Two people laughed and whispered something to each other when I walked by. They were probably saying that I looked unattractive. I *have* gained three pounds . . . "

"I am embarrassed when other people see me eat."

"When I see someone who is overweight, I worry that I will be like her."

Superstitious thinking, or believing in the cause–effect relationship of noncontingent events.

Examples:

"I can't enjoy anything because it will be taken away."

"If I eat a sweet, it will be converted instantly into stomach fat."

Note. From Garner and Bemis (1982, p. 137). Copyright 1982 by Plenum Publishing Corporation. Reprinted by permission.

sources of information from present, past, and anticipated experiences to fit the internal schematic representation. Beck (1976) has identified specific reasoning errors characteristic of depression, anxiety, and other emotional disorders; these have been adapted to patients with eating disorders (Garner, 1986; Garner & Bemis, 1982; Garner et al., 1982; Vitousek & Ewald, 1993; Vitousek & Hollon, 1990). Table 7.5 illustrates reasoning or processing errors that are common among eating disorder patients.

Throughout the course of therapy, the therapist needs to assist the patient in learning to identify dysfunctional thoughts and the processing errors that influence her perceptions, thoughts, feelings, and symptomatic behavior. Beliefs and behaviors that direct symptomatic behavior need to be connected to the more general and often implicit schemas referred to as "underlying assumptions" (Beck, 1976) or "higher-order implicit meanings" or "schematic models" (Teasdale & Barnard, 1993). Guidano and Liotti (1983) have described the progression in therapy from more superficial cognitive structures related to food and weight to "deep cognitive restructuring implying a modification of the personal identity" (p. 299).[3]

Developing Cognitive Restructuring Skills

Cognitive restructuring is a method of examining and modifying dysfunctional thinking. It consists of the following steps:

1. Monitoring thinking and heightening the awareness of thinking patterns.
2. Identifying, clarifying, distilling, and articulating dysfunctional beliefs or thoughts in their simplest form.
3. Examining the evidence or arguments for and against the validity and utility of dysfunctional beliefs.
4. Coming to a reasoned conclusion by evaluating the evidence for and against.
5. Making behavioral changes that are consistent with the reasoned conclusion.
6. Developing believable disputing thoughts and more realistic interpretations.
7. Gradually modifying underlying assumptions reflected by more specific beliefs.

Automatic thoughts, beliefs, and assumptions can be pinpointed by increasing awareness of the thinking process. They may also be accessed by observing behavioral patterns; for example, restricting eating to "fat-free" foods implies certain beliefs. In addition, an automatic thought may be identified by focusing on particular situations and replaying the thinking and feeling associated with that situation. Then the patient is encouraged to generate and examine the evidence for and against a particular dysfunctional belief. Most of the following cognitive strategies for implementing the steps listed above have been described in connection with the treatment of other emotional disorders; however, the content and style have been adapted for anorexia nervosa.

Helping Patients Articulate Beliefs

Normal verbalization in therapy tends to be complex, fragmented, disjointed, and often vague. Beliefs and dysfunctional thoughts are embedded in complicated accounts of current and past experiences. Even with some exposure to the cognitive model, patients require practice in "thinking about thinking" and help in distilling specific beliefs from their more complex stream of thought. The therapist serves an important function in clarifying, synthesizing, and condensing complicated ideas presented by a patient and translating them into brief summaries of dysfunctional thoughts in their simplest form. Sometimes simplifying or consolidating a belief may make the distortion highly apparent and lead to immediate attitude change.

Decentering

"Decentering" involves the process of evaluating a particular belief from a different perspective in order to appraise its validity more objectively. It is particularly useful in combating egocentric interpretations that the patient is central to other people's attention. For example, decentering may be useful for a patient who is afraid to go to the beach because others will notice her stomach or detect the fact that she has gained 5 pounds. The therapist can respond with the following types of comments:

How much do you really notice when other people gain or lose small amounts of weight? Do you remember whether my weight was up or down a week ago? Even if you did notice, would it have been a major event? It would be nice in a way to be the object of other people's preoccupations, but, realistically speaking, most people are pretty busy with their own personal concerns. What are the implications for you of your weight's going up or down? Do you really believe it is a reliable frame of reference for other people's worth?

Another patient may state, "I can't eat in front of others in the residence cafeteria, because others will be watching me." First, it needs to be established that the eating behavior is not indeed unusual. If not, the therapist might inquire: "How much do you really think about others' eating? Even if you are sensitized to their eating, how much do you really care about it except in the sense that it reflects back to your own eating? Even if your behavior was unusual, do others *really* care?" Through the technique of decentering, the patient may be encouraged to develop a more realistic idea of the impact that most of her behavior has on others.

Challenging Dichotomous Reasoning

"Dichotomous reasoning" (all-or-none or absolutistic thinking) is a common problem in anorexia nervosa. Examples are the beliefs that foods are either "good" or "bad," that deviation from rigid dieting is equivalent to bingeing, and that gaining a pound is a sign of complete loss of control. This style of thinking is applied to topics beyond food and weight. Patients commonly report extreme attitudes in the pursuit of sports, school, careers, and acceptance from others. People tend to be either deified or vilified. Similarly, all-or-none reasoning is applied to concepts such as happiness, morality, self-confidence, and success. This type of reasoning is particularly evident in patients' beliefs about self-control. Common examples include "If I am not in complete control, I will lose all control," "If I learn to enjoy sweets, I will not be able to restrain myself," "If I stop exercising for one day, I will never exercise," "If I enjoy sexual contact, I will become promiscuous," "If I become angry, I will devastate others with my rage." A major therapeutic task is to teach a patient to recognize this style of thinking, to examine the evidence against it, to evaluate its maladaptive consequences, and to practice adopting a more balanced lifestyle.

Decatastrophizing

Ellis (1962) originally described "decatastrophizing" as a strategy for challenging anxiety that stems from magnifying negative outcomes. It involves the therapist's asking the patient to clarify vague and implicit predictions of calamity, as follows: "What if the feared situation did occur? Would it really be as devastating as you imagined? How would you cope if the feared outcome did occur?" Ironically, catastrophizing can actually produce the feared outcome: In an attempt to avoid social rejection and isolation, patients can withdraw from all social interactions, thus becoming isolated. Fear of failure can lead to the scrupulous avoidance of risk, which results in failure. Moreover, there is no relief from catastrophic thinking. If patients believe that weight gain would be a catastrophe, it is clear why they would be fearful and anxious when they gain weight. What is less obvious is the fact that they are usually anxious when they do not gain because they can never be completely free of the risk. In addition to helping a patient temper dire forecasts about the future, the therapist can facilitate the development of coping plans for mastering feared situations if they were to occur.

Challenging Beliefs through Behavioral Exercises

A primary goal of cognitive therapy is helping patients alter behavior by modifying dysfunctional beliefs and underlying assumptions. However, the reciprocal effect of behavior on belief change is at least as important in the treatment of anorexia nervosa. Anxiety and fear are central to the maintenance of eating disorder symptoms. Even the most careful cognitive preparation does not eliminate the fear associated with changed eating patterns and weight gain. At some point, if patients are to recover, they must begin making behavioral changes in these areas. Behavioral changes provide the real opportunity to probe, challenge and correct faulty assumptions regarding eating, weight, and related self-attributions. It is difficult for patients to maintain the belief that they cannot eat dietary fat or sugar without losing control, if they indeed consume these substances without binge eating. Similarly, behavioral change can have a profound effect on beliefs unrelated to food and weight. Social interaction can attenuate the view of self as socially incompetent. Independent and self-reliant behavior interferes with personal and family schemas that foster overprotectiveness and excessive dependence. However, it is common for well-established beliefs to remain intact, despite undeniably contradictory behavior. It is important for the therapist to make sure that the implications of the behavioral change are integrated at the cognitive level.

Back-Translating Beliefs into Behavioral Exercises

Once tentative agreement can be achieved about the desirability of a paradigm shift, a patient should be strongly encouraged to "back-translate" the new schema into specific behaviors consistent with the new position. For example, once patients begins to recognize the flaws in inferring self-discipline from avoiding dietary fat, it is useful for them to arrange to consume foods with the "fat connotation" in a predetermined situation. Similarly, it is common for patients to claim that they really have made a commitment to recovery while persisting in symptomatic behavior. It is useful for the therapist to help these patients reaffirm the commitment and then back-translate it into specific behaviors consistent with presumed goals. A patient may want to make progress on a conceptual level, but then may engage in self-sabotage when it comes to daily food intake. Highlighting the dissonance between beliefs and behaviors, or beliefs on different schematic levels and behaviors, can be useful in dismantling behaviors maintained by habit rather than by firm convictions.

Employing Reattribution Techniques

There are no reliable methods for directly modifying body size misperception in anorexia nervosa. Instead of correcting the size misperception reported by some patients, it is useful simply to reframe the interpretation of the experience. This involves interrupting and overriding self-perceptions of fatness with higher-order interpretations, such as "I know that those with anorexia nervosa cannot trust their own size perceptions," or "I expect to feel fat during my recovery, so I must consult the scale to get an accurate reading of my size." The therapist asks the patient to attribute body self-perceptions to the disorder and to refrain from acting upon intrusive thoughts, images, or body experiences. This approach is contrary to the general thera-

peutic goal of encouraging self-trust in the validity and reliability of internal experiences.

Creating Dissonance between Incompatible Schematic Models

One of the aims of therapy is to increase dissonance between incompatible schematic models and to encourage shifts toward congruence in meanings, as well as in associated "downline" verbalizations and behaviors that are adaptive in the broader context. The integration of cultural and personal values concerning weight, shape, and eating is an example. Patients who evaluate their self-worth in terms of body weight, shape, and eating report feeling self-righteous, virtuous, "in control," safe, and superior when engaged in specific behaviors to control their eating and weight. These behaviors have been imbued with such strong positive valences that they elicit an almost involuntary flooding of positive thoughts, feelings, and images. Extremely negative thoughts and emotions are evoked by behaviors inconsistent with weight control. Nevertheless, the same patients may be able to recognize the shortcomings of using body weight in measuring human worth, particularly when this gauge is applied to others. The contradiction between the self-rating system and the system applied to others is minimized or lost altogether. The therapist may suggest that such patients invoke a scenario in which someone else (say, a person hiring a friend for a job) applies this weight stereotype in judging a friend's competence. Patients usually see the injustice immediately. They will admit that if human worth is judged at all, it should be based upon complex traits—benevolence, generosity, strength, perceptiveness, kindness, honesty, competence, and the like. Moreover, on one level, the same patients will recognize that current cultural pressures on women to diet are oppressive, superficial, dehumanizing, and destructive. If a patient is able to see this standard applied to others as superficial and inappropriate, then the therapist can direct attention back to the dissonance with her personal system. This process presumes sensitivity, good timing, and a trusting therapeutic relationship to guard against the patient's feeling depreciated in any way.

Modifying Self-Concept

"Self-concept" is a broad and multidimensional construct. Hall and Lindsey (1970) delineated two aspects of self-concept: "self-esteem" and "self-awareness." Self-esteem constitutes the appraisal or evaluation of personal value, including attitudes, feelings, and perceptions. In contrast, self-awareness relates to the perception and understanding of the internal processes that guide experience (Hall & Lindsey, 1970). The schematic content of self-concept deficits and the adaptive functions they serve have been central to the cognitive conceptualization of anorexia nervosa (Garner, 1986; Garner & Bemis, 1982, 1985; Garner et al., 1982; Garner & Rosen, 1990; Guidano & Liotti, 1983; Vitousek & Ewald, 1993; Vitousek & Hollon, 1990). Vitousek and Ewald (1993) have organized self-concept deficits characteristic of anorexia nervosa into three broad clusters of variables: the "unworthy self," the "perfectible self," and the "overwhelmed self." The unworthy self is characterized by (1) low self-esteem, (2) feelings of helplessness, (3) a poorly developed sense of identity, (4) a tendency to seek external verification, (5) extreme sensitivity to criticism, and (6) conflicts over autonomy versus dependence. The second cluster, the perfectible self, includes (1) perfectionism, (2) grandiosity, (3) asceticism, and (4) a "New Year's resolution" cognitive style. The third cluster, the overwhelmed self, is characterized by (1) a preference for simplicity, (2) a preference for certainty, and (3) a tendency to retreat from complex or intense social environments. Some of these tendencies have been addressed in examples in earlier sections. For example, it is easy to see how dichotomous thinking can conspire with and exacerbate most of these self-concept deficits. It is useful for the therapist to help the patient identify and address the different, but interrelated, elements of self-concept deficits.

Self-Esteem

It is well recognized that poor self-esteem often predates the appearance of eating disorder symptoms. The pride and accomplishment of weight control seem to alleviate this malady temporarily. The correction of low self-esteem, particularly if it is pervasive and long-standing, is a formidable task. Considering the amount of introspective energy devoted to self-evaluation, it is remarkable that so little formal education is devoted to the topic. At some point in therapy, patients usually reveal that they do not feel worthwhile or that they lack personal worth.

This assumption may emerge in discussing the meaning of dieting and weight control as markers for such constructs as competence, control, attractiveness, and self-discipline, which in turn reflect self-worth. It may be expressed in vague terms such as a general feeling of ineffectiveness, helplessness, or lack of inner direction.

It is useful for the therapist to help the patient distill vague assumptions about self-worth into a clear and simple statement, such as "I feel like a failure," "I do not feel like a worthwhile person," or "I must be liked by others in order to feel good about myself." Once the patient has expressed the view that she has low self-worth, it is useful to engage in a more general discussion about the basis for self-worth, and later to apply what has been learned back to particular index situations identified by the patient. It is often useful to begin by noting how much time and energy most people devote to trying to evaluate their self-worth. It is often a prominent topic commanding a significant portion of individuals' mental lives; however, most of us receive very little training in how to go about actually evaluating self-worth. For most patients, weight or shape has become the predominant gauge for inferring self-worth. It is possible to determine the pros and cons of this frame of reference, and then to extend this to other behaviors, traits, or characteristics employed in the process of self-evaluation, following the procedures described by Burns (1993). For example, what are the advantages and disadvantages of using support and acceptance from others as the standard for evaluating self-worth? This formula seems reasonable on the surface, and there is no question that it is more pleasant to be surrounded by accepting people; however, using this to infer self-worth can be a blueprint for anxiety and insecurity. The disadvantages of rejection are obvious. However, acceptance is problematic because it provides no insurance against ultimate rejection. Moreover, rating human worth in terms of performance or acceptance from others is problematic because outcomes can be ambiguous. Is a particular friend *really* a friend? How many friends are required for proof of acceptability? How does one analyze contradictory information? Is it justified to infer the abstract notion of human worth from particular performances? Is a B on an exam good enough? Can one lose or gain human worth on the basis of daily accomplishments? If so, how does one legitimately determine worth, based on an inventory of different traits and performances? How should relative weights or units of value be assigned for past, present, and future contributions?. What exactly are the definitions of a worthless or worthwhile person? What are the problems with defining self-esteem as conditional on traits and accomplishments?

Decentering can be used to analyze this "balance sheet" approach to human worth. Does the patient evaluate others in this same way? Are other people considered worthless or inferior if they make mistakes, are less intelligent, or do not perform well? The following example (from Garner & Bemis, 1985, p. 152) illustrates the process:

PATIENT. I am terrified I may do worse this year than last year in my studies.

THERAPIST. What would it mean if you did do worse?

PATIENT. Well, I guess it would mean that I am not very good as a person.

THERAPIST. You mean you are rating your worth as a person by your grades?

PATIENT. Yes, I guess that is right. It is important to do well in everything you attempt. I feel the same way about sports, hobbies, and my friends. In the last year losing weight has become the way for me to feel good about myself.

THERAPIST. The way that you are looking at your worth sort of relates to a philosophical question. How does one really evaluate or measure self-worth [i.e., how does the patient operationalize this belief]? You have implied that you base it on your daily performance, but this has some distinct advantages. [The therapist then outlines these as described above.]

PATIENT. Don't all people judge their worth by what they do?

THERAPIST. We may do this to some degree, but not as literally or as harshly as you seem to do, and not on a moment-to-moment basis. In fact, you might ask yourself if you rate others' worth by their performances. Do you rate your roommate's worth based on her grades? You haven't seemed particularly concerned about my grades in graduate school [decentering].

PATIENT. I just assumed that you did everything well.

THERAPIST. That is hardly the case. If you found that I did things poorly in several areas, would your evaluation of me decline?

PATIENT. Well, no, but you are different.

The aim of the approach is to help the patient gradually begin to question the utility of the "balance sheet" concept of self-worth. Although it is functional to rate performances, traits, and behaviors (since these have tangible consequences), it is not functional or legitimate to use these qualities to rate the abstract concept of human value. There is practical as well as philosophical merit in assuming that human worth is unconditional, unearned, and omnipresent (Burns, 1993; Ellis & Harper, 1975; Greiger, 1975). Gradual acceptance of the notion that there probably is no such thing as a worthwhile or worthless person makes continual self-evaluation less relevant. Patients often ponder: "If the aim of behavior is not to raise self-worth, then what is the point?" Ideally, the answer to this question is a shift toward pursuing activities and goals because they are intrinsically enjoyable or fulfilling, rather than because they are benchmarks for self-worth.

Patients may come to understand this idea, but may persist on another level in feeling flawed, defective, and inadequate. It is as if they feel their basic personalities are inherently defective, and the degree of self-loathing goes beyond poor self-esteem. This may indicate the operation of more fundamental and affect-laden patterns of self-appraisal, reflecting an implicit negative self-schema (Teasdale & Barnard, 1993). In these cases, simply presenting rational arguments to discredit, invalidate, or disprove negative automatic thoughts may be ineffective in reversing feelings of inadequacy. Changing the basic self-view of such patients involves going beyond specific evidence to restructuring overarching schematic models for inferring self-worth (Garner et al., 1982). For example, a common theme is the lack of acceptance of fundamental personality attributes in favor of idealized traits. Patients who tend to be socially dependent may view dependence with contempt and strive to be devoid of interpersonal needs. They repudiate the notion of deriving pleasure from nurturance, protection, affection, and interpersonal sharing, expecting themselves to be self-reliant in the pursuit of individualistic goals. Although these autonomous goals are not inherently negative, neither are those reflecting social dependence. The rejection of "social dependence" has to do with the perceived legitimacy or respectability of this trait. Rather than spurning this characteristic, a patient can be helped to redefine it to underscore the inherent strengths of "interdependence" (Gilligan, 1982). The process of self-acceptance is gradual and can be encouraged by the therapist's careful observation and reinforcement of the legitimacy of the patient's own traits.

It is common for patients to report an "anorexic identity," in that one source of inferring self-worth is the disorder itself. It is seen as a sign of self-control, self-discipline, and special status. Unfortunately, much of the coverage in the press has subtly reinforced this image of anorexia nervosa by associating it with celebrities and with such traits as intelligence, beauty, self-discipline, perfection, and fitness. Challenging the positive image the disorder may have acquired must be done with great care, to avoid directly confronting the patient in a destructive manner. It is useful for the patient to construct a detailed list of the pros and cons of this criterion for inferring worth. The therapist then can gently reframe the disorder in less than glamorous terms. Anorexia nervosa can be viewed as the antithesis of "control," since it involves conforming to rigid behavioral directives that allow few options and little control in life pursuits. As we have repeatedly argued, the disorder is functional at one level, but in broader terms it has been dysfunctional by setting an extremely low upper limit on social, vocational and overall functioning. Sometimes a patient can misinterpret the positive relationship with the therapist as support for the special "interest value" of the disorder. In this case, the therapist can provide direct feedback that it is not the basis for his or her judgment of the patient.

In sum, a significant aspect of Phase II of therapy is challenging dysfunctional self-schemas as models of self-evaluation and self-esteem. However, the maladaptive models of self-evaluation that are eroded through this process must be replaced with meaningful alternatives. Patients need to gradually develop other credible options for self-reinforcement that are inherently satisfying and more responsive to "real interests" than "idealized interests." This often requires exploring new vocational roles, recreational activities, and relationships. The movement away from earlier modes of self-definition to new alternatives is usually done with considerable trepidation. It can involve rejecting values and roles chosen by family members or friends. The result is self-doubt and sometimes significant interpersonal conflicts. The therapist plays a vital role in this process by encouraging and reinforcing the pursuit of more personally relevant and more adaptive new goals.

Interrelationships among Self-Concept Variables

Self-concept deficits tend to interact, blend together, and present as a somewhat confusing amalgam. It is useful for the therapist to help the patient to "unpackage" them and develop priorities for intervention, then collaboratively design interventions that address the identified problem areas. The following excerpt illustrates a characteristic potpourri of beliefs presented by a patient, as well as the process of breaking the components down so the patient can address them more effectively.

THERAPIST. So you were saying that you are really upset today. Tell me more about it.

PATIENT. All I have been doing is studying lately; I am frightened I will fail the exam [despite top marks]. I hate being less than best [perfectionism?]. I really think that it is necessary to be successful in everything I do [grandiosity?]. I sometimes feel so stupid [low self-esteem?]. The point is that I cannot disappoint my parents—they have such confidence in me [extreme sensitivity to criticism, tendency to seek external verification?]. I got so upset thinking about all of this that I just binged all evening [overwhelmed self?].

THERAPIST. It sounds like you are feeling overwhelmed on several fronts. Let's take a look at them and decide where to go first. You are worried about the exam and concerned about upsetting your parents. Do you remember what you were thinking about that precipitated the binge episode?

PATIENT. I really can't stand the pressure.

THERAPIST. What comes to mind when you think about the pressure?

PATIENT. My parents.

THERAPIST. What will your parents think?

PATIENT. They will see me as a failure, a fraud. My true self will be exposed.

THERAPIST. OK. Is it the feeling of being stupid, a fraud, that seems more upsetting, or is it your parents' reaction that you are most worried about?

PATIENT. I guess it is really feeling like a fraud. It really happens with everyone, not just my parents.

THERAPIST. OK, why don't we stick with feeling like a fraud for a moment? Are there other situations where you feel like a fraud and feel this pressure?

PATIENT. Yeah, it is even worse at school when I am with my friend Cathy.

THERAPIST. And how does Cathy make this feeling worse?

PATIENT. She is smart, and she can see that I am a fraud—that I am not very smart.

THERAPIST. And how do you feel around Cathy?

PATIENT. Inferior . . .

This line of questioning proceeded with other examples reinforcing the observation that the central issue was the patient's feeling inferior and inferring self-worth based on performance, while the initial comment about her parents was secondary. In such a case, a novice cognitive therapist might be tempted to intervene at the first sign of faulty thinking. However, it is worthwhile to exercise patience, gradually refining the questioning process, until the salient beliefs begin to emerge.

Self-Awareness: Labeling and Expressing Emotions

Bruch (1962, 1973) considered the "lack of interoceptive awareness"—inability to accurately identify and respond to emotions and other internal sensations—as fundamental to anorexia nervosa. She observed that patients with anorexia nervosa "behave as if they had no independent rights, [and seem to believe] that neither their bodies nor their actions are self-directed, or not even their own" (p. 39). The failure to identify and respond accurately to internal sensations has received some empirical support (Bourke, Taylor, Parker, & Bagby, 1992; Schmidt, Jiwany, & Treasure, 1993). The confusion surrounding internal state extends to mistrust of the validity and reliability of attitudes, motives, and behavior. The lack of confidence in thinking processes is reflected in exaggerated self-monitoring and rigidity.

Cognitive theorists have attributed this tendency to idiosyncratic beliefs, assumptions or schemas that anorexia nervosa patients use in evaluating their inner state (Garner & Bemis, 1985). These beliefs commonly center around attitudes about the legitimacy, desirability, acceptability, or justification of inner experiences. The following comments by patients are clues to the operation of this process: "I do not know how I feel; how should I feel?," "I do not experience pleasure," "I never feel angry," "I am always energetic and never get tired," "I admire others who don't show their feelings," "I can't stand these feelings—they are too strong," "I don't feel anything—I just binge." Asked about feelings in a family interview, one patient appeared confused and responded by pointing to her mother, stating, "Ask her. She knows me better than I do."

The conflict between "how one should feel" and "how one actually feels" is not always obvious. A patient may simply deny the existence of an emotion in the presence of precursors that could be expected to lead to a particular feeling state. Sometimes bingeing, vomiting, or intense exercise can interrupt feeling states that are considered "unacceptable." For example, one patient assumed that she could only experience anger if it had a "logical" basis. Rather than directly surveying inner experience, she applied the following reasoning: "I could only be angry at my mother if she were a bad person; my mother is not a bad person; therefore, I must not be angry at my mother." Another patient reported a similar inferential process related to depression: "I could only be depressed if I were weak; I am not weak; therefore, I must not be depressed." The correction of these types of dysfunctional rules for labeling and expressing emotions follows the steps described in the section on cognitive restructuring. The initial steps of this process are illustrated in the following interchange:

THERAPIST. How did you feel when your mother implied that you could not do it yourself?

PATIENT. Nothing. I really did not feel anything.

THERAPIST. What were you thinking?

PATIENT. That she was right—I can't do anything for myself.

THERAPIST. Were you thinking anything else about your mother?

PATIENT. Well, she should let me do things on my own.

THERAPIST. Did this make you feel angry?

PATIENT. No. I never get angry, I just get sick [vomit].

THERAPIST. Can you imagine getting angry at your mother?

PATIENT. Never. She is such a good person. And anger is not a good thing to feel toward people.

THERAPIST. "Never" is really extreme. I wonder if you have some beliefs about anger that make it so bad that you would cut any feelings off almost before they got started. What would it mean for you to get angry?

The thought that "she should let me do things on my own" could be expected to be accompanied by anger. Continued queries begin to elicit incipient feelings of anger. The affect was confirmed and "legitimized," leading to more clear articulation of this emotion. A later interchange made the beliefs about anger even more explicit: "I believe that if I get angry, my mother will retaliate with outrage or withdraw. I also fear that if I allow myself to experience anger, I will completely lose control, and this will devastate my mother." The procedures described for cognitive restructuring can be used to help such a patient crystallize her dysfunctional beliefs about anger and then examine the evidence supporting their validity. Since the denial of an emotion may be genuine, the therapist must proceed cautiously without prematurely implying that the patient's experience is distorted. When faced with an apparent discrepancy between affect and content, the therapist can explore the patient's thinking about the emotion in detail.

Similar convoluted thinking is applied by some patients to other internal experiences or sensations, leading to reliance on "rules" and intellectual strategies to determine what is happening inside the body. The experience of hunger and satiety provides an example. Historically, sensations of hunger have been interpreted by humans as unpleasant; food has acquired a positive meaning because of its role in alleviating distress. Eating disorder patients, as well as many strict dieters, reconstruct biological reality by applying a "higher-order" meaning to hunger. It is relabeled as an index of virtue and self-control, rather than a sign of distress; accordingly, food and fullness acquire negative-affect-laden connotations. Bruch (1978) described patients as "brainwashing" themselves into experiencing hunger as "pleasant and desirable" (p. 4), and Selvini-Palazzoli (1978) referred to "intrapersonal paranoia" replacing natural biological processes. Changing these firmly ingrained "antibiological" meaning systems associated with hunger and satiety is a slow process, partly because the meaning system applied to internal sensations is so positively reinforcing (i.e., the patients they feel virtuous). The therapist needs to help patients identify the faulty labeling process, recognize that it is functional on one level but maladaptive in light of other goals, and then slowly correct the mislabeling process.

Similar mislabeling can be applied to other sensations, such as pleasure, relaxation, or sexual feelings. Patients commonly interpret these sensations as "wrong," frivolous, or threatening. One patient reported, "If I give in to the urge to relax, I will become a degenerate." Once distorted meanings are revised, it is important for the therapist to encourage behavioral exercises to reinforce and legitimize the new interpretations.

Developing an Interpersonal Focus in Therapy

Interpersonal concerns are inevitably expressed by anorexia nervosa patients during the protracted course of therapy. The prominence of interpersonal schemas has been the basis for their inclusion in earlier cognitive approaches to the disorder (Garner et al., 1982; Garner & Bemis, 1985; Guidano & Liotti, 1983). Fairburn (1993) has cautioned that combining cognitive-behavioral and interpersonal therapy methods is "difficult, if not impossible, because their style and focus are so different" (p. 374) in the treatment of bulimia nervosa. He has suggested different pathways to explain the effectiveness of the two forms of therapy in bulimia nervosa:

Cognitive therapy	→	Improved eating habits and therapy	→	Improved interpersonal functioning
Interpersonal therapy	→	Improved interpersonal functioning	→	Improved eating habits and attitudes

Although there are stylistic differences in the two approaches, and it may be technically possible to exclude discussion of the interpersonal domain from cognitive therapy, the theoretical justification for this separation is not obvious. Self-schemas and interpersonal schemas both influence and are influenced by interactions with others. The literature on cognitive therapy has increasingly integrated interpersonal process and interpersonal schemas without compromising fidelity to cognitive theory (Baucom & Epstein, 1990; Beck et al., 1990; Safran & Segal, 1990; Liotti, 1993; Linehan, 1993). The interpersonal focus usually becomes more prominent in Phase II of therapy. Although this requires a shift in therapy content, the systematic reliance on standard cognitive procedures continues. Patients tend to apply the same types of schematic processing errors and dysfunctional assumptions to interpersonal relationships as those displayed in other areas.

An initial step in evaluating interpersonal relationships involves distinguishing between factors that appear to be secondary to the eating disorder and those that may be primary. Together, the therapist and the patient carefully review the nature of the patient's relationships prior to the onset of the eating disorder. What have been the satisfying and unsatisfying aspects of her relationships in the past? Is it possible to identify interpersonal strengths undermined by the eating disorder symptoms? Are there interpersonal fears or deficits that have been ameliorated by the eating disorder? Therapy sessions and homework need to be directed toward exposing the limitations the eating disorder places on social and intimate relationships. This leads to the inevitable conclusion that the social, emotional, and lifestyle restrictions created by a serious eating disorder preclude most healthy relationships. A healthy and informed partner rarely chooses to have a relationship with a person with an eating disorder; likewise, the strains of an eating disorder often lead to the destruction of a healthy relationship.

The next step is providing the patient with a cognitive conceptualization of interpersonal relationships. Baucom and Epstein (1990) distinguish five interrelated cognitive phenomena relevant to the development and maintenance of dysfunctional relationships: (1) perceptions (about what events occur), (2) attributions (about why events occur), (3) expectations (predictions of what will occur), (4) assumptions (about the nature of the world and correlations among events), and (5) beliefs or standards (about what "should" be). These cognitive variables are natural aspects of all relationships; however, each is subject to distortion. Persistent distortions can lead to emotional distress and dysfunctional relationships. It could be argued that the ideal format for changing dysfunctional interpersonal relationships involves direct participation by all parties. However, circumstances may preclude this, or it may be that the patient needs to alter dysfunctional thinking patterns in order to cultivate satisfying relationships.

The following are examples of common overlapping dysfunctional relationship themes in anorexia nervosa: (1) reinforcement of eating disorder symptoms or the "sick role" in relationships; (2) the patient's assumption of the caretaker role in relationships; (3) marked conflict or conflict avoidance; (4) difficulties in role transition (e.g., adolescence, leaving home, college, marriage); (5) lack of social support; (6) need for approval, fears of rejection, and excessive dependence; (7) lack of assertiveness; (8) repeated choices of unsatisfactory partners or sabotaging of relationships; (9) abusive relationships; (10) sexual conflicts; (11) inability to maintain intimate relationships; (12) jealousy; (13) grief.

Eating disorder symptoms often carry an interpersonal message or serve an interpersonal function. They may be a relatively "safe" way to communicate anger or elicit signs of support. Problematic interpersonal situations can also be triggers for eating disorder symptoms. These interpersonal markers can allow access to beliefs and assumptions about the relationships that may have been short-circuited in the past by symptoms. Then the process of identifying and changing dysfunctional interpersonal schemas is similar to that described earlier in the section on cognitive restructuring.

The focus on interpersonal relationships inevitably leads to the recognition that communication is complex and can occur on two or more levels. The content of an interaction may be congruent or discordant with communication occurring on another, higher-order or "metacommunication" level—a concept developed more fully in communication theory (Watzlawick et al., 1967) and applied to anorexia nervosa in the context of family therapy (Minuchin, Rosman & Baker, 1978; Selvini Palazzoli, 1978). A message sent on one level of meaning may be rejected, denied, or qualified on another level, in order to avoid directly confronting a threatening issue. For example, the mother of one patient relayed verbally that she loved her daughter dearly, but the sarcastic tone belied the content. Although these observations are derived from communication theory, their conceptual overlap with cognitive theory and application to anorexia nervosa have been noted for some time (Garner et al., 1982; Guidano & Liotti, 1983). Again, the different and sometimes contradictory levels of meaning are not specific to eating disorders. However, the eating disorder patient's inability to decode or interpret conflicting meanings can be a source of emotional distress that contributes to eating disorder symptoms.

Cognitive therapy generally eschews the exploration of historical material; however, this approach can be therapeutic in examining interpersonal schemas. First, it is sometimes necessary to examine historical relationships to find recurrent interpersonal patterns. Second, it can be useful for patients to develop some understanding of the historical events and relationships that may have made particular interpersonal schemas "adaptive." Understanding the earlier adaptive context can allow the patients to make sense of their current dysfunctional interpersonal schemas.

As discussed earlier in the section on the therapeutic relationship, the sessions provide *in vivo* opportunities to assess dysfunctional interpersonal schemas that may generalize outside of therapy. For example, a patient may be encouraged to examine beliefs that interfere with assertiveness and then to practice assertiveness in the therapy session. The therapist and the patient then need to plan out-of-session opportunities to apply this newly acquired skill outside of the therapy session.

Involving the Family in Therapy

Support for involving the family in the treatment of anorexia nervosa comes from a number of sources. First, as indicated earlier, there are ethical, financial, and practical grounds for including the parents in the treatment of younger anorexia nervosa patients. Second, recovered patients consider the resolution of family and interpersonal problems as pivotal to their recovery (Hsu et al., 1992; Rorty, Yager, & Rossotto, 1993). Third, there is evidence that family factors, such as levels of parental expressed emotion, are important predictors of outcome in

adolescent eating disorders (van Furth et al., 1996). Finally, though early reports may have overstated the effectiveness of family therapy (Martin, 1983; Minuchin et al., 1978; Selvini Palazzoli, 1974), this mode of intervention has had an enduring impact in the treatment of anorexia nervosa (Vandereycken, Kog, & Vanderlinden, 1989) and has received empirical support in controlled trials (Crisp et al., 1991; Russell, Szmukler, Dare, & Eisler, 1987). Comparing individual and family therapy, Russell et al. (1987) found family therapy superior for younger, less chronic patients. Crisp et al. (1991) reported that 3 months of outpatient individual and family psychotherapy sessions were as effective as intensive inpatient treatment at a 1-year follow-up on measures of weight gain, return of menses, and key psychosocial variables.

Practical factors are sufficiently compelling to justify the family approach with some patients; however, our primary impetus for integrating family and cognitive approaches to anorexia nervosa is the conceptual harmony that can be achieved in integrating these two treatment models (Garner et al., 1982; Garner, Garfinkel, & Irvine, 1986). On a fundamental level, there is agreement between models that "meaning" is the primary locus of clinical concern. Also, both models assume that symptoms are adaptive on one level of meaning and dysfunctional on another. Nevertheless, attempts to find common theoretical ground between cognitive and family therapy have revealed key differences as well as significant areas of overlap (Epstein, Schlesinger, & Dryden, 1988; Leslie, 1988). Some contrasts relate to intervention tactics and style, whereas others pertain to the language and conceptualization of the change process (Epstein et al., 1988). Epstein et al. (1988) define the role of the cognitive therapist as that of a consultant to clients, who generate, accept, or reject new cognitions based on rational evaluation of the evidence. This differs from the role of the systems and structural therapist, who provides new meaning to symptoms and prescribes behavioral change. However, the evolution of cognitive theory toward including different levels of meaning tends to blur these distinctions. The central question remains this: How is family therapy conducted from a cognitive perspective?

One issue that often bitterly divides the family and individual therapy camps may actually be illusory. It pertains to the mistaken assumption that family therapists rely exclusively on the family format for sessions. Although the point has not been widely publicized, Minuchin et al. (1978) recommended family therapy sessions only in the beginning for older adolescents; they advocated "moving quickly to separate the patient into individual sessions and the parents into marital sessions in order to foster disengagement" (p. 132). Family therapists argue that an eating disorder can maintain certain dysfunctional roles, alliances, conflicts, or interactional patterns within the family. Eating symptoms may be functional by directing attention away from basic conflicts in the family. For example, eating symptoms may prevent parents from addressing serious marital discord. Whether the format is individual or family, the conceptual framework offered by systems theorists can be directly translated into terms consistent with modern cognitive theory. Again, the cornerstone of systemic and structural family theory is the recognition that symptoms and behaviors function on different levels, and that they are adaptive at one level but maladaptive at another. In both cognitive and family therapy, the primary objective is to expose and alter meanings, generally by achieving shifts in interactional patterns. Another premise of both orientations to family therapy is that an eating disorder can deflect members of the family away from the developmental tensions that naturally emerge with the transition to puberty and the attendant preparation for emancipation. In this case, the eating disorder serves as a maladaptive solution to the child's struggle to achieve autonomy. Moves toward independence are perceived as a threat to family unity and activate behaviors aimed at preserving the status quo. This view is consistent with other major theories of anorexia nervosa including the cognitive formulations we have presented earlier. The only difference is the degree of emphasis on the individual's versus the family's reaction to this same predicament.

As they do in other interpersonal relationships, cognitive variables such as expectations, assumptions, and information-processing errors influence meaning and resulting interactions within the family. Cognitive schemas do not develop in isolation, but rather reflect repetitive family interactional patterns. Minuchin et al. (1978) identified four interactional patterns characteristic of families with anorexia nervosa: "enmeshment," "overprotectiveness," "conflict avoidance," and "rigidity." These interactional patterns reflect underlying assumptions about roles, conflict, and boundary rules in the family. In an enmeshed family, there is a low tolerance for independence because its connotation is threatening to one or more members of the family. Similarly, overprotectiveness in a family rests on the assumption that extreme protection is required. The family provides the primary context for the development of accurate interpretations of experiences, as well as unrealistic, erroneous, or dysfunctional ones. A pattern of distortions by one family member can create an escalating chain of dysfunctional interactions or conflicts in the family. Moreover, differences in rules, values, or the interpretation of events by various family members can be expected to lead to family conflicts.

The cognitive therapist does not assume the specific meaning behind interactional patterns, but tries to assist the patient and the family in identifying dysfunctional assumptions through questioning and the prescription of behavioral change. Some examples illustrate multilevel beliefs. One patient did not know why she was so angry at her mother's cheerful and congenial manner until she realized that it was really insincere. This same patient communicated her anger in her conflict-avoidant family by vomiting, claiming that her behavior was involuntary. The clue to the meaning of her behavior was that she always left the bathroom door open and retched so that all could hear. By defining her vomiting as involuntary, she denied its hostile intent and avoided reprisals.

Another adolescent began making moves toward independence by requesting more personal privacy. This threatened her mother, whose self-esteem was overly dependent on her role as a caretaker. In such a case, multiple meanings may lead to complicated responses. On one level the mother may believe that independence is legitimate, but on another level she may be so distressed that she responds with despondence, withdrawal, or rejection. In one family session, a mother tearfully described how proud she was that her daughter had decided to move out of the home. When asked why she was crying while describing her pride, she confessed that she did not know how she could cope now that her children were leaving. Everyone in the family may be aware of the predicament and respond to both aspects of the dilemma in different ways. The adolescent may feel drawn to independence and angered at steps to block her autonomy, but at the same time she may be fearful of rejection and withdrawal. The patient may even experience guilt associated with the wish for privacy or independence. She may engage in rebellious actions and deny that they are self-motivated. In some cases, this can apply to idiosyncratic eating patterns or vomiting. There are many possible scenarios. Since beliefs appear contradictory or are denied, behavioral experiments must be arranged to test hypotheses related to their presence and influence. This is where family therapists have been innovative in applying behavioral probes to test and challenge beliefs. In one family, simply legislating that the door to the patient's room should remain closed created such extreme responses that denial of the enmeshed pattern was no longer tenable. This is analogous to the behavioral probes we have recommended earlier for revealing the multiple levels and valences of meaning. An anorexic patient may profess to be following through on an eating plan while losing weight. In the same way, the results of the family experiment become the focus of cognitive interventions aimed at examining and revising dysfunctional beliefs underlying the enmeshed pattern. The challenge of therapy is in identifying and then altering the complex and multilevel meaning systems operating in the family.

In a minority of cases, the eating disorder is at least partially maintained by the assumption that it has resulted in increased caring on the part of others. Indeed, profound weight loss can be expected to result in intense worry, distress, and attentiveness on the part of family members. Family therapy in such a case would be concerned with two issues. The first is to identify the accurate meaning or function of the behavior for the entire family, and to prescribe more adaptive ways of achieving nurturance. The second is to challenge dysfunctional thoughts held by particular individuals in the family. The patient's assumption that the disorder is providing greater nurturance can be met with a detailed exploration of the pros and cons of maintaining the disorder. For example, questions along several lines of argument can be explored: (1) Even if the patient is receiving greater care for maintaining her disorder, what are the implications for the future? (2) Even if the disorder results in the initial intensification of family concern, what are the chances that this will be replaced by resentment, disaffection, and ultimate disengagement?

Although there are many areas of overlap, it is important to emphasize that certain interventions recommended by family therapists are inconsistent with the collaborative style of cognitive therapy. For example, the systemic family therapy approach does not focus on food refusal. Rather, eating disorder symptoms are given a positive connotation and relabeled as necessary in order to preserve the stability of the family system. The therapist usually evokes a "therapeutic paradox" by prescribing the continuation of symptoms (Selvini Palazzoli, 1978).

PHASE III: PREVENTING RELAPSE AND PREPARING FOR TERMINATION

The primary tasks of Phase III are preparing the patient for termination and developing specific strategies to reduce the likelihood of relapse (Vitousek & Orimoto, 1993). During this phase of treatment, the interval between meetings is extended to every other week or longer. In preparation for termination, patients need to develop confidence that they can cope with life's challenges on their own. There are several key aspects to this final phase of treatment.

Summarizing Progress

In preparation for termination, it is useful for the patient to "take stock" of the changes made during treatment. The therapist can guide the process of reviewing of improvements in eating disorder symptoms, self-esteem, thinking patterns, social functioning, vocational adjustment, and overall lifestyle. Patients sometimes remain wistful about certain aspects of their eating disorder. They may recollect the benefits of life's being much simpler when its focus was narrowed to food and weight. Some may even continue to view the disorder as having been a sign of self-control, discipline, and personal achievement. This is particularly true if it was associated with improved functioning in certain areas (e.g., school performance). Such patients need to be reminded that the positive outcomes of the disorder are limited, since they almost always lead to debilitation in the long run. At the same time, there may have been inadvertent benefits to having had anorexia nervosa. Some patients recognize that their premorbid value system, dominated by appearances, would have precluded their ever seeking treatment despite their underlying depression, low self-esteem, and troubled interpersonal relationships. In this sense, their disorder served an unforeseen purpose in their personal growth.

Reviewing Fundamentals of Continued Progress

It is useful for the therapist to summarize (repeatedly, if necessary) the aspects of treatment that have played a key role in symptomatic improvement. For example, it is essential to reinforce the absolute need to maintain regular patterns of eating. Ideally, patients should conclude treatment with a resolute "antidieting" stance. The personal sacrifices resulting from restrictive dieting can be bolstered by theoretical arguments for its broader social harm (Garner, 1995; Garner & Wooley, 1991; Wooley & Garner, 1991). Although patients should be discouraged from returning to obsessive checking of their body weight, they should agree to a plan for periodic weighings to safeguard against the tendency to drift downward. The cognitive-behavioral principles and tools that have been most helpful during treatment should also be reviewed. It needs to be emphasized that life will not be problem-free, but that knowledge of coping strategies is one key to future adjustment.

Summarizing Areas of Continued Vulnerability

Long-term follow-up studies of anorexia nervosa indicate that although some patients recover fully, others continue to experience a wide range of emotional problems—including anxiety, depression, personality disorders, and weight preoccupation—even if behavioral symptoms have ameliorated (Casper, 1990; Eckert, Halmi, Marchi, Grove, & Crosby, 1995; Schork, Eckert, & Halmi, 1994; Steinhausen et al., 1991; Stonehill & Crisp, 1977; Toner, Garfinkel, & Garner, 1986; Windauer, Lennerts, Talbot, Touyz, & Beumont, 1993). In an 8- to 10-year follow-up by Casper (1990), 25% of patients classified as having a good outcome were still weight-preoccupied and depressed.

It should be stressed that vulnerability to eating disorder symptoms can continue for many years. A valuable strategy in avoiding relapse is remaining alert to areas of potential vulnerability. These include vocational stress, holidays, and difficult interpersonal relationships, as well as major life transitions. Patients may become

distressed if they continue to gain weight. They may also be vulnerable during pregnancy. Patients without any overt symptoms may remain quite sensitive about weight and shape. They need to be prepared for encounters with people who may have seen them at a low body weight. During the termination phase of treatment, patients need to practice adaptive cognitive responses to well-meaning comments (e.g., "I see you have gained weight" or "My, how you have changed"). Patients may even need to be prepared for occasional callous comments about their weight. Vulnerability to relapse increases during periods of psychological distress. Susceptibility to relapse may also increase with positive life changes and enhanced self-confidence. Fresh relationships, career advancement, increased physical fitness, and overall improvement in self-confidence can activate latent beliefs: "Now that things are going so well, maybe I can lose a bit of weight and things will be even better." Patients need to be reminded that weight loss is enticing and insidious in its effects. Initial results may be positive; however, the adverse effects on mood and eating are inevitable over time.

Reviewing the Warning Signs of Relapse

It is useful to review early signs of relapse, with particular attention to weight or shape preoccupation, binge eating, precipitous weight gain, gradual or rapid weight loss, and loss of menstrual periods. Patients need to ask themselves periodically, "Am I thinking too much about weight?" Sometimes weight loss occurs for other reasons, such as depression or illness. Although the initial intention may not relate to weight or shape concerns, these may be activated later. Any significant change in body weight, whatever the reason, should be a matter of concern. The therapist should make early warning signs as concrete as possible. For example, depression should be identified by such signs and symptoms as poor sleep, loss of appetite, crying spells, restlessness, and dysphoria.

Clarifying When to Return to Treatment

The therapist should encourage the maintenance of a low threshold for returning to treatment. It is not uncommon for patients to believe that a return to treatment would be a humiliating or unacceptable admission of failure. Common beliefs that interfere with reinitiating therapy are "I should be able to do this on my own now," "If I am having problems again, it means recovery is hopeless," and "My therapist will be disappointed or angry." Since patients commonly delay the reinitiation of treatment too long, a conservative approach is a good policy. If patients are not sure whether they should return for a follow-up consultation, this means that they should. Sometimes it is useful for the therapist to define his or her role as a "family doctor" for eating disorders. Regular "checkups" are prudent, and meetings at the earliest sign of relapse are the best protection against escalation of symptoms.

What about Those Who Do Not Respond Favorably to Treatment?

Data from 67 follow-up studies from 1953 to 1989 attest to the variability in response to treatment (Steinhausen & Glanville, 1983; Steinhausen et al., 1991). The topic of terminating therapy for those patients who fail to make progress is often neglected. In this case, termination is commonly viewed as a sign of personal inadequacy and weakness on the part of the patient and the therapist alike. The ensuing frustration may lead to abrupt termination with inadequate follow-up plans. Patients are then reluctant to seek further assistance when their medical or psychological condition deteriorates. If careful evaluation leads to the conclusion (1) that the patient has had an adequate course of psychotherapy, (2) that she is not in imminent psychological or medical danger, (3) that she is sufficiently symptomatic to suggest ongoing potential medical risk, and (4) that there is no clear rationale for further psychotherapy, then termination from psychotherapy may be very appropriate as long as it is made conditional on the patient's agreeing to participate in ongoing "medical management" (Garner & Needleman, Chapter 5, this volume). The goal of "medical management" is very different from that of psychotherapy. Rather than focusing on overcoming the eating disorder, it is aimed at maintaining medical and psychological stability. It can be conducted in an individual or group format, meeting weekly with medical supervision. Body weight, electrolytes, and vital signs should be checked, with appropriate referral to medical specialists as needed. Patients derive the added benefits of group support and sharing with similarly afflicted patients. In some cases, these groups set the stage for renewed efforts to actively address the eating disorder symptoms.

A Final Comment on Hospitalization

A common reason for termination from outpatient treatment is the need for hospitalization. Criteria for hospitalization have been briefly reviewed in an earlier section on assessment and are elaborated elsewhere (Garner & Needleman, Chapter 5, this volume), as are the details of inpatient management (Anderson, Bowers, & Evans, Chapter 17, this volume; Garfinkel & Garner, 1982; Garner & Sackeyfio, 1993). However, we would be remiss in failing to underscore the point that inpatient or partial hospitalization remains a key component in the ongoing management of anorexia nervosa patients. Considering the emotional and financial expense of unproductive outpatient therapy, the structured hospital environment may be a desirable and humane alternative, even if it is not medically necessary. The therapist plays a vital role in encouraging the patient and family to pursue this treatment option. The decision to implement hospitalization often involves the delicate philosophical balance between free will and determinism (Crisp, 1980; Goldner, 1989; Tiller, Schmidt, & Treasure, 1993). On one hand, patients can be seen as free to maintain their eating disorder, even if it involves suboptimal functioning. On the other hand, it can be argued that the disorder so seriously impairs judgment that patients are unable to exercise free choice, particularly as it applies to appraisal of medical risks. Probably both points of view are correct, and there appears to be no consensus regarding the solution to the dilemma. Goldner (1989) suggests the following strategies to minimize treatment refusal: seeking a voluntary alliance, identifying the reasons for treatment refusal, carefully explaining the reasons for treatment recommendations, remaining flexible, showing respect for the patient's belief in the importance of thinness, minimizing intrusive interventions, weighing the risks and benefits of active treatment, avoiding punitive interventions, involving the family whenever possible, and considering involuntary treatment only when nonintervention constitutes an immediate and serious danger. The cognitive model described in this chapter echoes many of these recommendations and provides practical strategies for their implementation.

Once hospitalization is initiated, the duration

of treatment required to achieve the target weight needs to be realistic. High relapse rates are the unfortunate consequences of premature discharge (Baran, Weltzin, & Kaye, 1995). Finally, we want to stress that failure to respond to treatment does not always predict future failure. Some patients recover after multiple relapses that may include numerous hospitalizations. These patients may feel desperate and hopeless in the protracted struggle with anorexia nervosa; however, a stance of steadfast optimism is supported by published reports of recovered patients (Hsu et al., 1992; Windauer et al., 1993), as well as by our own clinical experience.

CONCLUSION

This chapter has refined and elaborated methods we have previously described. The cognitive procedures are presented in a manual format designed to facilitate teaching, clinical training, and controlled research. Cognitive-behavioral procedures for anorexia nervosa are divided into three treatment phases, with specific interventions at each stage. The manual is meant to complement theoretical formulations presented elsewhere (Garner & Bemis, 1982, 1985; Vitousek & Ewald, 1993; Vitousek & Orimoto, 1993). However, the etiological significance of cognitive mechanisms can be considered both conceptually and methodologically separate from the utility of cognitive-behavioral therapy in treating anorexia nervosa. As Hollon and Beck (1979) have noted, "there need be no necessary congruence between the factors that trigger a disorder and the factors that alleviate it" (p. 155). Variables of theoretical significance to the cognitive model, such as weight-related self-schemas, errors in information processing, and the operation of negative and positive self-reinforcement, merit continued investigation in their own right. Higher-order beliefs hypothesized to precede, to coexist with, and often to persist beyond the disorder itself have been the source of increasing investigation (Vitousek & Hollon, 1990).

Since anorexia nervosa was first recognized as a diagnostic entity, numerous etiological formulations have been proposed. However, at present, the cognitive model as well as other therapeutic approaches for anorexia nervosa must be considered tentative and provisional because of the paucity of controlled outcome research. A major obstacle to evaluative research is that descriptions of the conduct of outpatient psychotherapy lack sufficient detail to allow replication. Previous descriptions of the conduct of cognitive-behavioral therapy for anorexia nervosa (Garner & Bemis, 1982, 1985) have been applied unsystematically in clinical settings; however, they have not spawned research trials that could support or refute our favorable opinion of the efficacy of this form of treatment. Nevertheless, we do believe that clinical results are encouraging enough to warrant further examinations through more systematic clinical trials and comparative studies. Indeed, several rigorous research studies are currently in progress that will provide much-needed data bearing on the effectiveness of cognitive-behavioral therapy for anorexia nervosa. Thus, the tentative nature of our hypothesis about the applicability of cognitive-behavioral methods to this disorder cannot be overemphasized; however, we hope that the refinements presented here added to accounts elsewhere will stimulate testing of this model in research settings.

NOTES

1. Because the vast majority of patients with anorexia nervosa are female, feminine nouns and pronouns are used throughout the chapter (as in this quotation) to refer to these patients.

2. Minuchin, Rosman, and Baker (1978) observed: "With the child's entrance into adolescence, she finds herself in a crisis. Her wish to participate with a group of peers conflicts with her orientation to the family" (p. 60). Earlier, they note: "Eventually, the growth of the children must be met with change in the organization of daily life, a process that involves time and discomfort at best. The whole family must cope with the resulting sense of loss and strangeness" (p. 58). Selvini Palazzoli (1978) states that it "is in this precarious psychological situation that the physical developments associated with puberty suddenly overtake them [the anorexic patients]" (p. 68). Bruch (1978) identifies a treatment goal as the fear of "growing up and maturing." She states that "many [patients] will readily agree to this as their goal, that they want to be independent people, even though their total behavior reflects their fear of adulthood and grim determination not to grow up" (p. 139).

3. With reference to eating disorders, remarkable parallels have been noted between Bruch's (1973, 1978) recommendations for the conduct of psychotherapy and the principles advocated by cognitive

therapists (Garner & Bemis, 1982; Garner et al., 1982; Guidano & Liotti, 1983). Bruch (1978) described psychotherapy as "a process during which erroneous assumptions and attitudes are recognized, defined and challenged so that they can be abandoned. It is important to proceed slowly and to use concrete small events as episodes for illustrating certain false assumptions or illogical deductions" (1978, pp. 143–144). Although there is no indication that Bruch would confirm the correspondence we have observed between her methods and those proposed by cognitive theorists, Goldfried (1980) has argued that the existence of common clinical strategies across different therapeutic orientations should be reassuring, since they probably indicate the most durable methods for prompting behavior change.

REFERENCES

American Psychiatric Association. (1987). *Diagnostic and statistical manual of mental disorders* (3rd ed., rev.). Washington, DC: Author.

American Psychiatric Association. (1993). Practice guideline for eating disorders. *American Journal of Psychiatry, 150,* 212–228.

Baran, S. A., Weltzsin, T. E., & Kaye, W. H. (1995). Low discharge weight and outcome in anorexia nervosa. *American Journal of Psychiatry, 152,* 1070–1072.

Bachrach, L. K., Guido, D., Katzman, D., Litt, I. F., & Marcus, R. (1990). Decreased bone density in adolescent girls with anorexia nervosa. *Pediatrics, 86,* 440–447.

Baucom, D. H., & Epstein, N. (1990). *Cognitive-behavioral marital therapy.* New York: Brunner/Mazel.

Beck, A. T. (1976). *Cognitive therapy and the emotional disorders.* New York: International Universities Press.

Beck, A. T., Freeman, A., & Associates. (1990). *Cognitive therapy of personality disorders.* New York: Guilford Press.

Beck, A. T., Rush, A. J., Shaw, B. F., & Emery, G. (1979). *Cognitive therapy of depression.* New York: Guilford Press.

Bemis, K. M. (1983). A comparison of functional relationships in anorexia nervosa and phobia. In P. L. Darby, P. E. Garfinkel, D. M. Garner, & D. V. Coscina (Eds.), *Anorexia nervosa: Recent developments in research* (pp. 403–416). New York: Alan R. Liss.

Beutler, L. E., Machado, P. P. P., & Neufeldt, S. A. (1994). Therapist variables. In A. E. Bergin & S. L. Garfield (Eds.), *Handbook of psychotherapy and behavior change* (4th ed., pp. 229–269). New York: Wiley.

Biller, B. M., Saxe, V., Herzog, D. B., Rosenthal, D. I., Holtzman, S., & Klibanski, A. (1989). Mechanisms of osteoporosis in adult and adolescent women with anorexia nervosa. *Journal of Clinical Endocrinology and Metabolism, 68,* 548–554.

Bo-Lynn, G., Santa-Ana, C. A., Morawski, S. G., & Fordtran, J. S. (1983). Purging and calorie absorption in bulimic patients and normal women. *Annals of Internal Medicine, 99,* 14–17.

Bourke, M. P., Taylor, G. J., Parker, J. D. A., & Bagby, R. M. (1992). Alexithymia in women with anorexia nervosa: A preliminary investigation. *British Journal of Psychiatry, 161,* 240–243.

Braun, D. L., Sunday, R., & Halmi, K. A. (1994). Psychiatric comorbidity in patients with eating disorders. *Psychological Medicine, 24,* 859–867.

Brownell, K. D. (1982). Obesity: Understanding and treating a serious, prevalent, and refractory disorder. *Journal of Consulting and Clinical Psychology, 50,* 820–840.

Bruch, H. (1962). Perceptual and conceptual disturbances in anorexia nervosa. *Psychosomatic Medicine, 24,* 187–194.

Bruch, H. (1973). *Eating disorders: Obesity, anorexia nervosa and the person within.* New York: Basic Books.

Bruch, H. (1978). *The golden cage: The enigma of anorexia nervosa.* Cambridge, MA: Harvard University Press.

Burns, D. D. (1993). *Ten days to self-esteem.* New York: Quill/William Morrow.

Casper, R. C. (1990). Personality features of women with good outcome from restricting anorexia nervosa. *Psychosomatic Medicine, 52,* 156–170.

Casper, R. C., Eckert, E. D., Halmi, K. A., Goldberg, S. C., & Davis, J. M. (1980). Bulimia: Its incidence and clinical importance in patients with anorexia nervosa. *Archives of General Psychiatry, 37,* 1030–1034.

Channon, S., DeSilva, P., Hemsley, D., & Perkins, R. (1989). A controlled trial of cognitive-behavioural and behavioural treatment of anorexia nervosa. *Behaviour Research and Therapy, 27,* 529–535.

Cohler, B. J. (1977). The significance of the therapist's feelings in the treatment of anorexia nervosa. In S. C. Feinstein & P. L. Giovacchini (Eds.), *Adolescent psychiatry* (Vol. 5, pp. 352–384). New York: Jason Aronson.

Comerci, G. D. (1990). Medical complications of anorexia nervosa and bulimia nervosa. *Medical Clinics of North America, 74,* 1293–1310.

Cooper, P. J., & Fairburn, C. G. (1984). Cognitive behavioral treatment for anorexia nervosa: Some preliminary findings. *Journal of Psychosomatic Research, 28,* 493–499.

Crisp, A. H. (1970). Anorexia nervosa: 'Feeding disorder,' nervous malnutrition or weight phobia? *World Review of Nutrition, 12,* 452–504.

Crisp, A. H. (1980). *Anorexia nervosa: Let me be.* London: Academic Press.

Crisp, A. H., Callender, J. S., Halek, C., & Hsu, L. K. G. (1992). Long-term mortality in anorexia nervosa: A 20 year follow-up of the St. George's and Aberdeen cohorts. *British Journal of Psychiatry, 161,* 104–107.

Crisp, A. H., Norton, K., Gowers, S., Halek, C., Bowyer, C., Yeldham, D., Levell, G., & Bhat, A. (1991). A controlled study of the effect of therapies aimed at adolescent and family psychopathology in anorexia nervosa. *British Journal of Psychiatry, 159,* 325–333.

Dally, P. J., & Gomez, J. (1979). *Anorexia nervosa.* London: Heinemann.

Devlin, M. J., Walsh, B. T., Katz, J. L., Roose, S. P., Linkie, D. M., Wright, L., Vande Wiele, R., & Glassman, A. H. (1989). Hypothalamic–pituitary–gonadal function in anorexia nervosa and bulimia. *Psychiatry Research, 28,* 11–24.

Eckert, E. D., Halmi, K. A., Marchi, P., Grove, W., & Crosby, R. (1995). Ten-year follow-up of anorexia nervosa: Clinical course and outcome. *Psychological Medicine, 25,* 143–156.

Ellis, A. (1962). *Reason and emotion in psychotherapy.* New York: Lyle Stuart.

Ellis, A., & Harper, R. A. (1975). *A new guide to rational living.* Englewood Cliffs, NJ: Prentice-Hall.

Epstein, N., Schlesinger, S. E., & Dryden, W. (1988). Concepts and methods of cognitive-behavioral family treatment. In N. Epstein, S. E. Schlesinger, & W. Dryden (Eds.), *Cognitive-behavioral therapy with families* (pp. 5–48). New York: Brunner/Mazel.

Fairburn, C. G. (1981). A cognitive-behavioral approach to the management of bulimia. *Psychological Medicine, 141,* 631–633.

Fairburn, C. G. (1985). Cognitive-behavioral treatment for bulimia. In D. M. Garner & P. E. Garfinkel (Eds.), *Handbook of psychotherapy for anorexia nervosa and bulimia* (pp. 160–192). New York: Guilford Press.

Fairburn, C. G. (1993). Interpersonal psychotherapy for bulimia nervosa. In G. L. Klerman & M. M. Weissman (Eds.), *New applications of interpersonal psychotherapy* (pp. 353–378). Washington, DC: American Psychiatric Press.

Fairburn, C. G., Marcus, M. D., & Wilson, G. W. (1993). Cognitive-behavioral therapy for binge eating and bulimia nervosa. In C. G. Fairburn & G. T. Wilson (Eds.), *Binge eating: Nature, assessment, and treatment* (pp. 361–404). New York: Guilford Press.

Fairburn, C. G., Norman, P. A., Welch, S. L., O'Connor, M. E., Doll, H. A., & Peveler, R. C. (1995). A prospective study of outcome in bulimia nervosa and the long-term effects of three psychological treatments. *Archives of General Psychiatry, 52,* 304–312.

Favaro, A., & Santonastaso, P. (1996). Purging behaviors, suicide attempts, and psychiatric symptoms in 398 eating disordered subjects. *International Journal of Eating Disorders, 20,* 99–103.

Festinger, L. (1957). *A theory of cognitive dissonance.* Stanford, CA: Stanford University Press.

Fichter, M. (1995). Inpatient treatment of anorexia nervosa. In K. D. Brownell & C. G. Fairburn (Eds.), *Eating disorders and obesity: A comprehensive handbook* (pp. 336–343). New York: Guilford Press.

Fiske, S. T., & Taylor, S. E. (1984). *Social cognition.* Reading, MA: Addison-Wesley.

Flavell, J. H. (1963). *The developmental psychology of Jean Piaget.* (D. C. McClelland, Ed.). Princeton, NJ: Van Nostrand.

Frisch, R. E. (1983). Fatness and reproduction: Delayed menarche and amenorrhea of ballet dancers and college athletes. In P. L. Darby, P. E. Garfinkel, D. M. Garner, & D. V. Coscina (Eds.), *Anorexia nervosa: Recent developments in research* (pp. 343–364). New York: Alan R. Liss.

Frisch, R., & McArthur, J. (1974). Menstrual cycles: Fatness as a determinant of minimum weight for height necessary for their maintenance and onset. *Science, 185,* 941–951.

van Furth, E. F., van Strien, D. C., Martina, L. M. L., van Son, M. J. M., Hendrickx, J. J. P., & van Engeland, H. (1996). Expressed emotion and the prediction of outcome in adolescent anorexia nervosa. *International Journal of Eating Disorders, 20,* 19–31.

Garfinkel, P. E., & Garner, D. M. (1982). *Anorexia nervosa: A multidimensional perspective.* New York: Brunner/Mazel.

Garfinkel, P. E., Moldofsky, H., & Garner, D. M. (1980). The heterogeneity of anorexia nervosa. *Archives of General Psychiatry, 37,* 1036–1040.

Garner, D. M. (1985). Iatrogenesis in anorexia nervosa and bulimia nervosa. *International Journal of Eating Disorders, 4,* 701–726.

Garner, D. M. (1986). Cognitive therapy for anorexia nervosa. In K. D. Brownell & J. P. Foreyt (Eds.), *Handbook*

of eating disorders (pp. 301–327). New York: Basic Books.

Garner, D. M. (1988). Anorexia nervosa. In M. Hersen & C. G. Last (Eds.), *Child behavior therapy casebook* (pp. 263–276). New York: Plenum Press.

Garner, D. M. (1991). *Eating Disorder Inventory—2: Professional manual.* Odessa, FL: Psychological Assessment Resources.

Garner, D. M. (1992). Psychotherapy of eating disorders. *Current Opinion in Psychiatry, 5,* 391–395.

Garner, D. M. (1993). Binge eating in anorexia nervosa. In C. G. Fairburn & G. T. Wilson (Eds.), *Binge eating: Nature, assessment, and treatment* (pp. 50–76). New York: Guilford Press.

Garner, D. M. (1995). Measurement of eating disorder psychopathology. In K. D. Brownell & C. G. Fairburn (Eds.), *Eating disorders and obesity: A comprehensive handbook* (pp. 117–121). New York: Guilford Press.

Garner, D. M., & Bemis, K. M. (1982). A cognitive-behavioral approach to anorexia nervosa. *Cognitive Therapy and Research, 6,* 123–150.

Garner, D. M., & Bemis, K. M. (1985). Cognitive therapy for anorexia nervosa. In D. M. Garner & P. E. Garfinkel (Eds.), *Handbook of psychotherapy for anorexia nervosa and bulimia* (pp. 107–146). New York: Guilford Press.

Garner, D. M., & Friedman, L. L. (1994). Crisis intervention for eating disorders. In F. M. Dattilio & A. Freeman (Eds.), *Cognitive-behavioral strategies in crisis intervention* (pp. 137–160). New York: Guilford Press.

Garner, D. M., & Garfinkel, P. E. (1981). Body image in anorexia nervosa: Measurement, theory and clinical implications. *International Journal of Psychiatry in Medicine, 11,* 263–284.

Garner, D. M., Garfinkel, P. E., & Bemis, K. M. (1982). A multidimensional psychotherapy for anorexia nervosa. *International Journal of Eating Disorders, 1,* 3–46.

Garner, D. M., Garfinkel, P. E., & Irvine, M. J. (1986). Integration and sequencing of treatment approaches for eating disorders. *Psychotherapy and Psychosomatics, 46,* 67–75.

Garner, D. M., Garfinkel, P. E., Schwartz, D. M., & Thompson, M. M. (1980). Cultural expectations of thinness in women. *Psychological Reports, 47,* 483–491.

Garner, D. M., Garner, M. V., & Rosen, L. W. (1993). Anorexia nervosa "restrictors" who purge: Implications for subtyping anorexia nervosa. *International Journal of Eating Disorders, 13,* 171–185.

Garner, D. M., Olmsted, M. P., Davis, R., Rockert, W., Goldbloom, D., & Eagle, M. (1990). The association between bulimic symptoms and reported psychopathology. *International Journal of Eating Disorders, 9,* 1–15.

Garner, D. M., & Parker, P. (1993). Eating disorders. In T. H. Ollendick & M. Hersen (Eds.), *Handbook of child and adolescent assessment* (pp. 384–399). Elmsford, NY: Pergamon Press.

Garner, D. M., Rockert, W., Garner, M. V., Davis, R., Olmsted, M. P., & Eagle, M. (1993). Comparison of cognitive-behavioral and supportive-expressive therapy for bulimia nervosa. *American Journal of Psychiatry, 150,* 37–46.

Garner, D. M., Rockert, W., Olmsted, M. P., Johnson, C. L., & Coscina, D. V. (1985). Psychoeducational principles in the treatment of bulimia and anorexia nervosa. In D. M. Garner & P. E. Garfinkel (Eds.), *Handbook of psychotherapy for anorexia nervosa and bulimia* (pp. 513–572). New York: Guilford Press.

Garner, D. M., & Rosen, L. W. (1990). Anorexia nervosa

and bulimia nervosa. In A. S. Bellack, M. Hersen, & A. E. Kazdin (Eds.), *International handbook of behavior modification and therapy* (2nd ed., pp. 805–817). New York: Plenum Press.

Garner, D. M., & Rosen, L. W. (1994). Aggressive and destructive behavior in eating disorders. In M. Hersen, R. Ammerman, & L. Sisson (Eds.), *Handbook of aggressive and destructive behavior in psychiatric patients* (pp. 409–428). New York: Plenum Press.

Garner, D. M., & Sackeyfio, A. H. (1993). Eating disorders. In A. S. Bellack & M. Hersen (Eds.), *Handbook of behavior therapy in the psychiatric setting* (pp. 477–497). New York: Plenum Press.

Garner, D. M., & Wooley, S. C. (1991). Confronting the failure of behavioral and dietary treatments for obesity. *Clinical Psychology Review, 11,* 729–780.

Gilligan, C. (1982). *In a different voice.* Cambridge, MA: Harvard University Press.

Gladstone, R. (1974). Mind over matter: Observations on 50 patients with anorexia nervosa. *Journal of the American Academy of Child Psychiatry, 13,* 246–263.

Goldfried, M. R. (1971). Systematic desensitization as training in self-control. *Journal of Consulting and Clinical Psychology, 37,* 228–234.

Goldfried, M. R. (1980). Toward the delineation of therapeutic change principles. *American Psychologist, 35,* 991–999.

Goldfried, M. R. (1982). Resistance and clinical behavior therapy. In P. L. Wachtel (Ed.), *Resistance: Psychodynamic and behavioral approaches* (pp. 95–114). New York: Plenum Press.

Goldfried, M. R., & Davison, G. C. (1976). *Clinical behavior therapy.* New York: Holt, Rinehart & Winston.

Goldner, E. (1989). Treatment refusal in anorexia nervosa. *International Journal of Eating Disorders, 8,* 297–306.

Greiger, R. (1975). Self-concept, self-esteem and rational–emotive therapy: A brief perspective. *Rational Living, 10,* 13–17.

Guidano, V. F., & Liotti, G. (1983). *Cognitive processes and emotional disorders: A structural approach to psychotherapy.* New York: Guilford Press.

Hall, C. S., & Lindsey, G. (1970). *Theories of personality.* New York: Wiley.

Halmi, K. A., Eckert, E., Marchi, P., Sampugnaro, V., Apple, R., & Cohen, J. (1991). Comorbidity of psychiatric diagnoses in anorexia nervosa. *Archives of General Psychiatry, 48,* 712–718.

Heatherton, T. F., Nichols, P., Mahamedi, A. M., & Keel, P. (1995). Body weight, dieting, and eating disorder symptoms among college students, 1982 to 1992. *American Journal of Psychiatry, 152,* 1623–1629.

Hoek, H. W. (1993). Review of the epidemiological studies of eating disorders. *International Review of Psychiatry, 5,* 61–74.

Hollon, S. D., & Beck, A. T. (1979). Cognitive therapy for depression. In P. C. Kendall & S. D. Hollon (Eds.), *Cognitive-behavior interventions: Theory, research, and procedures* (pp. 153–204). New York: Academic Press.

Hollon, S. D., & Beck, A. T. (1994). Cognitive and cognitive-behavioral therapies. In A. E. Bergin & S. L. Garfield (Eds.), *Handbook of psychotherapy and behavior change* (4th ed., pp. 428–466). New York: Wiley.

Hsu, L. K. G. (1988). The outcome of anorexia nervosa: A reappraisal. *Psychological Medicine, 18,* 807–812.

Hsu, L. K. G., Crisp, A. H., & Challender, J. S. (1992). Recovery in anorexia nervosa: The patient's perspective. *International Journal of Eating Disorders, 11,* 341–350.

Jacobson, N. S. (1989). The therapist–client relationship in cognitive behavior therapy: Implications for treating depression. *Journal of Cognitive Psychotherapy, 3,* 85–96.

Katz, J. L., Boyar, R. M., Roffwarg, H., Hellman, L., & Weiner, H. (1977). LHRH responsiveness in anorexia nervosa: Intactness despite prepuberal circadian LH pattern. *Psychosomatic Medicine, 39,* 241–251.

Keesey, R. E. (1993). Physiological regulation of body energy: Implications for obesity. In A. J. Stunkard & T. A. Wadden (Eds.), *Obesity: Theory and therapy* (2nd ed., pp. 77–96). New York: Raven Press.

Keys, A., Brozek, J., Henschel, A., Mickelsen, O., & Taylor, H. L. (1950). *The biology of human starvation* (2 vols.). Minneapolis: University of Minnesota Press.

Kreipe, R. E., Churchill, B. H., & Strauss, J. (1989). Long-term outcome of adolescents with anorexia nervosa. *American Journal of Diseases of Children, 143,* 1322–1327.

Leslie, L. A. (1988). Cognitive-behavioral and systems models of family therapy: How compatible are they? In N. Epstein, S. E. Schlesinger, & W. Dryden (Eds.), *Cognitive-behavioral therapy with families* (pp. 49–83). New York: Brunner/Mazel.

Linehan, M. M. (1993). *Cognitive-behavioral treatment of borderline personality disorder.* New York: Guilford Press.

Liotti, G. (1987). The resistance to change of cognitive structures: A counter-proposal to psychoanalytic metapsychology. *Journal of Cognitive Psychotherapy, 2,* 87–104.

Liotti, G. (1993). Disorganized attachment and dissociative experiences: An illustration of the developmental–ethological approach to cognitive therapy. In K. T. Kuehlwein & H. Rosen (Eds.), *Cognitive therapies in action: Evolving innovative practice* (pp. 213–239). San Francisco: Jossey-Bass.

Mahoney, M. J. (1974). *Cognitive and behavior modification.* Cambridge, MA: Ballinger.

Markus, H. (1977). Self-schemata and processing information about the self. *Journal of Personality and Social Psychology, 35,* 63–78.

Markus, H. (1990). Unresolved issues of self-representation. *Cognitive Therapy and Research, 14,* 241–253.

Markus, H., Crane, M., Bernstein, S., & Siladi, M. (1982). Self-schemata and gender. *Journal of Personality and Social Psychology, 42,* 38–50.

Martin, F. (1983). Subgroups in anorexia nervosa: A family systems study. In P. L. Darby, P. E. Garfinkel, D. M. Garner, & D. V. Coscina (Eds.), *Anorexia nervosa: Recent developments* (pp. 57–63). New York: Alan R. Liss.

Meichenbaum, D. (1974). *Therapist manual for cognitive behavior modification.* Waterloo, Ontario: University of Waterloo Press.

Minuchin, S., Rosman, B. L., & Baker, J. (1978). *Psychosomatic families: Anorexia nervosa in context.* Cambridge, MA: Harvard University Press.

Mitchell, J. E. (1986). Anorexia nervosa: Medical and physiological aspects. In K. D. Brownell & J. P. Foreyt (Eds.), *Handbook of eating disorders: Physiology, psychology, and treatment of obesity, anorexia, and bulimia* (pp. 247–265). New York: Basic Books.

Orlinsky, D. E., Grawe, K., & Parks, B. K. (1994). Process and outcome in psychotherapy: *Noch einmal.* In A. E. Bergin & S. L. Garfield (Eds.), *Handbook of psychotherapy and behavior change* (4th ed., pp. 270–376). New York: Wiley.

Orimoto, L., & Vitousek, K. (1992). Anorexia nervosa and bulimia nervosa. In P. W. Wilson (Ed.), *Principles and practices of relapse prevention* (pp. 85–127). New York: Guilford Press.

Patton, G. C., Johnson-Sabine, E., Wood, K., Mann, A. H., & Wakeling, A. (1990). Abnormal eating attitudes in London schoolgirls—A prospective epidemiological study: Outcome at twelve month follow-up. *Psychological Medicine, 20,* 383–394.

Pike, K. M., Loeb, K., & Vitousek, K. (1996). Cognitive-behavioral therapy for anorexia nervosa and bulimia nervosa. In J. K. Thompson (Ed.), *Body image: Eating disorders and obesity* (pp. 253–302). Washington, DC: American Psychological Association.

Pirke, K. M., & Ploog, D. (1987). Biology of human starvation. In P. J. V. Beumont, G. D. Burrows, & R. C. Casper (Eds.), *Handbook of eating disorders: Part 1. Anorexia and bulimia nervosa* (pp. 79–102). New York: Elsevier.

Polivy, J., & Herman, C. P. (1985). Dieting and bingeing: A causal analysis. *American Psychologist, 40,* 193–201.

Prochaska, J. O., & DiClemente, C. C. (1983). Stages and processes of self-change in smoking: Toward an integrative model of change. *Journal of Consulting and Clinical Psychology, 5,* 390–395.

Prochaska, J. O., DiClemente, C. C., & Norcross, J. C. (1992). In search of how people change: Applications to addictive behavior. *American Psychologist, 47,* 1102–1114.

Ramos, R. H., & Warren, M. P. (1995). The interrelationships of body fat, exercise, and hormonal status and their impact on reproduction and bone health. *Seminars in Perinatology, 19,* 163–170.

Rastam, M., Gilberg, C., & Gilberg, I. C. (1995). Social avoidance, social negativism, and disorders of empathy in a subgroup of young individuals with anorexia nervosa. In H. C. Steinhausen (Ed.), *Eating disorders in adolescence* (pp. 69–81). New York: Walter de Gruyter.

Rogers, T. B., Kuiper, N. A., & Kirker, W. S. (1977). Self-reference and the encoding of personal information. *Journal of Personality and Social Psychology, 35,* 667–688.

Rorty, M., Yager, J., & Rossotto, E. (1993). Why and how do women recover from bulimia nervosa? The subjective appraisals of forty women recovered for a year or more. *International Journal of Eating Disorders, 14,* 249–260.

Russell, G. F. M. (1970). Anorexia nervosa: Its identity as an illness and its treatment. In J. H. Price (Ed.), *Modern trends in psychological medicine* (Vol. 2, pp. 131–164). London: Butterworths.

Russell, G. F. M., Szmukler, G. I., Dare, C., & Eisler, I. (1987). An evaluation of family therapy in anorexia nervosa and bulimia nervosa. *Archives of General Psychiatry, 44,* 1047–1056.

Safran, J. D., & Segal, Z. V. (1990). *Interpersonal process in cognitive therapy.* New York: Basic Books.

Schmidt, U., Jiwany, A., & Treasure, J. (1993). A controlled study of alexithymia in eating disorders. *Comprehensive Psychiatry, 1,* 54–58.

Schork, E. J., Eckert, E. D., & Halmi, K. A. (1994). The relationship between psychopathology, eating disorder diagnosis, and clinical outcome at 10-year follow-up in anorexia nervosa. *Comprehensive Psychiatry, 2,* 113–123.

Selvini Palazzoli, M. (1978). *Self-starvation: From individual family therapy to the treatment of anorexia nervosa.* New York: Jason Aronson.

Sharp, C. W., & Freeman, C. P. L. (1993). The medical complications of anorexia nervosa. *British Journal of Psychiatry, 162,* 452–462.

Siemers, B., Chakmakjian, Z., & Gench, B. (1996). Bone density patterns in women with anorexia nervosa. *International Journal of Eating Disorders, 19,* 179–186.

Srinivasagam, N. M., Kaye, W. H., Plotnicov, K. H., Greeno, C., Weltzin, T. E., & Rao, R. (1995). Persistent perfectionism, symmetry, and exactness after long-term recovery from anorexia nervosa. *American Journal of Psychiatry, 152,* 1630–1634.

Steinhausen, H.-C., & Glanville, K. (1983). Retrospective and prospective follow-up studies in anorexia nervosa. *International Journal of Eating Disorders, 2,* 221–235.

Steinhausen, H.-C., Rauss-Mason, C., & Seidel, R. (1991). Follow-up studies of anorexia nervosa: A review of four decades of outcome research. *Psychological Medicine, 21,* 447–454.

Stonehill, E., & Crisp, A. H. (1977). Psychoneurotic characteristics of patients with anorexia nervosa before and after treatment and at follow-up 4 to 7 years later. *Journal of Psychosomatic Research, 21,* 189–193.

Strober, M., Salkin, B., Burroughs, J., & Morrell, W. (1982). Validity of the bulimia–restrictor distinction in anorexia nervosa: Parental personality characteristics and family psychiatric morbidity. *Journal of Nervous and Mental Disease, 170,* 345–351.

Sullivan, P. F. (1995). Mortality in anorexia nervosa. *American Journal of Psychiatry, 152,* 1073–1074.

Teasdale, J. D., & Barnard, P. J. (1993). *Affect, cognition, and change: Re-Modelling depressive thought.* Hove, England: Erlbaum.

Theander, S. (1970). Anorexia nervosa. *Acta Psychiatrica Scandinavica, 214*(Suppl.), 1–194.

Theander, S. (1985). Outcome and prognosis in anorexia nervosa and bulimia: Some results of previous investigations, compared with those of a Swedish long-term study. *Journal of Psychiatric Research, 19,* 493–508.

Thompson, J. K. (1996). *Body image: Eating disorders and obesity.* Washington, DC: American Psychological Association.

Tiller, J., Schmidt, U., & Treasure, J. (1993). Compulsory treatment for anorexia nervosa: Compassion or coercion? *British Journal of Psychiatry, 162,* 679–680.

Toner, B. B., Garfinkel, P. E., & Garner, D. M. (1986). Long-term follow-up of anorexia nervosa. *Psychosomatic Medicine, 48,* 520–529.

Toner, B. B., Garfinkel, P. E., & Garner, D. M. (1988). Affective and anxiety disorders in the long-term follow-up of anorexia nervosa. *International Journal of Psychiatry in Medicine, 18*(4), 357–364.

Treasure, J. L., Wheeler, M., King, E. A., Gordon, P. A. L., & Russell, G. F. M. (1988). Weight gain and reproductive function: Ultrasonographic and endocrine features in anorexia nervosa. *Clinical Endocrinology, 29,* 607–616.

Ushakov, G. K. (1971). Anorexia nervosa. In J. G. Howells (Ed.), *Modern perspectives in adolescent psychiatry* (pp. 274–289). Edinburgh: Oliver & Boyd.

Vandereycken, W., Kog, E., & Vanderlinden, J. (1989). *The family approach to eating disorders.* New York: PMA.

Vitousek, K. M. (1995). Cognitive-behavioral therapy for anorexia nervosa. In B. D. Brownell & C. G. Fairburn (Eds.), *Eating disorders and obesity: A comprehensive handbook* (pp. 324–329). New York: Guilford Press.

Vitousek, K. B., & Ewald, L. S. (1993). Self-representation in eating disorders: A cognitive perspective. In Z. Segal & S. Blatt (Eds.), *The self in emotional disorders: Cogni-*

tive and psychodynamic perspectives (pp. 221–257). New York: Guilford Press.

Vitousek, K. B., & Hollon, S. D. (1990). The investigation of schematic content and processing in eating disorders. *Cognitive Therapy and Research, 14,* 191–214.

Vitousek, K. B., & Orimoto, L. (1993). Cognitive-behavioral models of anorexia nervosa, bulimia nervosa, and obesity. In P. Kendall & K. Dobson (Eds.), *Psychopathology and cognition* (pp. 191–243). New York: Academic Press.

Wachtel, P. L. (Ed.). (1982). *Resistance: Psychodynamic and behavioral approaches.* New York: Plenum Press.

Watzlawick, P., Beavin, J. H., & Jackson, D. D. (1967). *Pragmatics of Human communication.* New York: Norton.

Weltzin, T. E., Cameron, J., Berga, S., & Kaye, W. H. (1994). Prediction of reproductive status in women with bulimia nervosa by past high weight. *American Journal of Psychiatry, 151,* 136–138.

Williamson, D. A., Anderson, D. A., & Gleaves, D. H. (1996). Anorexia nervosa and bulimia nervosa: Structured interview methodologies and psychological assessment. In J. K. Thompson (Ed.), *Body image: Eating disorders and obesity* (pp. 205–223). Washington, DC: American Psychological Association.

Wilson, G. T. (1993). Binge eating and addictive behaviors. In C. G. Fairburn & G. T. Wilson (Eds.), *Binge eating: Nature, assessment, and treatment* (pp. 97–120). New York: Guilford Press.

Windauer, U., Lennerts, W., Talbot, P., Touyz, S. W., & Beumont, P. J. V. (1993). How well are 'cured' anorexia nervosa patients? An investigation of 16 weight-recovered anorexic patients. *British Journal of Psychiatry, 163,* 195–200.

Wooley, S. C., & Garner, D. M. (1991). Obesity treatment: The high cost of false hope. *Journal of the American Dietetic Association, 91,* 1248–1251.

CHAPTER 8

Psychoeducational Principles in Treatment

DAVID M. GARNER

Psychoeducation was originally proposed as one component of treatment for both anorexia nervosa and bulimia nervosa (Garner, Rockert, Olmsted, Johnson, & Coscina, 1985). There has been some variability in the content of treatments identified as "educational"; however, our approach provides specific information in several areas that are particularly important in the process of recovery (Garner et al., 1985). This approach is based on the assumption that eating disorder patients often suffer from misconceptions about the factors that cause and then maintain symptoms. It is further assumed that patients may be less likely to persist in self-defeating symptoms if they are made truly aware of the scientific evidence regarding factors that perpetuate eating disorders. The educational approach conveys the message that the responsibility for change rests with the patient; this is aimed at increasing motivation and reducing defensiveness. The operating assumption is that the patient is a responsible and rational partner in a collaborative relationship. The educational approach is also based on the merits of economy. Education is a relatively inexpensive initial option in the integration and sequencing model of treatment delivery.

Psychoeducational treatment has gradually become a standard component of cognitive-behavioral therapy. About 50% of early cognitive-behavioral treatment studies indicated that some form of psychoeducation was one ingredient of therapy (Garner, Fairburn, & Davis, 1987). This has changed with second-generation treatment studies that have fully assimilated psychoeducational content into standard treatment packages (Wilson & Fairburn, 1993). This is not surprising, since educational principles are consistent with the overall didactic goals of cognitive-behavioral treatment. Although cognitive-behavioral therapy is still the treatment of choice for most bulimia nervosa patients, there is evidence that brief educationally oriented treatments alone can lead to significant behavioral change in some patients. Ordman and Kirschenbaum (1986) compared cognitive-behavioral treatment to a "brief intervention wait-list" consisting of just three assessment sessions and minimal intervention. Cognitive-behavioral treatment was the superior treatment on most measures; however, the brief intervention led to a more than 30% reduction in vomiting frequency. Olmsted et al. (1991) compared individual cognitive-behavioral therapy and brief psychoeducational group treatment (five 90-minute sessions during a 1-month period, delivered in a group "classroom" format), and found brief psychoeducational group treatment to be as effective as cognitive-behavioral treatment with the least symptomatic 25–45% of a bulimia nervosa sample. Lassele et al. (1991) compared "nutritional management," defined by the same methods and goals as the psychoeducational approach above, and "stress management." They found that both treatments led to significant reductions in bingeing and vomiting, as well as lower scores on measures of psychopathology, at the end of treatment and at a 12-month follow-up.

However, nutritional management produced a significantly more rapid reduction in binge eating, higher abstinence rates, and greater improvements on some measures of psychopathology. Thus, some bulimia nervosa patients, particularly those with less severe pathology, seem to respond favorably to psychoeducation delivered in either a group or an individual format.

The aim of this chapter is to highlight psychoeducational content found to be useful to both clinicians and eating disorder patients. Much of the material originally designated as "psychoeducational" has now been directly imported into cognitive-behavioral treatment manuals (Fairburn, Marcus, & Wilson, 1993; Garner, Vitousek, & Pike, Chapter 7, this volume). Thus, the current approach does not follow the exhaustive reference style found in the original description (Garner et al., 1985). Rather, the current chapter presents a selective and abbreviated review of topic areas that are particularly useful in efforts to clarify and overcome eating disorder symptoms. There is some overlap with material presented elsewhere in this book, because this chapter is intended to provide a self-contained educational module that can be integrated with different approaches to therapy for eating disorders. Appendix 8.1 discusses the Eating Attitudes Test (EAT), an instrument that can be used to assess patients' eating concerns before, during, and after psychoeducation; it also provides a copy of the EAT-26, an abbreviated version of the EAT.

The reader should be cautioned that the information presented in this chapter should not be considered as a replacement for psychotherapy, but as a supplement to it. The information is intended to be used by individuals suffering from eating disorders, as well as by practitioners who want to know more about the psychological and physiological mechanisms that play a role in their perpetuation. The current chapter covers the following topics originally described by Garner et al. (1985):

1. Multiple causes of eating disorders.
2. The cultural context for eating disorders.
3. Set-point theory and the physiological regulation of body weight.
4. The effects of starvation on behavior.
5. Restoring regular eating patterns.
6. Vomiting, laxatives, and diuretics in controlling weight.
7. Determining a healthy body weight.
8. Physical complications.
9. Relapse prevention techniques.

MULTIPLE CAUSES OF EATING DISORDERS

Eating disorders are multidetermined; cultural, individual, and family factors contribute to their development in different ways for different individuals.

During the past several decades, single-factor causal theories have been replaced by the view that eating disorders are "multidetermined" (Garfinkel & Garner, 1982; Garner & Garfinkel, 1980; Garner, 1993a). The symptom patterns represent final common pathways resulting from the interplay of three broad classes of predisposing factors, as shown in Figure 8.1; cultural, individual (psychological and biological), and familial causal factors are presumed to combine with one another in different ways that lead to the development of eating disorders. The precipitants are less clearly understood, except that dieting is invariably an early element. Perhaps the most practical advancements in treatment have come from increased awareness of the perpetuating effects of starvation, with its psychological, emotional, and physical consequences (Figure 8.1).

THE CULTURAL CONTEXT FOR EATING DISORDERS

For several decades, the fashion, entertainment, and publishing industries have bombarded women with role models for physical attractiveness who are so gaunt as to represent virtually no women in the actual population; this has resulted in restrictive dieting and increased vulnerability to eating disorders.

Eating disorders involve an intense preoccupation with fatness, leading to extreme attempts to control body weight. Most cases of eating disorders occur among girls and women, and they have been linked to the intense pressure on women to diet in order to conform to today's ultraslender role models for feminine beauty (Garner & Garfinkel, 1980). A strong concern about physical appearance appears to predate

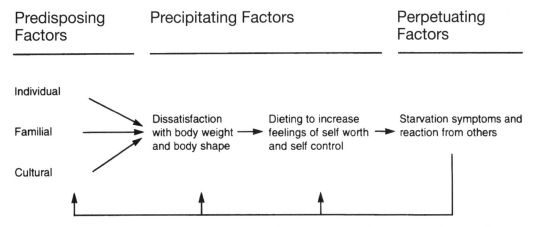

Predisposing Factors

Precipitating Factors

Perpetuating Factors

Individual

Familial

Cultural

Dissatisfaction with body weight and body shape → Dieting to increase feelings of self worth and self control → Starvation symptoms and reaction from others

FIGURE 8.1. Eating disorders as multidetermined disorders. From Garner (1993a, p. 1632). Copyright 1993 by the Lancet. Reprinted by permission.

the appearance of anorexia nervosa (Rastam, 1992). Research has shown that dieting to lose weight and fear of fatness are common in girls as young as 7 years old; these attitudes and behaviors escalate significantly during adolescence, particularly among those at the heavier end of the weight spectrum (Edlund, Halvarsson, & Sjödén, 1995). It has been shown that the risk of developing an eating disorder is eight times higher in dieting than in nondieting 15-year-old girls (Patton, Johnson-Sabine, Wood, Mann, & Wakeling, 1990). As young women from other more weight-tolerant cultures (e.g., Egyptian, Japanese, Chinese) are assimilated into "thinness-conscious" Western culture, they become more fearful of fatness, and eating disorder symptoms proliferate (Dolan, Lee, & Lee, 1996). In Western culture, those exposed to more pressure to diet, such as athletes participating in sports that emphasize leanness for performance or appearance, are at greater risk for eating disorders (Garner & Rosen, 1991). In North America, disordered eating patterns appear to be equally common among Caucasian and Hispanic females, less common among Black and Asian females and most common among Native Americans (Crago, Shisslak, & Estes, 1996).

One of the keys to overcoming an eating disorder is relaxing strict and extreme forms of dietary restriction. In order to accomplish this, there must be some understanding of the factors motivating individuals' attempts to control body weight. In some cases, the motivation involves complex emotional and interpersonal

problems that need to be addressed in order to make progress. In other cases, the primary motivation is the individual's acceptance of the cultural message that a thin body is crucial to personal happiness. Either way, recovery involves swimming against the cultural stream. Patients are continually barraged by messages from the media glorifying the virtues of dieting and thinness. It is impossible for most women to achieve the shape standard set by ultrathin fashion models portrayed in popular women's magazines. Garner, Garfinkel, Schwartz, and Thompson (1980) reported that just over 5% of female life insurance policy holders between the ages of 20 and 29 were as thin as the average Miss America Pageant winner between 1970 and 1978. Studies analyzing the content of women's magazines have documented the emphasis on thinness and dieting, and some of these studies indicate that increased exposure is linked to shape dissatisfaction and vulnerability to eating disorders (Andersen & DiDomenico, 1992; Garner et al., 1980; Nemeroff, Stein, Diehl, & Smilach, 1994).

There is evidence that pressures to diet have intensified over time. Garner et al. (1980) originally documented and quantified the changing expectations for thinness by reporting that *Playboy* centerfolds and Miss America contestants became significantly thinner between 1959 and 1979, and that there was a corresponding increase in diet for weight loss advertisements in popular women's magazines. These findings were extended by Wiseman, Gray, Mosimann, and Ahrens (1992), who found that the trends continued through 1988 (Figure 8.2). More-over, *Playboy* centerfolds and Miss America contestants hardly represent the bony-thin body frame typically promoted by the fashion and advertising industries.

Although women have indicated remarkable dissatisfaction with their shape for decades (Jourard & Secord, 1955), research has shown that there is a broadening gulf between actual and preferred shapes and that this has intensi-fied body dissatisfaction among young women. A 1988 National Adolescent Student Health Sur-vey (NASHS) of 8th- and 10th-grade students indicated that 61% of female students and 28% of male students reported dieting during the previous year (NASHS, 1989). The widespread efforts to lose weight have not translated into de-clining population weights in the United States. On the contrary, Figure 8.2 illustrates the grow-ing disparity between actual and "ideal" weights. The dotted line connects the average weight for

women in 1959 and the same standard in 1979, showing that there has been a steady *increase* in the actual weights for women the same age and height as the magazine models. This trend has continued, with the greatest weight increases for both women and men in recent years (Kucz-marski, Flegal, Campbell, & Johnson, 1994). Thus, the prevailing shape standards do not even remotely resemble the actual body shape of the average woman consumer.

The social norms for attractiveness presented in women's magazines have steadily woven the image of "fitness" into the slender shape ideal. Whereas the health benefits of exercise are un-deniable, its promotion as a weight loss strategy has been a growing theme (Wiseman, Gray, Mosimann, & Ahrens, 1992). Given the pro-found cultural pressures on women to diet, it is perhaps pertinent to ask why all women do not develop some level of disordered eating. An in-teresting yet largely unexplored area relates to

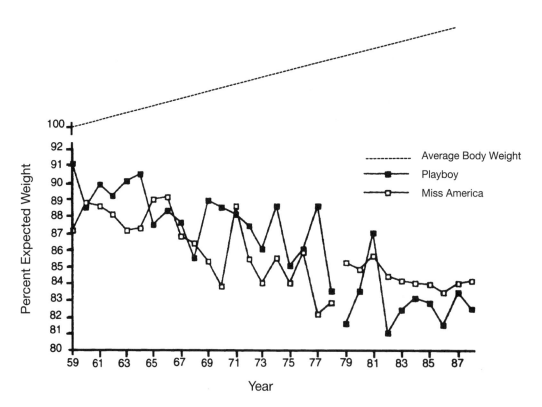

FIGURE 8.2. Changes in the average percentage of expected weight of *Playboy* centerfolds and Miss America contestants, 1959–1978 (data from Garner, Garfinkel, Schwartz, & Thompson, 1980) and 1979–1988 (data from Wiseman, Gray, Mosimann, & Ahrens, 1992). The broken line represents prorated changes in the average weights for women over the first 20-year period, based on the 1959 and revised 1979 Society of Actuaries' norms—a trend that has continued, according to later population studies (Kuczmarski, Flegal, Campbell, & Johnson, 1994).

protective factors that tend to prevent the expression of eating disorders. Other cultural risk factors, such as role conflicts experienced by women, may also be implicated in the development of eating disorders (Perlick & Silverstein, 1994).

The gradual recognition of the unreasonable stresses on women to conform to the contemporary "gaunt look" provides the basis for urging those suffering from eating disorders to reframe their disorder in cultural terms. The simple exercise of collecting appearance-oriented images from women's magazines can lead some women struggling with eating disorder symptoms to develop a healthy sense of indignation at the confining definitions of feminine attractiveness promoted in the media.

SET-POINT THEORY AND THE PHYSIOLOGICAL REGULATION OF BODY WEIGHT

Generally speaking, body weight resists change. Weight appears to be physiologically regulated around a "set point," or a weight that one's body tries to "defend." Significant deviations from this weight result in a myriad of physiological compensations aimed at returning the organism to this set point.

Set Point or Regulated Weight

The relative stability of body weight has been noted for many years. Hollifield (1968) observed that the "active man who remains the same weight over a period of 20 years must have balanced his food intake against energy expenditure to the nearest crumb" (p. 1471). However, a relatively constant weight can be maintained without monitoring food intake against energy output. Fox (1973) reported a personal weight range of between 72 and 77 kg (156 and 170 pounds) over 20 years, although he gave no conscious attention to the amount eaten or amount of exercise taken. The degree of precision in weight regulation is indicated by the fact that that a gain of 4.5 kg (10 pounds) in 1 year would require a consistent error of only about 100 calories daily. It has been shown that over a 6- to 10-week period, body weight varies by only 0.5% around an average weight (Robinson & Watson, 1965). This is a deviation of less than 280 g (10 ounces) for a 55-kg (120-pound)

woman, despite the fact that most adolescent women have as much as a fourfold variation in daily caloric intake (Lacey, Chadbund, Crisp, & Whitehead, 1978).

The concept of "set point" has been proposed to account for data from human and animal studies showing that there is remarkable stability in body weight over time. According to the set point concept, body weight is regulated by physiological mechanisms that oppose the displacement of body weight caused by either over- or underfeeding (Keesey, 1993; Nisbett, 1972; Powley & Keesey, 1970). From this perspective, body weight regulation operates much as a thermostat controls a furnace in stabilizing the heat level in a room. If the heat controls are set at a certain number, the system operates to maintain that temperature. If a window is opened and the room temperature drops, the thermostat automatically goes to work to increase the heat level. The machinery starts to churn and begins to pump out heat. If the room gets too hot, the furnace shuts off temporarily until the temperature returns to normal. This bidirectional sensing mechanism is altered automatically; it is extremely responsive to changes that displace the heat level from the temperature level that has been set.

Human bodies apparently work in much the same way, responding to deviations in body weight by turning the metabolic "furnace" up or down. There is some debate about the precise physiological mechanisms that influence the absolute levels at which weight regulation occurs. Nevertheless, there are impressive data indicating that (1) displacement of body weight, both upward and downward, usually results in metabolic adjustments designed to return to the body weight normally maintained; (2) this body weight "defense" occurs in obese as well as nonobese animals; (3) environmental factors, such as diet palatability, exercise, smoking, climate, and certain drugs, appear to influence the absolute levels (within certain limits) at which body weight is regulated; and (4) genetics are important in determining individuals' tendency to resist upward and downward regulation of body weight in response to these environmental influences. Thus, the terms "regulated weight" or "natural weight" have been favored over "set point'" since weight is not really defended around a precise point (Keesey, 1993). Nevertheless, body weight stability, the process of body weight defense, and physiological regulation of body weight are well established.

The principle of physiological regulation accounts for the remarkable stability of the organism in spite of wide variations in the external environment. It applies to the regulation of such conditions as heart rate, respiration rate, blood pressure, body temperature, blood glucose levels, and a host of other biological systems. The control of these biological conditions is not absolute; rather, they are maintained within particular limited range and at characteristic average levels. These average levels may be affected by environmental factors; daily, monthly, and seasonal cycles; gender; and stages of the life cycle. Nevertheless, they are regulated by active physiological defense and this leads to internal stability. For example, body temperature ranges between 97.0° and 99.1° F, with an average of 98.6° for a healthy adult (99.0° to 99.6° for the very young). Pulse rate is about 140 beats per minute at birth, and averages 72 beats per minute for males and 80 beats per minute for females over age 14. Respiration rate is 17 to 20 times per minute for the adult. Respiration is a particularly good example to use when trying to explain body weight regulation. Like body weight, respiration is biologically regulated and functions "automatically," yet it can come under voluntary control, within certain limits. All of these indices rise in response to increased physical activity, but they decline again when the organism returns to a normal resting state. In order to regulate these systems within the limits, the body must be able to monitor internal state continuously, as well as to initiate physiological compensatory mechanisms designed to restore the organism to a state of biological equilibrium.

Set Point and Obesity Treatment

The concept of set point has important implications for obesity. Nisbett (1972) argued that body fat, like all biological parameters, varies from one individual to another in the population. The absolute level of body fat determined by the set-point mechanisms may differ markedly in individuals of the same height and bone structure, depending on heredity and feeding experiences in childhood, when set point appears to be more malleable. According to this view, obesity for some individuals represents a "normal" or even an "ideal" body weight. Family and twin studies have shown that there is a strong genetic influence on who will be

obese and who will be thin (Meyer & Stunkard, 1993). Nisbett (1972) observed many behavioral parallels between obese humans and hungry or starving individuals. It was concluded that many obese people are genuinely hungry and in a chronic state of energy deficit, because they are desperately trying to hold their weight below their physiologically determined set point in response to social pressures to be thinner. Thus, many statistically overweight individuals who have responded by reducing their weight may actually be biologically underweight!

Thus, regardless of social pressures and medical advice to lose weight, there is biological resistance to permanent weight change. Dieters and people with eating disorders demonstrate the ability to suppress their body weight temporarily; however, they are not relieved of the constant physiological pressures to return to the natural weight their bodies prefer. As Bennett (1984) aptly put it, the effect of sustained caloric deprivation is "to pit the individual's 'will' against an untiring opponent, the set point mechanism" (p. 331). A good illustration of the remarkable stability of body weight comes from animal studies. Figure 8.3 presents the results from one study in which laboratory rats lost weight in response to caloric restriction (Mitchel & Keesey, 1977). When the animals were taken off the restrictive diet, they regained weight to levels very close to those of their nondeprived littermates. The advantage of animal studies is that this weight regain process cannot be blamed on lack of willpower, compulsive overeating, psychological disturbance, or poor parenting. The weights of these animals settled close to those of their nondieted lettermates without the aid of bathroom scales or peer pressure. As further illustrated in Figure 8.3, the same pattern of body weight defense occurred in a group of animals with lesions to the lateral hypothalamus, except that the absolute weight levels were lower. In these animals, the "set point" had been modified downward, but the weight regulation mechanism remained intact.

These conclusions are completely supported by decades of scientific research on obesity treatment. There is no question that most diets "work" in the short term, even though the clinical significance of the amount of weight loss has been questioned (Garner & Wooley, 1991). However, there can be little doubt that most treatments fail to reverse the obese state per-

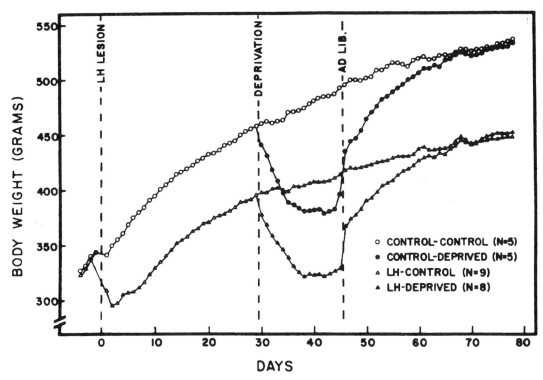

FIGURE 8.3. Recovery of body weight by control rats and rats with lateral hypothalamic (LH) lesions following a period of food restriction and return to an *ad libitum* feeding schedule. When allowed to feed *ad libitum,* the previously deprived rats from both groups quickly restored their body weights to the levels of their nondeprived reference group. From Mitchel and Keesey (1977, p. 1123). Copyright 1977 by Pergamon Press. Reprinted by permission.

manently: Long-term follow-up studies indicate that, regardless of the specific techniques used, 90–95% of those who lose weight will regain it within several years. Almost 20 years ago, Stunkard and Penick (1979) found that the majority of patients receiving both behavioral and traditional treatment regained most of the weight originally lost after 5 years. These findings have been consistently reaffirmed in subsequent long-term follow-up studies. The odds against maintaining long-term weight loss were dramatically illustrated by Kramer, Jeffery, Forster, and Snell (1989) in a study of 114 men and 38 women who had successfully completed a 15-week behavioral weight loss program. They reported that fewer than 3% of the patients maintained their posttreatment weight throughout the four yearly follow-up assessments. Figure 8.4 illustrates results from another carefully controlled study comparing behavior modification, a very-low-calorie diet, and the combination of these two approaches (Wadden, Sternberg, Letizia, Stunkard, & Foster,

1989). This pattern of findings has been well known for years and led Brownell (1982) to conclude that if "cure from obesity is defined as reduction to ideal weight and maintenance of that weight for 5 years, a person is more likely to recover from most forms of cancer than from obesity" (p. 820). Even earlier, Hirsch (1978) quipped that subjecting the obese to available dietary treatment is "the modern day equivalent of beating the insane to keep them quiet" (p. 2). It is difficult to justify the continued use of dietary treatments of obesity after reviewing the literature on their effectiveness (Garner, 1993b; 1995; Garner & Wooley, 1991). Regardless of the specific techniques used, most participants in weight loss programs regain the weight lost. The inevitability of this result is often obscured by the use of follow-up periods that are insufficient to capture the later phases of weight regain. Yet the failure of dietary treatments is to be expected, given what is known about the biology of weight regulation.

Weight loss leads to reduced metabolic rate

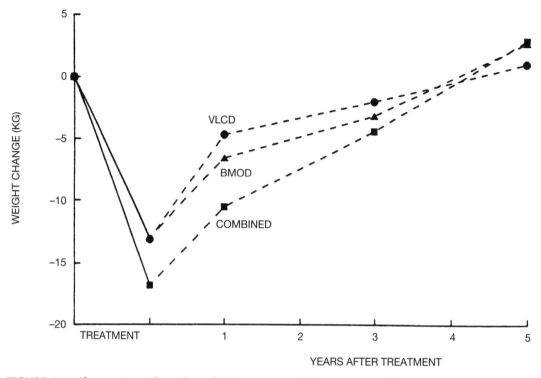

FIGURE 8.4. Changes in weight at the end of treatment and during a 5-year follow-up period for 67 women randomly assigned to a very-low-calorie diet (VLCD), behavior modification combined with a 1200-calorie-per-day diet (BMOD), and a combined treatment of VLCD and BMOD (COMBINED). Wadden (1993, p. 692) based on data from Wadden, Sternberg, Letizia, Stunkard, and Foster (1989, p. 692). Copyright by the American College of Physicians. Reprinted by permission.

which is one mechanism responsible for body weight regulation. Weight loss in the obese as well as the nonobese leads to reductions of 15–30% in energy requirements (see Garner & Wooley, 1991). Corbett, Stern, and Keesey (1986) reported that reducing the body weight of rats by 14.9% through caloric restriction led to a 24.6% decline in resting metabolic rate. As described later, comparable declines in metabolic rate have been demonstrated in humans exposed to semistarvation conditions (Keys, Brozek, Henschel, Mickelsen, & Taylor, 1950). Obese patients have been shown to make the same metabolic adjustments as, or greater ones than, their lean controls during reduced caloric intake and weight loss (Leibel & Hirsch, 1984). Leibel and Hirsch (1984) reported that obese humans who had lost a significant amount of weight (52 kg), but were still judged to be 60% overweight, had caloric requirements 28% below their pre-weight-loss levels. Even short-term restrictions involving small decrements in weight are accompanied by rather dramatic

metabolic adjustments (see Garner & Wooley, 1991, for details). Leibel and Hirsch (1984) reported that the reduced metabolic requirements endured in obese patients who had maintained a reduced body weight for 4–6 years.

Reducing body weight in the obese may make them superficially resemble those who are naturally lean, but basic differences in body fat stores persist. Tremblay, Despres, and Bouchard (1984) studied a group of men who, through a program of long-distance running, had lost an average of almost 40 kg and maintained a stable weight for at least 1 year. They found that the formerly obese runners were similar to sedentary controls on measures of body fat and fat metabolism, but that both groups differed significantly from elite runners. The tendency to defend body fat preferentially, at the expense of lean body mass, is illustrated by studies showing that both food restriction and jejunoileal bypass surgery are successful in keeping genetically obese rats at reduced body weight levels; however, they preserve elevated body fat levels at the expense of muscle mass and vital organs, such as the brain, heart, kidneys, and liver (Cleary & Vasselli, 1981; Greenwood, Maggio, Koopmans, & Sclafani, 1982). These findings suggest a powerful biological defense of fat. Results from human autopsy studies of emaciated patients are consistent with these findings, since the degree of wasting of vital organ mass (i.e., heart, liver, kidneys, and spleen) is proportional to the percentage of weight loss (Hill & Beddoe, 1986).

Set Point and Weight Gain

Just as the body resists weight loss by making metabolic adjustments, it also resists gain. In a classic experiment, prisoners volunteered to gain between 20% and 25% of their original body weight by eating about twice their usual caloric intake for about 6 months (Sims et al., 1968). Most of the men gained the initial few pounds with ease, but quickly became hypermetabolic and resisted further weight gain, despite continued overfeeding (Sims, 1976). One prisoner stopped gaining weight even though he was consuming close to 10,000 calories per day! With a return to normal amounts of food, most of the men returned to the weight levels that they had maintained prior to the experiment. The prisoners burned up much of the excess energy through increased metabolic activity; they perspired profusely and complained of oppressive body heat. The amount of weight gained only accounted for about 25% of the excess calories ingested. Moreover, the hypermetabolic state created by overeating meant that the men required 50% more calories to maintain their experimental obesity. The overindulgence became increasingly unpleasant; many of the men contemplated withdrawing from the experiment. Some became physically ill after meals, and their psychological state deteriorated. As soon as overeating was no longer required, the men rapidly began losing weight and ultimately stabilized at almost exactly their preexperiment weight levels. The only exceptions were the two men who initially gained weight rapidly, as well as two others with a family history of obesity or diabetes. The marked differences among individuals in the rate of weight loss and resistance to weight gain suggests differences in the biological propensity to overweight.

Metabolic rate appears to adapt to increased caloric intake by producing excess heat—a process termed "diet-induced thermogenesis." This phenomenon was first described over 80 years ago in a classic study by Neuman (1902), who set out to determine the effect of overeating over a prolonged period of time. During the first year of his experiment, he increased his intake by 430 calories per day; during the second year, he increased it by an additional 300 calories per day. If metabolic rate did not increase to accommodate the added calories, he should have gained about 18 kg (40 pounds) the first year and an additional 27 kg (60 pounds) the second. Neuman described only a modest weight increase during the 2-year period. He realized that his body was somehow able to burn off the surplus calories, and he called this "*Luxoskonsumption*" ("extra burning"). Gulick (1922) also reported a 10-month period during which he systematically overate; he, too, gained less weight than would have been predicted from the calories ingested. This amounted to 27–37% of the calories consumed. Brunner et al. (1979) overfed 26 agricultural workers (each ate 4,553 calories daily) for 7 months, but this resulted in an average weight gain of less than 3.2 kg (7 pounds). This accounted for only about 5% of the excess energy ingested! The fact that the agricultural workers "burned off" even more of the extra calories may be attributable to their physical activity and their genetic predisposition for leanness (Brunner et al., 1979).

THE EFFECTS OF STARVATION ON BEHAVIOR

One of the most important advancements in the understanding of eating disorders is the recognition that severe and prolonged dietary restriction can lead to serious physical and psychological complications. Many of the symptoms once thought to be primary features of anorexia nervosa are actually symptoms of starvation.

Given what we know about the biology of weight regulation, what is the impact of weight suppression on the individual? This is particularly relevant for those with anorexia nervosa, but is also important for people with eating disorders who have lost significant amounts of body weight. Perhaps the most powerful illustration of the effects of restrictive dieting and weight loss on behavior is an experimental study conducted almost 50 years ago and published in 1950 by Ancel Keys and his colleagues at the University of Minnesota (Keys et al., 1950). The experiment involved carefully studying 36 young, healthy, psychologically normal men while restricting their caloric intake for 6 months. More than 100 men volunteered for the study as an alternative to military service; the 36 selected had the highest levels of physical and psychological health, as well as the most commitment to the objectives of the experiment.

During the first 3 months of the experiment, the volunteers ate normally while their behavior, personality, and eating patterns were studied in detail. During the next 6 months, the men were restricted to approximately half of their former food intake and lost, on average, approximately 25% of their former weight. Figure 8.5 shows the Minnesota volunteers at mealtime, and Figure 8.6 reveals the physical results of the weight loss. Although this was described as a study of "semistarvation," it is important to keep in mind that cutting the men's rations to half of their former intake is precisely the level of caloric deficit used to define "conservative" treatments for obesity (Stunkard,

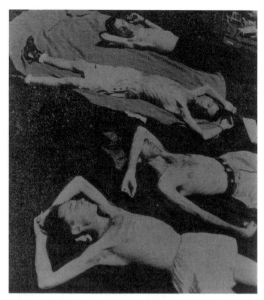

FIGURE 8.6. Minnesota volunteers after weight loss. Photo by Wallace Kirckland. Copyright 1950 by Life–Time–Warner.

1987). The 6 months of weight loss were followed by 3 months of rehabilitation, during which the men were gradually refed. A subgroup was followed for almost 9 months after the refeeding began. Most of the results were reported for only 32 men, since 4 men were withdrawn either during or at the end of the semistarvation phase. Although the individual responses to weight loss varied considerably, the men experienced dramatic physical, psychological, and social changes. In most cases, these changes persisted during the rehabilitation or renourishment phase.

What makes the "starvation study" (as it is commonly known) so important is that many of the experiences observed in the volunteers are the same as those experienced by patients with eating disorders. This section of this chapter is a summary of the changes observed in the Minnesota study. All quotations followed by page numbers in parentheses are from the original report by Keys et al. (1950) and are used by permission of the University of Minnesota Press.

Attitudes and Behavior Related to Food and Eating

One of the most striking changes that occurred in the volunteers was a dramatic increase in

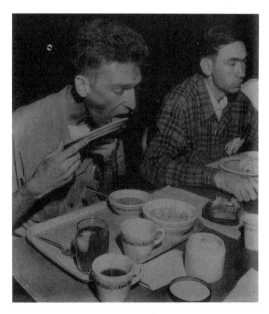

FIGURE 8.5. Minnesota volunteers at mealtime. Copyright 1950 by the University of Minnesota Press. Reprinted by permission.

food preoccupations. The men found concentration on their usual activities increasingly difficult, because they became plagued by incessant thoughts of food and eating. Figure 8.7 illustrates the increase in the average ratings of concern about food, as well as corresponding declines in interest in sex and activity, for 32 subjects at different stages of semistarvation and rehabilitation. Food became a principal topic of conversation, reading, and daydreams.

> As starvation progressed, the number of men who toyed with their food increased. They made what under normal conditions would be weird and distasteful concoctions. (p. 832) . . . Those who ate in the common dining room smuggled out bits of food and consumed them on their bunks in a long-drawn-out ritual. (p. 833). Cookbooks, menus, and information bulletins on food production became intensely interesting to many of the men who previously had little or no interest in dietetics or agriculture. (p. 833) . . . [The volunteers] often reported that they got a vivid vicarious pleasure from watching other persons eat or from just smelling food. (p. 834)

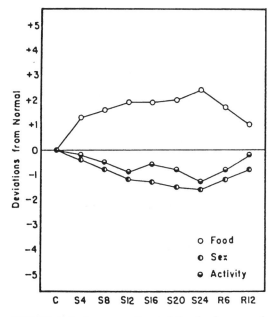

FIGURE 8.7. Average ratings of the food, sex, and activity drives for 32 participants in the Minnesota experiment. From Keys et al. (1950, p. 823). Copyright 1950 by the University of Minnesota Press. Reprinted by permission.

In addition to cookbooks and collecting recipes, some of the men even began collecting coffeepots, hot plates, and other kitchen utensils. According to the original report, hoarding even extended to non-food-related items, such as: "old books, unnecessary second-hand clothes, knick knacks, and other 'junk.' Often after making such purchases, which could be afforded only with sacrifice, the men would be puzzled as to why they had bought such more or less useless articles" (p. 837). One man even began rummaging through garbage cans. This general tendency to hoard has been observed in starved anorexic patients (Crisp, Hsu, & Harding, 1980) and even in rats deprived of food (Fantino & Cabanac, 1980). Despite little interest in culinary matters prior to the experiment, almost 40% of the men mentioned cooking as part of their postexperiment plans. For some, the fascination was so great that they actually changed occupations after the experiment; three became chefs, and one went into agriculture!

During semistarvation, the volunteers' eating habits underwent remarkable changes. The men spent much of the day planning how they would eat their allotment of food. Much of their behavior served the purpose of prolonging ingestion and increasing the appeal or salience of food. The men often ate in silence and devoted total attention to food consumption.

> The Minnesota subjects were often caught between conflicting desires to gulp their food down ravenously and consume it slowly so that the taste and odor of each morsel would be fully appreciated. Toward the end of starvation some of the men would dawdle for almost two hours over a meal which previously they would have consumed in a matter of minutes. . . . They did much planning as to how they would handle their day's allotment of food. (p. 833)

The men demanded that their food be served hot, and they made unusual concoctions by mixing foods together, as noted above. There was also a marked increase in the use of salt and spices. The consumption of coffee and tea increased so dramatically that the men had to be limited to 9 cups per day; similarly, gum chewing became excessive and had to be limited after it was discovered that one man was chewing as many as 40 packages of gum a day and "developed a sore mouth from such continuous exercise" (p. 835).

During the 12-week refeeding phase of the experiment, most of the abnormal attitudes and behaviors in regard to food persisted. A small number of men found that their difficulties in this area were quite severe during the first 6 weeks of refeeding:

> In many cases the men were not content to eat "normal" menus but persevered in their habits of making fantastic concoctions and combinations. The free choice of ingredients, moreover, stimulated "creative" and "experimental" playing with food . . . licking of plates and neglect of table manners persisted. (p. 843)

Binge Eating

During the restrictive dieting phase of the experiment, all of the volunteers reported increased hunger. Some appeared able to tolerate the experience fairly well, but for others it created intense concern and led to a complete breakdown in control. Several men were unable to adhere to their diets and reported episodes of binge eating followed by self-reproach. During the eighth week of starvation, one volunteer "flagrantly broke the dietary rules, eating several sundaes and malted milks; he even stole some penny candies. He promptly confessed the whole episode, [and] became self-deprecatory" (p. 884). While working in a grocery store, another man

> suffered a complete loss of will power and ate several cookies, a sack of popcorn, and two overripe bananas before he could "regain control" of himself. He immediately suffered a severe emotional upset, with nausea, and upon returning to the laboratory he vomited. . . . He was self-deprecatory, expressing disgust and self-criticism. (p. 887)

One man was released from the experiment at the end of the semistarvation period because of suspicions that he was unable to adhere to the diet. He experienced serious difficulties when confronted with unlimited access to food: "He repeatedly went through the cycle of eating tremendous quantities of food, becoming sick, and then starting all over again" (p. 890).

During the refeeding phase of the experiment, many of the men lost control of their appetites and "ate more or less continuously" (p. 843). Even after 12 weeks of refeeding, the men frequently complained of increased hunger immediately following a large meal:

> [One of the volunteers] ate immense meals (a daily estimate of 5,000–6,000 cal.) and yet started "snacking" an hour after he finished a meal. [Another] ate as much as he could hold during the three regular meals and ate snacks in the morning, afternoon and evening. (p. 846)

Such overeating took its toll:

> This gluttony resulted in a high incidence of headaches, gastrointestinal distress and unusual sleepiness. Several men had spells of nausea and vomiting. One man required aspiration and hospitalization for several days. (p. 843)

During the weekends in particular, some of the men found it difficult to stop eating. Their daily intake commonly ranged between 8,000 and 10,000 calories, and their eating patterns were described as follows:

> Subject No. 20 stuffs himself until he is bursting at the seams, to the point of being nearly sick and still feels hungry; No. 120 reported that he had to discipline himself to keep from eating so much as to become ill; No. 1 ate until he was uncomfortably full; and subject No. 30 had so little control over the mechanics of "piling it in" that he simply had to stay away from food because he could not find a point of satiation even when he was "full to the gills." . . . "I ate practically all weekend," reported subject No. 26. . . . Subject No. 26 would just as soon have eaten six meals instead of three. (p. 847)

After about 5 months of refeeding, the majority of the men reported some normalization of their eating patterns, but for some the extreme overconsumption persisted: "No. 108 would eat and eat until he could hardly swallow any more and then he felt like eating half an hour later" (p. 847). More than 8 months after renourishment began, most men had returned to normal eating patterns; however, a few were still eating abnormal amounts: "No. 9 ate about 25 percent more than his pre-starvation amount; once he started to reduce but got so hungry he could not stand it" (p. 847). Factors distinguishing men who rapidly normalized their eating from those who continued to eat prodigious amounts were not identified. Nevertheless, the main findings here are as follows: Serious binge eating developed in a subgroup of men, and this tendency persisted in some cases for months after free access to food was reintroduced; however, the majority of men reported gradually returning to eating normal amounts of food after about 5 months of refeeding. Thus, the fact that binge eating was experimentally produced in some of these normal young men should temper speculations about primary psychological disturbances as the cause of binge eating in patients with eating disorders. These findings are supported by a large body of research indicating that habitual dieters display marked overcompensation in eating behavior that is similar to the binge eating observed in eating disorders (Polivy & Herman, 1985, 1987; Wardle & Beinart, 1981).

Emotional and Personality Changes

The experimental procedures involved selecting volunteers who were the most physically and psychologically robust: "The psychobiological 'stamina' of the subjects was unquestionably superior to that likely to be found in any random or more generally representative sample of the population" (pp. 915–916). Although the subjects were psychologically healthy prior to the experiment, most experienced significant emotional deterioration as a result of semistarvation. Most of the subjects experienced periods during which their emotional distress was quite severe; almost 20% experienced extreme emotional deterioration that markedly interfered with their functioning.

Depression became more severe during the course of the experiment. Elation was observed occasionally, but this was inevitably followed by "low periods." Mood swings were extreme for some of the volunteers:

> [One subject] experienced a number of periods in which his spirits were definitely high. . . . These elated periods alternated with times in which he suffered "a deep dark depression." [He] felt that he had reached the end of his rope [and] expressed the fear that he was going crazy . . . [and] losing his inhibitions. (p. 903)

Irritability and frequent outbursts of anger were common, although the men had quite tolerant dispositions prior to starvation. For most

subjects, anxiety became more evident. As the experiment progressed, many of the formerly even-tempered men began biting their nails or smoking because they felt nervous. Apathy also became common, and some men who had been quite fastidious neglected various aspects of personal hygiene.

During semistarvation, two subjects developed disturbances of "psychotic" proportions. One of these was unable to adhere to the diet and developed alarming symptoms:

> [He exhibited] a compulsive attraction to refuse and a strong, almost compelling, desire to root in garbage cans [for food to eat]. He became emotionally disturbed enough to seek admission voluntarily to the psychiatric ward of the University Hospitals. (p. 890)

After 9 weeks of starvation, another subject also exhibited serious signs of disturbance:

> [He went on a] spree of shoplifting, stealing trinkets that had little or no intrinsic value. . . . He developed a violent emotional outburst with flight of ideas, weeping, talk of suicide and threats of violence. Because of the alarming nature of his symptoms, he was released from the experiment and admitted to the psychiatric ward of the University Hospitals. (p. 885)

During the refeeding period, emotional disturbance did not vanish immediately but persisted for several weeks, with some men actually becoming *more* depressed, irritable, argumentative, and negativistic than they had been during semistarvation. After two weeks of refeeding, one man reported his extreme reaction in his diary:

> I have been more depressed than ever in my life. . . . I thought that there was only one thing that would pull me out of the doldrums, that is release from C.P.S. [the experiment] I decided to get rid of some fingers. Ten days ago, I jacked up my car and let the car fall on these fingers. . . . It was premeditated. (pp. 894–895)

Several days later, this man actually did chop off three fingers of one hand in response to the stress.

Standardized personality testing with the Minnesota Multiphasic Personality Inventory (MMPI) revealed that semistarvation resulted in significant increases on the Depression, Hysteria, and Hypochondriasis scales. This profile has been referred to as the "neurotic triad" and is observed among different groups of disturbed individuals (Greene, 1980). The MMPI profiles for a small minority of subjects confirmed the clinical impression of incredible deterioration as a result of semistarvation. Figure 8.8 illustrates one man's personality profile: Initially it was well within normal limits, but after 10 weeks of semistarvation and a weight loss of only about 4.5 kg (10 pounds, or approximately 7% of his original body weight), gross personality disturbances were evident. On the second testing, all of the MMPI scales were elevated, indicating severe personality disturbance on scales reflecting neurotic as well as psychotic traits. Depression and general disorganization were particularly striking consequences of starvation for several of the men who became the most emotionally disturbed.

Social and Sexual Changes

The extraordinary impact of semistarvation was reflected in the social changes experienced by most of the volunteers. Although originally quite gregarious, the men became progressively more withdrawn and isolated. Humor and the sense of comradeship diminished amidst growing feelings of social inadequacy:

> Social initiative especially, and sociability in general, underwent a remarkable change. The men became reluctant to plan activities, to make decisions, and to participate in group activities. . . . They spent more and more time alone. It became "too much trouble" or "too tiring" to have contact with other people. (pp. 836–837)

The volunteers' social contacts with women also declined sharply during semistarvation. Those who continued to see women socially found that the relationships became strained. These changes are illustrated in the account from one man's diary:

> I am one of about three or four who still go out with girls. I fell in love with a girl during the control period but I see her only occasionally now. It's almost too much trouble to see her even when she visits me in the lab. It requires effort to hold her hand. Entertainment must be tame. If we see a

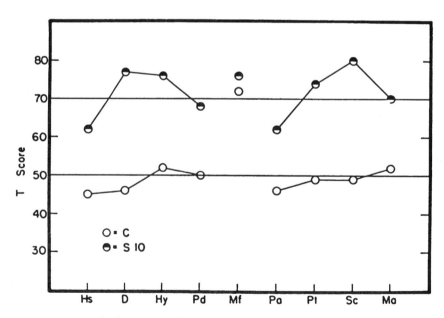

FIGURE 8.8. Minnesota Multiphasic Personality Inventory (MMPI) scores for one participant in the Minnesota experiment during the control period (C), and after 10 weeks of calorie restriction (S10) and weight loss of about 7% of his control weight. *T* scores between 50 and 70 are in the normal range. Hs, Hypochondriasis; D, Depression; Hy, Hysteria; Pd, Psychopathic Deviate; Mf, Masculinity–Femininity; Pa, Paranoia; Pt, Psychasthenia; Sc, Schizophrenia; Ma, Hypomania. From Keys et al. (1950, p. 856). Copyright 1950 by the University of Minnesota Press. Reprinted by permission.

show, the most interesting part of it is contained in scenes where people are eating. (p. 853)

Sexual interests were likewise drastically reduced (see Figure 8.7). Masturbation, sexual fantasies, and sexual impulses either ceased or became much less common. One subject graphically stated that he had "no more sexual feeling than a sick oyster." (Even this peculiar metaphor made reference to food.) Keys et al. observed that "many of the men welcomed the freedom from sexual tensions and frustrations normally present in young adult men" (p. 840). The fact that starvation perceptibly altered sexual urges and associated conflicts is of particular interest, since it has been hypothesized that this process is the driving force behind the dieting of many anorexia nervosa patients. According to Crisp (1980), anorexia nervosa is an adaptive disorder in the sense that it curtails sexual concerns for which the adolescent feels unprepared.

During rehabilitation, sexual interest was slow to return. Even after 3 months, the men judged themselves to be far from normal in this area. However, after 8 months of renourishment, virtually all of the men had recovered their interest in sex.

Cognitive Changes

The volunteers reported impaired concentration, alertness, comprehension, and judgment during semistarvation; however, formal intellectual testing revealed no signs of diminished intellectual abilities.

Physical Changes

As the 6 months of semistarvation progressed, the volunteers exhibited many physical changes, including gastrointestinal discomfort; decreased need for sleep; dizziness; headaches; hypersensitivity to noise and light; reduced strength; poor motor control; edema (an excess of fluid causing swelling); hair loss; decreased tolerance for cold temperatures (cold hands and feet); visual disturbances (i.e., inability to focus, eye aches, "spots" in the visual fields); auditory disturbances (i.e., ringing noise in the ears); and paresthesias (i.e., abnormal tingling or prickling sensations, especially in the hands or feet).

Various changes reflected an overall slowing of the body's physiological processes. There were decreases in body temperature, heart rate, and respiration, as well as in basal metabolic rate (BMR). BMR is the amount of energy (in calories) that the body requires at rest (i.e., no physical activity) in order to carry out normal physiological processes. It accounts for about two-thirds of the body's total energy needs, with the remainder being used during physical activity. At the end of semistarvation, the men's BMRs had dropped by about 40% from normal levels. This drop, as well as other physical changes, reflects the body's extraordinary ability to adapt to low caloric intake by reducing its need for energy. As one volunteer described it, he felt as if his "body flame [were] burning as low as possible to conserve precious fuel and still maintain life process" (p. 852). Recent research has shown that metabolic rate is markedly reduced even among dieters who do not have a history of dramatic weight loss (Platte, Wurmser, Wade, Mecheril, & Pirke, 1996). During refeeding, Keys et al. found that metabolism speeded up, with those consuming the greatest number of calories experiencing the largest rise in BMR. The group of volunteers who received a relatively small increment in calories during refeeding (400 calories more than during semistarvation) had no rise in BMR for the first 3 weeks. Consuming larger amounts of food caused a sharp increase in the energy burned through metabolic processes.

The changes in body fat and muscle in relation to overall body weight during semistarvation and refeeding are of considerable interest (Figure 8.9). While weight declined about 25%, the percentage of body fat fell almost 70%, and muscle decreased about 40%. Upon refeeding, a greater proportion of the "new weight" was fat; in the eighth month of rehabilitation, the volunteers were at about 110% of their original body weight but had approximately 140% of their original body fat!

How did the men feel about their weight gain during rehabilitation? "Those subjects who gained the most weight became concerned about their increased sluggishness, general flabbiness, and the tendency of fat to accumulate in the abdomen and buttocks" (p. 828). These complaints are similar to those of many eating disorder patients as they gain weight. Besides their typical fear of weight gain, they often report "feeling fat" and are worried about acquiring distended stomachs. However, as indicated in Figure 8.9, the body weight and relative body

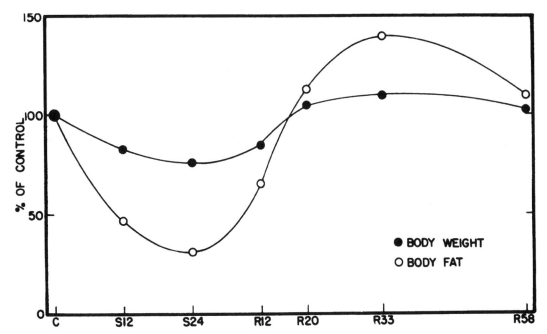

FIGURE 8.9. Body weight and body fat expressed as percentages of the control values for the volunteers in the Minnesota experiment. C, control; Sn, weeks of semistarvation; Rn, weeks of rehabilitation. From Keys et al. (1950, p. 117). Copyright 1950 by the University of Minnesota Press. Reprinted by permission.

fat of the Minnesota volunteers was at the pre-experiment levels after about 9 months of rehabilitation.

Physical Activity

In general, the men responded to semistarvation with reduced physical activity. They became tired, weak, listless, and apathetic, and complained of lack of energy. Voluntary movements became noticeably slower. However, according to Keyes et al., "some men exercised deliberately at times. Some of them attempted to lose weight by driving themselves through periods of excessive expenditure of energy in order either to obtain increased bread rations . . . or to avoid reduction in rations" (p. 828). This is similar to the practice of some eating disorder patients, who feel that if they exercise strenuously, they can allow themselves a bit more to eat. The difference is that for those with eating disorders, the caloric limitations are self-imposed.

Significance of the "Starvation Study"

As is readily apparent from the preceding description of the Minnesota experiment, many of

the symptoms that might have been thought to be specific to anorexia nervosa and bulimia nervosa are actually the results of starvation (Pirke & Ploog, 1987). These are not limited to food and weight, but extend to virtually all areas of psychological and social functioning. Since many of the symptoms that have been postulated to cause these disorders may actually result from undernutrition, it is absolutely essential that weight be returned to "normal" levels so that psychological functioning can be accurately assessed.

The profound effects of starvation also illustrate the tremendous adaptive capacity of the human body and the intense biological pressure on the organism to maintain a relatively consistent body weight. This makes complete evolutionary sense. Over hundreds of thousands of years of human evolution, a major threat to the survival of the organism was starvation. If weight had not been carefully modulated and controlled internally, early humans most certainly would simply have died when food was scarce or when their interest was captured by countless other aspects of living. The Keys et al. "starvation study" illustrates how the human being becomes more oriented toward food when starved and how other pursuits important to the survival of the species (e.g., social and sexual functioning) become subordinate to the primary drive toward food.

One of the most notable implications of the Minnesota experiment is that it challenges the popular notion that body weight is easily altered if one simply exercises a bit of "willpower." It also demonstrates that the body is not simply "reprogrammed" at a lower set point once weight loss has been achieved. The volunteers' experimental diet was unsuccessful in overriding their bodies' strong propensity to defend a particular weight level. Again, it is important to emphasize that following the months of refeeding, the Minnesota volunteers did not skyrocket into obesity. On the average, they gained back their original weight plus about 10%; then, over the next 6 months, their weight gradually declined. By the end of the follow-up period, they were approaching their preexperiment weight levels.

RESTORING REGULAR EATING PATTERNS

Restoring regualr eating involves meal planning and the following components: (1) mechanical eating, (2) spacing meals, (3) specifying the quantity of foodstuffs, and (4) specifying the quality of foodstuffs.

Meal planning consists of specifying the details of eating in advance of each meal. As described below, it involves prescribing specific foods and amounts to be consumed, and describing the context, such as place and time. The structure imposed by meal planning allows most patients to relax their rigid rules about food, and it assures them that they will not be allowed to go too far in the direction of either overeating or undereating. This structure may also help patients identify recurring situations or emotions that result in disturbed eating patterns.

Mechanical Eating

A patient should eat "mechanically," that is, according to set times and a predetermined plan. Food can be thought of as "medication" intended to "inoculate" the patient against future extreme food cravings and binge eating (Garner, Garfinkel, & Bemis, 1982). Removing the decision-making factor from eating is crucial early in treatment when patients are particularly likely to experience great anxiety and guilt in problematic eating situations. Any deviation from the eating plan, whether undereating or overeating, should be discouraged. Mechanical eating minimizes the sense of virtue for avoiding eating and guilt for giving in to the urge to eat. Patients need to realize that, at least temporarily, they cannot permit their eating behavior to be determined by "urges" and shifts in thinking and feeling. New rules for food intake need to be followed until eating can be more naturally regulated by internal signals. Promoting mechanical eating appears to conflict with the therapeutic goal of increasing patients' trust in their internal sensations, but it can take months or years for normal appetite to return. The analogy that mechanical eating is like a splint for a broken bone is useful: Firm support is needed while healing occurs.

Spacing Eating

Most patients try to "save" calories for later in the day or hope that they may be able to avoid eating altogether. However, growing hunger during the day often leads to overeating in the evening. This pattern of starving followed by overconsumption can actually lead to patients' establishing a higher body weight than they would without any dieting at all. Meals should be spaced throughout the day (Garner et al., 1985). Breakfast should never be skipped, and, ideally, there should be three meals and one or two snacks spread evenly throughout the day. Again, it is best for patients to confine eating to set times, rather than relying on internal sensations as guides. The reason for this type of plan is that it will lessen food cravings, urges to overeat or undereat, and loss of control.

Paying Attention to the Quantity of Foodstuffs

The number of calories that patients need to consume daily depends on their current weight, metabolic condition, eating patterns, and ability to tolerate change (Garner et al., 1985). Russell (1970) noted that some emaciated patients maintained their weight on a mere 600–900 calories per day. Slowly increasing caloric intake to achieve a weight gain of 1–2 pounds per week is ideal. For hospitalized patients, caloric intake should be adjusted to achieve a gain of 2–3 pounds per week. The prescribed diet for inpatients should never fall below 1,500 calories per day, and should generally be increased to 1,800 to 2,400 calories within the first week. All meals must be finished, so that patients can learn that the amount of food prescribed can be assimilated according to the plan for weight gain or weight stabilization. As patients shift from a hypometabolic to a hypermetabolic state, daily consumption may need to be increased still further, to as high as 3,500–4,000 calories. However, patients with a personal or family history of obesity will usually need fewer calories to achieve a desirable rate of weight gain. For outpatients, the speed of weight gain is not as important as gradual, steady progress toward weight gain.

Paying Attention to the Quality of Foodstuffs

At the beginning of treatment, most patients have little sense of what constitutes "normal" eating. They tend to divide food into "good" and "bad" categories, which are frequently based on nutritional myths (e.g., "Calories from dietary fat are stored as body fat, in contrast to calories from protein and carbohydrate, which are burned off"). Some of these ideas are extreme interpretations of sensible dietary guidelines. For instance, red meat may be excluded altogether, not just minimized; dietary fat and sugar can likewise be eliminated rather than reduced. Only foods considered "nonfattening" are permitted. The result is an unappealing dietary regimen, but it makes patients feel "safe."

One goal of treatment is for patients to become more relaxed about eating a wide range of foods. A weekly meal plan should begin to include small amounts of previously avoided or forbidden foods. Most patients who follow a vegetarian diet should be encouraged to abandon this food preference during their recovery. Foods that patients enjoyed before the onset of the eating disorder should serve as a guideline for more relaxed food choices. Patients should be encouraged to question their "good" and "bad" food categories by acknowledging that the calories of those foods previously labeled "bad" really have no greater impact on weight than those of the "good" food items. Patients who binge-eat should consume small amounts of the foodstuffs typically reserved for episodes of binge eating. Again, these foods should be redefined as "medication" that will help "inoculate" patients against binge eating by reducing

psychological cravings as well as by establishing new response tendencies to foods that formerly connoted loss of control. Even after considerable work has gone into refuting nutritional myths, patients are often overwhelmed with anxiety when they face certain food choices. This is why eating needs to be planned in advance, as described above. It can be helpful to construct a hierarchy of feared foods, and have a patient gradually move up this scale over time. These feared foods can be eaten in small amounts, but they should be included in every meal.

Helping patients combat specific food myths may call for specialized nutritional knowledge, and clinicians need to develop the necessary background in this area. Finally, persistent patterns of irrational thinking about food may reflect a more basic problem with flawed reasoning. Unwillingness or refusal to experiment with different types of foods may require the application of more formal cognitive-behavioral therapy methods (Garner et al., Chapter 7, this volume).

Using Self-Monitoring

Self-monitoring can be useful not only in establishing a regular eating routine but in gaining control over behaviors such as binge eating, vomiting, or laxative abuse. Self-monitoring consists of daily recording all food and liquid consumption and incidents of binge eating, vomiting, laxative abuse, and other extreme weight-controlling behaviors. Figure 8.10 illustrates a self-monitoring form. Patients are sometimes disinclined to complete self-monitoring forms, because they are embarrassed by their behavior or are afraid that self-monitoring will only increase their preoccupation with food. These concerns need to be dealt with by encouraging patients to acknowledge that self-monitoring can be extremely effective in gaining control over eating disorder symptoms. Self-monitoring is generally accepted as valuable, but recommendations related to timing and flexibility in implementing this procedure vary. In the early stages of treatment, some patients resist self-monitoring, even when they are presented with the rationale for its importance in recovery. A patient's reluctance to self-monitor is often related to overall low motivation to change or to commit to the goals of treatment. In such cases, discussing the patient's failure to comply with self-monitoring

Self-Monitoring & Meal Planning Form

Name: Date:

Time/ Place	Food and Liquid Consumed	B	V	Thinking, Feeling and Interpersonal Context

FIGURE 8.10. Self-monitoring form, which may also be used for meal planning. This form may be reproduced for personal use.

forms or reviewing the inaccurate forms may be pointless; instead, it may be necessary to adopt a more gradual and flexible approach.

VOMITING, LAXATIVES, AND DIURETICS IN CONTROLLING WEIGHT

Vomiting is not entirely effective in removing food from the stomach and it usually makes binge eating worse by perpetuating food cravings. Laxatives and diuretics are ineffective methods of weight control be-cause they do not cause malabsorption; they just cause temporary water loss. All of these symptoms have serious health conse-quences.

Most eating disorder patients begin vomiting, laxative, and diuretic abuse because these measures appear to be solutions to the predicament of their desire to eat on the one hand and their terror of weight gain on the other. Prior to the discovery of vomiting, overeating is generally avoided because it elicits so much anxiety and guilt. Vomiting usually occurs after eating large quantities of food (binge eating), but is also common after the consumption of smaller amounts of food. Paradoxically, it begins as a method to achieve "control" after eating, but it usually escalates in frequency, duration, and amount eaten until the person loses all sense of control. Vomiting not only perpetuates hunger by eliminating food, but it also tends to give the person permission to engage in binge eating. Over time, vomiting, binge eating, and dieting escalate into a self-perpetuating cycle (Figure 8.11). Moreover, vomiting is not entirely effective in removing food from the stomach (Kaye, Weltzin, Hsu, McConaha, & Bolton, 1993); thus, repeated episodes of binge eating and vomiting may actually lead to weight gain.

Laxative and diuretic abuse are also common methods used by eating disorder patients to prevent weight gain. Just like vomiting, they escalate and become self-perpetuating. Using laxatives for weight control is not only an extremely dangerous practice, but also an ineffective method of trying to prevent the absorption of calories. Laxatives primarily affect the emptying

of the large intestine, which occurs after calories have already been absorbed in the small bowel (Bo-Lynn, Santa-Ana, Morawski, & Fordtran, 1983). Weight change after laxative use is a result of diarrhea and water loss, not of calorie malabsorption. This was documented in a study where two bulimia nervosa patients each consumed 50 Correctol tablets after meals (Bo-Lynn, Santa-Ana, Morawski, & Fordtran, 1983). Although this large dosage of laxatives produced profuse diarrhea (over 6 liters or 6.3 quarts), it only led to a 12% decrease in caloric absorption; this amounts to less than 200 calories, or the equivalent of one small candy bar! As Bo-Lynn et al. (1983) point out, this is a small reward, considering the life-threatening effects of diarrhea plus the effort and expense involved. They reported that both bulimia nervosa patients participating in the study discontinued laxative abuse, partly in reaction to learning of these results. Thus, laxatives temporarily affect body weight by eliminating wa-

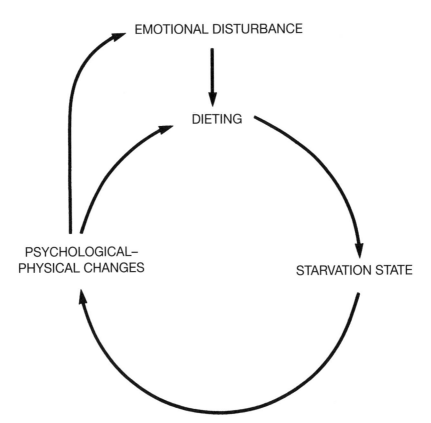

FIGURE 8.11. The vicious cycle whereby emotional disturbances can cause dieting and then can perpetuate an eating disorder through dieting, bingeing, or extreme forms of weight-losing behaviors. From Garner et al. (1985, p. 542). Copyright 1985 by The Guilford Press. Reprinted by permission.

ter, not fat. Dehydration is followed by rebound water rehydration.

Similarly, it is not uncommon for those with eating disorders to believe that body fat can be reduced with diuretics. This mistaken belief was shared by 25% of female physical education students in one study (Cho & Fryer, 1974). Diuretics have absolutely no effect on calories or body fat; they only change weight temporarily by changing water balance. Less often, people with eating disorders may resort to other dangerous weight control strategies, such as the use of appetite suppressants, the manipulation of medications (e.g., insulin or thyroid replacement hormone), or the ingestion of ipecac to induce vomiting. These symptoms can have very serious side effects. The misuse of ipecac can cause cardiotoxicity and sudden death.

DETERMINING A HEALTHY BODY WEIGHT

Weight tables should not be used to determine the desirable weight for an individual; "healthy body weights" naturally vary in the population and must be determined on the basis of each person's weight history and likely genetic background.

There is considerable confusion on the topic of how to determine one's desirable or ideal weight. This is a particularly sensitive topic for people with eating disorders. Part of the confusion stems from the convention of relying on weight norms or recommended weights provided by insurance companies or other agencies. The main problem with this practice is that it does not take into consideration that weight norms are statistical averages (based upon height and age) that reveal nothing about the natural variability in body weights around these midpoints. Body weight, like most other physical attributes, naturally varies among individuals in a population. Deriving desirable weights from an average weight table is as inappropriate as calculating expected heights from average height tables!

Figure 8.12 represents the theoretical normal distribution of body weights in the entire population of women. The "average weight," represented by vertical line A in the middle of the distribution, is the one that is recorded on the tables found in most doctors' offices. Some tables of "desirable weights" are even more unrealistic, since they recommend that people weigh 90% of average weight (line B in the distribution). As is evident from Figure 8.12, a range of body weights can be expected to occur in the population, and using the statistical average to determine a particular individual's "ideal" body weight is misguided. Rather than estab-

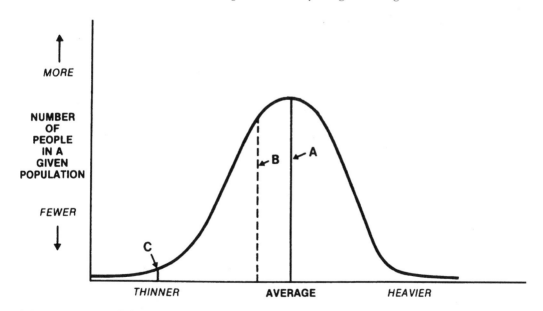

FIGURE 8.12. Normal distribution or natural distribution of body weights in the population. A, "average weight"; B, so-called desirable often recommended; C, the standard set for women by the fashion industry. From Garner et al. (1985, p. 544). Copyright 1985 by The Guilford Press. Reprinted by permission.

lishing an exact weight expectation, the most desirable approach to determining what one should weigh is to eliminate restrictive dieting, gain control over binge eating, engage in moderate exercise, and allow one's body to find its own "natural weight." Initially, most patients react negatively to this recommendation, since it usually means accepting a higher weight than the one they prefer. However, most people have been duped by the weight loss industry into believing that they can simply "choose" a body weight and then modify their diet to produce the desired result. The fact is that just as some people must cope with being shorter than average, those with a personal and family history of obesity must learn to cope with a body weight that is higher than average.

Another method recommended for establishing a realistic body weight is a "range" of about 2.3 kg (5 pounds) that is 10% below the individual's highest weight prior to the onset of an eating disorder (Garner et al., 1985). This recommendation is consistent with the findings of Abraham and Beumont (1982), who indicated that the "previous stable weight" for a group of bulimic patients was almost precisely 90% of their "highest weight ever attained." It is also consistent with findings from studies of both anorexia nervosa and bulimia nervosa that abnormalities in reproductive hormones tend to reverse themselves when patients return to a body weight that is closer to 90% of their own past highest weight rather than a weight determined by actuarial tables (Treasure, Wheeler, King, Gordon, & Russell, 1988; Weltzin, Cameron, Berga, & Kaye, 1994). The goal of about 10% below the previous highest weight is simply a guideline and may have to be modified, depending on a patient's weight and eating history. For example, some patients have had brief periods of rapid weight gain prior to the onset of their disorder, and 10% below their past highest weight may be unnecessarily high. Others may have always dieted, so that they have never allowed themselves to achieve a healthy or natural weight.

The general guidelines for establishing and monitoring body weight may be summarized as follows:

1. It is preferable for a patient to avoid choosing a specific goal weight; rather, the patient should simply concentrate on establishing appropriate eating patterns and discontinuing binge eating and purging.

2. Weight often varies because of daily fluctuations in water balance and the contents of the digestive tract; thus, the aim is a 5-pound weight range rather than an exact weight.

3. A goal weight range should take personal and family weight history into consideration.

4. A good estimate of a healthy weight is 10% below one's highest weight prior to the onset of eating problems.

5. As long as body weight is a matter of medical concern, it should be monitored once a week, preferably by a trusted therapist.

PHYSICAL COMPLICATIONS

Physical complications are common with eating disorders, and they can be life-threatening. Complications result primarily from starvation; vomiting; and abuse of laxatives, diuretics, and other medications. Risks can be reduced by understanding the complications and correcting eating disorder symptoms.

It is important for the patient as well as the clinician to be aware of the major medical complications of eating disorders. Reviewing potential complications and stressing the seriousness of certain symptoms can be helpful in enlisting motivation for change. In all cases, arrangements should be made for a medical consultation with a physician knowledgeable about the medical risks and complications associated with anorexia nervosa and bulimia nervosa. This section simply provides an overview of major complications; the reader is encouraged to consult more detailed and comprehensive reviews (Beumont, Russell, & Touyz, 1993; Comerci, 1990; Mitchell & Boutacoff, 1986; Mitchell, Pomeroy, & Adson, Chapter 21, this volume; Sharp & Freeman, 1993).

Mortality Risk

The risk of death from anorexia nervosa is significant. Anorexia nervosa can be chronic and it has the highest mortality rate of any psychiatric disorder (Theander, 1985; Sullivan, 1995). Table 8.1 shows the results from one long-term follow-up study of anorexia nervosa patients who probably received rather crude treatment, since their initial admission was during a three-decade period (1931–1960) when little was known about treatment of the disorder (Thean-

TABLE 8.1. Long-Term Outcome in
Anorexia Nervosa

	Years after onset of the disorder		
Outcome type	5 years	15 years	33 years
Good	55%	63%	76%
Intermediate	19%	17%	1%
Poor	18%	7%	6%
Death	8%	13%	18%

Note. Adapted from Theander (1985, p. 503). Copyright 1985 by Pergamon Press. Adapted by permission.

der, 1985). Table 8.1 shows the gradual filtering of patients into two outcome categories after 33 years: good (76%) and death (18%). One interpretation of these findings is that even people who manage to suppress their body weight by using extraordinary measures are ultimately worn down by the set-point mechanism and return to a normal weight. It is important to point out that more recent follow-up studies indicate better outcomes, probably associated with more adequate treatment (Crisp, Callender, Halek, & Hsu, 1992; Hsu, Crisp, & Callender, 1992; Herpertz-Dahlman, Wewetzer, Schultz, & Remschmidt, 1996; Steinhausen, Rauss-Mason, & Seidel, 1991). The long-term outcome of bulimia nervosa is less well established. In a 10-year follow-up, Collins and King (1994) found that 52% of patients had fully recovered, 39% had improved but had some symptoms, and 9% still had the full disorder. There was only one death, and this was apparently unrelated to the eating disorder.

Electrolyte Disturbances

Probably the most dangerous complication of vomiting and purgative abuse is the depletion of the electrolytes potassium, chloride, and sodium. These elements, among others, are called "electrolytes" because they have the property of carrying electrical charges when they are dissolved in solution. They are essential to the organism for metabolic processes, as well as for the normal functioning of nerve and muscle cells. Frequent vomiting, laxative abuse, and diuretic abuse can lead to the depletion of sodium, potassium, and chloride. Alkaline intoxication may result from the loss of sodium (hypoatremic alkalosis), chloride (hypochloremic alkalosis), or potassium (hypokalemic alkalosis). The mechanisms responsible for these changes are complex, and the

medical consequences are extremely dangerous (Mitchell, Pyle, Eckert, Hatsukami, & Lentz, 1983). Electrolyte abnormalities may cause weakness, tiredness, constipation, and depression. Moreover, they may result in cardiac arrhythmias and sudden death. Mitchell et al. (1983) found electrolyte disturbances in almost 49% of their bulimia nervosa sample.

Cardiac Irregularities

Deaths in anorexia nervosa and bulimia nervosa are most often attributed to cardiac abnormalities (Beumont et al., 1993; Sharp & Freeman, 1993). Cardiac abnormalities occur in as many as 87% of anorexia nervosa patients; these include bradycardia (heart rate less than 60 beats per minute), tachycardia, hypotension, ventricular arrhythmias, and cardiac failure (Schocken, Holloway, & Powers, 1989; Sharp & Freeman, 1993). Starvation seriously compromises cardiac functioning in many cases, and this, compounded by electrolyte disturbances, may result in serious irregularities in the heartbeat. Profound heart abnormalities have been observed during exercise, and these may be associated with sudden death. In a postmortem study of three women with anorexia nervosa, Isner, Roberts, Heymsfield, and Yager (1985) identified a potentially fatal slowdown in the electrical impulses that signal the heart to contract and relax. This particular electrical disturbance, called "QT internal prolongation," may result in one of the most lethal forms of irregular heartbeat. If not treated within several minutes, such an arrhythmia can result in sudden death. Occasionally patients attempt to induce vomiting by ingesting an emetic such as ipecac; this may have fatal consequences, as noted earlier. Adler, Walinsky, Krall, and Cho (1980) have described a bulimia nervosa patient who died of cardiac arrest following repeated use of ipecac.

Kidney Dysfunction

Kidney disturbances occur in up to 70% of anorexia nervosa patients (Brotman, Stern, & Brotman, 1986) and can include electrolytic abnormalities and edema, among other disturbances. In emaciated patients, care must be taken in refeeding to avoid sudden reduced phosphate levels and peripheral edema, which can have serious consequences. Russell (1979) described three patients who required treatment for urinary tract infections. Kidney damage has been reported in patients with potassium deficiencies (Russell, 1979). After 8 years of self-induced vomiting, one of Russell's patients developed kidney failure and ultimately required a kidney transplant.

Cerebral Atrophy

Brain scans are abnormal in more than half of patients with anorexia nervosa; they reflect cerebral atrophy, as indicated by enlarged cranial sulci, interhemispheric fissures, and dialation of the cerebral ventricles (Krieg, Pirke, Lauer, & Backmund, 1988; Touyz & Beumont, 1994). This finding is consistent with the animal studies of weight loss reviewed earlier in the section on set-point theory. Cerebral atrophy is also evident in some patients with bulimia nervosa (Krieg, Lauer, & Pirke, 1989; Touyz &

Beumont, 1994). Figure 8.13 illustrates a cranial computerized tomography (CT) scan for anorexia nervosa and Figure 8.14 shows scan for bulimia nervosa revealing structural brain changes in both eating disorders. In both eating disorders, this condition appears to reverse itself with renourishment.

Neurological Abnormalities

Abnormal electrical discharges in the brain are common in some patients with bulimia nervosa and usually associated with electrolyte disturbances (Mitchell & Pyle, 1982). Seizures have been reported in 4 of 30 cases described by Russell (1979). Muscular spasms (tetany) and tingling sensations in the extremities (peripheral paresthesia) have also been described by Russell (1979).

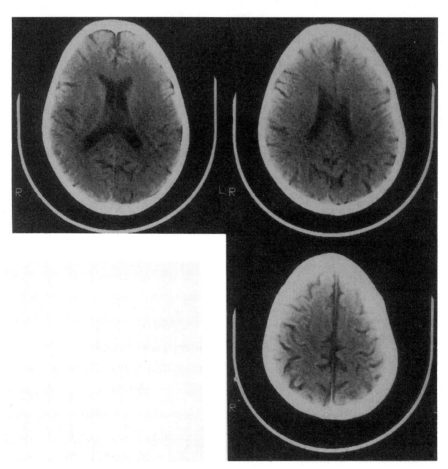

FIGURE 8.13. Computerized tomography (CT) scan of a 21-year-old female with anorexia nervosa showing mild cerebral atrophy and uniform prominence of the cerebral sulci. From Touyz and Beumont (1994, pp. 307, 319). Copyright 1994 by Academic Press. Reprinted by permission.

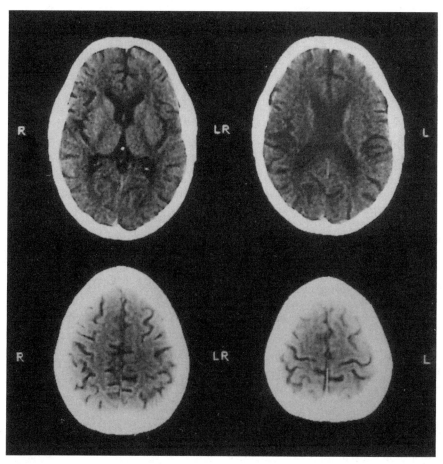

FIGURE 8.14. Computerized tomography (CT) scan of a 21-year-old female with bulimia nervosa showing dilated ventricles and enlarged cerebrospinal fluid spaces. From Touyz and Beumont (1994, pp. 307, 319). Copyright 1994 by Academic Press. Reprinted by permission.

Swollen Salivary Glands

A painless swelling of the salivary glands and accompanying facial swelling have been reported in about 25% of patients with bulimia nervosa, but also can occur in anorexia nervosa (Sharp & Freeman, 1993). This symptom is particularly distressing for patients, who are already sensitive about their shape. Salivary glands tend to return to normal when eating patterns are normalized and binge eating and vomiting are discontinued.

Gastrointestinal Disturbances

Frequently, patients complain of abdominal pain caused by the physical trauma of vomiting. Repeated self-induced vomiting occasionally results in the development of spontaneous regurgitation of food, which may perpetuate the disorder. Episodes of extreme binge eating can lead to severe abdominal discomfort. There have been rare case reports of extreme enlargement of the stomach (gastric dilatation) resulting from binge eating (Mitchell, Pyle, & Miner, 1982; Russell, 1966); in a few instances, this can lead to stomach rupture and death (Saul, Dekker, & Watson, 1981). Self-induced vomiting may also lead to serious tearing of tissue in the mouth and throat. Patients can choke on instruments used to attempt to induce vomiting, as well as on the vomitus itself. There is delayed gastric emptying in emaciated patients, leading to complaints of stomach bloating; however, this normalizes with renutrition. There can also be disturbances in the small intestine, liver, and pancreas. Russell (1979) has suggested the possibility of permanent loss of bowel reactivity with chronic abuse of laxatives. Some patients who have become dependent on laxatives for bowel functioning experience constipation once they discontinue the medication; however, in most instances bowel functioning returns with normal eating.

Dental Deterioration

The gastric acid from frequent vomiting can cause erosion of the dental enamel and underlying dentin (McComb, 1993). This erosion results in caries and periodontal disease. Tooth color changes from white to brown or grey, and complications may require extensive dental work or removal of teeth.

Finger Clubbing or Swelling

Finger clubbing or swelling has been observed in several cases as a consequence of chronic laxative abuse (Malmquist, Ericsson, Hulten-Nosslin, Jeppsson, & Ljungberg, 1980). This condition gradually reverses itself once laxatives are discontinued.

Edema and Dehydration

Dieting, vomiting, and laxative abuse or diuretic abuse often lead to alternating periods of dehydration and "rebound" excessive water retention. The dehydration is indicated by increased thirst and reduced urinary output. Many patients notice swelling or "puffiness" in their fingers, ankles, and faces as a result of edema. Edema is usually at its worst immediately after vomiting and laxative abuse have ceased. Some bulimic patients will gain between 2.3 and 4.5 kg (5 and 10 pounds) of water once they refrain from these abnormal weight control practices. Normalization of intake and discontinuation of vomiting and purgatives will gradually reduce the wide swings in water balance; however, patience is essential. Many bulimic patients become so alarmed at the sudden weight gain or swelling that they return to vomiting or laxatives before their bodies have had a chance to achieve balance, and this starts the cycle all over again.

Menstrual and Reproductive Functioning

Loss of menstrual periods is necessary for a diagnosis of anorexia nervosa, and menstrual irregularities and amenorrhea occur in about 50% of women with bulimia nervosa, even if body weight is within normal limits (Devlin et al., 1989). Menstrual dysfunction and infertility persist in some patients, even with weight gain; the incidence of prenatal complications is elevated in patients with eating disorders who become pregnant (Goldbloom, 1993).

Bone Abnormalities

Osteoporosis, vulnerability to fractures, and stunting of growth have been reported in anorexia nervosa (see Sharp & Freeman, 1993). Osteoporosis is evident within 2 years of the onset of anorexia nervosa, and is significantly correlated with duration of illness and degree of underweight (Sharp & Freeman, 1993; Siemers, Chakmakjian, & Gench, 1996).

Emotional Disturbance

As indicated in the earlier review of the Minnesota study (Keys et al., 1950), the range of emotional consequences of weight loss can include depression, anxiety, irritability, mood swings, and personality changes.

RELAPSE PREVENTION TECHNIQUES

When relapses occur, rather than becoming discouraged, patients should follow the "four R's" in reframing relapses: (1) reframing the episode as a "slip" rather than as "blown recovery"; (2) renewing the commitment to long-term recovery; (3) returning to the regular eating plan without engaging in compensatory behaviors; and (4) reinstituting behavioral controls to interrupt future episodes.

Patients need to be prepared for relapses in binge eating and vomiting, particularly during stressful period. After a binge, patients often chastise themselves with dysfunctional statements: "I have blown it, so it doesn't matter any more," "since I binged this morning, the rest of the day is ruined; I might as well continue bingeing," "All of my efforts are spoiled—now I must start all over again," "My binge eating proves that I will never recover." The hopelessness and despair that such statements generate can precipitate further symptomatic behavior, resulting in a vicious cycle. Patients need to be reminded that progress is rarely linear in nature. More commonly, it follows an irregular pattern, in which success can only be attained amidst intermittent setbacks. Patients need be encouraged to refrain from applying "all-or-none," perfectionistic thinking to relapses. They need to reframe such episodes by stepping back and evaluating them in light of the "big picture." On the other hand, episodes of binge eating and vomiting should not be dismissed lightly. Concern and trying to understand the factors that led to a "slip" constitute the optimal response. A common reaction to relapse is trying to compensate by skipping the next meal or undereating. This should be strongly discouraged, since it usually leads to increased food cravings and an escalation in binge eating.

If binge eating continues, the eating plan needs to be reviewed to ensure that the quantity of food it stipulates is sufficient to quell food cravings. In addition to the amount eaten, the quality of foods and the spacing of meals should be reviewed. Changes in a patient's weight may reveal a conscious or unconscious drift or bias toward undereating. Undereating may be viewed as providing "money in the bank" that can be used later if overeating does occur. However, the growing caloric deficits increase the biological basis for food cravings, and thus heighten the vulnerability to binges. In this situation, the person can be described as a "walking time bomb with a hair-trigger on eating." If this scenario applies, the biological basis for binge eating needs to be reviewed, with an emphasis on the need to adjust food intake appropriately to correct the state of undernutrition. With practice, patients usually learn how to interrupt a vicious cycle by monitoring and challenging their dysfunctional beliefs.

CONCLUSION

Bulimia nervosa and anorexia nervosa are complex disorders that are caused and then maintained by various social, psychological, and biological factors. The current chapter selectively reviews research findings related to semistarvation, weight regulation, dieting, obesity, and the cultural milieu that appear to bear upon the development and perpetuation of these disorders. However, it is important to emphasize two cautionary points.

First, this chapter is not an exhaustive review of all the scientific literature related to each of the points of emphasis. Each of the areas surveyed represents an enormous scientific literature, and this chapter has been intentionally selective. Evidence has been presented on the basis of its relevance to specific issues that patients have found useful in recovery.

Second, psychoeducational material should not be considered a substitute for psychotherapy. The present emphasis on the cultural context for eating disorders, the physiological regulation of body weight, and the effects of starvation on behavior is not intended to disavow the importance of psychological mediators in eating disorders. There is adequate evidence indicating that food and the body can become the battleground for a variety of psychological and interpersonal conflicts. Although some patients improve simply through learning more about the conflict between social and biological factors, the majority find some type of psychological intervention necessary. However, psychoeducational material forms the foundation for recommendations on altering eating patterns and attitudes toward food, weight, and the body.

REFERENCES

Abraham, S. F., & Beumont, P. J. V. (1982). How patients describe bulimia or binge eating. *Psychological Medicine, 12,* 628–635.

Adler, A. G., Walinsky, P., Krall, R. A., & Cho, S. Y. (1980). Death resulting from ipecac syrup poisoning. *Journal of the American Medical Association, 243,* 1927–1928.

Andersen, A. E., & DiDomenico, L. (1992). Diet vs. shape content of popular male and female magazines: A dose–response relationship to the incidence of eating disorders? *International Journal of Eating Disorders, 11,* 283–287.

Bennett, W. I. (1984). Dieting: Ideology versus physiology. *Psychiatric Clinics of North America, 7,* 321–334.

Beumont, P. J. V., Russell, J. D., & Touyz, S. W. (1993). Treatment of anorexia nervosa. *Lancet, 341,* 1635–1649.

Bo-Lynn, G., Santa-Ana, C. A., Morawski, S. G., & Fordtran, J. S. (1983). Purging and calorie absorption in bulimic patients and normal women. *Annals of Internal Medicine, 99,* 14–17.

Brotman, A. W., Stern, T. A., & Brotman, D. L. (1986). Renal disease and dysfunction in two patients with anorexia nervosa. *Journal of Clinical Psychiatry, 47,* 433–434.

Brownell, K. D. (1982). Obesity: Understanding and treating a serious, prevalent, and refractory disorder. *Journal of Consulting and Clinical Psychology, 50,* 820–840.

Brunner, D., Weissbort, J., Fischer, M., Bearman, J. E., Leoble, K., Schwartz, S., & Levis, S. (1979). Serum lipid response to a high caloric high fat diet in agricultural workers during 12 months. *American Journal of Clinical Nutrition, 32,* 1342.

Cho, M., & Fryer, B. A. (1974). Nutritional knowledge of collegiate physical education majors. *Journal of the American Dietetic Association, 65,* 30–34.

Cleary, M. P., & Vasselli, J. R. (1981). Reduced organ growth when hyperphagia is prevented in genetically obese (fa/fa) Zucker rats. *Proceedings of the Society of Experimental Biology and Medicine, 167,* 616–623.

Collings, S., & King, M. (1994). Ten-year follow-up of 50 patients with bulimia nervosa. *British Journal of Psychiatry, 164,* 80–87.

Comerci, G. D. (1990). Medical complications of anorexia nervosa and bulimia nervosa. *Medical Clinics of North America, 74,* 1293–1310.

Corbett, S. W., Stern, J. S., & Keesey, R. E. (1986). Energy expenditure in rats with diet-induced obesity. *American Journal of Clinical Nutrition, 44,* 173–180.

Crago, M., Shisslak, C. M., & Estes, L. S. (1996). Eating disturbances among American minority groups: A review. *International Journal of Eating Disorders, 19,* 239–248.

Crisp, A. J. (1980). *Anorexia nervosa: Let me be.* London: Academic Press.

Crisp, A. H., Callender, J. S., Halek, C., & Hsu, L. K. G. (1992). Long-term mortality in anorexia nervosa: A 20 year follow-up of the St. George's and Aberdeen cohorts. *British Journal of Psychiatry, 161,* 104–107.

Crisp, A. H., Hsu, L. K. G., & Harding, B. (1980). The starving hoarder and voracious spender: Stealing in anorexia nervosa. *Journal of Psychosomatic Research, 24,* 225–231.

Devlin, M. J., Walsh, B. T., Katz, J. L., Roose, S. P., Linkie, D. M., Wright, L., Vande Wiele, R., & Glassman, A. H. (1989). Hypothalamic–pituitary–gonadal function in anorexia nervosa and bulimia. *Psychiatry Research, 28,* 11–24.

Dolan, B. (1991). Cross-cultural aspects of anorexia nervosa and bulimia: A review. *International Journal of Eating Disorders, 10,* 67–79.

Edlund, B., Halvarsson, K., & Sjödén, P. (1995). Eating behaviours, and attitudes to eating, dieting, and body image in 7-year-old Swedish girls. *European Eating Disorders Review, 3,* 1–14.

Fairburn, C. G., Marcus, M. D., & Wilson, G. T. (1993). Cognitive behavior therapy for binge eating and bulimia nervosa: A comprehensive treatment manual. In C. G. Fairburn & G. T. Wilson (Eds.), *Binge eating: Nature, assessment, and treatment* (pp. 361–404). New York: Guilford Press.

Fantino, M., & Cabanac, M. (1980). Body weight regulation with a proportional hoarding response in the rat. *Physiology and Behavior, 24,* 939–942.

Fox, F. W. (1973). The enigma of obesity. *Lancet, ii,* 1487–1488.

van Furth, E. F., van Strien, D. C., Martina, L. M. L., van Son, M. J. M., Hendrickx, J. J. P., & van Engeland, H. (1996). Expressed emotion and the prediction of outcome in adolescent anorexia nervosa. *International Journal of Eating Disorders, 20,* 19–31.

Garfinkel, P. E., & Garner, D. M. (1982). *Anorexia nervosa: A multidimensional perspective.* New York: Brunner/Mazel.

Garner, D. M. (1991). *Eating Disorder Inventory—2: Professional manual.* Odessa, FL: Psychological Assessment Resources.

Garner, D. M. (1993a). Pathogenesis of anorexia nervosa. *Lancet, 341,* 1631–1635.

Garner, D. M. (1993b). Eating disorders and what to do about obesity [Editorial]. *International Review of Psychiatry, 5,* 9–12.

Garner, D. M. (1993c). Self-report measures for eating disorders. *Current Contents: Social and Behavioral Sciences, 25*(8), 8.

Garner, D. M. (1995). Dieting maelstrom or painful evolution? *American Psychologist, 50,* 944–945.

Garner, D. M., Fairburn, C. G., & Davis, R. (1987). Cognitive-behavioral treatment of bulimia nervosa: A critical appraisal. *Behavior Modification, 11,* 398–431.

Garner, D. M., & Garfinkel, P. E. (1979). The Eating Attitudes Test: An index of the symptoms of anorexia nervosa. *Psychological Medicine, 9,* 273–279.

Garner, D. M., & Garfinkel, P. E. (1980). Socio-cultural factors in the development of anorexia nervosa. *Psychological Medicine, 10,* 647–656.

Garner, D. M., Garfinkel, P. E., & Bemis, K. M. (1982). A multidimensional psychotherapy for anorexia nervosa. *International Journal of Eating Disorders, 1,* 3–46.

Garner, D. M., Garfinkel, P. E., Schwartz, D. M., & Thompson, M. M. (1980). Cultural expectations of thinness in women. *Psychological Reports, 47,* 483–491.

Garner, D. M., Olmsted, M. P., Bohr, Y., & Garfinkel, P. E. (1982). The Eating Attitudes Test: Psychometric features and clinical correlates. *Psychological Medicine, 12,* 871–878.

Garner, D. M., Rockert, W., Olmsted, M. P., Johnson, C. L., & Coscina, D. V. (1985). Psychoeducational principles in the treatment of bulimia and anorexia nervosa. In D. M. Garner & P. E. Garfinkel (Eds.), *Handbook of psychotherapy for anorexia nervosa and bulimia* (pp. 513–572). New York: Guilford Press.

Garner, D. M., & Rosen, L. W. (1991). Eating disorders in athletes: Research and recommendations. *Journal of Applied Sports Research, 5,* 100–107.

Garner, D. M., & Wooley, S. C. (1991). Confronting the failure of behavioral and dietary treatments of obesity. *Clinical Psychology Review, 11,* 729–780.

Goldbloom, D. S. (1993). Menstrual and reproductive function in the eating disorders. In A. S. Kaplan & P. E. Garfinkel (Eds.), *Medical issues and the eating disorders* (pp. 165–175). New York: Brunner/Mazel.

Greene, R. L. (1980). *The MMPI: An interpretive manual.* New York: Grune & Stratton.

Greenwood, M. R. C., Maggio, C. A., Koopmans, H. S., & Sclafani, A. (1982). Zucker fafa rats maintain their obese body composition ten months after jejunoileal bypass surgery. *International Journal of Obesity, 6,* 513–525.

Gulick, A. (1922). A study of weight regulation of the adult human body during overnutrition. *American Journal of Physiology, 60,* 371–395.

Herpertz-Dahlmann, B. M., Wewetzer, C., Schultz, E., & Remschmidt, H. (1996). Outcome in adolescent anorexia nervosa. *International Journal of Eating Disorders, 19,* 335–345.

Hill, G. L., & Beddoe, A. H. (1986). Dimensions of the human body and its compartments. In J. M. Kinney, K. N. Jeejeebhoy, G. L. Hill, & O. E. Owen (Eds.), *Nutrition and metabolism in patient care* (pp. 89–118). Philadelphia: W. B. Saunders.

Hirsch, J. (1978). Obesity: A perspective. In G. A. Bray (Ed.), *Recent advances in obesity research* (pp. 1–5). London: Newman.

Hollifield, G. (1968). Glucocorticoid-induced obesity: A model and a challenge. *American Journal of Clinical Nutrition, 21,* 1471.

Hsu, L. K. G., Crisp, A. H., & Callender, J. S. (1992). Recovery in anorexia nervosa: The patient's perspective. *International Journal of Eating Disorders, 11,* 341–350.

Isner, J. M., Roberts, W. C., Heymsfield, S. B., & Yager, J.

(1985). Anorexia nervosa and sudden death. *Annals of Internal Medicine, 102,* 49–52.

Jourard, S. M., & Secord, P. F. (1955). Body cathexis and the ideal female figure. *Journal of Abnormal and Social Psychology, 50,* 243–246.

Kaye, W. H., Weltzin, T. E., Hsu, L. K. G., McConaha, C. E., & Bolton, B. (1993). Amount of calories retained after binge eating and vomiting. *American Journal of Psychiatry, 150,* 969–971.

Keesey, R. E. (1993). Physiological regulation of body energy: Implications for obesity. In A. J. Stunkard & T. A. Wadden (Eds.), *Obesity: Theory and Therapy* (2nd ed., pp. 77–96). New York: Raven Press.

Keys, A., Brozek, J., Henschel, A., Mickelsen, O., & Taylor, H. L. (1950). *The biology of human starvation* (2 vols.). Minneapolis: University of Minnesota Press.

King, M. B. (1989). Eating disorders in a general practice population: Prevalence, characteristics and follow-up at 12 to 18 months. *Psychological Medicine,* Monograph Suppl. 14, 1–34.

King, M. B. (1991). The natural history of eating pathology in attenders to primary medical care. *International Journal of Eating Disorders, 10,* 379–387.

Kramer, F. M., Jeffery, R. W., Forster, J. L., & Snell, M. K. (1989). Long-term follow-up of behavioral treatment for obesity: Patterns of weight regain among men and women. *International Journal of Obesity, 13,* 123–136.

Krieg, J. C., Lauer, C., & Pirke, K. M. (1989). Structural brain abnormalities in patients with bulimia nervosa. *Psychiatry Research, 27,* 39–48.

Krieg, J. C., Pirke, K. M., Lauer, C., & Backmund, H. (1988). Endocrine, metabolic, and cranial computed tomographic findings in anorexia nervosa. *Biological Psychiatry, 23,* 377–387.

Kuczmarski, R. J., Flegal, K. M., Campbell, S. M., & Johnson, C. L. (1994). Increasing prevalence of overweight among U.S. adults. *Journal of the American Medical Association, 272,* 205–211.

Lacey, J. H., Chadbund, C., Crisp, A. H., Whitehead, J., & Stordy, J. (1978). Variation in energy intake of adolescent girls. *Journal of Human Nutrition, 32,* 419–426.

Laessle, R. G., Beumont, P. J. V., Butow, P., Lennerts, W., O'Connor, M., Pirke, K. M., Touyz, S. W., & Waadi, S. (1991). A comparison of nutritional management and stress management in the treatment of bulimia nervosa. *British Journal of Psychiatry, 159,* 250–261.

Lee, A. M., & Lee, S. (1996). Disordered eating and its psychosocial correlates among Chinese adolescent females in Hong Kong. *International Journal of Eating Disorders, 20,* 177–183.

Leibel, R. L., & Hirsch, J. (1984). Diminished energy requirements in reduced obese patients. *Metabolism, 33,* 164–170.

Malmquist, J., Ericsson, B., Hulten-Nosslin, M. B., Jeppsson, J. O., & Ljungberg, O. (1980). Finger-clubbing and aspartylglucosamine excretion in a laxative abusing patient. *Postgraduate Medicine, 56,* 862–864.

McComb, R. J. (1993). Dental aspects of anorexia nervosa and bulimia nervosa. In A. S. Kaplan & P. E. Garfinkel (Eds.), *Medical issues and the eating disorders* (pp. 101–144). New York: Brunner/Mazel.

Meyer, J. M., & Stunkard, A. J. (1993). Genetics and human obesity. In A. J. Stunkard & T. A. Wadden (Eds.), *Obesity: Theory and therapy* (2nd ed., pp. 137–149). New York: Raven Press.

Mitchel, J. S., & Keesey, R. E. (1977). Defense of a lowered weight maintenance level by lateral hypothalamically le-

sioned rats: Evidence from a restriction–refeeding regimen. *Physiology and Behavior, 18,* 1121–1125.

Mitchell, J. E., & Boutacoff, M. A. (1986). Laxative abuse complicating bulimia: Medical and treatment implications. *International Journal of Eating Disorders, 5,* 325–334.

Mitchell, J. E., & Pyle, R. L. (1982). The bulimic syndrome in normal weight individuals: A review. *International Journal of Eating Disorders, 1,* 61–73.

Mitchell, J. E., Pyle, R. L., Eckert, E. D., Hatsukami, D., & Lentz, R. (1983). Electrolyte and other physical abnormalities in patients with bulimia. *Psychological Medicine, 13,* 273–278.

Mitchell, J. E., Pyle, R. L., & Miner, R. A. (1982). Gastric dilatation as a complication of bulimia. *Psychosomatics, 23,* 96–99.

National Adolescent Student Health Survey: A report on the health of America's youth (NASHS). (1989). Oakland, CA: Third Party.

Nemeroff, C. J., Stein, R. I., Diehl, N. S., & Smilach, K. M. (1994). From the Cleavers to the Clintons: Role choices and body orientation as reflected in magazine article content. *International Journal of Eating Disorders, 16,* 167–176.

Neuman, R. O. (1902). Experimentelle Beitrage zur Legre von dem Taglichen Nahrungsbedarf des Menschen unter besonderer Berucksichtigung der notwendigen Eiweissmenge. *Archiv für Hygiene, 45,* 1–87.

Nisbett, R. E. (1972). Eating behavior and obesity in men and animals. *Advances in Psychosomatic Medicine, 7,* 173–193.

Olmsted, M. P., Davis, R., Garner, D. M., Rockert, W., Irvine, M. J., & Eagle, M. (1991). Efficacy of a brief group psychoeducational intervention for bulimia nervosa. *Behaviour Research and Therapy, 29,* 71–83.

Ordman, A. M., & Kirschenbaum, D. S. (1986). Bulimia: Assessment of eating, psychological adjustment, and familial characteristics. *International Journal of Eating Disorders, 5,* 865–878.

Patton, G. C., Johnson-Sabine, E., Wood, K., Mann, A. H., & Wakeling, A. (1990). Abnormal eating attitudes in London schoolgirls—a prospective epidemiological study: Outcome at twelve month follow-up. *Psychological Medicine, 20,* 383–394.

Perlick, D., & Silverstein, B. (1994). Faces of female discontent: Depression, disordered eating, and changing gender roles. In P. Fallon, M. A. Katzman, & S. C. Wooley (Eds.), *Feminist perspectives on eating disorders* (pp. 77–93). New York: Guilford Press.

Pirke, K. M., & Ploog, D. (1987). Biology of human starvation. In P. J. V. Beumont, G. D. Burrows, & R. C. Casper (Eds.), *Handbook of eating disorders: Part 1. Anorexia and bulimia nervosa* (pp. 79–102). New York: Elsevier.

Platte, P., Wurmser, H., Wade, S. E., Mecheril, A., & Pirke, K. M. (1996). Resting metabolic rate and diet-induced thermogenesis in restrained and unrestrained eaters. *International Journal of Eating Disorders, 20,* 33–41.

Polivy, J., & Herman, C. P. (1985). Dieting and bingeing: A causal analysis. *American Psychologist, 40,* 193–201.

Polivy, J., & Herman, C. P. (1987). Diagnosis and treatment of normal eating. *Journal of Consulting and Clinical Psychology, 55,* 635–644.

Powley, T. L., & Keesey, R. E. (1970). Relationship of body weight to the lateral hypothalamic feeding syndrome. *Journal of Comparative Physiology and Psychology, 70,* 25–36.

Rastam, M. (1992). Anorexia nervosa in 51 Swedish adolescents: premorbid problems and comorbidity. *Journal of the American Academy of Child and Adolescent Psychiatry, 31*, 819–829.

Robinson, M. D., & Watson, P. E. (1965). Day to day variations in body weight of young women. *British Journal of Nutrition, 19*, 225–235.

Russell, G. F. M. (1966). Acute dilatation of the stomach in a patient with anorexia nervosa. *British Journal of Psychiatry, 112*, 203–207.

Russell, G. F. M. (1970). Anorexia nervosa: Its identity as an illness and its treatment. In J. H. Price (Ed.), *Modern trends in psychological medicine* (Vol. 2, pp. 131–164). London: Butterworths.

Russell, G. F. M. (1979). Bulimia nervosa: An ominous variant of anorexia nervosa. *Psychological Medicine, 9*, 429–448.

Saul, S. H., Dekker, A., & Watson, C. G. (1981). Acute gastric dilatation with infarction and perforation: Report of fatal outcome in a patient with anorexia nervosa. *Gut, 22*, 978.

Schocken, D. D., Holloway, J. D., & Powers, P. (1989). Weight loss and the heart: Effects of anorexia nervosa and starvation. *Archives of Internal Medicine, 149*, 877–881.

Sharp, C. W., & Freeman, C. P. L. (1993). The medical complications of anorexia nervosa. *British Journal of Psychiatry, 162*, 452–462.

Siemers, B., Chakmakjian, Z., & Gench, B. (1996). Bone density patterns in women with anorexia nervosa. *International Journal of Eating Disorders, 19*, 179–186.

Sims, E. A. H. (1976). Experimental obesity, diet-induced thermogenesis and their clinical implications. *Clinics in Endocrinology and Metabolism, 5*, 377–395.

Sims, E. A. H., Goldman, R. F., Gluck, C. M., Horton, E. S., Kelleher, P. C., & Rowe, D. W. (1968). Experimental obesity in man. *Transactions of the Association of American Physicians, 81*, 153–170.

Steinhausen, C. H., Rauss-Mason, C., & Seidel, R. (1991). Follow-up studies of anorexia nervosa: A review of four decades of outcome research. *Psychological Medicine, 21*, 447–454.

Stunkard, A. J. (1987). Conservative treatments for obesity. *American Journal of Clinical Nutrition, 45*, 1142, 1154.

Stunkard, A. J., & Penick, S. B. (1979). Behavior modification in the treatment of obesity: The problem of maintaining weight loss. *Archives of General Psychiatry, 36*, 801–806.

Sullivan, P. F. (1995). Mortality in anorexia nervosa. *American Journal of Psychiatry, 152*, 1073–1074.

Theander, S. (1985). Outcome and prognosis in anorexia nervosa and bulimia: Some results of previous investigations, compared with those of a Swedish long-term study. *Journal of Psychiatric Research, 19*, 493–508.

Touyz, S. W., & Beumont, P. J. V. (1994). Neuropsychological assessments of patients with anorexia and bulimia nervosa. In S. Touyz, D. Byrne, & A. Gilandas (Eds.), *Neuropsychology in clinical practice* (pp. 305–326). New York: Academic Press.

Treasure, J. L., Wheeler, M., King, E. A., Gordon, P. A. L., & Russell, G. F. M. (1988). Weight gain and reproductive function: Ultrasonographic and endocrine features in anorexia nervosa. *Clinical Endocrinology, 29*, 607–616.

Tremblay, A., Despres, J. P., & Bouchard, C. (1984). Adipose tissue characteristics of ex-obese long-distance runners. *International Journal of Obesity, 8*, 641–648.

Wardle, J., & Beinart, H. (1981). Binge eating: A theoretical review. *British Journal of Clinical Psychology, 20*, 97–109.

Wadden, T. A. (1993). Treatment of obesity by moderate and severe caloric restriction: results of clinical research trials. *Annals of Internal Medicine, 119*, 688–693.

Wadden, T. A., Sternberg, J. A., Letizia, K. A., Stunkard, A. J., & Foster, G. D. (1989). Treatment of obesity by very low calorie diet, behavior therapy and their combination: A five year perspective. *International Journal of Obesity, 13*(Suppl.), 39–46.

Weltzin, T. E., Cameron, J., Berga, S., & Kaye, W. H. (1994). Prediction of reproductive status in women with bulimia nervosa by past high weight. *American Journal of Psychiatry, 151*, 136–138.

Wilson, G. T., & Fairburn, C. G. (1993). Cognitive treatments for eating disorders. *Journal of Consulting and Clinical Psychology, 61*, 261–269.

Wiseman, C. V., Gray, J. J., Mosimann, J. E., & Ahrens, A. H. (1992). Cultural expectations of thinness in woman: An update. *International Journal of Eating Disorders, 11*, 85–89.

APPENDIX 8.1
The Eating Attitudes Test (EAT)

In some circumstances, periodic assessment of the eating concerns typical of those with eating disorders may be desirable. For example, it is useful to track attitude change during the course of psychoeducational or other treatments. The EAT is probably the most widely used standardized measure of symptoms and concerns characteristic of eating disorders (Garner, 1993c). A factor analysis of the original EAT (Garner & Garfinkel, 1979) produced an abbreviated measure, the EAT-26 (Garner, Olmsted, Bohr, & Garfinkel, 1982), which consists of 26 forced-choice, 6-point items forming 3 subscales (i.e., Dieting, Bulimia and Food Preoccupation, and Oral Control). The EAT and the EAT-26 do *not* yield a specific diagnosis of an eating disorder, but studies have shown that the EAT-26 can be an efficient screening instrument as part of a two-stage screening process in which those who score above a cut off score of 20 are interviewed (King, 1989, 1991). It is also a useful global measure of eating concerns that may be used in treatment outcome studies.

Neither the EAT, the EAT-26, nor any other screening instrument has been established as highly efficient as the sole means for identifying eating disorders. This in large part is due to the relatively low prevalence of eating disorders in most populations of interest. A disorder must have a prevalence approaching 20% in order for the test to be efficient in detection. Thus, it is very difficult to achieve high efficiency in detecting eating disorders that have a prevalence between 2% and 4% in populations of adolescent or young adult women.

Surveys of adolescents or young adult women indicate that about 15% score at or above 20 on the EAT-26. Interviews of those who score *below* 20 on the EAT-26 show that the test produces very few false negatives (those with low EAT-26 scores who have eating disorders or serious eating concerns on interview). King (1989, 1991) analyzed data from 720 general practice respondents (534 women and 186 men) who completed the EAT-26 and other measures; 71 (13.3%) females and 5 (2.7%) males scored above the threshold of 20 on the EAT-26. Based on interviews, high scorers were divided into six groups: (1) persons with eating disorders who meet strict diagnostic criteria, 9.4%; (2) persons with "partial syndrome," who report marked dietary restriction, weight preoccupation, bingeing, vomiting, and other symptoms of clinical significance, but who fail to meet all of the diagnostic criteria for an eating disorder, 23.4%; (3) "obsessive dieters" or "weight-preoccupied" individuals, who express significant concerns about weight and shape, but who do not present the clinical concerns of those with the "partial syndrome," 20.3%; (4) "normal dieters," who are actively trying to lose weight, but who show no evidence of "morbid" or obsessive concern about weight and shape, 35.9%; (5) obese individuals, 4.7%; and (6) generally disturbed individuals, who respond positively on the EAT-26, but who do not have significant concerns about weight or shape on interview, 6.3%.

SCORING SYSTEM FOR THE EAT-26

On the EAT, respondents must rate whether each item applies "always," "usually," "often," "sometimes," "rarely," or "never." Responses for each item are weighted from zero to three, with a score of 3 assigned to the responses farthest in the "symptomatic" direction ("always" or "never" depending on whether the item is keyed in the positive or negative direction; *item 25 is the only negatively keyed item* on the EAT-26), a score of 2 for the immediately adjacent response, a score of 1 for the next adjacent response and a 0 score assigned to the three responses farthest in the "asymptomatic" direction. Thus, positively scored items are weighted as follows: always = 3, usually = 2, often = 1, sometimes = 0, rarely = 0, never =

Norms for the EAT-26

percentile	Patients with Eating disorders	Female controls
	EAT-26 Raw Scores	
99	69	37
90	58	23
80	50	18
70	46	14
60	42	9
50	36	6
40	32	5
30	28	4
20	21	2
10	11	1
1	1	0
Mean	36.1	9.9
(50)	(17.0)	(9.2)

Note. Cutoff score = 20. Adapted from Garner, Olmsted, Bohr, and Garfinkel (1982, p. 875) and Garner and Garfinkel (1979, p. 278). Copyright 1979 and 1982. Adapted by permission.

EATING ATTITUDES TEST-26 (EAT-26)

1. Age __ 2. Sex __ 3. Height____ 4. Current Weight____ 5. Highest Weight (excluding pregnancy)____

6. Lowest Adult Weight____ 7. Level of Education Completed: ☐ Grade School ☐ High School ☐ College ☐ Past College

•Please check a response for each of the following questions•	Always	Usually	Often	Sometimes	Rarely	Never
1. Am terrified about being overweight.	☐	☐	☐	☐	☐	☐
2. Avoid eating when I am hungry.	☐	☐	☐	☐	☐	☐
3. Find myself preoccupied with food.	☐	☐	☐	☐	☐	☐
4. Have gone on eating binges where I feel that I may not be able to stop.	☐	☐	☐	☐	☐	☐
5. Cut my food into small pieces.	☐	☐	☐	☐	☐	☐
6. Aware of the calorie content of foods that I eat.	☐	☐	☐	☐	☐	☐
7. Particularly avoid food with a high carbohydrate content (i.e., bread, rice, potatoes, etc.)	☐	☐	☐	☐	☐	☐
8. Feel that others would prefer if I ate more.	☐	☐	☐	☐	☐	☐
9. Vomit after I have eaten.	☐	☐	☐	☐	☐	☐
10. Feel extremely guilty after eating.	☐	☐	☐	☐	☐	☐
11. Am preoccupied with a desire to be thinner.	☐	☐	☐	☐	☐	☐
12. Think about burning up calories when I exercise.	☐	☐	☐	☐	☐	☐
13. Other people think that I am too thin.	☐	☐	☐	☐	☐	☐
14. Am preoccupied with the thought of having fat on my body.	☐	☐	☐	☐	☐	☐
15. Take longer than others to eat my meals.	☐	☐	☐	☐	☐	☐
16. Avoid foods with sugar in them.	☐	☐	☐	☐	☐	☐
17. Eat diet foods.	☐	☐	☐	☐	☐	☐
18. Feel that food controls my life.	☐	☐	☐	☐	☐	☐
19. Display self-control around food.	☐	☐	☐	☐	☐	☐
20. Feel that others pressure me to eat.	☐	☐	☐	☐	☐	☐
21. Give too much time and thought to food.	☐	☐	☐	☐	☐	☐
22. Feel uncomfortable after eating sweets.	☐	☐	☐	☐	☐	☐
23. Engage in dieting behavior.	☐	☐	☐	☐	☐	☐
24. Like my stomach to be empty.	☐	☐	☐	☐	☐	☐
25. Enjoy trying new rich foods.	☐	☐	☐	☐	☐	☐
26. Have the impulse to vomit after meals.	☐	☐	☐	☐	☐	☐

Note. Cutoff score = 20. Adapted from Garner, Olmsted, Bohr, and Garfinkel (1982, p. 875) and Garner and Garfinkel (1979, p. 278). Copyright 1979 and 1982. Adapted by permission.

0. The reversed-scored item (item 25) is weighted in the opposite manner (i.e., never = 3, rarely = 2, sometimes = 1, often = 0, usually = 0, always = 0). Items are assigned to the three subscales as follows:

Dieting subscale items: 1, 6, 7, 10, 11, 12, 14, 16, 17, 22, 23, 24, 25

Bulimia and Food Preoccupation subscale items: 3, 4, 9, 18, 21, 26

Oral Control subscale items: 2, 5, 8, 13, 15, 19, 20

Item scores contribute to only one subscale score. Subscale scores are computed by simply summing all item scores for that particular subscale. The Total EAT-26 score is the sum of all items (sum of the three subscales). The rationale for the 0–3 scoring system (rather than a 1-6 scoring system) is theoretical rather than empirical. It rests on the assumption that item scaling on the EAT-26 is continuous only for the responses weighted 1 to 3. Therefore responses in the non-symptomatic direction should not aggregate to contribute to a total subscale score reflecting psychopathology. With a 1–6 scoring system, it is possible for two responses in the nonsympto-matic direction to receive the same empirical weight (e.g. 3 + 3 = 6) as one extreme response in the symptomatic direction.

FAST TRACK FOR SCREENING

- The EAT-26 should not be used alone as a diagnostic instrument, but can be the first step in a two-stage screening process where high scorers are interviewed.
- A cutoff score of 20 on the EAT-26 is appropriate for many purposes; this score identifies approximately 15% of college and high school females, 10 to 40% of whom may be suspected as having clinically significant eating disorders.
- Cutoff scores may be adjusted to be higher or lower, depending on the purpose of screening.
- Addition of selected items from a measure such as the EDI-2 Symptom Checklist (Garner, 1991) may improve the discrimination of the EAT-26 and add information relevant to diagnosis.

CHAPTER 9

Nutritional Counseling and Supervised Exercise

PIERRE J. V. BEUMONT
CLAIRE CYNARA BEUMONT
STEPHEN W. TOUYZ
HAZEL WILLIAMS

Anorexia nervosa and bulimia nervosa are characterized by a complex pattern of behaviors directed at bringing about weight loss. For this reason, they are perhaps better termed "dieting disorders" than "eating disorders." Basic to anorexia nervosa are persistent undereating and the avoidance of high-calorie, fatty, or sweet foods. Some anorexic patients are also excessively active physically (Beumont, Arthur, Russell, & Touyz, 1994). These behaviors are termed "restrictive." In addition, many anorexics also use "purging" behaviors, such as self-induced vomiting, laxative abuse, and diuretic abuse (Beumont, George, & Smart, 1976). In contrast to anorexia nervosa patients, who are severely undernourished, bulimia nervosa patients are at an apparently normal weight or even overweight. They have a chaotic pattern of eating in which periods of severe restriction alternate with episodes of gorging, bulimia, or binge eating. They too may exercise excessively, albeit inconsistently. Most bulimic patients also use purging behaviors to compensate for overeating.

Although these behavioral abnormalities are basic to anorexia nervosa and bulimia nervosa, relatively little attention has been accorded in the literature to their direct management in treatment. The present chapter aims to provide a description of the role of nutritional counseling in restoring the nutritional state and improving the eating behaviors of patients with dieting disorders. In addition, the issues of overactivity and its management are discussed.

NUTRITIONAL COUNSELING IN THE TREATMENT OF ANOREXIA NERVOSA

Research and experience in the treatment of anorexia nervosa indicate that all of the physical symptoms and many of the psychological and social problems associated with the condition are secondary to the disturbance of nutrition. Unfortunately, it has also been found that a return to a healthy weight does not automatically dispel the abnormal eating behaviors and disturbed attitudes toward food commonly found in these patients (Windauer, Lennerts, Talbot, Touyz, & Beumont, 1993). Therefore, treatment regimes should focus initially on correcting nutritional status, but they should also provide counseling and education to normalize eating behavior, allay patients' fears about food, and provide accurate nutritional information. The appropriate person to direct nutritional rehabilitation and to provide dietary counseling is a dietitian, who should be an integral member of the treatment team (Beumont, O'Connor, Touyz, & Williams, 1987).

Unlike psychiatrists, physicians, psychologists, or nurses, dietitians have an expert knowledge of dietary matters, and their non-threatening status makes their advice more acceptable. On the other hand, they may be handicapped by their prior professional experience. Accustomed to dealing with overeating and the ingestion of diets that are too high in energy and relatively low in other nutrients, they may find anorexic patients paradoxical: such patients are actually practicing behaviors similar to those they encourage for obese patients. In order to be effective with anorexic patients, the dietitian must go beyond the prescription of an idealistic diet and promote instead a return to normal, sensible, "good enough" eating.

The Disorder of Eating

Excessive food restriction is the primary behavioral feature of anorexia nervosa. Patients typically follow current popular or faddish weight loss advice, as promoted by the mass media, their peers, or family members. They take their restrictive practices to unhealthy extremes, and usually start from a position of normal weight; they rarely have any real need to reduce.

Although the nutritional disturbance may be serious and complicated, with varying degrees of protein depletion, deficiencies in essential foodstuffs, and electrolyte imbalance, it is essentially a state of undernutrition resulting from a diet that is inadequate to meet energy demands.

The most common dietary pattern is first to decrease the consumption of foods containing fats and simple sugars, and then to avoid these foods altogether (Beumont et al., 1987). Low-fat dairy products are selected instead of whole-milk foods, and often milk and other dairy products are totally eliminated from the diet. Avoidance of red meat and a claim to be semi-vegetarian or lacto-ovo-vegetarian have become increasingly common (O'Connor, Touyz, Dunn, & Beumont, 1987). This has followed the "bad press" that red meats received in the 1970s and early 1980s in relation to saturated fats and heart disease.

There are also predictable changes in meal pattern and frequency in anorexic patients. Snacks eaten between meals (which normally contribute a valuable part of a teenager's energy and nutrient intake) are eliminated first, followed by breakfast and then lunch. The one re-

maining meal is usually dinner, because it is the time of day when eating is most visible to parents or spouse, and because it is perceived to be safer to eat at the end of the day, with few waking hours left to succumb to hunger.

Numerous abnormal eating behaviors, fears, and anxieties about food develop alongside food restrictions. Obsessional measurement of food to be eaten, cutting food into tiny mouthfuls, excessive chewing, and general anxiety at mealtimes are common and result in very slow eating. Patients are frequently observed to make strange mixtures of foods, to use excessive amounts of salt or other condiments, and to dispose surreptitiously of food at the table (e.g., by scraping butter under fingernails, pushing cake crumbs into pockets, and hiding uneaten food under table napkins). Such is their anxiety about eating that they focus their eyes and thoughts exclusively on their plates throughout meals and are unable to join in social conversation. Many inpatients have stopped eating in company altogether before being hospitalized.

The whole family may become enmeshed in an anorexic patient's food restrictions. All family members may change to eating the preferred foods of the patient; the patient may be allowed to decide what goes into the supermarket trolley, or permitted to take over the role of preparing family meals; and the family may cease to eat out in restaurants because the patient refuses to go.

Preoccupation with thoughts of food and eating is a result of any state of starvation, and anorexia nervosa is no exception. An anorexic patient may spend hours reading and collecting recipes, talking about meals, and preparing food. Moreover, such patients often select jobs that involve contact with food. This preoccupation may become most distressing for the patients when thoughts about food are so constant and strong that they interfere with sleep, study or work, and normal socializing.

Other weight-losing behaviors that are used by anorexia nervosa patients are induced vomiting; frequent use of laxatives, diet pills, and diuretics; and excessive exercise. Laxative and diuretic abuse are especially pernicious because of the medical dangers associated with their misuse and because of their intrinsic inefficacy. They bring about weight loss by causing a patient to lose fluids, not by reducing fat stores, and the weight loss they cause is quickly annulled when the patient is rehydrated. Excessive exercise is discussed separately later in this chapter.

Dietary Management

The principles of dietary therapy are the same for inpatient and outpatient treatment of anorexia nervosa. The goals of treatment, which should be established from the outset, are as follows:

1. To help patients attain and maintain normal nutritional status (in adults) and normal growth (in adolescents).
2. To assist patients in establishing normal eating behaviors.
3. To promote a normal attitude to food.
4. To help patients develop appropriate responses to hunger and satiety cues.

The Diet History

The skilled dietitian uses a diet history not just to obtain a detailed analysis of eating patterns and weight fluctuations from childhood to the present, but also to elicit information about the patient's nutritional beliefs and attitudes to food (Beumont, Chambers, Rouse, & Abraham, 1981). Of course, dietary histories are not infallible, as patients may be untruthful about their behavior; however, there is no reason to believe that they are any less reliable than other types of clinical data, such as medical or psychiatric histories. Nevertheless, it is also important to explore the beliefs and eating behaviors of the rest of the family. It is also usually appropriate to meet with at least one important family member (mother, father, or spouse) in the presence of the patient, to confirm the history, to ascertain whether other family members have problems with eating, and to ensure that the family is not condoning the patient's abnormal practices (Griffiths, Beumont, & Touyz, 1995).

During this initial interview, the dietitian begins to build a trusting relationship. This is essential if patients are to reveal the extent of their fears about eating and follow the advice they are given. Such trust is engendered by providing strictly accurate nutritional information; by being a sympathetic listener; by giving firm and consistent advice; and, importantly, by being a good role model. However, there is no room for compromise over a patient's beliefs and attitudes about food, and there is no point in trying to bargain over the goals of treatment.

Weight and Growth Expectations

The primary aim of nutritional management is restoration of normal body weight. For an adult, this may be defined as (1) the weight at which the patient is physically healthy and (2) the weight the person can maintain by eating a normal, healthy diet, without restrictions. It should be within the range of a body mass index (BMI) of 20–25. For a child or a younger adolescent, the target weight is one at which the patient is physically healthy and will continue to grow at a normal rate. A set BMI is not appropriate; instead, pediatric growth tables should be used, taking into account the growth stunting that may have already occurred. Perhaps an even better approach would be to refer to age appropriate BMI percentiles, as has recently been suggested (Hebebrand et al., 1996).

Weekly weight gain expectations are usually between 0.5 kg and 1.5 kg per week, depending upon the inpatient or outpatient status of the patient. Outpatients who are continuing with normal school or work and social activities should not be expected to gain weight as rapidly as more sedentary inpatients. If patients have been inducing vomiting, taking laxatives, or restricting fluids, they should be forewarned of a possible rapid initial weight gain because of rehydration.

Energy Level of the Recommended Food Intake

The recommended energy intake for normal-weight, healthy adolescents in Australia is between 8,400 kJ (2,000 kcal) and 10,000 kJ (2,400 kcal) for 13-18-year-old girls, and 9,800 kJ (2,300 kcal) and 13,500 kJ (3,200 kcal) for 13- to 18-year-old boys.

When a dietitian is recommending a therapeutic diet for an anorexic patient, the prescribed energy level depends initially upon the patient's intake prior to treatment and weight on presentation. If patients are extremely emaciated or have been eating minimally, an energy intake of as little as 5,000 kJ (1,200 kcal) is appropriate for the first few days. This will be adequate for some weight gain and will allow for gastric (and mental) readjustment to normal meal sizes. Less emaciated patients, who have been eating regular but small amounts, may be started on the recommended normal energy intake for their age.

Thereafter, dietary increases are made when weight gain slows down, but only if a patient is managing to complete each meal. Patients are consulted about each increase and given increasing autonomy in food selection and service as progress is made. Most female patients will require an energy intake in excess of 12,500 kJ (3,000 calories) daily to achieve full weight restoration. Once the recommended weight is achieved, food intake needs to be reduced to a level at which a patient is maintaining weight and eating a normal diet.

Food Content of the Recommended Diet

Since an anorexic patient's digestive tract is basically intact, except in the most severe of cases, the main obstacles to a return to normal eating are behavioral and psychological. It is not so much the management of the patient's diet that is difficult, but rather the management of the patient in taking that diet. The prescription of modified foods is unnecessary, other than gradual increases in bulk; indeed, it could be counterproductive, in that it may reinforce the patients' belief that they should not eat normal foods. It is our experience that tube feeding and total parenteral nutrition generally are not successful methods of refeeding these patients. Such procedures are invasive, not without physical danger, and do not help patients resume responsibility for their own health. They also fail to teach the patients about normal eating behavior and self-controlled weight gain. Similar criticisms may be made of high-energy liquid diets. These methods of refeeding should be used only when absolutely necessary—that is, when recalcitrant patients are at medical risk because of the severity of their undernutrition.

A regular meal pattern with a wide variety of normal foods is appropriate for most inpatients and all outpatients. They should be advised to avoid all "dietary" products aimed at weight loss, such as reduced-fat and artificially sweetened foods and drinks. These foods are counterproductive for weight gain and unnecessary for weight maintenance.

At the highest levels of energy intake for continued weight gain, the bulk of food can become uncomfortable for some patients. They may then be offered supplementary high-energy drinks as a temporary measure until the goal weight is reached.

Eating Behaviors

Eating behaviors should be the focus of specific attention, since abnormal behaviors are known to persist beyond weight normalization (Windauer et al., 1993). Eating in company is to be promoted, as other patients and staff members (or. in the case of outpatients, family members and friends) may provide useful role models. The previous practice of isolating anorexic patients at mealtimes was ill advised, as it merely reinforced their abnormal eating behaviors.

Actual eating behaviors should be carefully monitored in the hospital setting, so that encouragement and counseling to correct abnormal practices can be provided. Our Eating Behaviour Rating Scale provides a fairly objective means by which this may be done (Wilson, Touyz, Dunn, & Beumont, 1989). However, the conflicts that have taken place at home between patients and their families should not be reenacted. Confrontation should be avoided during mealtimes, and patients should be encouraged to interact socially in an appropriate way. Specific eating difficulties are addressed later in individual counseling sessions with a nurse or dietitian. Parents or spouses of outpatients should be similarly advised to avoid confrontation at meals and to leave the responsibility of choosing to eat to the patients. If a patient has persistent difficulties, these should be reported to the dietitian and discussed at the patient's next consultation with him or her.

In some instances, it is helpful to videotape patients during a meal and then use the tape in feedback sessions (Touyz, Williams, Marden, Kopec-Schrader, & Beumont, 1994). If the reasons for making such a tape are carefully explained to a patient, the procedure is usually well accepted.

Education

Patients with anorexia nervosa usually profess to have extensive knowledge about nutritional matters, and they are strongly opinionated about and extremely defensive of their nutritional beliefs and practices. However, their knowledge is highly selective, derived from dubious sources (such as popular magazines), often extreme, and usually incorrect (Abraham, Beumont, Booth, Rouse, & Rogers, 1981; Beumont, Chambers, Rouse, & Abraham, 1981). It is important that their misinformation be corrected and that they receive accurate information about their nutrient and energy requirements.

Educational issues should be addressed by the dietitian, either individually or in group sessions, throughout the treatment period. Topics that need to be explored are as follows: the physical and psychological consequences of excessive dieting and malnutrition; the nutrient content of foods; changes in dietary requirements with increasing weight; the dynamics of energy input, activity, and weight control; nutritional requirements for good health and weight maintenance; the dangers of purging behaviors; and, for older patients, practical advice about shopping and cooking.

The beliefs and attitudes of patients with anorexia nervosa do not change automatically with weight gain. Understanding based on correct information; personal experience of the benefits to health and energy that result from restored weight and nutrition; and continual support and reassurance are the most effective means of achieving change.

Weight Maintenance and Follow-Up

The dietary treatment of anorexia nervosa does not stop at the attainment of a healthy weight. Patients need continuing dietary guidance to help them adjust to a normal energy intake for weight stabilization, while maintaining a varied, nonrestrictive food intake. Many of their food fears and abnormal behaviors may return at this stage, when the security of having to gain weight under the dietitian's direction is removed.

Patients also need to develop a spontaneous, relaxed eating pattern, and to learn to cope with eating in restaurants, at school or work, or in friends' homes, instead of keeping to a rigid, unvaried pattern. None of these things comes easily to weight-restored patients, but much may be done with both inpatients and outpatients through discussions and practice sessions to prepare them for these challenges.

It is often beneficial for inpatients to stay in the hospital for a specified 2- or 3-week maintenance phase, during which they are given short periods of "leave" so as to provide an opportunity to practice eating at home prior to discharge. Occasional meals in restaurants are also useful in helping the patients adjust to eating outside the protective hospital environment.

Family members should be advised how to help patient readjust to a normal lifestyle after discharge. They should let the patient take responsibility for his or her own eating, since "stand-over" tactics at home are likely to be counterproductive. However, they must not condone anorexic practices or ignore evidence that the patient is relapsing. Without confrontation, they need to encourage the patient to return for further counseling sessions.

As eating behavior normalizes, and a patient's ability to maintain a healthy weight develops, sessions with the dietitian should be decreased. Continuing discussions and analyses of what patients eat will perpetuate dependence and an unnatural preoccupation with food matters. However, anorexia nervosa often persists for some years, and just as continued psychotherapy is required, so is persistent diet therapy necessary for long-term rehabilitation.

NUTRITIONAL COUNSELING IN THE TREATMENT OF BULIMIA NERVOSA

There are far more similarities than differences between the nutritional treatment of anorexia nervosa and that of bulimia nervosa (Beumont, O'Connor, Touyz, & Lennerts, 1988/1990). Just as energy deficiency has led to emaciation in anorexic patients, so has it led to a chaotic pattern of eating in bulimic patients, with periods of severe restriction alternating with episodes of compensatory hyperphagia or bulimia (binge eating). Bulimic patients are at an apparently normal weight and do not need to go on a weight gain program, but they do need to resume normal and relaxed eating, avoid restrictive practices, and learn to tolerate being at a weight that may be considerably higher than they wish.

Nutritional counseling should be undertaken early in the course of treatment. Patients need to regain control over their chaotic eating before they can be involved in meaningful psychotherapy. They view their problem as primarily one of overeating, and do not understand that the episodic gorging is largely a response to excessively restrictive eating. They have many fears and misconceptions about food and weight control, which must be identified and corrected. They firmly believe that they will get fat if they take regular meals or high-energy foods. And often their eating has been disordered for so long that they have lost the ability to eat normally. They need to learn the answers to such basic questions as these: "What is hunger? When should I eat? How much food is enough? And what is normal eating?" (Abraham & Beumont, 1982).

As with an anorexic patient, the dietitian first takes a detailed dietary history and fully explores the patient's eating behaviors, dietary knowledge, and attitudes toward food. In response to the patient's protestation that the problem is one of overeating, the dietitian emphasizes that this is but one aspect of a complex pattern of disordered eating, and that persistent and excessive dietary restraint is the primary trigger to the disorder. Binge eating is a response to unrealistic restraint, and the binge eater is really a "disinhibited dieter." If the patient can be persuaded to relinquish restrictive eating practices and resume normal eating, the urge to binge-eat gradually dissipates.

The line between bulimia nervosa and anorexia nervosa is very fine. Many bulimic patients are slightly underweight, although not so thin as to warrant a diagnosis of anorexia nervosa nor treatment on a refeeding program.[1] Others are overweight and have spent years attempting to lose weight by dieting. Continued dieting precludes the return to normal eating practices; for this reason, the dietitian should encourage bulimic patients not to focus on maintaining a particular weight, but rather to accept that a healthy weight is the weight they will maintain when they are eating a healthy diet and being reasonably active. Of course, this is difficult for weight-preoccupied patients to accept. Part of the skill of nutritional counseling is being able to present it persistently and persuasively.

Between binge-eating episodes, bulimia patients not only curtail the amount of food they eat, but completely avoid foods that they consider to be unhealthy or frightening—invariably, foods that have a high energy content (Touyz et al., 1994). (These often become the foods on which they binge.) The therapist tries to alter this misconceived perfectionism about food. Normal eating does not mean eating only "health" foods; it means taking a mixed and balanced diet containing the essential nutrients *and* sufficient calories for the body's needs. It also means accepting a "good enough" diet, rather than repeatedly failing to maintain an unrealistic, perfectionistic, "optimal" diet. The amount of food needed to meet daily energy demands is greater than that necessary for essential nutrient requirements, so that good health is achieved by supplementing a diet of "nutritionally sound" foods with a selection of some high-energy, less "nutritious" foods. If patients can be persuaded to take small amounts of high-energy foods every now and then, they are less likely to binge on them later.

Bulimic patients are persuaded to adhere to a defined meal plan and not to try to compensate for episodes of bulimia by further restriction or purgation. Each patient is also given accurate information about nutrition, and if possible, an appropriate, responsible family member is involved in these meetings.

Laxatives, both chemical and "natural," are frequently abused. The futility of this behavior in respect to true weight loss, and its dangers to physical health, need special emphasis.

If patients follow all of this advice for a few days, they begin to feel better. When this occurs, the dietitian should point out that many of the patients' symptoms were the direct results of poor eating. The resumption of normal meals and the cessation of purgation lead to only a slight gain of weight (usually between 1 and 3 kg), and this is attributable largely to rehydration. Patients are often amazed and delighted to realize that they can eat normally without becoming obese.

Most bulimic patients are treated as outpatients. They should be seen on a weekly basis to start with, then less frequently as they gradually resume control over their eating. The regular review of food diaries is a convenient means of providing support, reassurance, and education. Patients are advised of strategies to help regulate their eating, such as avoiding missing meals or snacks, using appropriate utensils, and not picking at food. They are also encouraged to introduce feared binge foods into their diet, and not to feel guilty about occasional, planned indulgences. They are told that minor relapses into bulimic behaviors are not total failure, but rather a stage in the process of recovery. Advice is given on meal planning, meal preparation, and eating in various situations so as to conform with social expectations. The use of alcohol or drugs such as marijuana is discouraged, as they are likely to induce a resumption of disrupted eating.

When therapy is terminated, the potential for relapse must be recognized; relapses may occur at times of stress or if a patient again embarks on a pursuit of thinness. When a relapse occurs, the patient should immediately return to a structured meal plan, and ready access to the dietitian should be assured.

Most anorexic patients are treated by a multidisciplinary team, of which a dietitian should be a valued member. On the other hand, the treatment of bulimic patients may sometimes be undertaken by a dietitian working alone. Of course, underlying psychological problems must not be overlooked, but these are not invariable, and for many patients sound nutritional advice and continued support constitute sufficient treatment (Laessle et al., 1981).

MANAGING THE EXCESSIVE ACTIVITY OF DIETING DISORDER PATIENTS

Excessive activity has long been recognized as a characteristic symptom of anorexia nervosa, and both Lasègue and Gull referred to overactivity in their descriptions of the disorder. Janet (1929), distinguishing between "hysterical" and "obsessional" presentations, compared the use of exercise to lose weight in the "obsessional" form to exercise as a denial in the "hysterical" form of the illness. Bruch (1973) described "obsessive hyperactivity" as being one of the four cardinal features of true anorexia nervosa.

Kron, Katz, Gorzynski, and Weiner (1978) surveyed the medical charts of female patients hospitalized for treatment over a 10-year period, and found hyperactivity in 25 out of 33 anorexia nervosa patients. Hyperactivity was judged to be present "when the patient clearly appeared to manifest a day-to-day level of physical activity that was far greater than [that of] most of her peers" (p. 434). The authors reported that excessive exercising was not merely a secondary symptom in hyperactive anorexic patients; rather, it usually preceded the onset of the illness, with 21 out of the 25 patients identified described as being extremely active well before they had ever dieted or lost weight. Kron et al. managed to follow up 15 of the original 33 patients, and found that for 11 of these, hyperactivity was still clearly present despite substantial weight recovery in 8. All of the hyperactive patients contacted at follow-up described their current activity level as being goal-directed, organized, planned, tightly scheduled, and rigidly carried out. The authors concluded that hyperactivity is "an early and enduring clinical feature of anorexia nervosa and not merely secondary to either a conscious attempt to lose weight or weight loss per se" (page 439).

Crisp (1965), in a retrospective analysis of the medical records of 102 anorexic patients, found excessive activity in 38, and King (1963) reported "intense athleticism" in up to 75% of anorexia nervosa sufferers.

We (Touyz, Beumont, & Hook, 1987) reviewed the clinical histories of 15 anorexia nervosa patients in whom overactivity had been noted as a cardinal feature. These patients were interviewed and compared to 17 anorexics in whom overactivity was not a predominant feature. We found that the initial motive for weight loss among the "exercisers" was a pursuit of *fitness* rather than a pursuit of *thinness*, and that 60% of the exercisers had commenced exercising excessively before engaging in dieting behaviors. All but one of the "exercisers" were engaged in strenuous physical activity for more than 2 hours per day prior to their hospital admission, compared to none of the "nonexercisers." There was a clear "debting" relationship between caloric intake and physical activity in all of the "exercisers." ("Debting" involves an attempt to regulate energy input through eating against energy output through exercise, so as always to remain in negative energy balance.) All the "exercisers" experienced marked withdrawal symptoms (e.g., irritability, guilt, or anxiety) when exercise was curtailed. A large number of the "exercisers" had sustained injuries as a result of their excessive activity, but continued to exercise regardless of pain. Many reported difficulty in controlling their activity when they returned home, and most were apparently unaware of the extent of their physical activity, tending to equate activity only with intense exercise. We (Touyz et al., 1987) concluded that for these exercising anorexia nervosa patients, overexercising was the major behavioral problem. We also suggested that "some subjects with 'exercise addiction' eventually progress to frank anorexia nervosa while in other anorexia nervosa patients who start with abstinence behaviors, excessive exercising develops later as the major behavioral problem" (pp. 145–146).

Implications for Treatment

Most behavioral programs for anorexia nervosa severely restrict activity, but some authors have made use of it in treatment. For example, Blinder, Freeman, and Stunkard (1970) used access to physical activity as a reinforcer of weight gain. In a series of three patients, they reported impressive weight gain with minimal confrontation when the patients were allowed

6-hour periods of unrestricted activity outside the hospital on any day on which the morning weight was at least half a pound up on that of the previous day. A similar approach was discussed by Liebman, Minuchin, and Baker (1974) and Garfinkel, Garner, and Moldofsky (1977).

Other authors have addressed the issue of specifically controlling exercise during the course of treatment. In a paper that has been much quoted, Mavissakalian (1982) used a response prevention strategy to treat two anorexia nervosa patients for whom overexercising was a major problem. He included an hour of bed rest after meals, to prevent the patients from attempting to neutralize the obsessionally feared consequence of overweight. The staff supervisors reported that the patients experienced great discomfort in complying with the rest period. Mavissakalian stressed how difficult it was for them to overcome the compulsive overactivity. Because the patients needed a very large number of sessions before they were able to adapt to the direction, it was only in the latter part of hospitalization that continuous supervision and response prevention could be eased. We (Touyz & Beumont, 1985) similarly included an hour of supervised bed rest after meals as part of a comprehensive treatment program, so as to prevent compulsive overexercising as well as self-induced vomiting.

The Clinical Assessment and Treatment of Overactivity

Theoretical, research, and therapeutic issues of the relationship of activity to anorexia nervosa are discussed by a number of authors from a variety of disciplines in a recent book edited by Epling and Pierce (1996). The assessment of overactivity and the use of supervised exercise in the treatment of dieting disorder patients have been discussed recently elsewhere (Beumont et al., 1994).

Many dieting disorder patients exercise excessively in response to media pressures that link self-worth and happiness to physical activity and fitness. This unrealistic view should be challenged in cognitive therapy. Families often play an important role in transmitting this influence. Parents who are themselves heavily involved in sporting activities may pass the commitment on to their children by their example. More damaging, perhaps, are those parents who get vicarious gratification from their child's sporting or dancing achievements, trying to relive their own lost youth. Such a child is enticed into meeting the parents' needs, perhaps in order to salvage a dysfunctional marriage by giving the parents a shared goal and sense of achievement. These sorts of problems should be addressed in family therapy.

Peer pressure is important, but perhaps more significant is the influence of teachers or coaches. Ill-considered comments concerning appearance, weight, body composition, or laziness assume great importance for an impressionable child, and may trigger harmful dieting and uncontrolled, excessive exercising.

In some cases, the increased physical activity helps screen the pathological aspects of the patients' weight-losing behavior. The patients' contacts are willing to condone their behavior when it is directed to becoming fit, whereas they would be alarmed if the patients admitted to the drive to lose weight. A level of activity that is reasonable for a healthy person who is eating an adequate diet is not appropriate for one who is already undernourished and on a severely restricted diet.

The salience assumed by the exercise is important. When exercise becomes so important as to interfere with interpersonal, social, educational, and vocational activities, it is excessive. Inability to abstain; intense anxiety when prevented from exercising; and a rigid, inflexible schedule of activities suggest an addictive quality to the exercising. Admission of chronic fatigue is further evidence that the level of activity is excessive.

Most patients show evidence of unhealthy activity when they are at very low body weights. It is unusual for patients who are severely emaciated (a BMI of 15 or below) not to be overactive, and usually the activity level increases as the patients continues to lose weight, until they reach a crisis when they are too weak to perform any but the most basic tasks. Even then, restless, aimless hyperactivity may persist. As weight is regained in treatment, the urge to engage in activity is usually reduced. Overactivity is less common and usually less severe in anorexic patients who are not markedly emaciated, or in those atypical eating disorder patients who have subclinical anorexia nervosa.

In some patients with bulimia nervosa, excessive exercising is also prominent. It often reflects the chaotic eating behaviors, with phases of hyperactivity alternating with inactivity. Excessive exercise is used as a means of compensating for disinhibited eating, together with (or in place of) laxative abuse and self-induced vomiting, and some patients refer to their exercising as self-punishment for bingeing. Other bulimic patients alternate between "good" phases (of adherence to a strict diet and exercise schedule) and "bad" phases (of binge eating and inactivity).

As Janet (1929) noted, there is considerable variation in the type of overactivity that different patients with dieting disorders display. Most striking is the restless activity seen in some anorexic subjects. They are unable to be still for even a few minutes, and are clearly distressed when their activity is restricted. Perhaps this presentation is the equivalent of Epling, Pierce, and Stefan's (1983) "activity-based anorexia," which occurs in laboratory animals that are put on a food deprivation cycle and given access to a running wheel. Instead of stabilizing at a lower weight, as other food-deprived animals do, these animals become more and more active and eat less and less until they die of starvation.

Other patients deliberately maximize their energy expenditure in undertaking everyday tasks. For instance, they will carry items up a stairway one at a time when a single trip with several articles would have sufficed, or they will perform other domestic duties at such a pace and in such a manner as to require maximum effort. Although such behavior would appear to be motivated by a desire to burn up calories, patients often rationalize the behavior to themselves and others, producing ingenious and far-fetched explanations.

A third form of overactivity is the adoption of a solitary exercise routine, closely resembling the excessive exercise of Yates, Leehey, and Shisslak's (1983) "obligatory runners." Many patients adopting this form of overactivity were previously involved in social or competitive sports, and although this involvement may continue for some time, there is a gradual shift toward activities that are repetitive and solitary. A patient's motivation changes from undertaking the activity predominantly for recreation, enjoyment, health, or fitness to a preoccupation with low body weight and slender shape. Many patients admit that they no longer enjoy the exercise, but are unable to stop.

In some patients, activity becomes clearly obsessive. They adhere strictly to a rigid exercise schedule and become distressed if they are unable to perform exactly the same routine each day (e.g., pass the same landmarks, do the same

or a greater number of laps, or perform their exercise at the same time on each occasion). If their routine is interrupted, they will repeat it from the beginning.

Although the effects of high levels of exercise are generally negative in respect to energy requirements and to the perpetuation of obsessional thinking and behavior patterns, there are also some positive aspects that must be considered. If exercise is regulated, it may contribute to the restoration of physical and mental health. One such possible beneficial effect is the suggestion that high activity levels may be a reason why anorexia nervosa patients maintain and restore their body protein more efficiently than do equally emaciated patients with medical diseases. However, in our own study of 32 patients with anorexia nervosa, we found no correlation between increase in body protein and documented exercise. Weight gain was the only determinant of protein repletion (Russell, Allen, Mira, Stewart, Vizzard et al., 1994).

Many treatment programs totally prohibit exercise, but we have found this to be both difficult to enforce and detrimental to recovery. Policing by staff members adds further strains to the therapeutic relationship, creating a battle of wills that distracts both the patients and the staff from the major goal of therapy—namely, to facilitate the patients' responsibility for themselves, rather than to increase feelings of helplessness, resentment, and dependence. For these reasons, we believe that a supervised program of exercise should be included in the treatment of anorexic and bulimic patients.

There is a basis of misinformation to these patients' behavior, which is as true for beliefs concerning exercise as it is for their distorted views about food. These false beliefs should be challenged by providing accurate information on the type and level of activity necessary for optimal health, with an emphasis on the deleterious effects of excessive exercise in the presence of undernutrition. It is important that such educational sessions be conducted by someone who has specific expertise in the area, such as a gymnasium teacher who also fully understands the nature of anorexia nervosa and bulimia nervosa.

The aim of therapy for dieting disorders is to return patients to a normal and healthy lifestyle. We believe that it is important to provide a model of healthy exercising that is not excessive while the patients are hospitalized; this model will serve as a basis for maintaining a reasonable and not excessive level of activity when they are discharged into the outside world, where high levels of exercise are portrayed as health-promoting. On these grounds, we have designed a special program of graded, supervised, mainly *anaerobic* activity during inpatient treatment. This program is summarized in the Beumont et al. (1994) article, and further details are available from us on request.

NOTE

1. It is the authors' view that patients who show bulimic behaviors, such as objective bulimia (uncontrolled gorging), simply eating more than they wish (subjective bulimia), or purging, but are also at such a weight that they need to be put on a weight gain program, should be diagnosed as "anorexia nervosa."

REFERENCES

Abraham, S. F., & Beumont, P. J. V. (1982). How patients describe bulimia or binge eating. *Psychological Medicine, 12,* 625–635.

Abraham, S. F., Beumont, P. J. V., Booth, A., Rouse, L., & Rogers, J. (1981). Nutritional Knowledge Questionnaire, Part Two. *Medical Journal of Australia, 1*(4), 39.

Beumont, P. J. V., Arthur, B., Russell, J. D., & Touyz, S. W. (1994). Excessive physical activity in dieting disorder patients: proposals for a supervised exercise programme. *International Journal of Eating Disorders, 15,* 21–36.

Beumont, P. J. V., Chambers, T., Rouse, L., & Abraham, S. F. (1981). The diet composition and nutritional knowledge of patients with anorexia nervosa. *Journal of Human Nutrition, 35,* 265–273.

Beumont, P. J. V., George, G. C. W., & Smart, D. E. (1976). 'Dieters' and 'vomiters and purgers' in anorexia nervosa. *Psychological Medicine, 6,* 617–622.

Beumont, P. J. V., O'Connor, M., Touyz, S. W., & Lennerts, W. (1990). Nutritional counseling in the treatment of bulimia. In M. M. Fichter (Ed.), *Bulimia nervosa: Basic research, diagnosis and therapy* (pp. 308–310). Chichester, England, Wiley. (Original work published 1988)

Beumont, P. J. V., O'Connor, M., Touyz, S. W., & Williams, H. (1987). Nutritional counseling in the treatment of anorexia and bulimia nervosa. In P. J. V. Beumont, G. D. Burrows, & R. C. Casper (Eds.), *Handbook of eating disorders: Part 1. Anorexia and bulimia nervosa* (pp. 349–359). Amsterdam: Elsevier/North-Holland.

Blinder, B. J., Freeman, D. M. A., & Stunkard, A. J. (1970). Behavior therapy of anorexia nervosa: Effectiveness of activity as a reinforcer of weight gain. *American Journal of Psychiatry, 126,* 1093–1098.

Bruch, H. (1973). *Eating disorders: Obesity, anorexia nervosa, and the person within.* New York: Basic Books.

Crisp, A. H. (1965). Clinical and therapeutic aspects of anorexia nervosa: A study of 30 cases. *Journal of Psychosomatic Research, 9,* 67–78.

Epling, W. F., & Pierce, W. D. (1996). *Activity anorexia: Theory, research, and treatment.* Mahcoah, NJ: Erlbaum.

Epling, W. F., Pierce, W. D., & Stefan, L. (1983). A theory of activity-based anorexia. *International Journal of Eating Disorders, 3*(1), 27–46.

Garfinkel, P. E., Garner, D. M., & Moldofsky, H. (1977). The role of behavior modification in the treatment of anorexia nervosa. *Journal of Paediatric Psychology, 2,* 113–121.

Griffiths, R., Beumont, P. J. V., & Touyz, S. W. (1995). Anorexie à deux: An ominous sign for recovery. *European Eating Disorders Review, 3*(1), 2–14.

Hebebrand, J., Himmelman, G. W., Heseker, H., Schaefer, H., & Remschmidt, H. (1996). Use of percentiles for the BMI in anorexia nervosa. *International Journal of Eating Disorders, 19,* 359–369.

Janet, P. (1929). *The major symptoms of hysteria* (2nd ed.). New York: Macmillan.

King, A. (1963). Primary and secondary anorexia nervosa syndromes. *British Journal of Psychiatry, 109,* 470–479.

Kron, L., Katz, J. L., Gorzynski, G., & Weiner, H. (1978). Hyperactivity in anorexia nervosa: A fundamental clinical feature. *Comprehensive Psychiatry, 19*(5), 433–439.

Laessle, R. G., Beumont, P. J. V., Butow, P., Lennerts, W., O'Connor, M., Pirke, K. M., Touyz, S. W., & Waadi, S. (1995). A comparison of nutritional management with stress management in the treatment of bulimia nervosa. *British Journal of Psychiatry, 159,* 250–261.

Liebman, R., Minuchin, S., & Baker, L. (1974). An integrated treatment program for anorexia nervosa. *American Journal of Psychiatry, 131,* 432–436,

Mavissakalian, M. (1982). Anorexia nervosa treated with response prevention and prolonged exposure. *Behaviour Research and Therapy, 20,* 27–31.

O'Connor, M. A., Touyz, S. W., Dunn, S., & Beumont, P. J. V. (1987). Vegetarianism in anorexia nervosa: A review of 116 consecutive cases. *Medical Journal of Australia, 147,* 540–542.

Russell, J., Allen, B., Mira, M., Stewart, P., Vizzard, J., Arthur, B., & Beumont, P. J. V. (1994). Protein repletion and treatment in anorexia nervosa. *American Journal of Clinical Nutrition, 59,* 98–102.

Touyz, S. W., & Beumont, P. J. V. (1985). A comprehensive multidisciplinary approach for the management of patients with eating disorders. In S. W. Touyz & P. J. V. Beumont (Eds.), *Eating disorders: Prevalence and treatment* (pp. 11–22). Sydney: Williams & Wilkins.

Touyz, S. W., Beumont, P. J. V., & Hook, S. (1987). Exercise anorexia: A new dimension in anorexia nervosa? In P. J. V. Beumont, G. D. Burrows, & R. C. Casper (Eds.), *Handbook of eating disorders: Part 1. Anorexia and bulimia nervosa* (pp. 143–157). Amsterdam: Elsevier/North-Holland.

Touyz, S. W., Williams, H., Marden, K., Kopec-Schrader, E., & Beumont, P. J. V. (1994). Videotape feedback of eating behavior in patients with anorexia nervosa: Does it normalize eating behavior? *Australian Journal of Nutrition and Dietetics, 51*(2), 79–82.

Wilson, A. J., Touyz, S. W., Dunn, S. M., & Beumont, P. J. V. (1989). The Eating Behavior Rating Scale (EBRS): A measure of eating pathology in anorexia nervosa. *International Journal of Eating Disorders, 8,* 583–592.

Windauer, U., Lennerts, W., Talbot, P., Touyz, S. W., & Beumont, P. J. V. (1993). How well are 'cured' anorexia nervosa patients? *British Journal of Psychiatry, 163,* 195–200.

Yates, A., Leehey, K., & Shisslak, C. M. (1983). Running: An analogue of anorexia? *New England Journal of Medicine, 308*(5), 251–255.

CHAPTER 10

Cognitive-Behavioral Body Image Therapy

JAMES C. ROSEN

THE IMPORTANCE OF BODY IMAGE IN EATING DISORDERS

Body Image Disorder: An Essential Feature of Eating Disorders

Abnormality of body image is one of the essential diagnostic criteria for both anorexia nervosa and bulimia nervosa (American Psychiatric Association [APA], 1994). Very few patients who seek assistance for bulimic episodes or starvation do not exhibit an overconcern with weight or body shape (Garfinkel, 1992; Herzog, Hopkins, & Burns, 1993). Although abnormality of body image is not among the research criteria for binge-eating disorder proposed for further study by the APA (1994), persons with this disorder also report significantly negative body image symptoms (Marcus, Smith, Santelli, & Kaye, 1992; Spitzer et al., 1993). Body dysmorphic disorder (BDD) is the only other diagnosis in the *Diagnostic and Statistical Manual of Mental Disorders* that is characterized by a disturbed body image. Patients can shift between BDD and eating disorders, the common element being excessive preoccupation with appearance (Hollander, Cohen, & Simeon, 1993; Jackman, Williamson, Funsch, & Warner, 1994; Pantano & Santonastaso, 1989; Phillips, McElroy, Keck, Pope, & Hudson, 1993; Sturmey & Slade, 1986).

Body Image and Risk for Eating Disorders

Of all psychological factors that are believed to cause eating disorders, body image dissatisfaction is the most relevant and immediate antecedent. Why would a future eating disorder patient attempt dieting unless she was dissatisfied with her weight?[1] Why would she resort to more drastic weight control unless body image was a desperate concern? Weight control is the patient's remedy for the defect she perceives in her appearance and is secondary to the body image problem. The importance of body image has been confirmed in longitudinal studies of at-risk populations (Killen et al., 1994; Rosen, 1992). Fluctuations in eating disorder symptoms over time in adolescent girls are best predicted by body image. Other variables, such as psychopathology, stress, and family dysfunction, are associated with symptoms concurrently but add less to the prediction of eating disorders over time after body image is controlled.

Body Image in Eating Disorder Treatment

Adequate treatment of an eating disorder should include assistance to change body image, not just eating behavior. Yet body image work appears to be greatly underemphasized in eating disorder treatment programs (Rosen, 1996). Recovery from anorexia nervosa or bulimia nervosa in terms of weight restoration and eating pathology does not guarantee improved body image. In fact, the degree of clinically significant change on standard questionnaires is much greater for eating, dieting, and purging behavior than for body image (Davis, Olmsted, & Rockert, 1990). Several follow-up studies of anorexic and bulimic patients who restored body weight and ceased binge eating and vomiting found that about one- to two-thirds of these success cases still worried excessively about their physical appearance (Deter & Herzog, 1994; Goldbloom & Olmsted, 1993; Ratnasuriya, Eisler, Szmukler, & Russell, 1991; Windauer, Lennerts, Talbot, Touyz, & Beumont, 1993). No matter how difficult it is to resist urges to binge, women with bulimia nervosa rate dealing with their desires to be thin as the hardest part of recovery (Rorty, Yager, & Rossotto, 1993). Clearly, body image work should be included, and even stressed, in the treatment of anorexia nervosa and bulimia nervosa.

CLINICAL FEATURES OF BODY IMAGE DISORDER

Types of Appearance Complaints

Eating disorder patients complain of being too fat, too big, or too wide all over or in specific body regions—typically in the stomach, thighs, buttocks, or hips. Feelings of fatness are often traced to cheeks, neck, breasts, and upper arms as well. Concerns about physique that sound like weight concern are often unrelated to weight per se. In particular, a larger hip circumference and higher waist-to-hip ratio, signifying a less proportioned or curvaceous physique, are associated with more body dissatisfaction (Bailey, Goldberg, Swap, Chomitz, & Houser, 1990; Thomas & Freeman, 1991; Davis, Durnin, Dionne, & Gurevish, 1994; Singh, 1994). Desire to have larger breasts is another common example of dissatisfaction in weight-preoccupied women (Thompson & Tantleff, 1992). Feelings of fatness can also relate to concerns about being too tall or too short.

About one-half of patients complain of non-weight-related appearance features—typically the size or shape of facial features; scars and other skin blemishes; sagging breasts; hands; thinning head hair; and excessive body hair (Rosen, Reiter, & Orosan, 1994). Fitness concerns have also become common (Ben-Tovim & Walker, 1991). Underlying complaints of body dissatisfaction in adults can reflect concern about aging (Gupta & Schork, 1993). Aging concern can masquerade as weight concern because people believe that weight reduction is a way to stay younger-looking. Clearly, dieting by eating disorder patients, even when it is accompanied by significant weight loss, may be ineffective in reducing total body dissatisfaction, which in part is focused on shape and other appearance features rather than on fatness.

Perceptual Disturbance

Eating disorder patients can experience distorted sensations or images of their physical appearance. They may imagine a defect in appearance that is completely imperceptible, or may exaggerate the appearance of existing physical features. A discrepancy between actual appearance and a patient's mental picture of herself suggests a perceptual disturbance. Misperception of sensory information about the body (visual, kinesthetic, tactile, olfactory) has been hypothesized to be responsible for these experiences (Bruch, 1962). The anorexic who firmly believes that she appears fat is the classic example of body image distortion. Following are some other typical examples. A bulimia nervosa patient with a premorbid history of obesity continued to view herself as obese despite weight loss. Another patient believed that her thighs should not touch when she was standing, indicating a distorted mental image of normal appearance. Feeling full was unpleasant for a third patient, because she had a distorted image of looking unattractive and having a protruding stomach after eating. One patient who felt that her breasts were too large seemed to ignore the remainder of her perfectly proportioned physique and described herself as "two breasts on a stick." An overweight patient imagined herself as much larger or more misshapen than was actually the case, indicating that real rather than imagined flaws can also be distorted. Finally, distortions may only surface during movement, such as in a patient who thought she looked foolish dancing.

At least half of eating disorder patients in a baseline, resting condition significantly overestimate their body size; nonpatients, by contrast, are much more likely to be reasonably accurate (Collins et al., 1987; Horne, Van Vactor, & Emerson, 1991). The validity of perceptual tests and even the construct of perceptual disturbance have been questioned, because size distortion overlaps between disordered and nondisordered subjects and has weak to moderate correlations with other body image measures (Hsu & Sobkiewicz, 1991). Instead of looking for simple group differences on size distortion, it may be more appropriate to examine body size distortion in challenging conditions. Cues that trigger size overestimation include negative moods (Taylor & Cooper, 1992), consumption of foods that are believed to be high in calories (Thompson, Coovert, Pasman, & Robb, 1993), viewing of thin women in media images (Hamilton & Waller, 1993), premenstruation (Carr-Nangle, Johnson, Bergeron, & Nangle, 1994), and instructions to estimate size on the basis of feelings (Crisp & Kalucy, 1974). Another consideration is that current perceptual assessment is not designed to capture nonvisual types of body image distortions.

Overall, it appears that eating disorder patients, especially those with great weight fluctuations (Collins et al., 1987) have unstable, reactive perceptions of their body size (Slade, 1994). Although body perception is a neurobiological process (Lacey & Birtchnell, 1986), its manifestation in eating disorder patients as currently assessed seems to be highly influenced by psychosocial stimuli relevant to physical appearance concerns.

Cognitive and Affective Features

Unlike normal self-consciousness about physical appearance, eating disorders involve a preoccupation that is time-consuming, distressing, and interfering. Although it can occur throughout the day, appearance preoccupation is even more intense after eating and in social situations in which a person feels self-conscious and expects to be scrutinized by other people (Haimovita, Lansky, & O'Reilly, 1993). This attention makes the patient feel anxious, embarrassed, and ashamed, because she believes that the defect reveals some personal inadequacy. Although a striking feature of anorexia nervosa or bulimia nervosa is the person's conviction about the existence (or severity) of the physical defect, this distortion is only the first step in a sequence of eating disorder beliefs. The typical thought pattern is as follows: "I look defective; other people notice and are interested in my defect; they view me as unattractive [ugly, deformed, deviant, etc.], and evaluate me negatively as a person; consequently, my appearance proves something negative about my character and worth to other people."

The importance given to physical appearance in self-evaluation is a better discriminator of women with eating disorders than perceived attractiveness is (Wilson & Smith, 1989). Patients who are subdiagnostic for anorexia nervosa of-

ten lack the required fear of gaining weight, probably because they have succeeded in losing weight, but meet the criterion for self-evaluation's being unduly influenced by physical appearance (Herzog et al., 1993). Moreover, persons with eating disorders can attach a wide range of connotations to physical appearance beyond the aesthetics of their looks. For example, a woman who felt too big all over was concerned that she appeared unfeminine and too assertive. Another patient wanted to lose weight in order to reduce the size of her buttocks; she thought her shape appeared indecent.

Beliefs in persons with body image disorder have been described inconsistently as either "obsessions," "overvalued ideas," or "delusions" (de Leon, Bott, & Simpson, 1989). It is difficult to distinguish among these, and there appears to be no single type of thought process that accounts for all patients. Rather than a single type of cognitive disturbance, thought processes in body image disorder probably vary on a continuum of insight from fair insight to delusion (Phillips & McElroy, 1993).

"Delusional thinking" about appearance refers to distortions of reality that are held with complete conviction. Beyond the delusional belief of having a defect, eating disorder patients can exhibit delusions of reference (e.g., a patient is convinced that people treat her in a certain way because of her appearance; Vitousek & Hollon, 1990). Delusional thinking in eating disorders is typically confined to circumstances that provoke attention to appearance, and although the person's life is significantly affected, thought processes outside such situations are nondelusional.

"Obsessional thinking" in body image disorder refers to repetitive, intrusive thoughts about appearance. Eating disorder patients can recognize obsessions and admit that their preoccupation is excessive, even if they are entirely convinced that their appearance is abnormal. A patient may complain, "I *know* my fat is hideous, but I just wish I could stop thinking about it all the time; I can't concentrate when I am with other people; I know they don't care about it as much as I do." "Overvalued ideas" in eating disorders fall somewhere between obsessions and delusions in terms of insight. That is, an overvalued belief is entrenched and sensible to the patient, but she can acknowledge the possibility that it may not be true (McKenna, 1984). A normal-appearing woman complained that people at work did not respect her because she was short and had fat cheeks. She said, "I look like an awkward teenager, not someone who knows what she is doing; I realize looks aren't everything to people, but it's how I feel about myself that really matters."

Clearly, not all negative body image attitudes are symptomatic of an eating disorder. What seems like excessive weight concern can be appropriate in women engaged in occupations such as dance, modeling, or athletics, which have strict physical standards. In general, physical beauty is a status symbol of success and other virtues. Moreover, it is common for people to use appearance as an excuse to explain some negative everyday occurrence. Thus, reduced to their basic form, eating disorder beliefs are not completely incomprehensible in appearance-conscious Western culture (McKenna, 1984). The difference is that eating disorder beliefs are unreasonable exaggerations of normal ideas and disrupt normal functioning.

Behavioral Features

Most eating disorder patients engage in some avoidance of social situations they believe might call attention to their appearance (Rosen, Srebnik, Saltzberg, & Wendt, 1991). In some cases, avoidance is extreme and the patients are housebound. More typically, a patient enters social situations, but finds ways to avoid full exposure of her appearance in public by wearing clothes, grooming herself, or contorting her body posture and movements in such a way as to hide the defect. These avoidance behaviors are more likely if the patient will be eating in public. For example, the patient might be able to wear a tight-fitting outfit, but only if she will not be eating. Alternately, she may simply avoid eating altogether so as to not attract attention to her appearance.

Various kinds of body checking behaviors are common, such as inspecting the defect in the mirror, weighing oneself repeatedly, engaging in grooming rituals, and asking others for reassurance. Comparing one's appearance to that of other people is another common form of checking behavior in eating disorder patients (Toro, Salamero, & Martinez, 1994). Although comparisons with female images in the mass media are frequent, weight-preoccupied women are most likely to compare themselves repeatedly to peers (Heinberg & Thompson, 1992). Like compulsions, these behaviors are difficult to resist, and in some extreme cases body checking

can last hours each day. Finally, eating disorder patients are convinced that the only way to improve their self-esteem is to improve they way they look. Dieting and exercise are viewed as the main beauty remedies. However, depending on the type of appearance concern, a patient may undertake cosmetic surgery or use unnecessary skin or hair treatments.

BODY IMAGE CHANGE: GUIDELINES FOR THERAPY

Format and Timing of Therapy

Body image therapy can be provided individually or in groups. In clinical trials, the standard format my colleagues and I used was eight 2-hour group therapy sessions with four to eight patients. In addition to women's eating disorder groups, we have mixed together persons with and without eating disorders; normal and overweight persons; men and women; anorexia nervosa and bulimia nervosa patients; and persons with weight-related and non-weight-related concerns. There seems to be no consistent advantage or disadvantage of these mixtures, though each presents unique challenges and opportunities. Although some people believe that gender of the therapist has an impact on body image work (Zunino, Agoos, & Davis, 1991), we have not been able to find any gender effect on treatment outcome in our clinic. With respect to the timing of body image therapy, ordinarily we would recommend waiting until a patient has made some progress in controlling eating behavior. Otherwise, we have been flexible about timing therapy concurrently with or separately from standard eating disorder treatment.

Finally, a frequent question about format that we are asked is "How do you handle sexual abuse in body image therapy?" We designed this program to help patients understand how traumas like these influence their body image attitudes and behaviors, but not to recall or process in detail recollections of the traumas themselves, or to deal with other symptoms resulting from them (e.g., posttraumatic stress disorder). We have had several patients who admitted to a sexual abuse history for the first time after undergoing emotionally charged exposure therapy assignments (e.g., being unclothed around other people; see below). In those instances, we arranged for the patients to receive additional therapy to deal with the sexual abuse more directly. On the other hand, many of our patients had undergone years of therapy for sexual abuse; although they succeeded in processing those experiences, they came to us because they still had unyielding and unpleasant feelings about their bodies and needed more direct help to change body image. In sum, the answer is that sexual abuse history is not a contraindication for body image therapy.

Initial Phase of Treatment

Prior to beginning therapy, a thorough examination of body image symptoms and appearance complaints is important. We use the Body Dysmorphic Disorder Examination, which taps into more severe and diverse types of body image dysfunction than most measures designed for eating disorder patients can assess (Rosen et al., 1995a).[2] Therapy should begin by addressing the goal of treatment and providing the patient with basic information on the psychology of physical appearance, the concept of body image, and the development of body image disorder (Cash & Pruzinsky, 1990; Feingold, 1992). In our group therapy program, we educate our patients and examine their body image history in the first two sessions, using minilectures, discussion, and homework from an audiotape series on body image therapy (Cash, 1991). Cash's self-help book is another useful companion to therapy (Cash, 1995).

It is helpful to have each patient write a brief developmental history of her body image. She should consider the following, separately: early childhood (up to age 7), later childhood (before puberty), early adolescence, later adolescence (later teenage years), early adulthood, and the present. For each period, she should be asked to describe her physical appearance and the important events or experiences that influenced her body image. For example, a patient may describe her later childhood thus: "I started to gain weight and was the tallest kid in class. Other kids called me 'the Whale.' " She should also be sure to note any incidents (if there *were* any) that made her feel confident in her appearance; however, being teased or given negative feedback from peers, friends, family members, or teachers is probably the most common experience that precipitates dieting in the future eating disorder patient (Cattarin & Thompson, 1994; Thompson & Heinberg, 1993) (see also case examples by Giles, 1988; Gislason, 1988; Yager & Smith, 1993). Others include being left

out or rejected because of overweight, failing in athletics, having an injury or illness, or being physically or sexually abused or assaulted (Rosen, Reiter, & Orosan, 1996). Later body image distress can be triggered by events or situations that resemble these earlier ones. Also, it is natural for people to try to make sense of experiences that cause them deep feelings of humiliation. Unfortunately, some people come to believe that a "defect" in their appearance means they are "defective" people.

The therapist will have to deal at the outset with typical forms of resistance to treatment, in order to gain the patient's cooperation and investment in therapy. Most notably, eating disorder patients believe upon entering therapy that they cannot feel any different about themselves until they eliminate their "defects." This must be countered at the beginning by stressing that the problem is how a person views herself from the inside, and that therapy is designed to change body image, not appearance. The patient must also understand that although cultural messages about appearance and personal historical events (e.g., being teased as a child) may have been important in her body image development, therapy will have to focus on overcoming the attitudes and behaviors that maintain the disturbances. Some other key points to stress are as follows: (1) Physical appearance is important in interpersonal perception, but mainly in initial impressions between unacquainted persons; and (2) body image is subjective and psychological, and the variables of body image and physical appearance can be independent (e.g., changes in appearance do not always lead to a changed body image; the relation between self-rated attractiveness and ratings by other people is weak [Feingold, 1992]; and body image can be altered without having to change physical appearance). These basic ideas about body image and the goal of therapy will need repetition as the therapist encounters resistance later and as the patient struggles to find evidence to counter her irrational beliefs.

Correcting Distorted Perceptions of Body Size

Perceptual distortion is a building block to other body image symptoms, but little information is available on how to change it directly. One technique is to turn the size estimation test into a corrective feedback exercise. To do so, the therapist demonstrates the discrepancy between the patient's actual size and her estimation by having the patient repeatedly correct her estimation until she is accurate. Any number of such exercises can be devised to fit a person's particular symptoms. For example, a real profile of the patient's face can be superimposed upon her own drawing. The patient who is preoccupied with the idea that her stomach protrudes after eating can be asked to examine herself in the mirror or to compare her actual stomach dimensions before and after eating. Instead of comparing herself to others subjectively, the patient can be asked to collect height and weight data on those individuals; this way, she can discover how close to or far from other people she truly is. Similarly, unrealistic complaints of overweight can be challenged with population weight norms (Najjar & Rowland, 1987) broken down by age and height.

Corrective exercises produce less distortion of appearance (Goldsmith & Thompson, 1989; Norris, 1984; Rosen, Saltzberg, & Srebnik, 1989), but not necessarily more satisfaction with appearance (Biggs, Rosen, & Summerfield, 1980; Fernandez & Vandereycken, 1994). Moreover, perceptual training does not add to the overall benefit of the basic cognitive-behavioral program (Rosen, Cado, Silberg, Srebnik, & Wendt, 1990). The main advantage of corrective feedback may be to facilitate insight into the disorder, rather than to alter body image per se (Garner & Bemis, 1982). Vandereycken, for example, shows his anorexia nervosa patients a videotape of how they looked in a bikini upon admission, in order to help break through their denial (Vandereycken, Probst, & Van Bellinghen, 1992). Although this confrontation has the potential to be therapeutic, the timing is important. To present a patient with objective feedback brings with it an implied demand that she accept the clinician's reality over her own. Confrontations about the reality of the defect at the outset of therapy can be counterproductive. It is often more effective to begin cognitive restructuring with beliefs that are less strongly held. As therapy progresses and the patient is more anxious to picture herself differently, size feedback exercises may become more useful.

Cognitive Restructuring

Basic Cognitive Procedures

Therapy requires a detailed behavioral assessment in order to pinpoint the dysfunctional attitudes and the situations in which they occur. A self-monitoring diary, like the one used with depressed patients (Beck, Rush, Shaw, & Emery, 1979), can greatly facilitate cognitive restructuring. The patient should record any situations that provoke self-consciousness about appearance—positive or negative, body image thoughts or beliefs, and the effects of these on mood or behavior. An example of a diary entry is the following:

Antecedent (situation): I walked into the shower room at the gym.

Belief: Everyone else seemed comfortable being undressed, but me. I felt like I stood out and looked like a freak. People were looking at the weight I needed to lose.

Consequence: I was embarrassed. I covered myself with the towel, dashed back to the locker room, and went home to shower.

Initially, self-statements in the body image diary may be superficial complaints of body dissatisfaction, such as "My thighs are really disgusting; they make me look like a penguin." These statements are just negative comments on the aesthetics of appearance, without implications of that appearance. In therapy, we call this "negative body talk." The cognitive assessment should proceed from this point by asking the patient to elaborate on her appraisal of situations in which the dissatisfaction occurred. For instance, if the patient thought, "I looked gross, weird," the therapist should encourage her to follow this thought to where it leads:

THERAPIST. What was upetting about looking "weird" in that situation?

PATIENT. People were looking at me.

THERAPIST. What did you imagine they saw or thought when they looked at you?

Typically, the sequence of thinking leads to beliefs that her appearance proves something negative about her character or desirability to other people. Examples are thinking that the defect is evidence of being unlovable, foolish, stupid, promiscuous, immoral, freakish, alien, offensive, weak, unfeminine, undisciplined, pushy, or the like. These are the types of beliefs that account for the deep feelings of shame and embarrassment in eating disorder patients. Finally, the therapist should consider other qualities of each cognition, such as unreasonableness, preoccupation (frequency of the thought), distress when dwelling on the thought, conviction (strength with which the belief is held), perceived controllability of the thought, and efforts to resist the thought (Lowe & Chadwick, 1990; Kozak & Foa, 1994).

Ideas that a patient considers to be facts are difficult to modify. At the beginning, instead, we typically intervene with the negative body talk, without questioning any of the related assumptions (such as that a defect really exists or that people judge the patient negatively.) To replace negative body talk or distract herself from it, the patient is asked to construct more objective, neutral, sensory self-descriptions that are free of emotionally loaded self-criticism, but are believable. For example, the patient with "penguin" thighs can rehearse describing them as "smooth" and "muscular." This patient can be asked to practice neutral self-talk during the day when she is reminded to do so by the sight of her thighs or by intrusive negative body talk. The new description should be rehearsed while carrying out the mirror exposure at home (see below). Positive self-descriptions are unnecessary at first and are generally rejected by the patient. The therapist should avoid arguing with the patient about the reality of the defect, and instead should try to eliminate the negative body talk that causes distress (e.g., "No matter how large your thighs may be, another problem seems to be the way you talk about them to yourself"). A slip back to self-criticism should be a cue to the patient to follow it with a corrective self-statement. The point is for her to distract herself from repeating the self-criticism over and over, rather than to stop the thought from occurring in the first instance. If the patient complains that she still doesn't like what she sees, the therapist should reassure her that some body dissatisfaction is normal and may be appropriate as long as she can overcome needless self-denigration.

Cognitive restructuring of the more unreasonable and distressing convictions about appearance can be accomplished with the standard techniques used in the treatment of depression and anxiety disorders (Barlow, 1988; Beck et al., 1979). Accordingly, the patient should be encouraged to evaluate the evidence for and against the belief; the evidence rather than the belief itself is questioned, at least in the beginning. For instance, a woman may worry that people think she is unattractive and slovenly, even though she dresses meticulously and looks classy. The discussion can center on comments about her appearance that people actually make, rather than what people may think. If she cannot recall any or seems biased, she should record in her body image diary any new feedback. Then the therapist should ask her whether this feedback or anything else that has happened between therapy sessions has altered her belief. Perhaps she will discover that people are complimentary or are not that interested in her appearance. Imagine that this patient also worries that her husband is "turned off" to her physically, and that she has to hide her nudity or he will leave her. To her, this belief seems more justified, because a husband should be more invested in his wife's appearance than strangers should be. The therapist can delve into these stronger convictions after the patient has made some progress with the others.

The patient should develop alternative self-statements that reflect the body image situation more accurately (e.g., "People really do think I look nice," "My husband told me he loves to see and touch my tummy"). These disputing thoughts should be written in the diary and rehearsed. Gradual changes in attitudes can be assessed by asking the patient to rate believability on a 0–100 scale next to the written disputing thought in the diary. For patients who have difficulty recognizing irrational beliefs or constructing alternatives, Cash (1991, 1995) lays out a model of the process in a self-assessment of typical cognitive errors and self-defeating assumptions.

Special Considerations

The therapist, to repeat, should not be overly distracted by protests that a defect is severe. As much as possible, the therapist should validate rather than discount the patient's perception ("I see what you're pointing to. Your stomach isn't flat like you want; it's curved and rounded"). Therapy should build the patient's tolerance to admitting physical imperfections, but, more importantly, should challenge the perceived implications of the defect.

Eating disorder patients can fear that learning to accept themselves will cause them to abandon their self-control and develop more of a weight problem. By implication, the corollary is that a patient must dislike herself in order to remain acceptable-looking. To handle this resistance to cognitive change, the therapist should focus on its logical inconsistency or maladaptiveness. Also, regular weighing or an eating/exercise diary in conjunction with the cognitive change assignments can be a behavioral test of the feared prediction. Does the patient really gain weight as her body image improves? (Overweight women who undergo body image therapy do not gain weight; see Rosen, Orosan, & Reiter, 1995.)

Some patients need to realize that weight reduction will not solve their body dissatisfaction, because weight is just a proxy for concerns attributable to body proportion, height, skin, facial features, or the like. The main concern may not be clear until the patient examines the issue closely in her body area hierarchy (see below). At that point, she may be more agreeable to abandoning weight reduction.

Ironically, anorexia nervosa patients can be free of body dissatisfaction and preoccupation because they have achieved the weight loss they desire (Garner, Garner, & Van Egeren, 1992). In such cases, cognitive restructuring should focus on problems the patients anticipate with weight restoration. Often these predictions are difficult for a patient to dispute; otherwise, she would not resist weight gain so vigorously in the first instance. However, weight regain presents a tangible opportunity for the patient to test her beliefs through her own body image experiences. The patient should carefully monitor body image thoughts in the diary in conjunction with weight change. The same issue applies to those women with bulimia nervosa for whom weight gain is inevitable.

Like patients with somatoform disorders, persons with eating disorders attribute most of their troubles to their perceived physical defects. Recovery from an eating disorder will be facilitated if a patient can identify explanations for her distress other than her appearance. For example, the patient who feels that her obesity makes people reject her should be asked whether there is any other way in which she may discourage interest from other people. Maybe she does not know how to maintain conversations or to self-disclose to others. She should be asked to weigh these factors against appearance as being important for developing relationships. Arriving at other explanations may allow the patient to abandon the idea that she must change her appearance in order to be more happy and successful. Although it may be distressing to admit to another dysfunction, at least it may be one that is more modifiable than physical appearance.

Coping with Stereotypes and Prejudice

Overweight patients with eating disorders, may be confronted with situations in which they are discriminated against. Realistic thoughts about these encounters should not be discounted. However, such patients can be helped to learn more self-enhancing ways to respond to discrimination and to cope with the stigma of obesity. First, the patients should be discouraged from always looking for defects within themselves to explain negative attitudes from other people. Rather than accepting criticism as being personally relevant, the patients should recognize it as prejudice and as unfair and ignorant treatment of an entire segment of society. Moreover, because most obese persons buy into obesity stereotypes and blame themselves excessively for their overweight, it is important to bolster their resistance by providing information on the nonbehavioral, genetic, and physiological causes of obesity. The patients can also be encouraged to find examples from their own experience to counter stereotypes (e.g., they cannot be weak and undisciplined, because they are strong-willed and competent in many other areas of life).

Second, obese patients will have to learn to reduce the importance of the characteristics on which they are judged—that is, their overweight appearance. Although overweight persons are judged by peers as less attractive, peer ratings do not show obese–nonobese differences in amount of liking or in perceived social competence (Jarvie, Lahey, Graziano, & Farmer, 1983; Miller, Rothblum, Felicio, & Brand, 1995).

Third, obese persons should be discouraged from only comparing themselves to people who are thinner than they. Lopsided comparisons perpetuate feelings of alienation. Instead, they should compare themselves to people with a more diverse and representative range of body types. As long as these do not become excessive, social comparisons should be made to other overweight persons.

Behavioral Procedures

Exposure to Avoided Situations

We recommend that before facing anxiety provoking situations in public, a patient should begin with exposure to the sight of her body, unsupervised and in the privacy of her own home. A hierarchy of body parts from satisfying to most distressing can be created by interviewing the patient or using a simple body satisfaction scale, such as the Body Cathexis Scale (Secord & Jourard, 1953) or the Body Areas Satisfaction scale of the multidimensional Body-Self Relations Questionnaire (Brown, Cash, & Mikulka, 1990). The patient should practice viewing each step in the hierarchy for up to a minute or two until she is able to do so without significant distress. The exposure should be carried out clothed and then unclothed in front of a full-length mirror. A patient may benefit from relaxation training in order to progress through the hierarchy using systematic desensitization (Cash, 1991; Giles, 1988).

The patient should be sure to view both her satisfying and mildly dissatisfying areas in order to take in the whole picture of herself, rather than focusing immediately on the offensive locations. Many eating disorder patients avoid looking at their defects and will find this assignment to be extremely challenging. The exposure may need to be conducted over several weeks. Other patients already scrutinize themselves in the mirror. In those cases, the exposure assignment should be conducted anyway; however, the patients should be instructed to practice neutral, objective body talk while viewing themselves.

The avoidance techniques of eating disorder patients can be subtle, so a thorough assessment is needed. The more avoidance habits that can be identified, the more opportunities the therapist can concoct for the patient to unlearn self-consciousness. The body image self-monitoring diary can give evidence of avoidance (see the example given earlier, in which the patient wrote that she covered herself with a towel and could not shower at the gym). The Body Dysmorphic Disorder Examination asks about general categories of avoidance (e.g., social and public places, clothing, nudity, physical activities, touching the body). Detailed examples of these types of avoidance should be obtained. Observation of the patient may reveal disguising types of nonverbal behaviors or dress (e.g., not removing her coat, keeping her hands folded over her stomach) that the patient is unaware of or does not volunteer. Contextual cues that influence the difficulty, such as familiarity of people, physical proximity to others, and type of social interaction (e.g., speaking to a group vs. speaking to an individual), should also be taken into account in developing a hierarchy of distressing situations.

Examples of exposure assignments we have used include the following: wearing a form-fitting outfit instead of baggy clothes; undressing in front of one's spouse; not hiding facial features with hands or combed-down hair; dressing to reveal scars; exercising in public wearing workout clothes; showering at the health club rather than at home; drawing attention to appearance with more trendy clothes or makeup; accentuating a distressing feature (e.g., wearing a necklace around a fat neck); standing closer to people; and trying on clothes or make up in stores and then asking sales clerks for feedback.

An example of a graded exposure hierarchy with a patient who was overly self-conscious about her chubby cheeks and fleshy upper shoulders was as follows: wearing her long hair pulled back rather than combed over her face; applying rouge to her cheecks; wearing a blouse with a scooped neck instead of a turtleneck; wearing her hair up; wearing a necklace and earrings; and, finally, having her husband give her a neck massage with the lights turned on.

Marks and Mishan (1988) reported five cases of body dysmorphic disorder that were treated with exposure techniques. A patient preoccupied with her reddish complexion and lips gradually reentered avoided social situations, from riding on buses to sitting close to others to (eventually) leaving bits of toothpaste on her lips to call more attention to them! Neziroglu and Yaryura-Tobias (1993a, 1993b) described several BDD patients with hair concerns who were required to go into public with their hair messed up, while thoughts of needing to be perfect and approved were challenged by the therapist.

A self-defeating aspect of avoidance in eating disorders is that efforts to camouflage or hide a defect can actually worsen appearance by locking the patient into a rigid lifestyle of inhibited dressing, grooming, nonverbal behavior, and physical activities. Many of our patients who fear being viewed as unattractive, uninteresting, ugly, odd, and so on, create their own reality by avoiding the very behaviors that might make them more attractive. In the course of exposure therapy, patients typically discover not only that they can tolerate the anxiety, but that they experience a sense of liberation when they incorporate new styles of dress and physical activity into their repertoires.

Response Prevention of Checking and Grooming

Most eating disorder patients engage in some form of body checking that involves deliberate efforts to inspect, scrutinize, measure, or correct their appearance. Typical behaviors are inspecting oneself in the mirror, weighing, pinching skinfolds, and measuring body parts with a measuring tape. Excessive grooming behavior coupled with checking is common. Examples are checking oneself in several outfits before finishing dressing in the morning, straightening hair repeatedly, applying makeup many times in one day, showering after eating, and adjusting clothes to cover body parts. These behaviors may sometimes resemble compulsions, in that an eating disorder patient may engage in body checking as a ritual to undo a distressing thought about a defect. For example, a patient may run to the mirror and scrutinize herself upon having the thought that she looked hideous to someone with whom she just spoke. In other instances the behaviors lack compulsive features, but nonetheless the checking perpetuates a negative preoccupation with appearance. For example, a patient may berate herself while she checks her weight three times a day.

Checking and grooming behaviors can generally be decreased by means of simple self-management techniques. Examples include reducing the frequency of weighing, covering mirrors, leaving home without the makeup kit, setting a fixed time for dressing, allowing oneself only two changes of clothes, refraining from inspecting skin blemishes, and so forth. A situational assessment of these behaviors, recorded in the body image self-monitoring diary, is helpful to identify the cues that trigger checking behavior and to incorporate these into the behavior change plan. For example, a patient may report weighing herself after every meal, in addition to morning and evening weighings. Depending on the strength of the urge to engage in the behavior, the patient can start by eliminating weighings at night and morning, and later practice eating without weighing. Generally these interventions can be conducted without supervision by the therapist. Afterwards, the therapist should debrief the assignment by asking the patient about the actual effect of not checking, as compared with the effect she feared. For instance, the weight-checking patient may be relieved to discover that her weight remains stable even though she does not

monitor it closely. Or another patient may find that people treat her no differently even when she ventures out without makeup. Cash (1991) has provided a monitoring form on which a patient can identify the behavior, her plan to manage without it, and the effect of not engaging in the behavior. A worksheet such as this doubles as a cue for change in the patient and a means of assessing progress for the therapist.

In cases when the frequency of a behavior is high or the urge to engage in the behavior is strong, supervised exposure plus response prevention procedure will be necessary. Marks and Mishan (1988) described a woman with BDD who worried that her sweat smelled terrible; they accompanied her at first to help her go on public outings without bathing or applying deodorant. To strengthen resistance to a behavior, it may be useful first to accentuate the desire to correct the defect and then to prevent the behavior. For example, Neziroglu and Yaryura-Tobias (1993b) had a woman exaggerate the vascular markings around her nose with a red pen and then refrain from applying makeup while she viewed herself in the mirror. Messing up hair and then refraining from grooming in front of the mirror was used in several other cases (Neziroglu & Yaryura-Tobias, 1993a).

Reassurance Seeking

Another form of checking behavior is seeking reassurance from other people, usually by asking whether a defect is noticeable or worse than before. Reassurance seeking can reach high frequencies (e.g., a patient may ask her spouse dozens of times whether she looks OK before leaving home). This behavior is another example of negative body talk, except that it is verbalized aloud to others. Reassurance seeking is self-defeating because it does not eliminate the preoccupation (the patient does not believe the reassurance); it inadvertently trains other people to take even more interest in the patient's appearance; and it can strain relationships with partners and family members.

Generally, it is possible and desirable to eliminate this behavior completely. The patient may need to be convinced to cooperate with the intervention by emphasizing the negative consequences of reassurance seeking on her relationships. Also, it helps to explain how therapy is designed to make her feel more self-confident, and that to do so, she must learn not to depend on the opinions of others. In most cases, the patient can simply be instructed to stop asking for feedback. Indirect attempts to elicit reassurance need to be eliminated as well. For example, a patient should refrain from saying aloud, "Honey, I'm looking so fat today." Exposure plus response prevention may be required. For example, the patient may need to practice walking in front of her spouse, dressing imperfectly, and refraining from asking his opinion. Medical reassurance seeking, such as repeated dermatology consultations, should be eliminated as one might do in the cognitive-behavioral treatment of hypochondriasis (Warwick & Salkovskis, 1989).

Related to reassurance seeking is the problem of eating disorder patients' discounting positive feedback they receive on a spontaneous basis. Unfortunately, because of their distorted cognitive processes, these patients typically overlook or refuse any feedback that is discrepant from their negative body image. Because other people can be more objective, and usually more positive, about a patient's appearance, it is desirable for the patient to attend to such information and incorporate it into her self-image. To attack this problem on a behavioral level, we use role-played conversations to train patients not to make discounting statements (e.g., "Oh, you can't mean that; I really look terrible today"). Instead, the patients practice accepting a compliment (e.g., "Thank you very much; it *is* a new hair style") and rehearsing it subvocally to allow it to be absorbed.

Comparing

A final type of checking behavior is comparing oneself with others. Some patients try to reassure themselves by comparing their defects to the corresponding body parts in other people. The frequency of comparing can reach high levels, to the point at which a patient is unable to look at other people without focusing on her own appearance. Looking at pictures in fashion and fitness magazines is another common cue for comparing (Toro et al., 1994). These comparisons are usually flawed, because a patient's distorted body image perception makes the comparisons nonobjective. Also, the patient selectively focuses on people who are more perfect-looking than she is, rather than comparing herself to a normal range of people. Finally, comparing is another body image situation that provokes negative body talk.

Because it is so self-defeating, an effort should be made to control this form of checking. Behavioral self-control strategies can be devised to suit the patient's habit. For instance, the patient can be asked not to buy fashion magazines or to stand at the front of her aerobics class, where she will not be able to watch the other participants; or not to make comparison statements aloud to other people (e.g., "How do you stay so thin? I wish I had your genes"). A difficulty in reducing comparing is that it is typically manifested more cognitively than behaviorally. Cognitive strategies include focusing on an aspect of the other person's appearance besides the one related to the patient's defect (e.g., looking at her smile rather than the size of her waist); interrupting negative comparisons ("I wish I had her shape") with self-accepting statements; appreciating the beauty in others ("What a lovely figure she has") instead of dwelling on hostile, jealous thoughts ("I can't stand these skinny women"); and focusing on non-appearance-related features in other people ("How friendly she seems"). Because comparing is a subjective experience, it may be difficult for the patient to recognize the extent of the problem. To facilitate assessment, the therapist can administer the Physical Appearance Comparison Scale, a simple self-report inventory of comparing (Thompson, Heinberg, & Tantleff, 1991), or can ask the patient to begin recording cognitive and behavioral comparisons in her body image self-monitoring diary.

Pleasurable Bodily Experiences

Positive body image is not a matter of just feeling physically attractive, but also feeling physically effective. To help patients get in touch with their bodies, Vandereycken (see Vandereycken et al., 1992) provides exercises such as breathing, massage, movement, and sensory awareness training. His body image work is like dance therapy and is designed to help patients experience their bodies as pleasurable instruments. Cash (1991, 1995) also recommends sensory experiences. No information is available on the effectiveness of nonverbal body therapies in eating disorders. However, there is some evidence that weight training and aerobic exercise can improve body image in weight-preoccupied women (Fisher & Thompson, 1994). In addition to increasing pleasure, these activities can double as cues for exposure therapy.

CONCLUSION

Body image disturbance is a distressing and disabling component of eating disorders and is important in their onset and maintenance. Accepted eating disorder treatments, especially the multi-component cognitive-behavioral programs described elsewhere in this volume, are somewhat effective in reducing body image symptoms. However, body image change is a continuing struggle for eating disorder patients, and standard treatment produces only modest change. There has been an explosion of literature on body image since the late 1970s as eating disorders have gained more attention. Most of this information concerns the assessment, pathology, and development of body image; by contrast, little attention has been given to its modification. Nonetheless, a new technology is emerging for body image change, developed mainly with non-eating-disordered patients, that is applicable to patients with anorexia nervosa, bulimia nervosa, and binge-eating disorder. More systematic body image work in eating disorder treatment programs is needed. Systematic treatment depends upon systematic assessment. Too often, current body image assessment for eating disorders is limited to variables such as body dissatisfaction. The clinician needs to determine all facets of body image disturbance, including situational cues and specific attitudes and behaviors. Determining a set of problematic situations will enable the clinician to focus treatment and make the problem less overwhelming for the patient. Because of the effect of body image on the development of eating disorders, further knowledge about its modification will benefit not only persons who already have such disorders, but other persons who are at risk.

NOTES

1. Because the great majority of patients with eating disorders are female, I use feminine nouns and pronouns throughout the chapter to refer to such patients.
2. The Body Dysmorphic Disorder Examination (interview and self-administration versions) and the cognitive-behavioral body image therapy manual are available from me.

REFERENCES

American Psychiatric Association (APA). (1994). *Diagnostic and statistical manual of mental disorders* (4th ed.). Washington, DC: Author.

Bailey, S. M., Goldberg, J. P., Swap, W. C., Chomitz, V. R., & Houser, R. F. (1990). Relationships between body dissatisfaction and physical measurements. *International Journal of Eating Disorders, 9,* 457–461.

Barlow, D. H. (1988). *Anxiety and its disorders: The nature and treatment of anxiety and panic.* New York: Guilford Press.

Beck, A. T., Rush, A. J., Shaw, B. F., & Emery, G. (1979). *Cognitive therapy of depression.* New York: Guilford Press.

Ben-Tovim, D. I., & Walker, M. K. (1991). The development of the Ben-Tovim Walker Body Attitudes Questionnaire (BAQ), a new measure of women's attitudes towards their own bodies. *Psychological Medicine, 21,* 775–784.

Biggs, S. J., Rosen, B., & Summerfield, A. B. (1980). Video-feedback and personal attribution in anorexic, depressed, and normal viewers. *British Journal of Medical Psychology, 53,* 249–254.

Brown, T. A., Cash, T. F., & Mikulka, P. J. (1990). Attitudinal body-image assessment: Factor analysis of the Body-Self Relations Questionnaire. *Journal of Personality Assessment, 35,* 134–144.

Bruch, H. (1962). Perceptual and conceptual disturbances in anorexia nervosa. *Psychosomatic Medicine, 24,* 187–194.

Carr-Nangle, R. E., Johnson, W. G., Bergeron, K. C., & Nangle, D. W. (1994). Body image changes of the menstrual cycle in normal women. *International Journal of Eating Disorders, 16,* 267–273.

Cash, T. F. (1991). *Body image therapy: A program for self-directed change* [Audiocassette series including client workbook]. New York: Guilford Press.

Cash, T. F. (1995). *What do you see when you look in the mirror?: Helping yourself to a positive body image.* New York: Bantam Books.

Cash, T. F., & Pruzinsky, T. (Eds.). (1990). *Body images: Development, deviance, and change.* New York: Guilford Press.

Cattarin, J. A., & Thompson, J. K. (1994). A three-year longitudinal study of body image, eating disturbance, and general psychological functioning in adolescent females. *Eating Disorders: The Journal of Treatment and Prevention, 2,* 114–125.

Collins, J. K., Beumont, P. J. V., Touyz, S. W., Krass, J., Thompson, P., & Philips, T. (1987). Variability in body shape perception in anorexic, bulimic, obese, and control subjects. *International Journal of Eating Disorders, 6,* 633–638.

Crisp, A. H., & Kalucy, R. S. (1974). Aspects of the perceptual disorder in anorexia nervosa. *Journal of Medical Psychology, 47,* 349–361.

Davis, C., Durnin, J. V. G. A., Dionne, M., & Gurevish, M. (1994). The influence of body fat content and bone diameter measurements on body dissatisfaction in adult women. *International Journal of Eating Disorders, 15,* 257–263.

Davis, R., Olmsted, M. P., & Rockert, W. (1990). Brief group psychoeducation for bulimia nervosa: Assessing the clinical significance of change. *Journal of Consulting and Clinical Psychology, 58,* 882–885.

de Leon, J., Bott, A., & Simpson, G. M. (1989). Dysmorphophobia: Body dysmorphic disorder or delusional disorder, somatic subtype? *Comprehensive Psychiatry, 30*, 457–472.

Deter, H. C., & Herzog, W. (1994). Anorexia nervosa in a long-term perspective: Results of the Heidelberg–Mannheim study. *Psychosomatic Medicine, 56*, 20–27.

Feingold, A. (1992). Good-looking people are not what we think. *Psychological Bulletin, 111*, 304–341.

Fernandez, F., & Vandereycken, W. (1994). Influence of video confrontation on the self-evaluation of anorexia nervosa patients: A controlled study. *Eating Disorders: The Journal of Treatment and Prevention, 2*, 135–140.

Fisher, E., & Thompson, J. K. (1994). A comparative evaluation of cognitive-behavioral therapy (CBT) versus exercise therapy (ET) for the treatment of body image disturbance. *Behavior Modification, 18*, 171–185.

Garfinkel, P. E. (1992). Evidence in support of attitudes to shape and weight as a diagnostic criterion of bulimia nervosa. *International Journal of Eating Disorders, 11*, 321–325.

Garner, D. M., & Bemis, K. M. (1982). A cognitive-behavioral approach to anorexia nervosa. *Cognitive Therapy and Research, 6*, 123–150.

Garner, D. M., Garner, M. V., & Van Egeren, L. F. (1992). Body dissatisfaction adjusted for weight: The Body Illusion Index. *International Journal of Eating Disorders, 12*, 263–271.

Giles, T. R. (1988). Distortion of body image as an effect of conditioned fear. *Journal of Behavior Therapy and Experimental Psychiatry, 19*, 143–146.

Gistason, I. L. (1988). Eating disorders in childhood (Ages 4 through 11 years). In B. J. Blinder, B. F. Chaitlin, & R. Goldstein (Eds.), *The eating disorders: Medical and psychological bases of diagnosis and treatment* (pp. 285–293). New York: PMA Publishing Group.

Goldbloom, D. S., & Olmsted, M. P. (1993). Pharmacotherapy of bulimia nervosa with fluoxetine: Assessment of clinically significant attitudinal change. *American Journal of Psychiatry, 158*, 770–774.

Goldsmith, D., & Thompson, J. K. (1989). The effect of mirror confrontation and size estimation feedback on perceptual inaccuracy in normal females who overestimate body size. *International Journal of Eating Disorders, 8*, 437–444.

Gupta, M. A., & Schork, N. J. (1993). Aging-related concerns and body image: Possible future implications for eating disorders. *International Journal of Eating Disorders, 14*, 481–486.

Haimovita, D., Lansky, L. M., & O'Reilly, P. (1993). Fluctuations in body satisfaction across situations. *International Journal of Eating Disorders, 13*, 77–84.

Hamilton, K., & Waller, G. (1993). Media influences on body size estimation in anorexia and bulimia: An experimental study. *British Journal of Psychiatry, 162*, 837–840.

Heinberg, L. J., & Thompson, J. K. (1992). Social comparison: Gender, target importance ratings, and relation to body image disturbance. *Journal of Social Behavior and Personality, 7*, 335–344.

Herzog, D. B., Hopkins, J. D., & Burns, C. D. (1993). A follow-up study of 33 subdiagnostic eating disordered women. *International Journal of Eating Disorders, 14*, 261–267.

Hollander, E., Cohen, L. J., & Simeon, D. (1993). Body dysmorphic disorder. *Psychiatric Annals, 23*, 359–364.

Horne, R. L., Van Vactor, J. C., & Emerson, S. (1991). Disturbed body image in patients with eating disorders. *American Journal of Psychiatry, 148*, 211–215.

Hsu, L. K., & Sobkiewicz, T. A. (1991). Body image disturbance: Time to abandon the concept for eating disorders? *International Journal of Eating Disorders, 10*, 15–30.

Jackman, L. P., Williamson, D. A., Funsch, C. L., & Warner, M. S. (1994). *Body dysmorphic disorder in female college athletes*. Manuscript submitted for publication.

Jarvie, G. J., Lahey, B., Graziano, W., & Farmer, E. (1983). Childhood obesity and social stigma: What we know and what we don't know. *Developmental Review, 3*, 237–273.

Killen, J. D., Taylor, C. B., Hayward, C., Wilson, D. M., Haydel, K. F., Hammer, L. D., Simmonds, B., Robinson, T. N., Litt, I., Varady, A., & Kraemer, H. (1994). Pursuit of thinness and onset of eating disorder symptoms in a community sample of adolescent girls: A three-year prospective analysis. *International Journal of Eating Disorders, 13*, 227–238.

Kozak, M. J., & Foa, E. B. (1994). Obsessions, overvalued ideas, and delusions in obsessive-compulsive disorder. *Behaviour Research and Therapy, 32*, 343–353.

Lacey, J. H., & Birtchnell, S. A. (1986). Body image and its disturbances. *Journal of Psychosomatic Research, 30*, 623–631.

Lowe, C. F., & Chadwick, P. D. J. (1990). Verbal control of delusions. *Behavior Therapy, 21*, 461–479.

Marcus, M. D., Smith, D., Santelli, R., & Kaye, W. (1992). Characterization of eating disordered behavior in obese binge eaters. *International Journal of Eating Disorders, 12*, 249–255.

Marks, I., & Mishan, J. (1988). Dysmorphophobic avoidance with disturbed bodily perception: A pilot study of exposure therapy. *British Journal of Psychiatry, 152*, 674–678.

McKenna, P. J. (1984). Disorders with overvalued ideas. *British Journal of Psychiatry, 145*, 579–585.

Miller, C. T., Rothblum, E. D., Felicio, D., & Brand, P. (1995). Compensating for stigma: Obese and nonobese women's reactions to being visible. *Personality and Social Psychology Bulletin, 21*, 1093–1106.

Najjar, M. F., & Rowland, M. (1987). *Anthropometric reference data and prevalence of overweight: United States, 1976–80* (Vital & Health Statistics, Series 11, No. 238; PHS Publication No. 87-1688). Hyattsville, MD: U.S. Department of Health and Human Services.

Neziroglu, F. A., & Yaryura-Tobias, J. A. (1993a). Body dysmorphic disorder: Phenomenology and case descriptions. *Behavioural Psychotherapy, 21*, 27–36.

Neziroglu, F. A., & Yaryura-Tobias, J. A. (1993b). Exposure, response prevention, and cognitive therapy in the treatment of body dysmorphic disorder. *Behavior Therapy, 24*, 431–438.

Norris, D. L. (1984). The effects of mirror confrontation on self-estimation in anorexia nervosa, bulimia and two control groups. *Psychological Medicine, 14*, 835–842.

Pantano, M., & Santonastaso, P. (1989). A case of dysmorphophobia following recovery from anorexia nervosa. *International Journal of Eating Disorders, 8*, 701–704.

Phillips, K. A., & McElroy, S. L. (1993). Insight, overvalued ideation, and delusional thinking in body dysmorphic disorder: Theoretical and treatment implications. *Journal of Nervous and Mental Disease, 181*, 699–702.

Phillips, K. A., McElroy, S. L., Keck, P. E., Pope, H. G., & Hudson, J. I. (1993). Body dysmorphic disorder: 30 cases of imagined ugliness. *American Journal of Psychiatry, 150*, 302–308.

Ratnasuriya, R. H., Eisler, I., Szmukler, G. I., & Russell, G. F. M. (1991). Anorexia nervosa: Outcome and prognostic factors after 20 years. *British Journal of Psychiatry, 158,* 495–502.

Rorty, M., Yager, J., & Rossotto, E. (1993). Why and how do women recover from bulimia nervosa? The subjective appraisals of forty women recovered for a year or more. *International Journal of Eating Disorders, 14,* 249–260.

Rosen, J. C. (1992). Body image disorder: Definition, development, and contribution to eating disorders. In J. H. Crowther, D. L. Tennenbaum, S. E. Hobfoll, & M. A. P. Stephens (Eds.), *The etiology of bulimia: The individual and familial context* (pp. 157–177). Washington, DC: Hemisphere.

Rosen, J. C. (1996). Body image assessment and treatment in controlled studies of eating disorders. *International Journal of Eating Disorders, 20,* 331–343.

Rosen, J. C., Cado, S., Silberg, S., Srebnik, D., & Wendt, S. (1990). Cognitive behavior therapy with and without size perception training for women with body image disturbance. *Behavior Therapy, 21,* 481–498.

Rosen, J. C., Orosan, P., & Reiter, J. (1995). Cognitive behavior therapy for negative body image in obese women. *Behavior Therapy, 26,* 25–42.

Rosen, J. C., Reiter, J., & Orosan, P. (1995a). Assessment of body image in eating disorders with the Body Dysmorphic Disorder Examination. *Behaviour Research and Therapy, 33,* 77–84.

Rosen, J. C., Reiter, J., & Orosan, P. (1996). Cognitive behavioral body image therapy for body dysmorphic disorder. *Journal of Consulting and Clinical Psychology, 63,* 263–269.

Rosen, J. C., Saltzberg, E., & Srebnik, D. (1989). Cognitive behavior therapy for negative body image. *Behavior Therapy, 20,* 393–404.

Rosen, J. C., Srebnik, D., Saltzberg, E., & Wendt, S. (1991). Development of a Body Image Avoidance Questionnaire. *Psychological Assessment: A Journal of Consulting and Clinical Psychology, 3,* 32–37.

Secord, P. F., & Jourard, S. M. (1953). The appraisal of body-cathexis: Body-cathexis and the self. *Journal of Consulting Psychology, 17,* 343–347.

Singh, D. (1994). Ideal female body shape: Role of body weight and waist-to-hip ratio. *International Journal of Eating Disorders, 16,* 283–288.

Slade, P. D. (1994). What is body image? *Behaviour Research and Therapy, 32,* 497–502.

Spitzer, R. L., Yanovski, S., Wadden, T., Wing, M. D., Stunkard, A., Devlin, M., Mitchell, J., Hasin, D., & Horne, R. L. (1993). Binge-eating disorder: Its further validation in a multisite study. *International Journal of Eating Disorders, 13,* 137–153.

Sturmey, P., & Slade, P. D. (1986). Anorexia nervosa and dysmorphophobia. *British Journal of Psychiatry, 149,* 780–782.

Taylor, M. J., & Cooper, P. J. (1992). Experimental study of the effect of mood on body size perception. *Behaviour Research and Therapy, 30,* 53–58.

Thomas, C. D., & Freeman, R. J. (1991). Body-image marking: Validity of body-width estimates as operational measures of body image. *Behavior Modification, 15,* 261–270.

Thompson, J. K., Coovert, D. L., Pasman, L. N., & Robb, J. (1993). Body image and food consumption: Three laboratory studies of perceived calorie content. *International Journal of Eating Disorders, 14,* 445–457.

Thompson, J. K., & Heinberg, L. J. (1993). Preliminary test of two hypotheses of body image disturbance. *International Journal of Eating Disorders, 14,* 59–63.

Thompson, J. K., Heinberg, L., & Tantleff, S. (1991). The Physical Appearance Comparison Scale (PACS). *The Behavior Therapist, 14,* 174.

Thompson, J. K., & Tantlif, S. (1992). Female and male ratings of upper torso: Actual, ideal, and stereotypical conceptions. *Journal of Social Behavior and Personality, 7,* 345–354.

Toro, J., Salamero, M., & Martinez, E. (1994). Assessment of sociocultural influences on the aesthetic body shape model in anorexia nervosa. *Acta Psychiatrica Scandinavica, 84,* 147–151.

Vandereycken, W., Probst, M., & Van Bellinghen, M. (1992). Treating the distorted body experience of anorexia nervosa patients. *Journal of Adolescent Health, 13,* 403–405.

Vitousek, K. B., & Hollon, S. D. (1990). The investigation of schematic content and processing in eating disorders. *Cognitive Therapy and Research, 14,* 191–214.

Warwick, H. M. C., & Salkovskis, P. M. (1989). Hypochondriasis. In J. Scott, J. M. G. Williams, & A. T. Beck (Eds.), *Cognitive therapy: A clinical casebook* (pp. 78–102). London: Routledge & Kegan Paul.

Wilson, G. T., & Smith, D. (1989). Assessment of bulimia nervosa: An evaluation of the Eating Disorders Examination. *International Journal of Eating Disorders, 8,* 173–179.

Windauer, U., Lennerts, W., Talbot, P., Touyz, S. W., & Beumont, P. J. V. (1993). How well are 'cured' anorexia nervosa patients? An investigation of 16 weight-recovered anorexic patients. *British Journal of Psychiatry, 163,* 195–200.

Yager, J., & Smith, M. (1993). Restricter anorexia nervosa in a thirteen-year old sheltered Muslim girl raised in Lahore, Pakistan: Developmental similarities to Westernized patients. *International Journal of Eating Disorders, 14,* 383–386.

Zunino, N., Agoos, E., & Davis, W. N. (1991). The impact of therapist gender on the treatment of bulimic women. *International Journal of Eating Disorders, 10,* 253–263.

III

PSYCHODYNAMIC, FEMINIST, AND FAMILY APPROACHES

CHAPTER 11

Eating Disorders: A Self-Psychological Perspective

ALAN GOODSITT

It is my intention in this chapter to present what a self-psychological perspective has to offer toward the understanding and treatment of those who suffer from eating disorders. I begin by discussing theories of self psychology and comparing these to other psychodynamic theories in their view of symptoms in general and of eating disorders in particular. I then discuss psychotherapy, management issues, and finally specific therapeutic issues, including transference and countertransference.

PSYCHODYNAMIC THEORY

Psychodynamic theorists of different persuasions have attempted to explain and make meaningful the strange behaviors and the complex inner lives of patients with eating disorders. This first section of the chapter is organized around the three primary derivatives of psychoanalytic theory: the drive–conflict model, the object relations model, and the self-psychological perspective.

Drive–Conflict Model

The first major psychoanalytic attempt to comprehend an eating disorder utilized Freud's (1923/1961) drive–conflict model. Freud developed this model of the mind in the patriarchal, well-defined, well-structured, but sexually oppressive society of late 19th- and early 20th-century Vienna. His patients were conflicted

about sexuality, and his drive–conflict theory was serviceable in understanding and treating his patients.

Drive–conflict theorists believe that pathology derives from an internal conflict among three agencies of the mind: id, ego, and superego. There is an assumption of the relative intactness of the mind, as opposed to deficits in structure. Symptoms represent symbolic expressions of sexual and/or aggressive aims and defenses against these aims. The root of pathology is the intrapsychic conflict between biological aims seeking discharge and culturally influenced constraints against this discharge. Treatment emphasizes cure through interpretation and the development of insight.

The drive–conflict model of the mind works best for the neurotic patient with a well-structured psyche. It works less well for borderline patients or for patients with deficits in psychic structure.

Object Relations Theories

The object relations model is based upon an alternative developmental theory. Mahler's (1968) theory, derived from observations of infants, postulates several stages of object relations. The child moves from infantile autism to symbiosis to separation–individuation, and then on to object constancy.

For the object relations theorist, the emphasis shifts from the mind's seeking biological discharge of aims to the mind's seeking to integrate various representations of the self and objects. Some object relations theorists invoke sexual or aggressive aims as driving behavior and relationships, but others do not emphasize such aims; instead, they stress deficiencies and/or distortions in the development of object relationships and their psychic representations. Nevertheless, symptoms represent symbolic expressions of these self- and object representations. Cure comes through interpretation of these distorted representations.

Theories of Self Psychology

For the self psychologist, psychic incapacities or deficiencies and immature or undeveloped psychic structure are more prominent. The consequences of these incapacities are painful experiential states of the mind or self-states of devitalization (emptiness and numbness; a sense of going through the motions, not feeling alive, and not really living), dysphoria, and tension. Thinking may be disrupted and disorganized. Symptoms are viewed more as desperate or emergency measures to restore a sense of vitalization, wholeness, or effectiveness. Symptoms may convey symbolic meaning, but their invocation derives more from an emergent need to drown out painful self-states. Object relationships are emphasized, since it is through human relationship that one experiences vitalization and develops mature capacities to self-vitalize and self-regulate. Cure may emphasize interpretation that moves toward insight, but the content of these interpretations focuses on legitimate and previously unmet needs for human connection that are vitalizing or self-enhancing. Some self psychologists would argue that provision of unmet needs in a therapeutic relationship, with the ultimate aim of righting a derailed psyche or mobilizing an undeveloped one, is more important than insight via interpretation.

For Kohut (1971), the capacity to tolerate separation without some form of psychic decompensation depends upon the internalization of certain mental functions and structure. Important functions, called "selfobject functions," include the capacity to provide (more or less) one's own cohesiveness, soothing, vitalization, narcissistic equilibrium (sense of well-being and security), tension regulation, and self-esteem regulation.

Kohut viewed these regulatory functions as initially being provided by an external caretaker, such as the mother. It is the caretaker who initially provides soothing and protects the infant from stimulus overload. Later these functions are transferred to a transitional object, such as a blanket (M. Tolpin, 1971). It is then the transitional object, which the child totally controls, that provides a sense of well-being and security. The transitional object is cognitively perceived as external, but is experienced as a part of the self. If "good enough" mothering (Winnicott, 1965) occurs, these functions are internalized (M. Tolpin, 1971) and become part of the child's mental structure (the selfobject).

Kohut (1971) defined a "selfobject" as an intrapsychic object or function that references the caregiving functions originally provided by caregivers. A person who provides these functions in lieu of deficient internalization of these functions is experienced as a part of oneself, not as a separate human being with his or her own initiatives, interests, or qualities.

Developmentally, if caregiving is not traumatically frustrated but is sufficiently responsive to needs, a healthy and mature organization of the self results. With this maturity of the self-organization, one should be relatively skilled at providing one's own regulation of tension, self-esteem, and self-cohesion. Kohut identified three pathways to this result: mirroring of the child's archaic but developmentally normal grandiosity; idealization of an idealized object; and twinship, or the experience of validation that occurs when another is like oneself and thus reflects oneself. One may say that an environment that allows idealization or that provides mirroring or twinship experiences is responding to selfobject needs that build, maintain, or restore the self-organization. Other selfobject needs that have been identified are those for validation and self-delineation (Stolorow & Atwood, 1992).

If caregiving is not responsive to developmental needs, the capacities to provide vitalization, cohesion, and tension and self-esteem regulation are relatively deficient, and a disorder of the self results. In this case, the connection with another person who triggers selfobject experiences is vital.

Conflict or Deficit?: An Illustration

It can be difficult to discern whether eating disorder pathology is driven by conflict over sexual/aggressive aims, by distortions of the self and objects, or by impaired capacities to vitalize oneself. The following case illustrates what appeared to be a straightforward sexual conflict in an anorexic girl, but proved upon careful exploration to be more complex.

Mary was 13 years old when she was hospitalized for anorexia nervosa.[1] She presented during sessions as a passive, empty shell. She said little unless asked. When asked for feelings and reactions, she appeared puzzled, would not respond at all, or would respond with a gesture or a one-word statement such as "lost." When I would press her for her feelings, she would at times refer me to her parents for the answer—reflecting a mental function, the capacity to identify and articulate self-states, as outside of herself. She did express feeling "lost" and "like dying" in reaction to the separation from her parents that was the result of her being hospitalized. When I would open the door to the interview room, the door would hit the doorstop and invariably bounce back and hit her unless I stopped it. It was as if I was expected to understand, protect, and cure her without her having to speak or exert any effort to participate in the treatment. From a self-psychological perspective, she experienced me as an aspect of herself, and she relied upon my mental functions to maintain her well-being. I functioned for her as an idealized, omnipotent selfobject.

She responded well to benign, supportive, and exploratory therapy, and to the implicit hope that she would eat and gain weight. Early in treatment I took a week's vacation, which coincided with the wedding of her brother. It was also at this time that she resumed menstruation. On her brother's wedding night, she became psychologically fragmented and delusionally proclaimed that her father was dead. Associative material revealed a pregnancy fantasy and a feeling of being too close to her father. She believed her father would die if he knew how "wild"—that is, sexual (in her own fantasy)—she was.

From this associative material, we were then able to reconstruct what initiated her self-starvation in the first place. Her father had previously had a heart attack. It was her fantasy that her developing sexuality had so disturbed him that it brought on his heart attack. As with me in the transference, she had an idealized relationship with her father and relied upon him for her mental functions. Just as one cuts off a gangrenous leg to save the body, she sacrificed her sexuality to save her father and his availability as a vital selfobject.

In the context of two sexually stimulating events (her brother's wedding and her resumption of menstruation), and a separation from me because of my vacation, Mary's psychic intactness (cohesion) was disrupted. She was delusional. The experience of herself as sexual threatened her selfobject bond with her father. The separation from me disrupted her stabilizing selfobject bond with me.

Sexuality was feared not because it was taboo or a transgression against superego precepts, as in a typical neurosis, but rather because it threatened the selfobject bond with her father that was vital for her psychic cohesion. Mary's anorexia reflected a profound disorder in her self-organization. Her central anxieties were those of disintegration with disruption of the self-organization, rather than guilt related to sexual transgression. Seemingly sexual anxiety and conflict functioned to deal with more primary self-organization and self-intactness issues.

APPLICATIONS OF THEORETICAL MODELS TO EATING DISORDERS

Eating disorders are symptomatic expressions that can occur in a relatively intact or structured psyche and reflect an internal conflict, or can occur in an undeveloped or incomplete mental structure and reflect a disorder of the self. The symptoms of an eating disorder can be either symbolic expressions of psychic aims and defenses (drive–conflict model); symbolic expressions of distorted self and object representations (object relations model); or nonsymbolic, restitutional emergency measures used to stem the tide of disrupted self-states threatened with the loss of cohesion of the self (self-psychological model).

Applications of the Drive–Conflict Model

The early theories about anorexia nervosa were of the drive–conflict type. Moulton (1942), Rowland (1970), and Waller, Kaufman, and Deutsch (1940) all postulated that self-starvation is a defense against sexual fantasies of oral impregnation. Berlin, Boatman, Scheimo, and Szurek (1951) and Masserman (1941) saw the refusal of food as a defense against ambivalent oral sadistic fantasies. Blitzer, Rollins, and Blackwell (1961), Grimshaw (1959), Margolis and Jernberg (1960), Masserman (1941), and Tustin (1958) all emphasized either ambivalent oral impregnation or oral sadistic fantasies.[2]

Applications of the Object Relations Model

Selvini Palazzoli (1978) sees the future anorexic as having unresolved problems in the oral incorporative stage, which impede separation–individuation. The anorexic fantasizes an oral incorporation of a maternal, bad, and overcontrolling object. This maternal introject is then equated with the anorexic's body. The anorexic experiences an identity of her body as her mother.[3] Self-starvation is thus the adolescent's attempt to end the feminization of her body, and thus to minimize the confused, ambivalent identification with her mother. Selvini Palazzoli explains anorexic behavior as resulting from these distorted mental representations of body, self, and object.

For Masterson (1978), the anorexic is plagued by an array of introjects. There is a hostile, rejecting, withdrawing maternal introject in response to the anorexic's attempt at separation. There is also a supportive, rewarding maternal introject in response to the anorexic's regressive, clinging behavior. There are thus two corresponding self-representations—one that is inadequate, bad, guilty, and empty, and another that is passive, compliant, and good. Although Masterson speaks of arrested development at symbiosis and separation–individuation, with corresponding ego defects, his theory points primarily to the distorted self and object representations as the sources of anorexic behavior.

In a more recent paper, Masterson (1995) describes a case of bulimia as representing a "closet narcissistic personality disorder." A child's (pathological) grandiosity undergoes a traumatic disappointment and is then hidden behind defensive idealization of the other. The latter results in these patients' defensively focusing on others instead of themselves.

Sours (1980) stresses defects in the ego and the self, as well as symbolic, dynamic conflicts and distortions. He refers to defects in the ego,

sense of self, poor differentiation between the self and objects, and the failure to develop self and object constancy. For Sours, treatment is aimed at developing a therapeutic alliance by understanding the nature of the fixated, deviational, and atypical development of ego functions, self representations, and object representations. The main barrier to the development of the alliance—primitive defenses of denial, negation, disavowal, splitting, and omnipotence—must be dealt with by confrontation and interpretation.

Selvini Palazzoli (1978), Masterson (1978), and Sours (1980) emphasize distortions in representations of the body, the self, or objects. Sugarman and Kurash (1982) are object relations theorists who propose an ego defect as a central causative factor. Restricting themselves to a consideration of bulimic patients, Sugarman and Kurash assert that these patients lack the ego function of object constancy. Thus, when separated from the symbiotic mother, they are unable automatically to evoke a mental representation of the mother and become soothed. Since eating is a sensorimotor activity associated with the childhood feeding experience with the mother, bingeing becomes a means of evoking the sensorimotor object representation of the symbiosis.

Sugarman (1991) proposes a developmental failure in the bulimic woman to communicate her needs, wishes, and affects in verbal symbolic form. The bulimic's body is the vehicle of communication, and bulimic symptoms express unconscious conflicts. The body self is not integrated into the psychological self. Affect regulation is either defensively attributed to the maternal representation or is never integrated into the self-representation.

Kernberg (1994) understands eating disorder pathology as a "relentless sadistic attack on the patient's body." For these patients, the body symbolically represents conflictual pleasure per se, mother, femininity, and/or heterosexuality.

Applications of Self Psychology

Self psychologists have attempted to understand eating disorders from various perspectives. In this subsection, I address self-psychological viewpoints on development, the (restorative) function of symptoms, the meaning of the patient's body, interoceptive deficits, needs, and fantasies.

Developmental Considerations, Needs, and Fantasies

Self psychologists emphasize developmental failures in the provision of mirroring, idealizing, and validating needs leading to deficits in capacities to maintain self-esteem, cohesion, and various self-regulating functions. The result is a vulnerability to developing an eating disorder (Geist, 1985, 1989; Goodsitt, 1977, 1983, 1985; Sands, 1989, 1991).

Sands (1989) notes that developing girls are presented with particular obstacles in both the mirroring and idealizing dimensions. In contrast to boys, little girls are discouraged from exhibitionist "showing off, being cocky, acting smart or aggressive" (p. 77). Instead, they are supposed to be "lady-like." Only in the sphere of physical appearance are developing girls encouraged, albeit ambivalently, to obtain exhibitionistic (mirroring) gratification. Thus, later in life, women are predisposed to reveal their psychopathology through bodily symptoms such as eating disorders.

The failure to provide appropriate, affirming selfobject needs may occur when parents are themselves self-absorbed, anxious, needy, overwhelmed, depressed, or psychotic. When this is the case, children may decide that reliance upon others to supply selfobject needs is too risky. A facade of pseudo-self-sufficiency (Modell, 1975) may be adopted—more so among anorexic than among bulimic patients. Furthermore, such a child, interpreting that she is the cause of a parent's overwhelmed condition, may commit herself to never being a burden on others. Her goal becomes maintaining others' well-being or narcissistic balance. She becomes the compliant model child who has turned off her own needs. By devoting herself to the care, feeding, and well-being of others, she functions as a selfobject for them while thereby negating her own selfobject needs.

As a result, the maturation of the anorexic's own selfobject and self-regulatory capacities is thwarted. On some level, the girl is aware of her limitations and is unconsciously afraid to grow up. Pubertal bodily changes and adolescence may terrify the young girl, because it means becoming a self-sufficient adult woman and doing without another who provides vital selfobject functions. Growing up means loss, loneliness, isolation, emptiness, helplessness, and coming apart. Thus, the prospect of doing or being well or of gaining weight is dreaded.

With the onset of the illness, these thwarted needs and wishes break through. For the anorexic, her emaciated body and her sickness make dramatic exhibitionistic statements to others: "Take notice. Don't ignore me. I'm here. Getting some attention and responsiveness, even if it is negative, is better than none and feeling like nobody." The illness permits the expression of these wishes to be the center of all things and to be in omnipotent control of at least a narrowly defined world. The anorexic's environment is made to dance to her tune. It cannot now ignore or be indifferent to her demands or needs.

Nevertheless, the psychological consequences of impaired selfobject capacities are profound. The absence of reliable internal self-regulation results in the anorexic's feeling inadequate, ineffective, and out of control—expressed as feeling fat. Anorexics feel excessively influenced and exploited because they are deficient in self-regulatory structure and are therefore dependent upon others for their well-being (Goodsitt, 1977, 1983).

The typical picture of the young bulimic girl prior to the onset of bulimia is of a child who is more tension-ridden, conflicted, and impulsive than the anorexic child. Her self-esteem is unstable. She is conflicted between pursuing her own life and maintaining the psychic equilibrium of an unhappy parent whose life has been disrupted by, for example, divorce, alcoholism, or mental instability. The bulimic enters puberty and adolescence poorly equipped to regulate her moods, tensions, self-esteem, and cohesion. She turns to bodily manipulation in the form of bingeing, purging, and weight control to temporarily restitute a sense of vitalization and effectiveness.

Symptoms as Restorative

Eating disorder pathology often reflects restitutional attempts to restore cohesion or vitalization when these are threatened or damaged (Barth, 1988; Geist, 1985, 1989). Subjective meanings of these symptomatic experiences are present, but these are not the source of a need for emergency self-management (Gehrie, 1990).

Lacking reliable self-soothing, tension regulation, and mood regulation, and feeling restlessly bored, empty, and aimless, the anorexic is driven to constant activity and strenuous physical exertion to drown out these painful internal conditions. By focusing on food and weight, by rigidly counting calories and regulating ingestion, by turning off her need of others and turning inward to herself, and by filling up her life with rituals that help her feel a sense of predictability and control, she narrows down her world to something she feels she can manage. Feeling her self-organization to be out of control, she insists on meticulous control of her body self. By starving herself, she feels strengthened and temporarily superior to others. This is the antidote to her feelings of weakness, shame, and inadequacy related to her true need of others.

Once anorexia nervosa (or bulimia) develops and becomes a chronic condition, it provides the patient with a pathological, compensatory identity or selfhood that allows some contrived sense of having a significant and meaningful presence in the world: "I am an anorexic. I don't know what I'd feel if I weren't an anorexic." The illness then is defended as all that stands between the patient and nothingness or insignificance.

Lichtenberg, Lachman, and Fosshage (1992, pp. 143–144) state that in individuals whose basic motivational needs have been consistently frustrated, intense alternative affective states (selfobject experiences) that temporarily enliven or vitalize are invoked despite their otherwise maladaptive aspects. An individual whose hunger signals were ignored during infancy may be drawn to self-starvation as a familiar, valued, intense affect-laden experience. Another individual may self-starve or overexercise because of the inherently intense quality of these experiences, which effectively blot out other painful affective states. Another individual may use symbolic elaboration of fantasy to achieve vitalization and cohesion. An example of this would be the equation of thinness with beauty or superiority.

The Meaning of the Patient's Body

Both object relations and self-psychological theorists have attempted to explain the peculiar relationship eating-disordered patients, particularly anorexics, have with their bodies. My formulations regarding this were developed primarily in my work with anorexics.

As I see it, anorexics view their bodies in multiple ways. Many anorexics experience their bodies as the battleground of the separation–individuation war. Who owns their bodies is a matter of contention (Goodsitt, 1977). Adolescent anorexics perceive their bodies to be the last vestige of their infantile, archaic grandiosity. Grandiose individuals need to be the center of all things around which the world revolves, to feel they are in total control of everything, and to experience themselves as perfect. Anorexics focus all of these needs on their bodies. Now their bodies must be perfect and unchanging, and they must be in total and absolute control of them. The changes of puberty in a child, then, threaten this grandiosity and thereby threaten the adolescent's fragile psychic equilibrium.

Furthermore, the problem with the body in such a patient seems to be its lack of integration into the self-organization (Rizzuto, Peterson, & Reed, 1981).[4] Anorexics are often indifferent to their bodily needs. They fail to take adequate care of their bodies. They ignore nutritional needs. They are strangely unconcerned about dangerous changes in the heart and other organs. They are out of touch with their inner bodily experiences and feelings. They seem not to cathect or invest in their bodies in a wholesome manner.

In this regard, it should be noted that the self is at its core a body self (Goodsitt, 1977, 1983, 1985; Krueger, 1988, 1989). Developmentally, the nucleus of the self consists of bodily sensations. Freud (1923/1961) stated, "The ego is first and foremost a bodily ego" (p. 26). This applies to the self, which is first and foremost a body self. As Kohut (1971) has pointed out, when the cohesive self becomes unstable, bodily symptoms (hypochondriasis) result. The anorexic's failure to invest appropriately in the body, and the resulting bodily distortions and delusions, are all symptomatic of a lack of cohesiveness of the self-organization. The body is poorly integrated into the self-organization.

When the integrity or cohesion of the self is threatened, eating-disordered patients experience this threat concretely in terms of loss of control of the body (Goodsitt, 1977, 1983, 1985). Excessive attempts to control the shape of one's body derive from a terrible sense that one's body, as an aspect of the self-organization, is out of control—easily influenced, invaded, exploited, and overwhelmed by external forces, whether these are peers, parents, or food. Anorexics complain that if they take one bite of food, they will not be able to stop; if they eat a meal, they will gain 10 pounds immediately or they will suddenly blow up and look like an elephant. One anorexic complained to me that if she ate chicken breasts, it would give her breasts. Another anorexic experienced food as sitting in her stomach in its preingestion form. Such patients experience eating as being occupied by a foreign force. What is missing is the conviction that their bodies are active agents that metabolize food, break it down into component parts, and transform it into a part of their own bodies. In their conception of the relationship between their bodies and food, their bodies are strangely passive, impotent, and unable to regulate metabolic activities.

It is only with the attainment of a stable, cohesive self that such a patient can process an external stimulus, be it food or information, and maintain a sense of wholeness and integrity. Furthermore, it permits her to confront external influences, digest or process them, and assimilate them into the self or reject them with equanimity. It is a well-integrated self that allows a person to fell effective and in control, not just an empty receptacle subject to foreign occupation. The anorexic's experience of bodily helplessness indicates a lack of integrity of the self (Goodsitt, 1977).

When the integrity of the self is threatened, an eating-disordered patient attempts to stave off further disruption by hypercathecting, stimulating, and obsessively focusing on the body (Goodsitt, 1983, 1985). The anorexic's constant activity and exercise are her attempts to feel herself within her body. They are restitutional attempts at feeling alive, whole, and cohesive.

If the anorexic's strange relationships with her body reflects the lack of integration of her body into her core self, then therapeutic interventions will be guided by this formulation. Rather than interpreting to the anorexic that she symbolically equates her body with her mother (i.e., that she has distorted self- and object representations), or interpreting the oral incorporative fantasy, the therapist should attempt to heal the disintegrated self. In contrast to the object relations therapist's emphasis on the interpretation of distorted self- and object representations, the self-psychological therapist emphasizes deficits in psychic structure, unmet selfobject needs, and derailed self-development, which can be remobilized with the establishment of a selfobject transference or even with provision or responsiveness to selfobject needs.[5]

Interoceptive Deficits

Sours (1980) accurately notes that the difficulty these patients have in discussing their own affects, memories, and fantasies is in part secondary to starvation and a lack of a therapeutic alliance. This explanation does not go far enough, however (Goodsitt, 1982). For some time, anorexics have been observed to be alexithymic and have been described as nonverbal (Bruch, 1962; Eissler, 1943; Goodsitt, 1969; Jessner & Abse, 1960; Scott, 1948; Wall, 1959). I believe that their difficulty in relating inner experiences is yet another manifestation of deficits in the self-organization. These patients fail to relate to inner experiences because they have an impaired capacity to live within the body self. They are out of touch with their core experiences. There is a failure to integrate bodily, cognitive, and affective experiences into an organized core self (Goodsitt, 1983, 1985; Sands, 1989, 1991; Dellaverson, 1994).

Therapists like Garner, Garfinkel, and Bemis (Garfinkel & Garner, 1982; Garner & Bemis, 1982; Garner, Garfinkel, & Bemis, 1982) have called our attention to the cognitive defects that constitute one aspect of this phenomenon. Bruch (1962) has long emphasized the need to help these patients get in touch with their feelings. Levenkron (1983) points out that these patients do not have a language for talking about themselves. As a therapist, he takes an active role in providing and teaching them a vocabulary for the self. In my opinion, all of these therapists recognize the deficits in the self-organization; moreover, they have all devised treatment techniques to deal with these deficits.

Hostile, Vindictive Fantasies

For the most part, these patients find it difficult to be angry. Anger is disavowed. Nevertheless, an observer may see it written on a patient's face or expressed in her behavior. For example, an anorexic frequently stops eating when her mother or anyone else is pleased by her eating. In the anorexic's profound stubbornness, negativism, and oppositionalism, anger is apparent.

A central unconscious fantasy at play in the anorexic's self-starvation is for her to become a concentration camp victim, a vision of (impending) death, a walking cadaver. This can occur in response to a parent's having identified the future anorexic with an ambivalently loved relative who died. In the mind of this parent, the future anorexic is a replacement for the dead relative (Falstein, Feinstein, & Judas, 1956; Goodsitt, 1969). Fearing the realization of unconscious death wishes now directed at the child, this parent anxiously overprotects the child and fosters an overly controlling symbiosis. The parent acts as if death is always just around the corner. The anorexic's appearance is her cruel, vindictive parody of the parent's worst fears (Goodsitt, 1969).

A variation on this theme is illustrated by one patient, Ann. Ann had a fantasy of her parents grieving over her dead body. She could then gloat that her parents finally realized the wrong they had done her, but now it was too late. Another patient, Beth, went further: She kept her bedroom darkened except for candlelight, and created an altar in front of which she prayed. She fantasized herself as her parents' human sacrifice upon the altar. This gloomy, sacrificial room, permeated with the sense of death, was meant to deliver a vindictive accusation to her parents: "You have killed me." Beth reveled in the knowledge that when her mother embraced her, she would be aghast with horror in feeling only bones. Beth hoped that her appearance evoked shock in others as well. She wanted to be sick, ugly, pitiful, and freakish.

This pursuit of ugliness is an often-overlooked phenomenon. In contrast, much has been said about sociocultural standards that equate thinness with beauty. On a conscious level, anorexics claim they are striving to be perfectly beautiful by becoming thin. On a less than conscious or unconscious level, just the opposite is found, as described above: The goal is to achieve a degree of emaciation that is repulsive, ugly, and shocking. This not only fulfills fantasies of revenge, but represents an attempt by the anorexic to awaken her parents to her dreadful plight and perhaps to make them responsive to her needs for recognition, significance, and validation.

Self-Guilt: Guilt for Occupying Psychological Space

The concept of separation anxiety as a significant impediment to separation–individuation has been thoroughly elucidated by Mahler (1968). Individuals who remain symbiotically bound experience annihilation anxiety, psychic disruption, or fragmentation during separation. Those individuals who have progressed to the level of separation–individuation are more able to remain structurally intact or cohesive. These individuals are more aware of their dependence, and are thus more vulnerable to experiencing separation anxiety than to experiencing psychic disruption.

In working with these patients, I have found another factor that I believe significantly impedes the separation–individuation process. These patients suffer profound guilt for the wish to separate and for acts of separation and individuation. This guilt is manifested in different ways from the guilt expressed by neurotics who are conflicted over specific or focal taboo drives or impulses.

Self-guilt, in contrast to neurotic guilt, is experienced by a patient as a more ill-defined but pervasive sense of discomfort for simply being or existing. She generally cannot articulate this experience. Nevertheless, the patient feels guilty for occupying both physical and psychological space—that is, for having a vigorous and vital presence. She minimizes her presence in a variety of physical and psychological ways. In dance therapy, an anorexic uses a smaller portion of the room than a bulimic or a non-eating-disordered person. Psychologically, the patient is in constant fear of burdening others. She refrains from making demands and expressing wishes, desires, and needs. She allows others to use and abuse her. She does not confront those who do abuse her. She does not represent herself (her selfhood) well with others. She feels uneasy and guilty when given to. She turns away gifts and compliments. She acts as if she is undeserving. Nevertheless, she considers herself selfish.

The anorexic negates her selfhood. She extols the virtues of self-denial, discipline, and asceticism (Mogul, 1980), while abhorring anything that smacks of indulgence. Unlike the neurotic, who feels guilty for indulging specific taboo desires, the anorexic feels guilty for the act of indulgence itself. Pleasure per se is taboo. The emaciated body shape is an ideal that graphically portrays this moral value of self-negation.

Self-negation is evident in the anorexic's devotion to meeting the expectations of others. Duty, obedience, and obligation occupy high positions in the anorexic's hierarchy of values and ideals. By leading a highly regimented, ritualized life, regulated by rules, taken up by schedules and obligations, the anorexic precludes any chance to look inward and consider her own wishes and needs. She thereby negates her selfhood. Instead, she directs her attention to pleasing, accommodating, and being sensitive to others. The guiding rule for life is to serve others by meeting their needs. She strives to become a selfobject (i.e., a function for others) and not a self.

It is as if the future anorexic has a hard time justifying her existence. Modell (1965) first described a type of patient who suffers separation guilt. He noted that such patients are arrested in the phase of separation–individuation. They experience a vague yet pervasive and ill-defined type of guilt. He aptly stated that these patients do not feel they have a right to a life (of their own).

Friedman (1985), also influenced by Modell and by similar concepts developed by Weiss and Sampson (Weiss, Sampson, & Modell, 1983), has presented a thesis remarkably parallel to my conceptualization of self-guilt in eating-disordered patients. Working with anorexics, in whom this phenomenon is most prominent, Friedman described two forms of survivor guilt in these patients. "Separation guilt" refers to a child's experiencing her growth and separation as destructive to her mother or others. "Depletion guilt" refers to the experience that whatever the child receives, obtains, or gets is at the expense of someone else. I concur that both of these types of guilt are rampant phenomena in anorexics. Anorexics not only are afraid to grow up (separation anxiety), but experience guilt for growing up and thereby abandoning their parents. Anorexics feel disloyal for having feelings, wishes, needs, interests, values, and goals that are different from those of their parents. They feel guilty for wanting or having a separate identity or selfhood.

Ann, described earlier, reported that she would feel herself "click off" in the presence of her mother and "click on" in her mother's absence. Another patient, Debbie, told her depressed mother that she would never leave her mother as her older brothers had; they had left home to marry and establish lives of their own. A third anorexic described how she had always felt she owed her mother her life. This patient struggled to feel that her life was her own to live. Beth spoke of her being the center of her mother's life; she felt that her mother could "never be happy without me." Any time Beth felt happy, she proceeded to "kill the happiness." She explained, "I am not supposed to be happy. I should leave all that to Mother."

These illustrations demonstrate both the anorexic's self-guilt and the belief that her role in life is to be a selfless selfobject. Often she feels she is a special or precious child, born to fill an emptiness or the needs of a parent. She sees herself as compensating her parent for a disappointing spouse or sibling. This goal thus intensifies the anorexic's need to be perfect—to be a model child for the parent. Feeling, thinking, and doing in the world represent a disloyal betrayal of her obligation to be a selfless selfobject. Any act of occupying psychological space is experienced as an immoral, hostile, and destructive act that deprives others of their psychological space. Since it is her obligation to be a selfobject, she experiences self-guilt when she does not fulfill this role. She cannot say "no," refuse to accommodate others' demands and needs, or obtain gratification or fulfillment of her needs unless she does so in a disguised or unacknowledged fashion. The symptoms of anorexia nervosa (and bulimia nervosa) serve this purpose. They provide a vehicle for the expression of anger, while at the same time fulfilling selfobject needs for soothing, vitalization, recognition, validation, self-definition, specialness, self-confirming responsiveness, and a sense of effectiveness.

The need to be a selfobject may also be evident in the transference to the therapist. Ann would begin each session by scrutinizing the therapist's face for any sign of fatigue. She could not begin to talk about herself until she had been reassured that the therapist was "OK" or in a good mood.

A conceptualization of self-guilt makes meaningful some aspects of self-starvation. To eat means to give to oneself. It means that one responds to inner sources of need, as opposed to outer expectation, duty, or obligation. To eat means one has made a decision that one has a right to consider oneself a priority vis-à-vis others. Self-interest is legitimate. Thinking of oneself and giving to oneself are legitimate; they have their place—and, in fact, their priority—in the scheme of things. For the anorexic, eating means depriving another of sustenance. It is also an act of unjustifiable self-indulgence. It is a betrayal of the function of being a selfobject. Any act that indicates or suggests self—self-indulgence, self-direction, self-caring, self-interest—is pejoratively labeled and experienced as selfish, and is therefore considered illegitimate. By starving herself, the anorexic creates a self-defining self-space that defeats, renders helpless, and excludes all outside influences. In this restitutional act, she reverses her obligation to be a selfless caregiver to others. In the solitary,

secretive acts of bingeing and purging, the bulimic steals a self-space that is solely her own;
these are often the only moments in her busy
day devoted to (restitutional) self-experience.

Anorexics and bulimics have slightly different
adaptations to the dilemma of their selfobject
neediness and their fear and guilt with regard to
pursuing these needs. Anorexics attempt to regard themselves as beyond ordinary human
neediness (i.e., as selfless). The anorexic says,
"All that is for mere mortals. If I am beyond
needs, I will not be traumatically injured by others' failure to meet my needs. Furthermore, I
won't feel guilty for depriving others of their sustenance and psychological space." Bulimics have
not as completely attempted to negate their
needs for selfobject responsiveness from human
beings. But because they have been traumatically injured, disappointed, and disillusioned, their
neediness is expressed interpersonally in archaic
and maladaptive ways. A bulimic has difficulty
identifying, accepting, and owning her need of
others. When these needs present themselves in
a relationship, they take the form of self-defeating demands, manipulations, or self-defeating
and disguised sarcastic expressions. This leads to
further injury and eventually to seeking nonhu-
man sources of self-restitution—that is, bingeing and purging (Sands, 1991).

When presented with self-guilt, the therapist
takes the position that it is the patient's
birthright to have a life of her own. Self-interest
is differentiated from selfishness. Clarification,
insight, and being responsive to the patient's
selfobject needs are crucial in working through
this issue.

THE PSYCHOTHERAPEUTIC PROCESS

In this section, I discuss the process of dynamic
individual psychotherapy with patients with eating disorders. The stages of treatment are considered, as are the therapist's role and the role
of transference. Symptom management, hospitalization, family involvement, and transference–countertransference issues are also addressed.

Stages of Therapy

The Beginning Stage

Certain problems are more or less germane to
specific stages of therapy. In the first stage of

therapy, the main issue is the patient's reluctance to be a patient. The disavowal of illness
must be addressed during the initial consultation. Frequently the patient appears to have
been pushed into the consultation room. She
looks as if the therapist and his or her office are,
respectively, the last person she would rather
see and the last place on earth she would rather
be. When such resistance appears, it should be
addressed immediately, or the patient will be
gone.

The therapist carefully explores the patient's
motivation for therapy. If she presents with
considerable disavowal of illness or a facade of
self-sufficiency, it is important to find and make
contact with the part of the patient that hurts or
experiences psychic pain. The therapist should
actively solicit how miserable, hopeless, and de-
spairing the patient feels. The therapist needs
to determine whether the patient believes she
is entitled to help and whether she feels it is
permissible to seek help for her misery. The
therapist must surely advise her that it is precisely because people feel the way she is feeling
that they seek and in fact do obtain relief within
a psychotherapeutic process. The therapist
should explore what myths the patient harbors
about the process of therapy.

The therapist should keep in mind that, as a
rule, anorexic women are withdrawn, distrust-
ing, frequently alexithymic, and proudly independent. They are terrified of intimacy, closeness, and being in an office alone with another
person. They are ashamed of longings and selfobject needs. The therapist should also be
aware that anorexic patients are performance-
oriented and therefore feel panicked about the
expectation that they carry the conversation.
The therapist must have minimal expectations
that these alexithymic patients can verbalize
their inner feelings. The responsibility for establishing meaningful contact and rapport thus
rests with the therapist. The therapist psychologically reaches out to such a patient and tries
to anticipate and allay her misperceptions and
anxieties about therapy. The therapist does not
allow silences to continue so long that both participants feel terribly uncomfortable. Eating-
disordered patients must be taught how to explore their feelings and how to utilize therapy.

During the initial consultation, the therapist
verbally anticipates that the patient may not
feel comfortable with therapy and may wish to
run from it. The therapist tells the patient that
when this happens, the therapist wants her to

address this important feeling. If the patient is there under duress, the therapist makes it clear that his or her mission is to help the patient feel better about herself. The therapist is her agent—not anyone else's. The therapist attempts to establish a verbal contract with the patient to help her with the specific problems that have been identified. These issues are central to developing a therapeutic alliance, which is vital to the therapeutic process.

The Middle Stage

The middle stage of therapy involves the establishment of a selfobject transference, within which selfobject needs are identified, experienced, and fulfilled. Two processes occur simultaneously: insight into the developmental origins of the fundamental pathology, and the experience of being understood. It is the latter experience that provides a selfobject experience of validation. In the area of traumatic frustration, understanding or insight is achieved. In the area of unmet selfobject needs, a new experience of provision occurs, which enhances the self-organization. The following case illustrates this process, and further articulates treatment goals within the self-psychological paradigm. The relationship between the achievement of these goals and symptomatic remission is also noted.

Ellen, a married woman, the mother of two children, and a competent professional in a caregiving field, was referred to me by a colleague who had treated her unsuccessfully for 1½ years. Ellen, now in her mid-40s, had had one other therapeutic endeavor, which occurred in her 20s.

Ellen had been obese as early as second grade, dieted in 8th grade, and weighed 200 pounds (at a height of 5'7") in high school until she began to restrict her food intake severely. Her weight dropped to 150 pounds in her last year of high school. In the context of an abusive first marriage in her 20s, she began bingeing and purging; this was continuing to occur up to six times daily, with purging after each ingestion of food, at the time of her referral to me. Weighing 125 pounds at referral, she met the diagnostic criteria for bulimia nervosa. She had overcome earlier body image distortions, but she continued to dread becoming fat with the ingestion of normal amounts of food. She either avoided

breakfast and lunch or purged after eating these meals. She structured her life to provide space for her binges and purges, and she bought food specifically to binge on.

Ellen understood her symptoms as blunting her feelings. She noted that she was more responsive and more fully present in the world when she was not symptomatic. For the most part, she experienced an emptiness and a life not fully lived. She stated, "My feelings are withered. I don't live my life to the fullest. I'm not completely real." Often she felt lost and aimless. At times she felt alive, but she recognized that she was dependent upon others to create this within her: "I'm a candle lit from the outside. I glow and have enthusiasm, but I can't light myself." She described herself as a busy professional whose life was taken up by pleasing and taking care of others, duty, and responsibility. She organized her life around reacting to others' needs and to crises, and she did not assert her own needs nor consider her own feelings. She saw herself as a nice person who was sensitive, shy, and afraid of conflict and anger. She understood her bulimia not only as blunting feelings, but also as releasing tensions.

Ellen's early years were troubled. Her father was absent for the most part, but critical and angry at her when present. Her early memories of him were of being yelled at for intruding on his work and getting spanked by him for getting stuck in some mud. She reported that he would chastise her so as not to bother her mother. Ellen described her mother as critical, negative, judgmental, and invalidating. Consequently, Ellen felt inadequate, not good enough, not valued, and (given her obesity) an embarrassment to her mother. Her mother focused on Ellen's faults and incapacities. For years, she would remind Ellen that Ellen almost got her sister killed when Ellen, who was 4 at the time, fell asleep in the car and her 2-year-old sister wandered off. It was only in the course of this therapy that Ellen recognized the inappropriateness of her mother's leaving her, at age 4, in charge of her 2-year-old sister in a car. Ellen received no praise for her almost straight-A grades, but she got an earful for the occasional B grade. The major sins for the mother were pride, such as Ellen's being excited and proud about a good report card, and selfishness. Ellen recalled being reprimanded for crying at her grandfather's funeral because her crying was making others feel worse. This telling incident was just one of many illustrating the messages Ellen received—that who she was and how she felt were bad and burdensome to others.

When Ellen was 2 and her sister was born, her mother was ill for several months afterward. In addition to her parents' not addressing Ellen's deprivation of her mother, Ellen was repeatedly admonished both not to bother her mother and not to leave her mother alone. With the birth of a calf on her grandmother's farm, Ellen's excited whoops and hollers were met with "Don't. Your mother is tired." Her feelings and vitalized states were bad, and she was to be muffled or silenced. Her very nurturing and loving grandmother was the only figure during her early years who made her feel special and valued. Her experience with her mother often left her feeling inadequate and "crushed." As she reported, "I felt empty and lonesome and wanted to be told I was loved."

During the initial phase of treatment, I met Ellen's shame and sense of failure and inadequacy for being symptomatic with nonjudgmental inquiry and the following attitudinal posture: "There is a good reason for these symptoms. They have helped you in some important way. When and where they occur constitute valuable information. I am keenly interested in you, your experience, and your feelings." Ellen's response was to declare her reluctance to give up her bulimia. Her metaphor for herself as sick was that of a "derailed train," relieved of responsibility. She ambivalently saw her bulimia as effectively containing her anger and as having allowed her to remain in her disastrous first marriage, without having to face the pain.

Evidence that my acceptance of Ellen as a person with or without her symptoms was reflected in new self-revelatory behavior. She revealed to her new husband of 1½ years the shameful secret of her eating disorder. She also revealed to a friend a "weakness" and was delighted to discover that she didn't lose her friend. She entertained ideas of being more visible and present with her longings and feelings. She dreamed of being a child and angrily yelled at by her parents, but in the dream, she got angry in return.

We identified a pattern: Bingeing and purging occurred when Ellen ignored a self-state of tiredness or a longing to drop her responsibilities, curl up in bed, and read a book. She had a guilt-ridden fantasy of spending money on a tan at a tanning spa. She revealed to me that the secretive bingeing and purging were the only activities for which she allowed herself time and space in her busy day. I affirmed the importance of identifying her self's needs and tending to them, and the heavy price she paid for ignoring these needs. It was her birthright to have a self. Tending to her self's needs was as vital as providing food and water for her body. As long as she ignored or negated herself, she would need to be bulimic. We explored her longings, fantasies, wishes, and needs as legitimate expressions of her self. Thus the focus was not just on what had gone wrong in her past, but also on identifying her unfulfilled longings and on providing validating understanding and affirming legitimization of her selfobject needs. Clearly, it was healing and integrating for Ellen to reveal to me the worst aspects of herself or her most secret desires and to find I was still on her side.

Ellen was interested both in using Prozac to contain her binge–purge impulses and in doing some goal setting in regard to her symptoms. I agreed to prescribe Prozac and to assist her with the goal setting. Prozac was initiated in the second week of therapy. She reported some decrease in her binge–purge impulses within 1 week. Her dosage was increased from 20 mg to 40 mg 1 month after starting the Prozac. Over the next 2 months, she experienced some days free of bingeing and purging, but for the most part her frequency was reduced from several times daily (prior to the beginning of therapy) to once daily (at this time). The symptoms were less urgent and more dystonic, and were experienced as less of an intrinsic expression of herself. When I increased the dosage of Prozac, I also helped Ellen set a goal of not bingeing or purging before 4 P.M. daily, and this intervention was fairly effective. Between 3 and 9 months of therapy, without any change in the dosage of Prozac, her binge–purge frequency was reduced to several times a week.

Since psychotherapy and psychopharmacology were done concomitantly, I cannot assert which contributed more to Ellen's improvement. My sense of it is that the Prozac provided a "jump start" in diminishing the urgency of her binge–purge impulses, but that reduction of her binge–purge episodes and her greater sense of freedom from and control over her impulses evolved gradually alongside her increasingly stronger sense of self and the experience of her self as in charge of her life.

At one point after her bingeing and purging were diminished, Ellen informed me that she also suffered from daily rumination of food (involuntary eructation). This symptom was rather remarkably controlled by the use of Propulsid (cisapride), which increases (tightens) pressure of the lower esophageal sphincter, increases lower esophageal peristalsis, and accelerates gastric emptying. Propulsid was used for 1 month. Rumination remained infrequent after this medication was discontinued.

Ellen and I developed an understanding of her central dynamics. In order to be tolerated or not abused by significant others, she (defensively) idealized them; accommodated and deferred to them; and did her best to negate, nullify, and muffle her self and her self object needs. Viewing her ordinary self as an out-of-control train, she spoke of needing to "derail herself" in order to be liked. She saw her husband as a stronger person to whom she needed to accommodate. She did her best to nullify any differences she had with him, and she dreaded his disapproval for significant aspects of herself, such as her wish to read and be less productive at times.

I interpreted her shame over her wishes to indulge herself as related to the self-negating messages and ethic in her childhood home. Her view of herself as a runaway train was interpreted as reflecting her conflict over having a vigorous presence that occupied psychological space (i.e., that was visible and had significance and impact). She struggled and moved back and forth between trying out a new more assertive and present self and retreating from this into blaming herself or feeling "diminished." She noted that she came to therapy to get rid of her symptoms, but that her new goal was to truly live her life. Her symptoms were significantly reduced, despite the only behavioral interventions' being the requirement to examine her feelings and the context prior to a binge and the one instance of goal setting.

The therapeutic process was unlabored and quiet, and without intense anger or empathic derailments that required repair. Ellen experienced our work together as helpful and facilitating. She was not overly deferential. She had no difficulty in cancelling or rescheduling sessions when she needed to. My interventions were well received. I looked forward to our sessions, as I believed she did. I saw the central transference issue as one of validation and affirmation of her having a self with presence. A dream depicted some of this. In the dream, she and a man were on horses. He was leading her toward Valley Forge. She was aware she was leaving her children behind, but she felt it was necessary and knew that what she was doing was time-limited. She realized she had a poncho on to protect her from the rain. She did not see the imagery of Valley Forge as I anticipated: as relating to hardship, a bitter winter, and starvation or deprivation. Instead, she saw the man as leading her in her struggle to fight for an important cause. Despite the presence of conflict and hardship, she felt protected and focused on achieving her goal or ideal. The cause we understood was her self—and, as I later learned, a self that was centrally committed to the pursuit of her convictions and ideals, rather than centrally committed to accommodating others.

Changes in the way Ellen experienced herself and her world were profound. Besides becoming more revealing, honest, and forthright with others, she began to experience others and especially her husband as separate human beings with their own qualities, and not just as people she needed to please. In her work, she was more engaged and listened more to her own feelings. At the cost of losing a client who had made a demand upon her, she realized that she could not agree to it and instead followed her own convictions. She experienced herself as living more in the world. She discovered that she could choose to be authentic and that the choice was hers; she experienced this as a "new way of being." She no longer dreaded making a mistake, but saw imperfections and mistakes as part of life and as opportunities to learn. She found herself enjoying her own children more, as well as other kids she taught at church. She was no longer trying to simply keep them busy to get through the Sunday school hour; rather, she was really devoted to teaching them and sharing herself with them. Instead of passively accepting an assigned room that did not facilitate the educational goal, she creatively altered the room. All of this was done with a newfound sense of pride for herself and an enthusiasm for life: "I can tell the difference. I'm living more inside of myself." She began to take classes, not just to fill the time so she wouldn't binge, but rather because the subject interested her. She devoted herself to causes that gave expression to her wish to give to others, her morality, and her compassion for the needy and the helpless.

These results were of course well beyond symptom reduction, but symptom reduction did occur. These changes reflected a central shift in the way Ellen experienced herself and her relationship to the world she now lived in. They illustrate the types of goals and changes that can occur with intensive psychotherapy.

Relapse and Termination Issues

Issues of symbiotic or selfobject bond loss, separation anxiety, and guilt over progress and the development of a vigorous self are manifested via negative therapeutic reactions. The term "negative therapeutic reaction" refers to an impasse or regression that occurs when least expected. Solid therapeutic work and insight have been achieved, and the patient has made good progress. Then, without warning, the patient acts out self-destructively, falls apart psychologically, or relinquishes hard-earned previous gains. What has happened?

Both pre-Oedipal and Oedipal determinants have been observed to be the root causes of negative therapeutic reactions. For example, doing well, growing up, and being successful may precipitate guilt because it means surpassing, replacing, or defeating the Oedipal rival. In most anorexics, however, this is not the issue. Rather, for anorexics, growing up and being successful mean giving up the symbiotic object or selfobject bond that they feel is vital for their existence, cohesion, or well-being (Goodsitt, 1969, 1977). Growing up means to the anorexic that, in a very concrete sense, she must be totally self-reliant and never depend or rely upon anyone again. It means being sentenced to a life of isolation. This is illustrated in the following case.

Ann, aged 18, was in the termination phase of a successful 10-month hospitalization. She had been hospitalized the day after her high school graduation, when she weighed 60 pounds at 5'2" tall. With five-times-weekly psychotherapy, she gained weight (to 90% of her ideal weight) and made solid psychological progress.

While on a 24-hour pass at home, Ann was able to eat meals without conscious concern for calories. Feeling proud of her accomplishment, she contemplated discharge from the hospital. That night she dreamed that her parents took in a boarder at home. She consoled herself that since she was younger than the boarder, she might still obtain some small share of parental attention. We understood several things from this dream. Her progress and her growing up in general meant loss—loss of attention and loss of attachment to the pre-Oedipal nurturer and symbiotic object. Furthermore, Ann was also the boarder. She would return home and no longer have the only role she had known—that of the dependent, symbiotic child. Progress and adulthood meant becoming an isolated boarder or stranger in her own home.

Self-guilt, described earlier, plays an important role in negative therapeutic reactions in anorexic patients. As opposed to guilt about an Oedipal victory, this guilt is more related to becoming a person, developing a selfhood, experiencing pleasure, and separating from parents.

Like Ann, Beth was in the termination phase of a successful hospitalization (in Beth's case, of 3 months' duration). She too had regained to 90% of her ideal weight, after entering the hospital very ill, extremely dehydrated, and 35% under ideal weight. She responded immediately to our taking over the management of her eating and to five-times-weekly psychotherapy. She had an intensely symbiotic relationship with her mother.

Beth was feeling both pleasure and great pride about her recent accomplishments in the hospital. She was boldly and maturely addressing the differences between herself and her mother directly with her mother. After having essentially dropped out of life and living almost totally in her room at home prior to hospitalization, she was now planning to enter college and to live away from home for the first time.

At this point, while on a group excursion from the hospital, she very obviously attempted to steal pills at a drugstore and was caught. In explaining her action to me, she stated that she had been feeling "too happy" and felt she had to "kill the happiness. It didn't feel natural or right. I shouldn't be happy." Beth felt guilty for her happiness while she was planning to establish a life of her own apart from her mother. Enjoying life apart from her mother was an act of disloyalty and betrayal. Beth stated that she had been the center of her mother's life and that her mother could never be happy without her.

The issues of symbiotic and selfobject loss, separation anxiety, and self-guilt occur throughout the therapy. Each new incident allows the patient and the therapist to view the issue from a slightly different perspective. It is then observed and analyzed in all its ramifications. For the patient to complete the therapy successfully, these issues, often intensified during the termination phase, must be modified or resolved.

The Role of the Therapist

The therapist responds in many ways and is many things: a parent, teacher, guide, and coach (Levenkron, 1983). The therapist is available as a committed, caring professional and is actively involved; he or she relates, encourages, cajoles, and exhorts. The therapist also provides expert knowledge and experience. He or she empathically anticipates and cares about the patient's subjective experience, welfare, and well-being. He or she patiently explains and clarifies the patient's cognitions and significant issues. Most important, the therapist is often the carrier of hope for a future for the patient, while at the same time truthfully acknowledging her present shortcomings. Instead of criticizing her defensive adaptations, the therapist conveys that there are good reasons for all her behavior, incapacities, and feelings. By doing all this and more, the therapist lends the patient his or her self-organization—his or her capacity to anticipate; delay gratification; use sound judgment; relate to another person; care for and forgive oneself; regulate tension and moods; and integrate affect, cognitions, and behavior.

The therapist creates a therapeutic space in which the patient is encouraged to take risks. These patients are patients because they have suffered disappointments and psychic injuries; as a consequence, they have developed defenses against reinjury. It is the therapist's role to understand this and to establish a helpful, respectful, reliable, and safe therapeutic space

where a patient feels helped, accepted, understood, responded to, and encouraged to be.

If the patient suffers incapacities to regulate tensions (Swift & Letven, 1984), affects, and basic physiology (the latter being secondary to disrupted and chaotic eating or purging), then some form of external provision is often indicated (see note 5). Provision or "filling the deficit" (Goodsitt, 1983, 1985), or "managing the transference" (Goodsitt, 1985) in contrast to interpreting the transference, are all types of intervention that acknowledge some degree of deficit or incapacity in the patient. The following discussion illustrates these concepts.

Bulimic patients may require behavioral management of their disordered, chaotic eating patterns as well as their bingeing and purging. Eating-disordered patients in general may require the therapist to function as a tension or affect regulator. This may take the form of anything from a psychopharmacological intervention to educating the patient on the management of tensions and affects (Gehrie, 1990) or affirming the patient's nascent efforts at self-management (Swift & Letven, 1984).

The therapist may actively reassure or calm the patient. If the anorexic patient is panicked that her stomach will balloon up when she eats or drinks, the therapist provides reassuring knowledge about the digestive process (Levenkron, 1983). Moreover, the therapist should not wait until the patient is actively panicking; the therapist should empathically anticipate the panic and dose out the preventive medicine of reassuring information.

As a tension regulator, the therapist not only soothes the patient, but anticipates her distress and teaches her how to manage it herself. When asking a patient to eat more, the therapist explains that he or she knows that this is most difficult. The therapist explains that he or she is asking her to give up a major adaptive defense that has served important protective functions for her. The therapist expects her to feel anxious. The therapist asks her to sit with her anxiety while the therapist sits with her. The therapist explains that asking her to give up an adaptive defense (anorexia or bulimia) is like asking a person who cannot swim to let go of the life preserver and try swimming. The person's fear is that she will drown, but she will not be left alone to sink or swim. The therapist may point out that it is really a choice she must make. She may continue to desperately hold on to what seems like a life preserver (i.e., her illness) and continue to feel some temporary relief in not eating. She can also expect to continue her lonely, miserable, suffering life unchanged. On the other hand, the therapist continues, she can choose to let go and take a chance on eating—and life. Clearly, by doing so, she is entering a forbidding unknown. The therapist knows that the patient has little faith in her capacity to relate to others or to live an enjoyable or satisfying life of her own. She may indeed have good reason, based on past experience, not to be optimistic about her future. If this is the case, the therapist should acknowledge that. But the therapist tells the patient that he or she is committed to helping the patient learn the skills (the functions of ego and self) she needs to make her life better. Until now, she has been trying to learn to swim with one hand tied behind her back. No wonder it is difficult!

This approach is quite different from simply analyzing the unconscious symbolic meanings of eating and gaining weight. The therapist is providing physiological and reassuring tension regulation, while implicitly conveying an understanding of these selfobject needs and limitations in a nonjudgmental manner.

Growth of the self and enhancement of the self-organization are facilitated by knowing oneself. It is the therapist's job to help the patient to direct her attention to inner experience. The therapist values her feelings and takes them seriously. When the patient denies that anything is wrong, the therapist asks her to look inward to find out what she is feeling. When she explains her bingeing or vomiting as simply habit, the therapist asks her to examine carefully what was occurring and how she was feeling immediately prior to the binge–purge episode.

The therapist's role is to build up and enhance the patient's sense of self. The therapist does this by truly listening to and taking seriously her feelings and thoughts. The therapist must also be prepared to actively help the patient find her own feelings and to elicit the expression of them. By helping the patient to get in touch with her inner experience, the therapist is helping her to ground or center herself, and to integrate her external behavior with her inner feelings and beliefs. This enriches the personality and solidifies the self-organization. When this is accomplished, the patient will no longer experience herself as empty, bored, passive, dead, indecisive, and aimless. When this is not accomplished, behaviors are often reactions to the inner dysphoric states of a disrupted self, and not active expressions of initiative from the depth of the self—its values and goals. If the patient is constantly trying to extinguish internal emotional fires, she is in no condition to change, learn, or develop. It is the therapist's job to help the patient find her true self, her values and goals, for only then is fulfillment possible.

The Role of Transference

For many patients, the establishment of a selfobject transference results in symptom relief (Gehrie, 1990). The selfobject transference not only provides background support that buttresses the psychotherapeutic work, but may also provide the central elements of change and healing. Some self psychologists (see M. Tolpin, 1994) have elaborated on the therapeutic endeavor as addressing, strengthening, and responding to previously unmet selfobject needs or undeveloped sectors of the psyche, with the aim of mobilizing a derailed self-structure or developing new self-structures and capacities. This is in contrast to previous notions of psychoanalytic cure, which focused on a remobilization or a reworking in the transference of past traumatic experiences and the resultant pathological psychic structures. Healing is accounted for and comes less from an analysis of what went wrong than from having a new experience with another person, within which selfobject needs are mobilized, understood, and/or responded to.

As noted by many clinicians who work with eating-disordered patients, the patients often seem to experience the empathic connection of therapy as a first-time phenomenon (Barth, 1988; Rizzuto et al., 1981). These patients complain that no one has ever really taken them seriously and that no one has ever listened to them before. The provision of selfobject needs and relationship that is part and parcel of a psychotherapeutic engagement allows such a patient to feel that she counts, and that her experience and her feelings matter to and even have impact upon another person. Unmet selfobject needs for validation, mirroring, idealizing, twinship, self-delineation (Stolorow, Atwood, & Brandchaft, 1992), affect attunement (Bacal, 1985; Lichtenberg et al., 1992; Stolorow et al., 1992), self-esteem regulation, mood and tension regulation, soothing, and vitalization are brought into the therapeutic setting for response and/or interpretation. When appropriate responsiveness occurs and a selfobject transference is engaged, the patient's self-organization is enhanced or strengthened and is experienced as whole and vitalized, resilient and directed. Symptomatic improvement will occur through this healing of the self.

Symptom Management

Although transference has a powerful impact in relieving symptoms, I do not ignore directly addressing the symptoms. Viewing the obsessive preoccupation with an imperfect body as the concrete bodily expression of a damaged self, I translate these expressions into understandable feelings and cognitions.

Eating-disordered patients frequently focus insightfully on their psychology to the exclusion of their symptomatic behaviors, or on their symptoms to the exclusion of their psychodynamics. For psychologically minded patients, the place and function of the symptoms in the patients' lives may never be examined. These patients need direction to discuss these activities.

On the other hand, certain patients will isolate the symptoms from the context of their lives by discussing only their weight, body, and food preoccupations. These patients need encouragement to look at the context of the symptoms in their lives. How a therapist does this is crucial. The therapist must respect the importance of the symptoms for each patient. The patient's present (albeit misguided) mode of feeling in control, effective, and powerful is tied up in the symptoms. It is useful for the therapist to acknowledge from the start that the symptoms serve an important function and may be the best current solution to the patient's dilemma.

The therapeutic work with Carol illustrates these concepts. Carol was an 18-year-old woman who was hospitalized when she was 30% under ideal weight. Her parents were divorced. Her home environment was chaotic and destructive. She had nothing in her life to point to with pride, and truly nothing to look forward to. She felt weak, ineffective, incapable, unlikable, and defeated. Her bodily obsessions and compulsions made her feel strange and freakish. Unlike other anorexics, who attempt to burn off calories with exercise, she would rather sit in one place and hold or press her stomach in. She could not tolerate any expansion of her abdomen. She sat because she felt that if she stood up, she would more or less "hang out." Any attempt to use reality testing by pointing out her thinness or the flatness of her abdomen resulted in her feeling crushed. Reality testing meant that people were telling her she was crazy, and she would then hold on to her stomach even more intensely.

Her therapist reassured Carol that her symptoms were meaningful. Carol eventually was able to say that if she did not continue to hold her stomach in, she would be overwhelmed by intense despair and depression. She would feel empty and would have to face the "nothingness" inside. The therapist acknowledged that to remove the symptoms meant, to Carol, taking away her life preserver and allowing her to drown in her depression. She needed to feel that she had something else to hold on to, and she needed to learn how to swim. The therapist would let her hold on to him until he could teach her to swim, but she would have to take the risk of letting go of her current life preserver.

A therapist may approach a body image distortion, such as Carol's by acknowledging that food and water do in fact expand the abdomen; this is especially noticeable to the patient, since her abdominal muscles are atrophied and she has no abdominal fat. However, rather than arguing with Carol that her stomach was not fat, her therapist explored why she could not tolerate any bodily or other imperfection. Furthermore, the therapist acknowledged her concern and listened for the underlying significance of her obsession.

Carol berated herself because all she talked about were food and her body. The therapist told her that when one has a toothache, all one can think about is the ache; the mind addresses itself to problems that demand attention. Together, the therapist and Carol had to find the good reason why carol was so preoccupied. Carol continued to belabor the point that she was fat, her eating was uncontrollable, her body was distorted, and she could not do anything about it. The therapist acknowledged her concerns and said, "I hear you are not in charge, unable to regulate, feel good, or like yourself. You feel weak, ineffective, and helpless." Here the therapist took what the patient tendered—the concrete bodily expressions of a damaged self—and translated these into understandable feelings and cognitions.

Hospitalization and Symptom Management

In this subsection, I address the problems I have found with shortened inpatient care and with inpatient care that is not individualized. Either of these problems leads to not engaging the patient on her own terms, and thus repeats an earlier psychic injury.

Hospitalization was often an efficacious, irreplaceable, and invaluable therapeutic intervention. In the 1990s, however, the full utilization of this intervention has been limited by the restrictions imposed in particular by managed care, and in general by a lack of commitment in U.S. culture to the health of its people, as evidenced by diminished funding and stringent insurance limitations.

Today, hospitals can be used to reverse dangerously abnormal nutritional, biochemical, and physiological abnormalities, but not to establish a relationship with a patient that is aimed at correcting the equally dangerous pathological self-states. These self-states include not only severely impaired capacities for self-regulation and self-care (see Khantzian, 1978, and Krystal, 1978, for discussions of the capacity for self-care), but also severely impaired capacities to participate truly and fully in a treatment process. Some of these patients will comply, or "eat their way out of the hospital," but they have not engaged the treatment process in any real fashion. Patients with disturbances severe enough to require hospitalization have usually experienced traumatic selfobject injuries and have adopted defenses that protect themselves from human engagement. They instead turn to bodily manipulation for some momentary sense of vitalization or effectiveness. They have given up on obtaining satisfaction in human relationships via an engagement of their true or real selfobject needs. They have traded competence in relationships for the illusion of effectiveness, control, mastery, and competence that comes with self-starvation or with purging to be thin. Yet they are not capable of healthily managing their own needs. They are prone to "fake it" in treatment, and the therapist is prone to settling for the illusion of a successful treatment, as measured by laboratory data improved, weight restored, or bingeing and purging lessened. Hospitalization begs the crucial question of

how to provide external management without thereby creating a passive, accommodating patient who is not truly participating or engaged in her own treatment. In other words, the more one does for and to the patient, the less one is asking the patient to accept responsibility for her own care and for what happens to her and her body. Is the message to the patient "No, you are not allowed to have a self"? Many of these patients are quite capable of surrendering an aspect of themselves, their bodies, to the therapist. The result then is a "person who suffers as before, but looks normal—an anorectic [sic] clothed in weight" (Goodsitt, 1977, p. 311).

These questions first occurred to me with some poignancy in the 1980s, when I had what initially appeared to be quite remarkable success with hospitalized eating-disordered patients. Anorexics gained weight and bulimics stopped having binge–purge episodes, and the patients were discharged. The problem was that these apparent successes were not sustained once the patients were out of the hospital. Despite good psychotherapeutic follow-up, significant relapses were the rule, not the exception. One needs to understand the treatment milieu and philosophy I worked in to comprehend why this occurred.

The milieu was established with the notion that these patients could not self-regulate well and needed a controlled environment that would assume much of the responsibility for their welfare or health. Thus the management of the health of the patients' bodies was the responsibility of the treatment team. Simultaneously, a strong milieu and group therapy program, coupled with individual psychotherapy four to five times weekly, attended to the psychological health of these patients. A level system was established, with varying degrees of responsibility given to a patient as she showed herself capable. Each patient and her peers participated in the decision-making process by providing input. All patients entered the program at Level I and worked toward higher levels of self-responsibility. Patients in Level I were rather completely managed as to what, where, how, and when they ate, as well as when they used the bathroom, sat in the day room, took walks, and so on. In this system, most patients did remarkably well; as stated earlier, however, their gains were not well maintained upon discharge from this environment.

When my colleagues and I explored what was going wrong, we realized that the patients experienced the program, despite its emphasis on individual and group therapy, as a strong, authoritarian one that did not truly engage their individuality. The fact that patients were met at the door with a well-established or preformed program applied uniformly to all new patients meant to them that the importance of them as unique individuals with unique needs was given only lip service. They could easily plug themselves into the program, and could just as easily unplug themselves at the time of their release from the hospital. What was missing was a true engagement of their selves in the treatment process.

The question remained as to how to do this while simultaneously not letting a patient psychologically drown in her symptoms. The therapeutic stance should be one that respects the vital importance of the symptom for the patient and yet does not abandon the patient to struggle unassisted with an illness that controls her. To my mind, it is crucial to work collaboratively with the patient on establishing treatment goals and a treatment plan, rather than simply prescribing the goals and plan. If the patient is not truly "on board" and is just "going along for the ride," treatment will fail. The treatment plan is the product of a real engagement with the patient that bears her stamp. As such, it is not a formula applied equally to all patients, but is custom-tailored to suit this particular person who has an eating disorder. Individualized treatment plans are the hallmark of high-quality treatment programs even in this era of restricted care.

This stance does not mean that life-saving measures such as tube feeding will not be considered or utilized. A decision to institute tube feeding is not necessarily incompatible with the principle that treatment does not exist without the patient's meaningful involvement in the process. This involvement may be as limited as the patient's giving permission to the therapist for tube feeding. This permission must be given as a result of a process between the patient and the therapist. The therapist may forgo his or her goals and therapeutic ambition, and instead negotiate a goal the patient can agree to. Furthermore, the therapist may need to inform the patient of his or her impotence to help the patient without her participation in the process. Responsibility for the treatment outcome is shared by the patient and the therapist. The therapist cannot do it by himself or herself. This philosophical approach means that treatment gains are less dramatic, more hard-earned, and slower to come, but are also more real. The gains are integrated ones, rather than "grafts" to be sloughed off when the patient leaves the hospital.

Family Involvement

Self psychology illuminates two important issues that must be addressed for treatment to go forward. The first is the patient's selfobject neediness, which can be experienced by family members as the patient's provocative, tyrannical control of them. The second is the family's use of the patient as a needed selfobject, which interferes with the patient's having a life of her own.

When individuals have an impaired capacity to provide their own selfobject functions and experiences, they either utilize others or resort to pathological means to experience vitalization or achieve soothing, self-esteem, and cohesion. The utilization of others to provide vital selfobject functions can be and often is experienced by family members as a form of tyrannical control (Goodsitt, 1977). When one person utilizes and depends upon another in place of one's own selfobject capacities, one relates to the other as a repository of required functions, and not as a separate person with his or her own initiatives, interests, and goals. The other person may feel used, disregarded, controlled, exploited, and abused.

Similarly, when developing children are relied upon by parents for the parents' own mirroring and other selfobject needs, the children are likely to experience themselves as not having a right to live their own lives. Such children, who devote themselves to the well-being of others while neglecting and negating their own inner needs, are prone to develop an eating disorder.

Both an eating-disordered patient and her family need to work on these issues of use of the other, to lay the groundwork for healthy psychological individuation and separation. Family therapy,[6] especially with the younger patient who continues to reside in the parental home, is a good vehicle for this. Individual psychotherapy may occur concurrently.

As I have noted throughout this chapter, it is my premise in working with eating-disordered patients that it is their birthright to have lives of their own. Work either within the family or individually is aimed at achieving this goal. When a parent needs a developing child as an extension of himself or herself, this parent may need considerable support and/or psychotherapy to let this happen. It is not unknown for a "symbiotic parent" to develop a psychosis as a child achieves healthy individuation. When the eating-disordered patient is in individual psychotherapy as an outpatient or inpatient, the family members should not be ignored or excluded. Their guilt, shame, anger, and need for support and guidance must be attended to, or the treatment may be undermined.

Transference and Countertransference

Eating-disordered patients present with typical psychological configurations that challenge a therapist's equanimity and are likely to produce responses of overmanagement or undermanagement. These are as follows: (1) A patient exercises tyrannical control over her world, including the therapist; (2) a patient is committed to defeating hope and the therapy; (3) a patient does not relate to others, including the therapist, as separate human beings; (4) a patient adopts the psychological position of selflessness and engages in a "selfless transference" (this pattern is typical of anorexics); and (5) a patient engages the therapist as a withholding, omnipotent other (this pattern is more typical of bulimics).

Within the context of these typical transference configurations, I have found that the more life-threatening and maladaptively out-of-control a patient's disorder is, the more likely it is that countertransference responses to the patient, in the form of over- or undermanagement of her symptoms, will be present. For the therapist who relies upon empathy and introspection, or who adopts a position that the patient's (and his or her own) subjectivity is the only relevant data, the risk of undermanaging is present. Overmanagement is the risk for the therapist who relies upon extrospection (i.e., observable data and "reality") as a means of relating to the patient.

To elucidate, I use the example of an anorexic patient who presents with a typical transference configuration of selflessness. This patient acts as if she is without selfobject need and asks little of others. She is consumed with fears of growing up and having a (vigorous) presence, and she experiences guilt for having a self. This patient buries her needs and devotes herself to being a caregiver to others. For a variety of reasons, she will not address her feelings, problems, or symptoms with the therapist. Besides not having access to her inner life, this patient utilizes therapy poorly because she feels guilty about the attention given to her as part of therapy, and because she doesn't want to burden the therapist with her suffering. In therapy, she is not fulfilling her obligation to be a selfless selfobject.

What problems may the "empathic" therapist have with the selfless transference? This therapist, not wanting the patient to feel badly about herself and wanting to support the patient's fragile self-regard, may then collude in the avoidance of addressing the symptoms. This becomes more problematic when the symptom (starvation) is out of control and requires active management. Another reason why this therapist may avoid addressing the symptom and managing it is his or her own grandiosity. This may take the form of unconsciously believing that his or her love, caring, and empathy should be curative by itself. This unconscious dynamic may be buttressed by self-psychological theory, which emphasizes the importance of empathic attunement; however, empathic attunement does not provide the data (i.e., the patient is starving) that mandates external management. A third reason for undermanaging by the therapist has to do with his or her aversion to the kind of aggression and intrusiveness required to take this type of action. The fourth reason relates to this therapist's capacity to be empathic. He or she is then vulnerable to becoming "infected" with the patient's helplessness and impotence via projective identification. The therapist does not take appropriate action because he or she feels helpless.

In contrast, the therapist who relies more on extrospection is more likely to overmanage. This therapist tends to emphasize his or her knowledge of external "reality" and to make judgments about whether the patient's behavior is in accord with this reality. In confronting the alexithymia of the selfless anorexic patient, this therapist is likely to tell the patient how she is supposed to feel, instead of helping her find and identify her own feelings. This may derive from this therapist's grandiosity in believing that his or her reality is the more relevant one. An authoritative posture may also derive from the therapist's narcissistic need to hear his or her own voice. The therapist's own selfobject needs for mirroring or validating may be intensified when the patient negates her need of him or her, and/or when the patient uses the therapist as a function or a selfobject while neglecting the therapist's own individuality. Furthermore, the patient's need for tyrannical control over herself and her environment may threaten the therapist's own grandiose need to be in control. This therapist may then meet control with a sadistic countercontrol. Treatment is prescribed, and the already voiceless patient is given the message that her participation (and voice) in the treatment process is not wanted. Treatment programs with a rather totalitarian bent are established not to be controlled by patients, who feel desperately out of control themselves and then attempt to control their environment.

When a therapist examines the manner in which he or she responds to a patient's out-of-control or maladaptive behaviors, countertransference experiences can be identified and themselves managed therapeutically.

CONCLUSION

In 1966, I undertook the intensive treatment of Mary, the 13-year-old anorexic girl described early in this chapter. I was told that Mary's condition, anorexia nervosa, was quite a rare illness. I was intrigued and challenged to make sense of this baffling phenomenon in which an occasional young girl would voluntarily starve herself. Five days a week over the next year, I sat and tried my best to listen carefully and thoughtfully to Mary, her experience, her inner life, while at the same time trying to be helpful to her. I also reviewed the literature. The psychoanalytic formulations of conflict over oral sexual and aggressive fantasies did not match my understanding of what Mary was describing to me about her inner life. Nor did it explain the peculiar manner in which she related to me and how I experienced her use of me. Hilde Bruch's down-to-earth descriptions of anorexics did match my experience of Mary, but Bruch's work was essentially atheoretical. I hungered for a theory that would attempt to explain this condition in some sensible and comprehensible fashion.

Margaret Mahler's (1968) exposition on symbiosis and separation–individuation, a theory developed in her work with psychotic children, was helpful. This work spoke to an understanding of the symbiotic quality of Mary's attachment to me. I was not a target of Mary's sexual or aggressive fantasies. I was experienced as a vital, not separate, stabilizing aspect of her self. When separated from me, she experienced psychotic fragmentation. I utilized Mahler's concepts to explain anorexia nervosa as reflecting arrested development at symbiotic or separation–individuation levels (Goodsitt, 1969). Since then, object relations theorists have elaborated on these formulations. Many of the object relations theorists have maintained that conflict over sexual and aggressive aims is central to the development of an eating disorder. This was not my finding. Instead of guilt over drive impulses, I saw what appeared to be central experiences of annihilation anxiety, fragmentation, emptiness, depletion, and devitalization. Furthermore, object relations theories do not, in my opinion, adequately address the sense of incomplete psychic structure and functioning of these patients.

In this chapter, I have attempted to clarify what a self-psychological perspective offers toward the understanding and treatment of an eating disorder. My self-psychological orientation includes the idea that some eating disorder pathology may represent, in any particular patient, a symbolic expression of a compromise between a drive aim and defenses. Nevertheless, much of the pathology I have seen is better understood as related to patients' insufficiently developed capacities to provide their own vitalization, validation, cohesion, and self-regard, as well as regulation of self-esteem, mood, and tension. Given these incapacities, symptoms reflect nonsymbolic emergency measures aimed at stemming the rising tide of anxiety that accompanies a disrupted self, or they are restitutional measures aimed at vitalizing an empty, depleted self. Compounding the woes that are by-products of these incapacities is the patients' belief that they do not have a right to have a self that vigorously occupies physical and psychological space.

Given the incompleteness of the psychic structure, these patients face the choice of (1) continuing to look toward others for maintenance and regulation of their self-esteem, moods, and tensions, and for the vitalization and stabilization of their self-organization, despite past traumatic disappointments in human relationships; or (2) turning toward these emergency symptomatic attempts at restitution. The problem with the latter is that these measures provide only temporary surcease from these painful self-states.

Therapy is an endeavor that offers a patient a new opportunity to invest in herself and another person, with the aim of developing a more effective and vitalized self—a self that enthusiastically occupies psychological space. This healthy result occurs when the therapist adopts a certain view of his or her role. Symptoms are seen less as hostile and adversarial attempts to control him or her than as desperate attempts at self-restitution. Given the patient's incapacities, the therapist thinks more in terms of psychological holding and provision of unmet need than simply in terms of insight (which itself can provide needed validation). Therapy may be the patient's first experience of an empathic relationship focused on self-enhancement rather than analysis. The therapist takes the position that it is the patient's birthright to have a self. In therapy, responsiveness to the mobilization of unmet selfobject needs may prove more beneficial than the remobilization and analysis of past traumatic relationships. If all of this goes well, the therapist will see the patient develop a vigorous presence and a life authentically and truly lived. Then the therapist will have the distinct pleasure of having participated in the psychological birth of his or her patient.

NOTES

1. For the full case report, see Goodsitt (1969).
2. For more recent versions of the utilization of this model and the object relations model for the treatment of eating disorders, see Wilson, Hogan, and Mintz (1983) and Schwartz (1988). For a more eclectic psychodynamic perspective, see Johnson (1991).
3. Since most eating-disordered patients are female, I utilize feminine nouns and pronouns in reference to them.
4. For previous and more elaborate discussions of the relationship between the body and the self-organization, see Goodsitt (1977, 1983, 1985). For a very similar and quite comprehensive and sophisticated discussion, see Krueger (1988, 1989).
5. See Bacal (1985), Bacal and Newman (1990), Shane and Shane (1994), Terman (1988), M. Tolpin (1983, 1994), and P. Tolpin (1988) for discussions of optimal responsiveness and optimal provision.
6. See Humphrey (1991) for a discussion of family psychodynamics and therapy.

REFERENCES

Bacal, H. A. (1985). Optimal responsiveness and the therapeutic process. In A. I. Goldberg (Ed.), *Progress in self psychology* (Vol. 1, pp. 202–226). New York: Guilford Press.

Bacal, H. A., & Newman, K. M. (1990). *Theories of object relations: Bridges to self psychology.* New York: Columbia University Press.

Barth, F. D. (1988). The treatment of bulimia from a self psychological perspective. *Clinical Social Work Journal, 16,* 270–281.

Berlin, I. N., Boatman, M. J., Scheimo, S. L., & Szurek, S. A. (1951). Adolescent alternation of anorexia and obesity. *American Journal of Orthopsychiatry, 21,* 387–419.

Blitzer, J. R., Rollins, N., & Blackwell, A. (1961). Children who starve themselves: Anorexia nervosa. *Psychosomatic Medicine, 23,* 369–383.

Bruch, H. (1962). Perceptual and conceptual disturbances in anorexia nervosa. *Psychosomatic Medicine, 24,* 187–194.

Dellaverson, V. (1994). *The desomatizing selfobject transference from body self to psychological self: Analysis of an eating disorder.* Paper presented at the 17th Annual Conference of the Self, Chicago. (This paper is available on audiotape from Audio Archives International, Inc., 3043 Foothill Boulevard, Suite 2, LaCrescenta, CA 91214.)

Eissler, K. R. (1943). Some psychiatric aspects of anorexia nervosa, demonstrated by a case report. *Psychoanalytic Review, 30,* 121–145.

Falstein, E. I., Feinstein, S. C., & Judas, I. (1956). Anorexia nervosa in the male child. *American Journal of Orthopsychiatry, 26,* 751–772.

Friedman, M. (1985). Survivor guilt in the pathogenesis of anorexia nervosa. *Psychiatry, 48,* 25–39.

Freud, S. (1961). The ego and the id. In J. Strachey (Ed. and Trans.), *The standard edition of the complete psychological works of Sigmund Freud* (Vol. 19, pp. 3–66). London: Hogarth Press. (Original work published 1923)

Garfinkel, P. E., & Garner, D. M. (1982). *Anorexia nervosa: A multidimensional perspective.* New York: Brunner/Mazel.

Garner, D. M., & Bemis, K. J. (1982). A cognitive-behavioral approach to anorexia nervosa. *Cognitive Therapy and Research, 6,* 123–150.

Garner, D. M., Garfinkel, P. E., & Bemis, K. M. (1982). A multidimensional psychotherapy for anorexia nervosa. *International Journal of Eating Disorders, 1,* 3–46.

Gehrie, M. J. (1990). Eating disorders and adaptation in crisis: A hypothesis. In A. Tasman, S. M. Goldfinger, & C. A. Kaufman (Eds.), *Review of psychiatry* (Vol. 9, pp. 369–383). Washington, DC: American Psychiatric Press.

Geist, R. A. (1985). Therapeutic dilemmas in the treatment of anorexia nervosa: A self psychological perspective. In S. W. Emmett (Ed.), *Theory and treatment of anorexia nervosa and bulimia* (pp. 268–288). New York: Brunner/Mazel.

Geist, R. A. (1989). Self psychological reflections on the origins of eating disorders. *Journal of the American Academy of Psychoanalysis, 17,* 5–27.

Goodsitt, A. (1969). Anorexia nervosa. *British Journal of Medical Psychology, 42,* 109–118.

Goodsitt, A. (1977). Narcissistic disturbances in anorexia nervosa. In S. C. Feinstein & P. Giovacchini (Eds.), *Adolescent psychiatry* (Vol. 5, pp. 304–312). New York: Jason Aronson.

Goodsitt, A. (1982). [Review of *Starving to death in a sea of objects* by J. A. Sours]. *International Journal of Eating Disorders, 1,* 70–76.

Goodsitt, A. (1983). Self-regulatory disturbances in eating

disorders. *International Journal of Eating Disorders, 2,* 51–60.

Goodsitt, A. (1985). Self psychology and the treatment of anorexia nervosa. In D. M. Garner & P. E. Garfinkel (Eds.), *Handbook of psychotherapy for anorexia nervosa and bulimia* (pp. 55–82). New York: Guilford Press.

Grimshaw, L. (1959). Anorexia nervosa: A contribution to its psychogenesis. *British Journal of Medical Psychology, 32,* 44–49.

Humphrey, L. L. (1991). Object relations and the family system: An integrative approach to understanding and treating eating disorders. In C. L. Johnson (Ed.), *Psychodynamic treatment of anorexia nervosa and bulimia* (pp. 321–353). New York: Guilford Press.

Jessner, L., & Abse, D. W. (1960). Regressive forces in anorexia nervosa. *British Journal of Medical Psychology, 33,* 301–312.

Johnson, C. L. (Ed.). (1991). *Psychodynamic treatment of anorexia nervosa and bulimia.* New York: Guilford Press.

Kernberg, O. F. (1994). *Technical approach to eating disorders in patients with borderline personality disorder.* Paper presented at the 14th Regional Conference of the Chicago Psychoanalytic Society, Chicago.

Khantzian, E. (1978). The ego, the self, and opiate addiction. *International Review of Psychoanalysis, 5,* 189–198.

Kohut, H. (1971). *The analysis of the self.* New York: International Universities Press.

Kreuger, D. W. (1988). Body self, psychological self, and bulimia: Developmental and clinical considerations in bulimia. In H. J. Schwartz (Ed.), *Bulimia: Psychoanalytic treatment and theory* (pp. 55–72). Madison, CT: International Universities Press.

Krueger, D. W. (1989). *Body self and psychological self: A developmental and clinical integration of disorders of the self.* New York: Brunner/Mazel.

Krystal, H. (1978). Self representation and the capacity for self care. *Annual Review of Psychoanalysis, 6,* 209–246.

Levenkron, S. (1983). *Treating and overcoming anorexia nervosa.* New York: Warner Books.

Lichtenberg, J. D., Lachmann, F. M., & Fosshage, J. L. (1992). *Self and motivational systems: Toward a theory of psychoanalytic technique.* Hillsdale, NJ: Analytic Press.

Mahler, M. (1968). *On human symbiosis and the vicissitudes of individuation.* New York: International Universities Press.

Margolis, P. M., & Jernberg, A. (1960). Anaclitic therapy in a case of extreme anorexia. *British Journal of Medical Psychology, 33,* 291–300.

Masserman, J. H. (1941). Psychodynamics in anorexia nervosa and neurotic vomiting. *Psychoanalytic Quarterly, 10,* 211–242.

Masterson, J. F. (1978). The borderline adolescent: An object relations view. In S. C. Feinstein & P. L. Giovacchini (Eds.), *Adolescent psychiatry* (Vol. 6, pp. 344–359). Chicago: University of Chicago Press.

Masterson, J. F. (1995). Paradise lost—bulimia, a closet narcissistic personality disorder: A developmental, self, and object relations approach. In R. C. Marohn & S. C. Feinstein (Eds.), *Adolescent psychiatry* (Vol. 20, pp. 253–266). Hillsdale, NJ: Analytic Press.

Modell, A. H. (1965). On having the right to a life: An aspect of the superego's development. *International Journal of Psycho-Analysis, 46,* 323–331.

Modell, A. H. (1975). A narcissistic defense against affects

and the illusion of self-sufficiency. *International Journal of Psycho-Analysis, 56,* 275–282.

Mogul, S. L. (1980). Asceticism in adolescence and anorexia nervosa. *Psychoanalytic Study of the Child, 35,* 155–175.

Moulton, R. (1942). A psychosomatic study of anorexia nervosa including the use of vaginal smears. *Psychosomatic Medicine, 4,* 62–74.

Rizzuto, A.-M., Peterson, R. K., & Reed, M. (1981). The pathological sense of self in anorexia nervosa. *Psychiatric Clinics of North America, 4,* 471–487.

Rowland, C. V., Jr. (1970). Anorexia nervosa: A survey of the literature and review of 30 cases. *International Psychiatric Clinics, 7,* 37–137.

Sands, S. H. (1989). Eating disorders and female development: A self-psychological perspective. In A. I. Goldberg (Ed.), *Progress in self psychology* (Vol. 5, pp. 75–103). Hillsdale, NJ: Analytic Press.

Sands, S. H. (1991). Bulimia, dissociation, and empathy: A self-psychological view. In C. L. Johnson (Ed.), *Psychodynamic treatment of anorexia nervosa and bulimia* (pp. 34–50). New York: Guilford Press.

Schwartz, H. J. (1988). *Bulimia: Psychoanalytic treatment and theory.* Madison, CT: International Universities Press.

Scott, W. (1948). Notes on the psychopathology of anorexia nervosa. *British Journal of Medical Psychology, 21,* 241–247.

Selvini Palazzoli, M. (1978). *Self-starvation.* New York: Jason Aronson.

Shane, E., & Shane, M. (1994). *In pursuit of optimal frustration, optimal responsiveness and optimal provision.* Paper presented at the 17th Annual Conference on the Psychology of the Self, Chicago. (This paper is available on audiotape from Audio Archives International, Inc., 3043 Foothill Boulevard, Suite 2, LaCrescenta, CA 91214.)

Sours, J. A. (1980). *Starving to death in a sea of objects.* New York: Jason Aronson.

Stolorow, R. D., & Atwood, G. E. (1992). *Contexts of being: The intersubjective foundations of psychological life.* Hillsdale, NJ: Analytic Press.

Stolorow, R. D., Atwood, G. E., & Brandchaft, B. (1992). Three realms of the unconscious and their therapeutic transformation. *Psychoanalytic Review, 79,* 25–30.

Sugarman, A. (1991). Bulimia: A displacement from psychological self to body self. In C. L. Johnson (Ed.), *Psychodynamic treatment of anorexia nervosa and bulimia* (pp. 3–33). New York: Guilford Press.

Sugarman, A., & Kurash, C. (1982). The body as a transitional object in bulimia. *International Journal of Eating Disorders, 1,* 57–67.

Swift, W. J., & Letven, R. (1984). Bulimia and the basic fault: A psychoanalytic interpretation of the bingeing–vomiting syndrome. *Journal of the American Academy of Child Psychiatry, 23,* 489–497.

Terman, D. (1988). Optimal frustration: Structuralization and the therapeutic process. In A. I. Goldberg (Ed.), *Progress in self psychology* (Vol. 4, pp. 113–125). Hillsdale, NJ: Analytic Press.

Tolpin, M. (1971). On the beginnings of a cohesive self. *Psychoanalytic Study of the Child, 26,* 316–352.

Tolpin, M. (1983). Corrective emotional experience: A self psychological reevaluation. In A. I. Goldberg (Ed.), *The future of psychoanalysis* (pp. 363–379). New York: International Universities Press.

Tolpin, M. (1994). *Compensatory structures: Paths to the restoration of the self.* Paper presented at the 17th Annual Conference of the Self, Chicago. (See, in particular, the discussions to this paper by J. L. Fosshage, F. M. Lachmann, M. Tolpin, and E. Wolf. This paper is available on audiotape from Audio Archives International, Inc., 3043 Foothill Boulevard, Suite 2, LaCrescenta, CA 91214.)

Tolpin, P. (1988). Optimal affective engagement: The analyst's role in therapy. In A. I. Goldberg (Ed.), *Progress in self psychology* (Vol. 4, pp. 160–168). Hillsdale, NJ: Analytic Press.

Tustin, F. (1958). Anorexia nervosa in an adolescent girl. *British Journal of Medical Psychology, 31,* 184–200.

Wall, J. H. (1959). Diagnosis, treatment and results in anorexia nervosa. *American Journal of Psychiatry, 115,* 997–1001.

Waller, J. V., Kaufman, M. R., & Deutsch, F. (1940). Anorexia nervosa: Psychosomatic entity. *Psychosomatic Medicine, 2,* 3–16.

Weiss, J., Sampson, H., & Modell, A. (1983). *Narcissism, masochism and the sense of guilt in relation to the therapeutic process* (Bulletin No. 6, Psychotherapy Research Group). San Francisco: Department of Psychiatry, Mount Zion Hospital and Medical Center.

Wilson, C. P., Hogan, C. C., & Mintz, I. L. (1983). *Fear of being fat: The treatment of anorexia nervosa and bulimia.* New York: Jason Aronson.

Winnicott, D. W. (1965). *The maturational processes and the facilitating environment.* New York: International Universities Press.

CHAPTER 12

Consultation and Therapeutic Engagement in Severe Anorexia Nervosa

MICHAEL STROBER

Anorexia nervosa is a bewildering form of human suffering. It has few rivals in evoking morbid curiosity—not simply as the image of death imbuing life, but also as a stark example of how impotent we can be rendered as would-be helpers. It confounds our sensibilities in many different ways. To the most seasoned of clinicians, it is a daunting challenge; parents and friends, and the novice therapist who confronts its stark images and ruthless intensity for the first time, are kept in thrall. If anyone steps too heavily on the patient's sensitivities, opportunities for intervention fade with astonishing speed, as many health workers and loved ones learn with dismay. The disorder is eerily compelling because it is utterly beyond comprehension—this precipitous descent into weird rituals, uncharacteristically intemperate manner, and shrill, absurdly trivial complaints about the unfairness of being implored to eat. How does the therapist even dare attempt to mitigate the suffering of a person whose self-perceptions and avowed personal goals are distorted well beyond the realm of common sense? It is a conundrum that Gull (1874) and Lasègue (1873) found themselves struggling with and writing thoughtfully about over a century ago.

This chapter is prepared as an instructional guide of sorts for the "student." But its focus is a limited one; little is said of the many different facets or stages of intervention per se. There is a dearth of rapid, specifically effective cures for the severe or chronic form of anorexia nervosa, and rarely does its treatment follow a smooth, predictable line. Instead, the chapter's principal focus is on the initial consultation—specifically, on the process of establishing connection and intimacy with the patient and assessing her accessibility to treatment.[1] The initial consultation is doubtless the most important encounter between patient and therapist; it constitutes the cornerstone of the treatment that follows. Yet, with rare exceptions, it receives only perfunctory treatment, and typically greater attention is paid to how the clinician should gather history and review systems to establish the objective character of the patient's symptoms and distress. But consider how frequently it is that initial treatments of this disorder do not work out, and how large the psychological and physical toll is if the opportunity for treatment is irrevocably lost. Crisp (1980) and Bruch (1988) have duly stressed how the treatment of anorexia nervosa creates its own unique conundrums: If the patient's physical health is restored—the undeniable hope of all who gaze upon her with revulsion and panic—she is left feeling profoundly inadequate and psychologically imperiled by comparison. As therapist and physician keep striving to add one more small increment of weight gain, the patient shudders, feeling vanquished and cowed as she loses the one facet of her life where she misguidedly thinks she excels. She may genuinely come to treatment seeking relief from the misery created by malnourishment and distorted self-perceptions, but she may not always grasp the forces working to actively discourage her from realizing this goal. There is thus an inevitable and vexing tension of conflicting agendas hanging over the initial consultation, and this tension must be addressed early if impasse and confusion are to be minimized. If this consultation is to end meaningfully, either the patient must feel she has been witness to an experience that gives her reason to hope for a less painful alternative to the forbidding prospect of continuing her life as it is; or the patient and therapist must reach a consensus that opportunities for effective therapeutic work do not presently exist, and that the resources needed to undertake such treatment will be protected should conditions appear more favorable in the future.

Against this backdrop, the present chapter discusses key parameters of the initial consultation with severely ill anorexic patients. In addition to considering specific technical issues, it has several broadly related objectives: (1) to provide the student with knowledge of the intrapsychic and interpersonal psychological terrain to be sifted by therapist and patient in establishing the background and context for intensive long-term treatment; (2) to show how intuitive appreciation of these matters is the key to building the therapeutic alliance; and, of greatest importance, (3) to illustrate how the therapist profitably draws on his or her skill in bringing evocative language, imagery, and affectivity into the therapeutic dialogue. Not only the spoken word, but the therapist's physical presence as well, must be imbued with perceptible emotional intensity and texture for the purpose of rousing the patient's desire for understanding, affiliation, sustenance, and protection, and drawing her attention away from the feverish intensity of dieting rituals to something more compelling.

WHAT CONSULTATION WITH A SEVERELY ILL PATIENT DEMANDS OF THE THERAPIST

Although the treatment of severe anorexia nervosa is, under usual circumstances, painfully slow, its impasse can be reached very quickly. A patient who is not adequately prepared for the demands of treatment, or who commences treatment with deep suspicions about the ideology, therapeutic values, or human qualities of the therapist, will soon be dancing in endless, unavailing circles around questions about the true seriousness of her illness, or discussing the minutiae of her feeding behavior to the neglect of substantive matters. That it is not always possible to avoid this is self-evident to experienced clinicians. Even so, it underlines the crucial importance of the therapist's preparation for understanding and articulating the contradictory images of suffering and restitution that are inherent to this disease and that give shape and force to its symptoms. Simply put, the therapist must bring to the consultation a cogent frame of reference for understanding these different currents, and a firm, unalterable commitment to sharing it with the patient—especially in those moments (and there will be many) when reason slips and resistance prevails.

The psychopathology of anorexia nervosa is a complex story of how the patient is drawn into new psychological arrangements that effectively sustain her avoidance of maturational fears, thus stifling conflicts and reducing intrapsychic "dis-ease" (Crisp, 1980). Baffling as this story frequently is to the patient, it must be unraveled and then retold with deep empathic understanding if her accessibility to treatment is to be gauged accurately. If by the end of the consultation the patient senses or is somehow aware of the therapist's uniquely intuitive ability to decode the hidden meaning of her illness, a prerequisite for establishing therapeutic partnership will have been met, and both parties will better understand the shared commitment that is needed to confront the daunting tasks that lie ahead. If not, the chances of making any real progress are greatly lessened.

Of course, there are severely ill patients whose malnourished physical state and psychological depletion are too advanced or refractory for the work of psychotherapy to proceed. But this is true only for a minority. Most, even when profoundly impaired, retain the capacity for human connection. Unfortunately, this essential point is not always appreciated by clinicians. If a patient feels that she is being spoken down to, as if she were feeble-minded, it becomes difficult and sometimes impossible to create a viable therapeutic alliance. The indignation is often brooked in silence, but the patient nonetheless feels dehumanized and humiliated, and she reaches out once again for the illusions of safety that surround her illness. I have consulted with numerous patients—some incapacitated by their wasted state, others deemed treatment failures—who, though in urgent need of hospital care and not immediately accessible to psychotherapy, still registered clear emotional responsiveness to the consultation and made a successfully commitment to treatment at a later date. Thus, I return to the point just made: The factor of distinctive importance in work with this patient group is the therapist's readiness, even at the very outset of the consultation, to give compelling emotionally expression to a patient's suffering and to shed new light on the forces underpinning her weird symptoms and the suffocating terror rising up as she contemplates even the idea of "normal" eating.

A person afflicted with anorexia nervosa is thus aptly viewed as an extraordinary icon of conflict and suffering. Indeed, one essential objective of the consultation is to help the patient see the paradox and conundrum of her illness at its many different levels. Just as surely as she is trapped in a life made up of flat, repetitive rituals and hobbled by an exasperating, numbing resistance to meaningful change, the therapist who brings sense to non-sense, clarity to bewilderment, tenderness and compassion to ruthless discipline and self-abnegation, will be viewed as having an almost magical understanding of the human condition and the uncommon ability to describe the most twisted of psychological issues with compelling, poetic eloquence. For the patient living such a painfully restricted and emotionally depleted life, this view of her withered self and recognition of her desperate, unspoken need for sustenance constitute medicine of extraordinary power. If the therapist is lacking in these qualities or is of rigid bearing, the initial encounter will be deprived of vital elements. Discussions of the treatment of anorexia nervosa do not often take up this issue; however, I believe that it is an issue to be reckoned with. The treatment of this illness is slippery and time-consuming, and the stakes are very high. Not all therapists are prepared to begin such undertakings, and some will be poorly suited for work with this population.

UNSPOKEN THEMES AND CURRENTS IN THE INITIAL CONSULTATION

It is thus plainly evident that the therapist must bring into the arena of consultation and treat-ment an awareness of the role he or she plays in an infinitely deep existential drama. Reduced to its bare, morbid essence, this drama centers around the question of whether or not chaos, chronicity, or death will ultimately defeat the fragile therapist–patient partnership. Precisely because the drama is so profound, and the patient's entry into treatment is so steeped in suspicion and desperation, the therapist must embrace his or her "gifts" of insight and interpretive psychological prose with self-assurance, as they are vital commodities—tools the therapist will use to divert the patient from the menacingly seductive authority of dieting rituals, and to give her security and license to discover what is afoot and how to put it right. It now becomes evident why the psychological anatomy of anorexia nervosa deserves a full and reasoned exposition.

Clinicians familiar with this illness have long recognized that patients typically approach treatment not only with profound dread, but often without any clear understanding of the particulars of their *psychological* illness. Few human maladies seem as unfathomable and frustrating, with so many twisted, deeply etched tensions played out in raw physical imagery and underlying psychological motives. As already stated and as illustrated in the sections that follow, how, and at what depth of clarity and intensity, the therapist first compels the patient's attention, reinterprets the obscure language of her symptoms, and finally moves her gently but persuasively to unravel these conflicting tensions are the most crucial elements of psychotherapeutic engagement. But how does a therapist forge coherent understanding of an illness that stokes an uncommon appetite for "self-determination" and obstinacy in an otherwise submissive, compliant young woman who may have but the dimmest understanding of what summons and transfixes her rage against "fatness" and the psychological needs served by it? The illness is embraced by the patient with inexplicable fervor and mindlessly upbeat determination, even as it strips away nuances of character and reduces time and experience to uncounted days of futile rituals. It causes flesh to melt away from underlying bone even as it goads its host into greater exertion and more frantic dieting. The illness provides refuge from the imperiling strains of adolescent maturation—unbridled egotism, emotional fury, strange new impulses, and pressures to leave the securities of home—but leaves suffering, shame, and arrested development in its wake for years to come if it continues unhindered. Slowly but surely, it will leave a person of rock-solid discipline and a gentle nature disabled by her unbending pursuit of skeletal efficiency and absolute restraint of human impulse and need.

Each passing day is idle witness to this senseless, uninterrupted march of symptoms, bringing the patient ineluctably closer to abject listlessness and passivity. Yet this same crippling illness is restitutive—a disease, if you will, precipitated by developmental crisis (see Crisp, Chapter 13, this volume), and then covering over the patient's mounting and unmanageable inner feelings of "dis-ease." To all outward appearances, she is crazed (indeed, madly inspired, so it seems) by some feverish, unnamable urge to participate in her own demise. But only rarely is she so degraded by malnutrition and stupor as to be truly oblivious to the terror gripping those who offer her solace and who implore her to seek treatment for her malady. How, then, can she face the devastation wrought by this illness with apparent equanimity? How can a person of apparently solid upbringing and promising future (it is acknowledged that the early background of some patients is one of appalling neglect, trauma, or chaos) be so terribly derailed as to wind up in this strange place of demented ideas and shocking lack of civility with loved ones? A 28-year-old woman, ill since age 16 and treated minimally until the time of her consultation with me, put it this way:

> Intellectually, I see the absurdity of brooding about my weight and the things I eat. I see how easy and natural it is for my friends, even my sister, to be fulfilled in life, and to accept the fact that a body needs nourishment as fuel. But even after all I have been through, I still fail to relate any of this to me. I still believe, without really knowing why, that being thin is a barometer of moral superiority.

Here, then, is the paradox and conundrum of anorexia nervosa, to be wrestled with as the consultation unfolds: It can leave the patient bruised and devitalized, retreating from friendships and family, but is still "defended" with tenacity as a trusted expression of self-respecting discipline and the patient's only effective antidote to the strains of her development and deeply rooted personal fears. Resolving this conundrum is a daunting challenge, but the therapist must see it through, using measured judgments about the patient to identify psychological resources she barely recognizes (indeed, whose very existence she questions), and remaining confident that with time she will see the advantage to challenging the illness that now seems too puzzling and frustrating to comprehend. If the consultation fails to bring light to the subtle, insidious nature of this conundrum, or if the therapist accedes to the patient's many demands for greater autonomy in managing her symptoms, there will be a risk of an even steeper slide into chronicity from which full recovery will be more difficult.

A THEORETICAL MODEL

It is impossible to deny that anorexia nervosa is a multidetermined condition. Most who treat it, or research it in the laboratory, are reconciled to the need to approach it broadly and flexibly. The model I use for clinical work is but one approach, although it is receiving more attention of late because of its power to account implicitly for core features of the disorder, and because it is provides a perspective on the maturational crisis inherent in anorexia nervosa (Crisp, 1980) that is acceptable to the vast majority of patients. The model is scientifically defensible, but its main value is in giving patient and therapist common ground for a psychological understanding of this disorder. It is a means of translating its strange symptoms and emotional currents into therapeutically workable concepts; as such, it provides support for the difficult work that lies ahead. A more detailed exposition of this model can be found elsewhere (Strober, 1991, 1995). Here it is presented in abbreviated form.

Prompted by evidence that the major structures of personality are part of our genetic heritage and interact with experience in shaping not only the character of normative development but the symptoms of psychological illness as well (see Cloninger, 1986, 1987), the model sees anorexia nervosa as originating in inherited extremes of personality that severely restrict a young woman's adjustment to the challenges of pubertal growth and development. Implicating genetic factors in a disorder like anorexia nervosa is a sensitive matter, and the potential for misunderstanding and misuse of such theoretical concepts is very real. Psychiatry has a long, unfortunate history of misconstruing and pathologizing female behavior, and only recently has there been broader theoretical appreciation of the power of gender differences in self-development and the adverse effects of stereotyping children too rigidly by sex or gender. And even though science is shedding new light on how different facets of human behavior are strongly rooted in inheritance, it also demonstrates the equally important role of developmental experience in this process. The point is that in clarifying this confluence of heredity and experience for the patient, and helping her to see that these influences are neither fixed nor unchanging, the therapist informs her understanding not only of why she was ill prepared to meet the strains of her development, but of why, in a world of more prosaic realities, her harsh self-judgments are misdirected and undeserved.

The model's emphasis on heritable personality traits does not conflict with the incontrovertible facts that anorexia nervosa is a culture-bound or culture-driven syndrome, and that cultural factors influence the different trajectories shown by males and females for problem areas in which disorders of weight and shape are core. Nor does it negate the importance in anorexia nervosa of early failures in parenting, trauma, or other psychological experiences that interfere with development of the self. However, culture alone is an unsatisfactory groundwork for explaining anorexia nervosa to patients or exploring the complex forces that sustain it. Dieting and the pursuit of thinness are commonplace in Western society, to be sure. But the majority of young women who diet are not panic-stricken as they face the onset of adolescence, or desperate to avoid being irreparably trapped by its force. Anorexia nervosa is not a favored cultural norm.

The model thus draws attention to three streams of causal influence underpinning the maturational crisis and the regression precipitating from it: (1) temperament and personality traits common to, if not universally present in, individuals with anorexia nervosa; (2) the psychological dynamics of pubertal growth; and (3) the familial environment.

Personality

As noted, the heritability of temperament and personality is well documented. Likewise, the idea that certain qualities of personality may confer vulnerability to anorexia nervosa is hardly novel (Strober, 1995). Indeed, one "fact" about this illness that patients and parents come to respect strongly with time is the remarkable consistency with which these personality traits appear in those who suffer from it. They are evident prior to the onset of weight loss, but are often accentuated by it and persist after weight recovery, as research has demonstrated (Casper, 1990; Strober, 1980). The traits include the following:

- High emotional reserve and cognitive inhibition.
- Preference for routine, orderly, and predictable environments, and poor adaptability to change.
- Heightened conformity and deference to others.
- Risk avoidance and dysphoric overarousal by appetitive or affectively stressful events.
- Excessive rumination and perfectionism.

In short, the anorexic carries with her a disposition to avoid whatever is novel, intense, or unfamiliar; to have nagging self-doubt and to ruminate; to shun intimate ties with others, especially those outside her immediate family; and to persevere, even in the absence of tangible reward.

The Nature and Demands of Puberty

Consider, against the backdrop of these personality traits, the essential nature of puberty and the new demands it requires of the developing child:

- Increasing instinctualization of behavior.
- A widening and intensification of affective experience.
- A shift from reliance on family and external structure as regulators of behavior to greater self-direction and self-interest.
- Stronger drives for affiliation and intimacy.
- Changes in body morphology.

How these various elements of pubertal growth and development will challenge the emotional reticence and persevering steadiness of these young girls requires a knowledge of the rearing environment and its interaction with these personality traits.

Family Environment

The complex nature of psychological illnesses easily hampers efforts to parse the separate effects of nature and nurture in their etiology. Genes, and the behavioral propensities they express, appear to play the larger role in determining who is susceptible to disease; however, the significance of environmental effects cannot be ignored. Concerning anorexia nervosa, although there is no convincing evidence that a single common family portrait exists (Vandereycken, Kog, & Vanderlinden, 1989), certain features are notable:

- Limited tolerance of disharmonious affect or psychological tension.
- Emphasis on propriety and rule-mindedness.
- Parental overdirection of the child or subtle discouragement of autonomous strivings.
- Poor skills in conflict resolution.

That these patterns bear some relationship to the personality descriptors noted previously is not unanticipated, given the genetic resemblance of parents and children for behavioral tendencies.

The Maturational Crisis

For most teens, puberty is a period of stumbling awkwardness, embarrassment, and angst. But for the young woman who is prone to nagging self-doubt, who is inclined to a life of predictable order, who obtains self-validation largely through external reward, and who has little tolerance of affectively charged experience, puberty is an insidious process triggering feelings of dread and "dis-ease." Suddenly she is in a new and unfamiliar place, vastly different from the world of understandable concepts and clear expectations. Simply put, she is terribly out of sorts. She examines her body, and where straight, angular features once prevailed, she now finds roundness and curves—uninvited and thus unwelcome. Her social world is in equally disturbing flux: Her friends are giving themselves freely to what seem wasteful and loathsome appetites for excitement, selfish needs, kinship outside of their families, and sexual intrigue. Her natural self and the imperatives of development are hopelessly and dangerously irreconcilable; she is now in the throes of maturational crisis.

For the anorexic, then, maturation is the shattering of an innocent child's covenant that safety, steadiness, and esteem will always come to those who are respectful, compliant, and emotionally reserved. Suddenly, she is adrift in life changes that take on more menacing and sinister implications with each passing day. She is unhinged, as though she is being bluntly and grimly uprooted by unrecognizable (but surely undisciplined) forces, from which she must take hasty retreat if she is to avoid the devastations she fears they bring.

That this crisis is concretized in anomalous perceptions of the body is not difficult to understand. The body is as natural and vital a conduit of growth, pleasurable gratification, and constructive energies as it is a potent metaphor and symbol of illness and distress. For the anorexic, existential safety now requires her to separate body from self, so that each may exist in entirely different spheres. Her body is not like other teenage bodies—an embarrassment to tolerate or a source of giddy pleasures. Rather, it is odious—a lurking, cancerous blight whose growth must be arrested, depleted of energy, then vanquished.

Though it was never intended to do so, dieting has given expression to the anorexic's desperate need for regression, for a return to simpler times. She soon realizes that she is wondrously capable of sustaining it—effortlessly, so it seems—by relying on her natural capacities for rigid discipline and ritualized actions. Even if she has a visceral awareness that her appearance has turned ghastly, her anxiety goads her into ever-strengthening vigilance and further weight loss. Finally, the disquieting emotions and needs are muzzled, and the once familiar patterns of discipline, predictable routine, and tangible reward are blessedly restored; the crisis has been turned back.

Of course, the patient is never alone in illness. As experience with these families shows, it is quite common for parents and anorexic children to share a discomfort with arousing and dysphoric affect, and to favor rigid patterns and conformity with social expectations. These similarities are "felt" by all, though rarely is this acknowledged so openly. Thus, it is not only the anorexic who is threatened by the sudden disquiet of adolescent growth; her family experiences the threat as well. This is surely the case, as clinical experience with anorexic families frequently shows that certain members intuitively perceive other members as they experience themselves—as exquisitely sensitive to change and easily prone to psychological injury. Moreover, just as frequently, certain members harbor the secret conviction that they are, in some vague way, indispensable to other members' well-being and safety. In short, as surely as it brings hardship and suffering, anorexia nervosa silences needs, yearnings, and emotional tensions that the patient fears (accurately, in many cases) will bring too great a burden for loved ones to bear, or that she secretly fears they will fail to recognize, thus leaving her sensitive nature exposed to bitter disappointments.

My colleagues and I also know of families in which there are experiences of a radically different sort: abuse, gross neglect, ridicule, and hostile criticism. In these cases, experiences of emotional relatedness, affect expression, and the desire for need gratification are, for the patient, forbidding triggers of calamity, *malevolent* intrusion, and the anticipation of painful letdowns. The character of family life in these cases may differ, but the role served by the anorexic's biological and psychic regression is much the same: It enables her to move from impending dread and entrapment to psychological "safety" and restitution.

Ultimately, the regression of anorexia nervosa unmasks profound despair and self-loathing—an intense suffering ultimately brought into even sharper relief, as it must be, by the patient's treatment. As she reflects on a life of rigid conformity, timidity, and avoidance of self-interest, she feels justified in brutally harsh criticism of her "powerlessness" and shameful lack of vigor. Convinced that her life is a sham and that the qualities others admire in her were obtained deceptively through compliance, she is convinced that she is plain and lacking in distinctiveness. She withholds the content of her inner mental life to avoid exposure and mockery, only to feel further ineptitude and an even more urgent need to steady herself through more restrictive dieting and unrelenting exercise. The line demarcating self and disease is now hopelessly blurred, and she is unremittingly beholden to maniacal rituals, mercurial moods, and misdirected energies. It is against this backdrop that therapist, patient, and family contemplate entering into a long and costly relationship to seek a way out of the maelstrom.

PREPARING FOR CONSULTATION: PROSPECTS AND CAVEATS

The overarching goal of consultation is to determine whether meaningful change is possible. But this is a deceptively simple objective, considering the seductively complex psychology and physiology of anorexia nervosa. Only a very small minority of anorexic patients—those who are truly demented by prolonged life-threatening malnutrition—are unable to see that their lives have been choked by dreadful behaviors, whether they state so or not. Indeed, it is hardly necessary for the consultant to declare that the patient needs treatment (this is self-evident, and she has heard it before), or to put forward heroic efforts to convince her that this is so. The true goal of consultation is to provide a concentrated moment of drama, at the end of which the patient can answer the all-important question: Will I allow *this* person to make a difference in my life? Thus, rarely should the consultant have any particular reason to argue the need for treatment with the patient. Indeed, doing so deprives the consultation of its dramatic essence and may blur the distinction between previous failed treatments—often experienced as coercions and as violations of her "free will"—and the current moment. And remember, what is for most a bluntly objective issue (i.e., people who are ill need treatment) is for the patient a raging existential conundrum, because she believes that freedom from the tyranny of her illness will plunge her into a world of ineffable terror. The issue is complicated even further by the fact that for the most brittle patients, being asked to inhabit this new and oddly ordered emotional world can precipitate levels of regression that render effective treatment impossible. And, of course, *enforced* treatment is an oxymoron, because in such cases there can be no shared responsibility in the quest for change.

This leads us to another critical point of the consultation, but one that is rarely clearly articulated: The decision to undertake treatment is a responsibility shared by patient *and* clinician. Accordingly, consultation has the purpose of determining whether treatment is even feasible, or whether potentially greater benefits might be obtained if treatment is postponed to a later date. Rarely is it so clear that clinicians must at times exercise the right to decline treatment of a particular patient, especially a patient who seems less then decidedly committed. In such cases the consultant does indeed have to declare, "I am reluctant to work with you at this time, not because of any negative feeling toward you or intimidation by the seriousness of your condition, but because the search for important and very painful truths hidden behind the disguises of compliance, denial, and feeding rituals can only succeed if you are committed to working with me as a partner." Vandereycken and Meerman (1984) present a very lucid discussion of this matter, arguing that to delay or refuse treatment can be informative and salutary in the following ways:

- It can protect patient and family alike from potentially disruptive and nontherapeutic regression.
- It can prevent a wasteful expenditure of emotional and financial resources.
- It can allow for the initiation of treatment at a more propitious moment in the patient's life.
- It can allow the patient to contemplate more deeply the true extent of her misery and the ultimate futility of a life encumbered by her symptoms.
- Finally, it can avoid the illusion of treatment when truly effective psychotherapy is neither possible nor applicable.

Managing treatment refusal on the part of either patient or therapist is admittedly a complex medico-legal process, and is beyond the scope of this chapter. An excellent discussion of these matters can be found elsewhere in this volume (see Goldner, Birmingham, & Smye, Chapter 26).

Contact with a severely ill anorexic patient and her family can easily evoke deep pity and understandable impulses to act quickly and decisively. Yet there are other reasons for not moving ahead with treatment without careful reflection and preparation. Even when patients are intellectually vibrant and charming, treatment can grind on with such terrible monotony and heart-breaking suffering that even skilled therapists are pushed to their limits of endurance. To the degree that this treatment will require a therapist to have patience, alertness, intellectual clarity, and unfailing empathy, the dangers of accruing too many severely ill patients in a practice are real and should be averted. Likewise, undertaking treatment without adequate resources for skilled management of the patient in a hospital (should this be neces-

sary) carries its own unique risks and burdens, including iatrogenic effects of coercively managed weight gain; the patient's exposure to demeaning and disrespectful attitudes harbored by medical personnel who have contempt for such willful behavior; excessive medicalization of the treatment; and inadequate lengths of stays. Already prone to rapid shifts in their resolve to persevere with treatment, patients hardly need additional reasons for disdain or mistrust of health professionals or the treatment environment.

Thus, therapists should consider declining treatment, or at least delaying its start, in the following circumstances:

- Unremitting refusal to follow through with basic elements of a treatment plan, including nutritional stabilization.
- Malignant dependence, evidenced by abrogation of personal responsibilities for change, or harshly critical attitudes toward health professionals and the "value" of psychotherapy as means of healing and renewal.
- Repeated relapses following high-intensity treatment programs known to be of high quality.

Sadly, it has been my experience that attempts to engage patients with long-standing severe illness in treatment when any one of these circumstances is present rarely meet with success.

PREPARING THE PATIENT AND FAMILY FOR CONSULTATION

Timing and Logistics

As previously alluded to, a consultation that dwells too long on the patient's symptom history, or is too easily beset by the pleas of loved ones for urgent intervention, will leave the patient uninspired. Likewise, a consultation that is too brief affords little opportunity to arouse the patient's interest in the therapist or galvanize her into action. Thus, logistics and timing of the consultation, as well as instructions given to the patient and her family on how they will need to prepare for it, are highly important parameters with intended therapeutic effects.

The patient and family (family members are included if the patient is still living at home, has regular contact with them, or is financially dependent on them) are told that the consultation will normally require two 3- to 4-hour sessions, to be spread over 7 to 10 days. The enormous burden on their time is acknowledged, but they are told that it must be this way because the issue before them is important; they surely will have many questions and repeated needs for reassurance or clarification, especially if they now find themselves reaching their limits of patience and understanding. It is also pointed out that if they are uninformed about the nature of psychiatric treatment, or generally scornful of those who practice it, they will need added time to form opinions of the consultant: whether he or she is a person of sufficient intelligence and competence to meet this challenge, and has the right blend of warmth, compassion, and unperturbed directness the patient will require to feel sufficiently safe and adequately challenged. This is not a trivial matter, especially in regard to family members. If there is one critical omission in consultations with adult patients, it is the failure to give time and attention to the concerns of their families (except, of course, when contact with a family is not allowed). It is an omission that can seriously jeopardize treatment at a later date, especially if progress is slow and family members come to question the therapist's competence or the seriousness of the patient's commitment to change.

The labor-intensive duration of this consultation has other intended purposes, though they are not acknowledged directly. One is to convey that the consultant/therapist is a person of formidable strength and patience who can remain firm and clear-headed, day after dreadfully monotonous and hard day. Another is to show that the therapist can translate the patient's jangled behavior into a language that reconciles the seemingly divergent forces operating within her. The therapist is tolerant of her forbidding appearance, but is committed nevertheless to the need for change and to helping her see that her troubles are human and understandable. The extended consultation also allows patient and therapist sufficient time to grow more at ease with each other, to share and reflect upon moments of pain and humor, and to hit upon moments when the therapist can communicate more expressively through gestures, shifts in posture, facial displays, and the touch of a gentle hand on shoulders hunched over in tears or embarrassment. In short, everything about the consultation and its structure conveys in some small way something important about the therapist and the psychotherapeutic process.

Instructions Given to Patient and Family

For an illness in which challenges to treatment loom large and financial costs are high, the importance of gauging the patient's and family's potential for sustaining involvement and investment in this process cannot be overestimated. Nevertheless, in too many cases preciously little time is devoted to preparing severely ill patients for the demands that lie ahead, just as therapists are insufficiently frank about the danger that results from a patient's abdicating personal responsibility for her treatment. Accordingly, to prepare all parties for the consultation, I now routinely offer an introduction—usually by way of a letter that outlines the consultation, its purpose, and the information I will need to prepare helpfully for it. (This form of initial communication has become necessary of late, because of the increasing demand on my time for consultation.) The letter, which is addressed separately to the patient and (when relevant) to family members, contains (but is not limited entirely to) the following passages. The excerpts here are from one letter, sent to a highly educated 26-year-old patient.

> I cannot overstate how difficult the treatment of this problem can be. Maybe you already recognize how your head is filled with so many confusing and opposing pressures. You may concede how much you suffer because of anorexia nervosa, but still have crushing ambivalence about letting it go. Actually, this is very common. Whether or not treatment can succeed depends partly on the ability of patient and therapist to form an attachment—a trust that will encourage the patient to share inner thoughts and feelings with the therapist. But you may wonder how this can happen for you, given your desire to remain aloof and perfectionistic, without any hint of neediness. You may already sense that an important goal of this treatment is to help you live a more natural and spontaneous life, but if you're firmly convinced that you lack truly admirable traits or self-confidence, you question whether this can ever be achieved. You may also think that being "normal" means you will always lack the kind of unique and special qualities that people take note of; in-

deed, you may already fear that you are such a person—merely average, whose inner thoughts and needs are of no possible interest to others, and for this reason undeserving of consideration. If this is the case, then the temptations to stay put—to continue life as it is—are understandably great. The purpose, then, of our meeting together in this consultation is to see whether these opposing forces can be worked with.

To ask a patient whose self-confidence is shaky at best and whose energies are dwindling to ponder what *she* can bring to this treatment may seem strangely out of place—a callous, if not cruel, request. But this really is not the case at all. Recall for the moment the risks of imposing treatment on individuals who regard anorexia nervosa as an immutable fact of life, or in whom pathology of the self is so pervasive and developmental trauma is so malignant that they become dangerously unhinged by the psychic turmoil precipitated by weight gain. The consultant needs critical information from patient and family to determine whether these ominous conditions prevail, or whether the prospects for long-term change appear reasonably favorable. The letter of introduction continues as follows:

Anorexia nervosa brings something to you that is very important. Why else would you hold on to it so fiercely? Its importance to you and the role that it serves must be respected. Even so, it is nothing if not a symptom of troubled development; because it is both a cause of suffering and a means of lightening your fears of developing, its treatment will take time and will requires much of me as the therapist and you as the patient. Little good will come out of our meeting if you feel that treatment is being imposed on you, or if your motivation to deny conflicts and keep them under wraps is stronger than the wish for a better vision of yourself. If this turns out to be the case, you may not be ready for treatment at this time. Given that treatment of this problem requires several years, we also have to decide whether we are compatible together. Finally, I have come to accept the fact that a small number of people with anorexia nervosa will not tolerate a life without this illness. If you are such a person, it may be unwise to push you into treatment; instead, we can use our meeting to discuss

how you might find ways of living with it more comfortably. So you can see why there is much I need to know about you and your background. But it will be equally important for me to offer you a viewpoint on what causes your suffering and why it is so hard for you to imagine being any different. At the end of the consultation, you must decide if what I have to say about all of this makes sense.

With this introduction, the patient (and, when appropriate, her family) is asked to prepare an "autobiography," which is to be mailed to the consultant in advance of the first meeting. The patient is told that although she may genuinely question the value of her self-statements or feel tempted to exclude details of her life she deems trite or undeserving of special attention, any temptation to censor this autobiography or avoid answering a particular question must be avoided. First, background information pertaining to the illness per se is requested:

- Current physical exam, including full blood and urine analyses and electrocardiogram.
- A time line detailing (1) course of symptoms and weight changes; and (2) the presence and severity of exercise, purging behaviors, laxative/diuretic use, and use of prescription, over-the-counter, and illicit anorectic agents.
- Course of anxiety and depressive symptoms, and instances of intentional self-injurious behaviors.
- A detailed account of all past treatments, the frequency of these contacts, aspects of the treatment thought to be most helpful and those believed harmful, and qualities of the therapist(s) that were responded to favorably or felt to be objectionable. (This information is of special importance. Unfortunately, many patients with anorexia nervosa have received treatment that is deeply offensive to their sensibilities, if not patently iatrogenic. As these are often perceived as unpardonable acts, and patients recover slowly from them, their harmful elements must be frankly acknowledged by the consultant.)

Concerning personal development, the patient is asked to provide sufficient information in the autobiography to give the consultant a better understanding of the following:

- The quality of childhood and adolescent relationships with parents, other caregivers, and peers, as well as the quality of current ties.
- Academic history, including favored subjects and areas of greatest proficiency.
- Experiences with early separation and any difficulties encountered.
- Approaches to problem solving and conflict resolution, including patterns displayed by other family members.
- Perceptions of parental child rearing and capacities of each parent for emotional expressiveness.
- Experiences with puberty and sexual development, and adjustment of parents to her adolescent growth strains.
- Perceptions of her parents' marital relationship and their capacity for intimacy.
- Specific childhood apprehensions or phobias, and those areas of current worry.
- Satisfaction with current vocation or future career goals.
- Hobbies or special interests.

With respect to her illness, the patient is asked to provide answers to the following questions (adapted in part from Crisp, Joughin, Halek, & Bowyer, 1989):

- Did you ever think that your illness helped to resolve certain anxieties about your development or inner discontent?
- Has the illness been soothing or reassuring to you in any way, then or now?
- What would your life be like today if anorexia nervosa never existed?
- How do you wish you could communicate differently with others, and what would you like others to see in you?
- What emotions, both positive and negative, have been silenced by anorexia nervosa, and what presently unexpressed feelings do you wish to tolerate better?
- Are there aspects of human nature that you hope to experience in a more natural and spontaneous way at some point in the future?
- Do you hope to have a more mature adult sexual life?
- What aspects of weight gain and change in body shape will be most distressing to you?
- What good, if any, will arise from the effort to overcome this illness?

- Do you believe that meaningful change is possible? If so, what resources do you have to promote beneficial change?
- Do you have reason to believe you can form a close and effective therapeutic relationship? If not, why? And if so, what qualities in a therapist are most important to you?

With respect to the consultation itself, both patient and family are asked to answer these questions:

- What is your purpose in requesting consultation at this time, and what do you believe are others' perceptions of the need for treatment?
- What are your immediate and long-term treatment goals?
- Are you being forced to participate in this consultation against your will? If so, what are your specific reasons for not wishing to undertake treatment at this time?
- What factors might lead you to be more open to treatment at a later date?

Finally, the patient is asked to bring to the consultation (or to send in advance if at all feasible) photographs, videotapes, artistic works, or other tangible expressions of her unique interests or talents. Many respond to this request with perceptible reluctance; some consider it oddly intrusive, others are outwardly offended, and still others approach the sharing of this material with dreadful embarrassment. Nevertheless, the consultant insists on this—of course, with gentle and sensitive persuasion—and for very good reason: Much is often revealed about the passionate convictions, gritty spirit, originality, curiosity, and vivacity of the patient through such material. This reason is stated explicitly to the patient.

With autobiography in hand, the consultant is prepared to move swiftly to bring specific focus to the first meeting; the economy of effort afforded by having the patient prepare the background for her consultation in advance of the initial session is easy to see. As terribly shattered as the patient is in her notion of herself, the request for this information signifies the consultant's undeterred commitment to genuine and deep understanding of the ways in which she defines herself, and it declares that she too powerfully shapes how this relationship is to work. On the other hand, the material may reveal a history of illness so chronic and unremitting, and a patient so severely arrested in her development, that treatment options are sadly limited.

THE PROCESS OF CONSULTATION

Enabling the Patient to Consider New Possibilities

The consultant now prepares to use the autobiographical material to galvanize the patient by creating an experience that enables her to consider new possibilities. The transcript presented below,[2] from the first session of a consultation with a 20-year-old woman, is illustrative of the process. The reader should take note of how interactive the dialogue is; how strong a presence the consultant is in this process; and how issues of deep affective significance can be taken up even in a first encounter, in spite of the discomfort engendered.

> K had been ill since age 13, but this was her first serious consideration of treatment. She had seen three therapists up to this time, but little was accomplished. She described her previous treatment as little more than "being asked over and over again" why she didn't want to grow up, and her responding by shrugging her shoulders. At 5'6", she weighed 81 pounds. She had no history of purging or drug use of any type, but she exercised for more than 6 hours a day, stopping only when she was in agonizing physical pain. She was very articulate, at least when she allowed herself to speak freely. In their letter to the consultant, the parents stated that they had always felt left out of their daughter's treatment and had never come to a true understanding of how her emaciated state was evidence of psychological illness.
>
> K described herself as straightlaced and reticent, if not painfully shy. She was orderly (to the point of meticulously organizing her daily activities with elaborate schedules), intolerant of change, and uncomfortable with any hint of intense emotion (which she took to be a sign of imperfect control). She admitted that her personality traits had cost her many friendships. She was now humiliated that her controls had slipped to the point of now having to take medical leave from the prestigious university she attended, where she was excelling academically in her joint major of mathematics and music (K was a concert pianist). These two interests, it turned out, revealed a good deal about her inner world and the conflicts within her that were increasing in intensity.
>
> K wrote that she was a carbon copy of her father, who was described as stoical (a man of few words) and as sharing her quiet temperament. It was a close relationship, she said, but she later acknowledged that rarely had either one of them known what the other thought or felt about things of importance. Her mother, on the other hand, was a person K held in contempt and viewed with disdain. "She has always embarrassed me," K wrote, describing her as emotionally fragmented, prone to fits of foolishness, "lacking control," and frequently making statements about K in public that K deemed too revealing. K wrote that she grew up determined never to be like her mother in any way.
>
> This section of the transcript came roughly 2 hours into the first session, immediately after K and the consultant had watched a video (taken by her father) of one of her recent musical performances.

THERAPIST. Can you anticipate my reaction to watching your performance?

PATIENT. Not really.

THERAPIST. Try. I have a strong reaction to this tape, and it has everything to do with what you said about yourself in the autobiography.

PATIENT. That I play with so much feeling and passion.

THERAPIST. Exactly. So you must be very much aware of this extraordinary contrast to your normally restrained and controlled daily life.

PATIENT. My music teacher was always frustrated with me because I was too inhibited when I played. He said I could never be a great pianist if I couldn't find the passion in my music.

THERAPIST. Did it concern you that you might never reach your full potential as a pianist because of this? Actually, maybe the issue is even more complicated; music may be the one vital avenue for expression of the same emotional drives that trouble you so much. Ironic, isn't it?

PATIENT. I guess it is. I always feel embarrassed after playing very strong pieces, like I'm losing myself and making a spectacle. I think people are sitting there ridiculing me.

THERAPIST. But it isn't surprising to me that you would feel this. How would you avoid it, believing as you do that emotions should be tightly controlled, just as your daily routine is so tightly and impossibly controlled down to the very last waking minute? By their very nature, emotions resist control, and this is what gives our life drive and color. By knowing our emotions, we have greater connection to things that have deep meaning. You cannot succeed in your efforts to control feelings; maybe that is why you have tried so hard to stifle them. Why you try so hard to do just this is an important question to seek answers to, should you decide to follow through with treatment.

PATIENT. But why is it bad to control feelings?

THERAPIST. This is a very important question. Let me try answering it by posing a question of my own for you to consider: How do you avoid being so uncomfortably stressed when you sit at the piano, thinking—as I suspect you do—that "If this performance is not flawless, it has no merit and I have little true ability"? Let me try an answer for you, because it will be important for you to consider whether or not my way of looking at these things makes sense. The answer to both questions is: Because it is impossible to do, and attempting such control prevents you from being in the moment. When you clamp down on your inner life, not only does your music turn flat, but so do you. You may have the illusion of being safe and secure, but in reality you are turning lifeless and listless. You have a wonderful talent, but your emotional conflicts make it difficult for you to breathe life into it.

PATIENT. But I will lose self-control.

THERAPIST. By that you mean what exactly?

PATIENT. That I will, I don't know, be weak and selfish and get lazier.

THERAPIST. And scattered and poorly disciplined? Everything you feared you might turn into if you let your guard down as you went through your teenage years?

PATIENT. Sort of like that.

THERAPIST. The parallels to the conflicts you've described in relation to your mother are also obvious.

PATIENT. Well you've seen her; don't you think she is loud? She's embarrassing.

THERAPIST. I see how the two of you come from different personalities. She is unlike you in many ways, and I have no doubt that over the years her presence has been more unsettling than it has been soothing. But the silent language that passes between you and your father is no less helpful. No, I do not think that you will become like your mother if you are more open to your feelings.

PATIENT. My father and I are just more comfortable together.

THERAPIST. I can see why, but there is nothing helpful or fulfilling in the way the two of you communicate, if you can call it that. It maintains the false belief that more natural and intimate relations are unnecessary or that they are dangerously uncomfortable.

PATIENT. My boyfriend has said the same thing to me.

THERAPIST. What is he like?

PATIENT. He's shy and quiet, like me. But he wants me to talk more about myself. It bothers him that I don't say much about how I feel about him.

THERAPIST. Is this an unreasonable desire? What are his feelings about you?

PATIENT. He says he loves me.

THERAPIST. And you wonder how this can possibly be, since you share so little of your true feelings. It's as though he is in love not with your true self, but rather with qualities that you express out of compliance and the belief that they will be received favorably by others.

PATIENT. Yes, exactly. That's why I am so uncomfortable. I think it was a mistake to get involved.

THERAPIST. Don't come to conclusions about important things so quickly. When you think about it, this relationship is very much like the push-and-pull struggle with your music. Here you are, a person with deep but hidden interests, sensitivities, and feelings. You are obviously drawn to something about this young man—which shows that you are every bit as human as the rest of us—but you now prepare to do battle against every wonderfully exciting and, yes, nerve-wracking and embarrassing thing that young people experience when they approach intimacy and sexual curiosity.

PATIENT. But I don't like feeling this way.

THERAPIST. Of course not, but only because the rigid nature of your personality has equated these feelings with danger and alarm, or maybe even with qualities that you found so objectionable in your mother. But give your mother credit for being connected to things and valuing her emotions. What you are being asked to consider now as you get ready to come back next week is whether or not you desire to understand more about this struggle, to become less estranged from your inner life, and to live with fewer punishing rituals and routines.

Explaining Maturational Crisis to the Patient

Along with the consultant's approach and demeanor, providing an explanation of the patient's maturational crisis is an important means of engaging the patient. Frightened and bewildered by the strangeness and dangerousness of her condition, she needs an anchor or she will surely continue to drift aimlessly and without direction. Because the large majority of patients who present for consultation have had previous treatment, and because many describe this treatment as lacking a clear focus, the consultant's perspective on the nature of the patient's illness is a matter of prime importance and should be articulated with force and clarity. As stated earlier, if she is to become attentive to someone more grounded than she, and accepting of a cognitive discourse more rational than her own distorted convictions, she must be intrigued about the prospect of being understood and of being given tools to effectively reinterpret the meaning of her actions.

Finishing up K's first session, the consultant summarized her crisis as follows. (Because of space limitations, ongoing comments by the patient and other dialogue between therapist and patient have been deleted.)

Having read through your autobiography, and now having spent this time with you, I can see how you came to recoil from the changes brought on by adolescence. For a person as disciplined as you are, and comfortable only in a world of perfect structure and predictability, growing into womanhood was a rude and uncomfortable challenge—one that you wanted no part of. Unfortunately, neither your mother's excitable nature nor your father's emotional reserve made this transition any easier; you were convinced that neither of them could truly grasp the panic inside, or make sense of it. Perhaps you also thought that because you breezed through school so effortlessly and were seen by others as having many talents, your worries and insecurities would never be taken seriously. It can be hard to understand why a person such as yourself now struggles with self-doubts and insecurities. But consider how difficult it is for a person who shuns new and intense experiences, and who believes that everything in life must be subject to perfect control, to adjust to the demands of adolescence. You sense new urges and impulses that are discomforting, and you are encouraged by teachers and friends to communicate your ideas more openly and assertively. But you are more comfortable respecting others before yourself and in being restrained. So, suddenly, you find yourself feeling uncomfortably challenged, as if rudely exploited by your own development. No longer are compliance and emotional reserve automatically rewarded, or something you can count on.

What you have shared with me leads me to think that you are repeatedly dismayed in your efforts to fit in. Even your body has deserted you, turning into something you do not wish it to be. Being the natural organizer that you are doesn't seem to do you much good now. This dieting ritual may be hard to make sense of, but consider how it has given you a protection of sorts against this terrible agitation: Your life turns once again around very predictable rituals, as if the success achieved in losing weight is proof of your control and discipline. But this deprivation and restraint—which are a big part of the dieting and weight loss—also quiet down the needs and feelings that haunt you. By denying yourself as you do, you express a deeply rooted belief that you are not as special as people think—that you have deceived people into thinking that you have admirable abilities, but your skill really is in the ability to follow rules and other people's expectations. Dieting is your way of saying, "I must get along on less, because I deserve so little."

So you can see why people find your behavior so mystifying and challenging. Many different and competing feelings and thoughts play themselves out in this illness. It is punishment for your conviction that you are shamefully undeserving of the positive things said about you. But you are also drawn to the rigid discipline, as though it fills a gaping hole; it leaves you feeling strong and invincible because you think you now control parts of your inner life that upset you. However, it weakens you to the point that you must leave school. Your appearance is truly alarming, but you marvel at the fact—maybe you are even touched emotionally—that your parents are more tuned in to your emotional needs than ever before. Remember, you made the point earlier that this was the first time in your entire life that you saw your father cry. (*The patient is crying at this point, the first sign of perceptible emotion in the session; offering her a tissue, the consultant continues.*) You may be uncomfortable with this, but emotional bonds between parent and child and between yourself and others outside your home are absolutely essential to your physical and emotional health.

The first session ended with the consultant asking K about the experience, noting that many patients feel a bit overwhelmed and exhausted by the process. She acknowledged feeling both of these things, but said she was curious about many of the things discussed, and surprised that so much of what the consultant said touched upon matters that she had been unable to comprehend fully up to this point. In spite of the fact that she had been ill over 7 years and well below normal body weight this entire time, the consultant felt that the prospects for treatment were favorable. K did agree to treatment, and its outcome, after a 2-month hospitalization and 29 months of biweekly outpatient individual and group therapy, was excellent.

"Sparring" with Patients

In some cases, the consultant will need to "spar" gently with patients, especially those who

present as if they were boxers, bound and determined to knock the consultant out of the ring.

E was one such patient. At 24, she had been ill with anorexia nervosa for 11 years; had been hospitalized four times for a total of 9 months; and had seen seven different therapists, all of whom she detested. She characterized her four male therapists as "arrogant pricks, for the most part," and was hardly more charitable in her descriptions of the three female therapists: "well-meaning but rather sappy women who I could never really respect." She was the second of three children from an exceedingly wealthy and socially prominent family. E was a brilliant woman, an artist, and an exceptional beauty (at least in earlier photographs). She had no close female friends and had never sustained a heterosexual relationship for more than several months. At the time of the consultation she weighed 98 pounds at 5'9".

Although E's background would be considered privileged by many, it was emotionally bleak. According to her description, her father was rude, volatile, and pompous, and as unpleasant as he was demanding. E described of her mother as a "showpiece"—very beautiful, but forced to tolerate her father's boorish behavior without complaints. She was "pathetically lacking in character, completely timid and submissive in my father's presence," in E's words. E said that she could never really love her mother because she pitied her too much; in addition, her mother had abused alcohol and various barbiturates throughout E's childhood and adolescence. For her father, E had only scorching contempt. She detested his hypocrisy, for the family's wealth was passed down from the grandparents. As she commented in her autobiography, "My father liked to strut his importance in the high society circles he traveled in, but my family's money is from inheritance; if we had grown up having to depend on his ingenuity, intelligence, or drive to support us, we would have been paupers." Neither of her parents ever read to her as a child, took serious interest in things that interested her, or displayed genuine physical or emotional affection.

E described herself as a difficult child—impossibly temperamental, difficult to please, and easily brought to explosive rage over little things. She was aloof from her parents, but remembered being terribly insecure and jealous of those who had a more balanced upbringing. She found many things difficult about her home life, especially the sense of disorder that came from seeing her parents taking so little responsibility for things that mattered. She, on the other hand, craved orderliness and regularity in her routines; she was mocked repeatedly for this by her brother and sister, both of whom she described as "on the shallow and dim-witted side" and completely indifferent to the family's hypocrisy. Her older sister, who (E always suspected) was easily intimidated by E's intelligence and physical beauty, took particular pleasure in introducing E to friends and relatives as "the congenitally oppositional and bratty sister."

E never was able to state what she hoped to gain from the consultation. She agreed to meet with the consultant only at the instigation (indeed, the insistence) of her gynecologist, a woman E had some respect for. And the consultant only agreed to meet with E out of respect for E's physician, who was also a colleague. At the juncture in the first session from which the following transcript is taken, patient and therapist had been discussing the nature of anorexia nervosa and its relevance to E's background. Throughout the consultation, E was challenging, skeptical, and cynical beyond reason, barraging the consultant with question after question. She was clearly uncomfortable with the process and was defensive out of all proportion to the consultant's manner. Yet not once did the consultant comment on this behavior.

PATIENT. Why is it then that so few women develop anorexia nervosa if we are all so crazed about the desire to lose weight?

THERAPIST. Have you ever wondered why yourself? It's an excellent question. I suspect it has something to do with the extremes of personality I spoke of earlier as showing up repeatedly in the background of people who develop this problem. It's my hunch that whatever shapes these personality traits is also what turns dieting into an unbending obsessional ritual. People who naturally find comfort in order and routine will just as naturally strive to restore ritual, discipline, and routine when

confronted with psychological challenges. Because of individual differences in temperament, biology, and emotional experience, the development of this illness comes easier for some than others. And then there are a host of emotional factors that reinforce the behavior once it develops.

PATIENT. So my asshole father and dumbbell sister were right all along: I'm biologically deficient. They would relish hearing you say this, you know.

THERAPIST. But I wouldn't put it this way. You are not deficient, but you have been hampered in your efforts to adjust comfortably to your development. Your adjustment has been compromised by self-defeating and misguided efforts to resolve these tensions and to maintain self-integrity in the face of disappointments and suffering. Unfortunately, it hasn't been easy for you to face up to any of this.

PATIENT. What makes you think I still suffer from these things? You shrinks have a habit of finding neuroses wherever you look to justify your professional existence and to pay the mortgage. (*There is no attempt at humor here; E states this mockingly and with contempt.*)

THERAPIST. E, really, that is absurd; why would you want to waste time with these ridiculous assertions? Just look at these drawings (*referring to the artwork brought by E to the consultation*). The figures are dark and muscular, and they fill the page. They have a bold presence, but their faces are either blank or burdened by sadness. I know little about art, but certainly artists express what is within. It's so self-evident that it surprises me that you would so easily deny this.

PATIENT. So what is the point about all this? I have to want to change, and I really do not want to be part of this world of feelings, attachments, and needs.

THERAPIST. But I have no intention of convincing you that you must. That never was the point of the consultation, which I was careful to point out at the very beginning. If remaining distant from others, living a life devoid of meaningful and nurturing friendships, and communicating mainly with razor-sharp cynicism are desired virtues, so be it; I concede your virtues. But I do think this is terribly tragic.

PATIENT. (*Smiling*) And why is it tragic?

THERAPIST. I can think of many reasons. Because as you continue to spurn intimacy and falsely boost your self-esteem through punishing restraint, you will deteriorate physically and become even more isolated and unhappy; because your creative energies are directed mostly by your troubling conflicts; because you are so busy trashing everything you believe your family valued that you have little time to explore what in life is genuinely meaningful to you; because you avoid receiving things any human being needs, out of fear that your life will repeat the same affectionless, loveless, and controlling relationships you grew up with. Your present and future are your past. This is why I think that it is terribly tragic.

This was the only point in the consultation when E was without a retort. The session ended shortly afterward. E said that although she appreciated the therapist's time, she knew she wasn't ready for such deep self-examination, but if this changed she would be in touch. She did not wish to return for the second session.

Eight months later, the consultant ran into E at a local shopping mall. This time, she greeted him warmly and reported that she had gained 10 pounds. She apologized for the "rudeness" displayed at the earlier meeting, and said that the consultation was more helpful than she imagined it would be. Asked what proved most helpful, she said it was partly the consultant's steady, unflappable way of relating to her, as if there was little she could do to be offensive or outrageous. It was exasperating, she said, because she had wanted so much for this meeting to end like her meetings with other therapists—that is, with the consultant being overwhelmed by her impossibly difficult style. The consultant told her that he never really did find her difficult, only uncomfortable, and that he was sorry she had decided she was not ready for treatment. E left saying that she knew she was getting closer to making such a commitment, and to doing so for the first time on her own initiative.

The Second Session

The time between sessions serves several purposes. The patient is asked to think deeply about what has transpired; to consider whether the issues dealt with in the first session encourage her to move ahead with long-term treatment; and, if so, to consider whether she prefers to work with the consultant or with another therapist. Likewise parents and other family members are asked to consider whether and in what ways they are prepared to assist this process, including keeping a respectful distance from it if this seems necessary. The patient is also told that if treatment is desired, an immediate question will be whether it should begin in an inpatient setting, ideally in a specialized program for the treatment of eating disorders. It has been my own experience that this is preferable when body weight is 30 pounds or more from the ideal; it isn't that very emaciated patients can never restore normal body weight in outpatient treatment alone, but rather that the process of doing so can drag on interminably. Accordingly, the patient is given a maintenance diet of between 1,000 and 1,200 calories per day and told that the decision will rest on how well she tolerates this regimen until her return to the second session. Likewise, patients who are purging or using laxatives or other substances are given a taper-down schedule to determine whether the frequency of these behaviors can be reduced so that treatment can begin with less immediate risk. If a patient cannot tolerate the diet or reduce the frequency of compensatory behaviors between the first and second sessions, acceptance of inpatient care is a prerequisite for the consultant to agree to her treatment.

WHEN ONLY MANAGEMENT IS POSSIBLE

Telling a patient or her family that she must learn to live within her illness is not pleasant, but it is foolish to deny that this is a reality for some. It is just as difficult to know when management is to be emphasized over treatment, since no "threshold" of chronicity can be identified that, when surpassed, increases a patient's refractoriness to change. But the adult patient with long-standing illness who has passed through adolescence and young adulthood completely asocial and asexual is, sadly, a poor risk for treatment; in this case, management of illness is a viable alternative to intensive therapy. Such patients' chronically low body weight (as opposed to rapidly deteriorating body weight, which poses far greater medical risk) allows them to adapt metabolically to prolonged malnutrition, even though they are at risk for significant bone disease and depressed immune function. If they concur, a management plan with the following components is then presented:

- Working up to a maintenance diet of at least 1,000 calories per day.
- Biweekly monitoring of vital signs and electrolytes.
- Very limited, passive, mild exercise.
- Attempts at some form of social contact, however minimal, to blunt the effects of isolation and invalidism.
- Weekly supportive counseling.

A POSTSCRIPT ON LONG-TERM TREATMENT

If the consultation succeeds, it is the first step in what will be a long, painfully slow process. Since anorexia nervosa arises from maturational crisis, the therapist, as Crisp writes in chapter 13 of this volume, must return her to the source of this conflict, but this time with her hand held securely. As the illness originates in a personality marked by extreme need for restraint and avoidance of things uncomfortably new and intense, the psychotherapist must lead the patient in directions opposite to those she feels most secure moving in—that is, toward experiences of deeper emotion, reflection without action, tolerance of growth and change, and nourishment (both physical and emotional). And in this same regard, if we believe that the coming together of drives for self-expression and interrelatedness is the cornerstone of identity formation, then surely psychotherapy is the setting in which this integration must be fostered. But this will be possible only to the extent that the therapist brings to the arena of treatment a deep understanding of the illness and its complexity, a keen sense of intuition, and the ability to remain steady and committed in the face of formidable challenges. Over time, this treatment must kindle in the patient an appetite for change that steadily grows stronger and becomes more compelling than the safety her illness affords. It is a new resolve—one that allows her to shed defenses that are destructive to her spirit, to explore hidden aspects of her mental life, to face up to her abilities without self-devaluation, and to permit the return of her body's natural form.

The success of this process is ultimately measured not only by the patient's commitment to a mature body shape, but by the strengthening of her desire to be sustained in her thoughts, feelings, needs, and self-directed actions, as well as of her willingness to face up to new experiences with greater curiosity and vigor. If she has trust in the therapist and in this process, there is greater hope of her living a life free of extreme vigilance and unnatural suppression of the body's vital energies. The present chapter offers a perspective on setting this process in motion.

NOTES

1. Throughout the chapter, female-gender nouns and pronouns are used in reference to patients with anorexia nervosa.

2. All consultations were recorded, and transcribed for use in this chapter, by permission of the patients. Some aspects of the patients' histories have been altered to maintain their anonymity.

REFERENCES

Bruch, H. (1988). *Conversations with anorexics.* New York: Basic Books.

Casper, R. A. (1990). Personality features of women with good outcome from restricting anorexia nervosa. *Psychosomatic Medicine, 52,* 156–170.

Cloninger, C. R. (1986). A unified biosocial theory of personality and its role in the development of anxiety states. *Psychiatric Developments, 3,* 167–226.

Cloninger, C. R. (1987). A systematic method for clinical description and classification of personality variants. *Archives of General Psychiatry, 44,* 573–588.

Crisp, A. H. (1980). *Anorexia nervosa: Let me be.* New York: Grune & Stratton.

Crisp, A. H., Joughin, N., Halek, C., & Bowyer, C. (1989). *Anorexia nervosa and the wish to change.* London: St. George's Hospital Medical School.

Gull, W. W. (1874). Anorexia nervosa (apepsia hysterica, anorexia hysterica). *Transactions of the Clinical Society of London, 7,* 22–89.

Lasègue, C. (1873). On hysterical anorexia. *Medical Times Gazette, 2,* 265–266.

Strober, M. (1980). Personality and symptomatological features in young, non-chronic anorexia nervosa patients. *Journal of Psychosomatic Medicine, 24,* 353–359.

Strober, M. (1991). Disorders of the self in anorexia nervosa: An organismic–developmental perspective. In C. Johnson (Ed.), *Psychodynamic treatment of anorexia nervosa and bulimia* (pp. 354–373). New York: Guilford Press.

Strober, M. (1995). Family–genetic perspectives on anorexia nervosa and bulimia nervosa. In K. D. Brownell & C. G. Fairburn (Eds.), *Eating disorders and obesity: A comprehensive handbook* (pp. 212–218). New York: Guilford Press.

Vandereycken, W., Kog, E., & Vanderlinden, J. (1989). *The family approach to eating disorders: Assessment and treatment of anorexia nervosa and bulimia.* New York: PMA.

Vandereycken, W., & Meerman, R. (1984). *Anorexia nervosa: A clinician's guide to treatment.* Berlin: de Gruyter.

CHAPTER 13

Anorexia Nervosa as Flight from Growth: Assessment and Treatment Based on the Model

ARTHUR H. CRISP

No one doubts that anorexia nervosa is difficult to treat. It is physically, psychologically, and socially crippling, and carries the heightened prospect of an early death: Mortality at 20-year follow-up of the core population of severely ill anorexics stands at around 15–20% (Seidensticker & Tzagournis, 1968; Ratnasurya, Eisler, Szmukler, & Russell, 1991; Theander, 1985). Yet the youthful, not to say childlike, anorexic individual seems unconcerned and desperately resists intervention, sometimes even preferring suicide. The individual is convinced that she will never "recover."[1] The disorder invites comparisons with other deeply self-destructive human conditions—for instance, the more severe substance dependence syndromes. It can lay claim to being the most severe of all mental illnesses.

As members of the health care professions, we seem to divide neatly into a minority of us who become deeply interested in anorexia nervosa and the rest, some of whom have little patience with these afflicted individuals and families. For those frustrated by anorexic individuals' resistance to change, their disorder may invite the dismissive and face-saving label of being self-inflicted. The weighting of the condition toward those of higher socioeconomic status can lead to further disapproval.

As might be expected, I have long pondered the source of my own fascination with this disorder. It cannot be my attempt as a medical practitioner to escape from the real world of suffering. The blighting, hopeless, and destructive nature of the condition ensure that this is not so. Can it be an undue preoccupation with the female form? (If so, how "undue" is undue?) I can say at least that it is not embedded in an actual eating disorder within myself; such a disorder would prove an insurmountable handicap to being helpful to an anorexic. Is it then a more benign but projected preoccupation with nurturing and growth, or even an omnipotent belief in my powers of resurrection of others? The ability sometimes to help a 25-kg near-comatose anorexic who is not responding to intravenous therapy to turn the corner and recover is deeply satisfying. Is it a fascination with puberty as a major and unavoidable life event (unless one develops anorexia nervosa!)—the first brush with the full extent of the real world and personal mortality? Or is it an attachment to the belief that a person's conception—the point when the parents first incorporate themselves biologically and experientially into the person, which can lay claim to being the first and most important life event—is laid bare for inspection when the condition is studied? In my case, the potential for better understanding of both conception and puberty, and of their impact on adolescence, has provided the impetus for my interest.

The inevitable consequent recapitulation of our own adolescence in that of our children, occurring before our very eyes, and the challenges and opportunities this provides for our own personal growth, are perhaps the outstanding properties of the family and the potential rewards that come from having offspring, if the basis of our own conception has been sound enough. I have found it a privilege to extend such experiences into the caring role in relation to other families and their offspring in the framework of anorexia nervosa. Moreover, recovery from anorexia nervosa often requires that some degree of depression and related self-awareness be experienced. I regard the ability to tolerate such depression—a state of mind wherein problems are acknowledged, although they may be daunting—as a sign of maturity and a potential gateway to a "sadder but wiser" position. No wonder I feel at home when working with anorexics and their families, so long as I have the security that comes with being the carer! And with anorexia nervosa, there are numerous physical as well as psychological and social markers to chart any progress.

Such thoughts both underpin and derive from the model of the psychopathology of anorexia nervosa that my colleagues and I have developed and used since 1960 in our efforts to help successive generations of anorexics. Indeed, our work has always been fueled by this need to try to help anorexics and their families. In the present chapter on our treatment methods, the model is briefly described, but detailed references to its experimental exploration are not included. Our ideas are elaborated in detail in the book *Anorexia Nervosa: Let Me Be* (Crisp, 1980/1995), which includes a relevant (and recently updated) bibliography.

THE MODEL OF THE PSYCHOPATHOLOGY

Anorexia nervosa, at the level of psychopathological mechanism, is construed as a phobic avoidance disorder. The phobic objects are normal adult body weight and shape, which are themselves markers for females' perceptions of their "fatness." In the fully fledged syndrome, the avoidance mechanism involves the pursuit and maintenance thereafter of a subpubertal weight, wherein this pubertally driven normal "fatness" is banished. The fear of any greater obesity within anorexia nervosa is not specific to it but such a fear is commonplace within the general population. However, maintenance of body weight at a subpubertal level is inherently unstable; the bodily imperative to ingest food and grow is unrelenting and powerful. Further weight loss may be the necessary insurance. In early-onset cases, the feared objects are less clearly experienced as full normal adult body weight and shape (which will never have been achieved); the fear is more attached to the need to avoid the level of body weight gain and shape change that would be associated with any further growth.

The typical anorexic's fear is of loss of control over this avoidance position, which, in the average and once fully grown female, is reflected in any weight gain above about 95–100 pounds (the biological point at which puberty usually begins). The avoidant position in anorexia nervosa is therefore a profoundly psychosomatic one, rooted in the seemingly miraculous and certainly unique capacity to reverse the pubertal process and hence all of its social and psychological impacts. The anorexic posture divorces the individual biologically from the aspect of her life that, sooner or later, has become the mainspring of her panic. It is no longer meaningful for her except as a receding memory, and is simply collapsed into and experienced as a fear of weight gain above the threshold. In very chronic anorexia nervosa, the specific details of the phobic objects themselves may be lost to sight. Most often, however, they are simply *denied,* especially to others. The revelation of the phobia may require reexposure to a fully normal adult weight, within which the pubertal process is reactivated.

For females (and a few males), the "fatness" that goes with normal adult body weight will always have had a sexual dimension, serving as it does both direct reproductive and related social and biological purposes, such as its attraction for males. The attempted regulation and control of weight and shape are commonplace among teenage females searching for a greater sense of ownership of the body and its impulses; the success of such attempts leads to enhanced self-esteem.

Pubertal development is not only sexual in the narrow sense, however. It heralds a spectrum of challenges as large as life itself. For the majority of males, such teenage bodily preoccupations center mainly on lean body mass—

often, the wish to be bigger and stronger—which also has biological and social purposes. The male's search for self-regulation more often targets this domain of the self. "Fatness" to him more often signals just obesity, and sometimes its potential stigmata of self-indulgence, poor self-regulation, and passivity. (Occasionally, when there is gender identity doubt, it also takes on a sexual connotation; it may then become a source of panic for that particular male, with the potential through flight for the emergence of the anorexic avoidant stance. However, the remainder of the present discussion is confined to females.)

Puberty is a lengthy process. In the female it starts well before the menarche, often at the ages of 9, 10, or 11. The first noticeable changes are often experiential and behavioral, having a concurrent impact on the individual and her parents. Puberty, like conception, is hardly "elective." It may immediately be experienced as unwanted, threatening, and destructive, either to the individual or to some part of the family system. Such impact, on the other hand, may be delayed until much later in life, when related conflicts (which may have been dealt with previously by social avoidance or reacted to with depression) are now reactivated or even prompted for the first time by events such as the first sexual experience, childbirth, death of parents, or even menopause. Puberty, as has been suggested, is sometimes also the first experiential brush with death. It is, after all, only necessary because of death. The greatest task in becoming adult is surely to render unasked-for puberty (and its antecedents) ego-syntonic. For the anorexic, it is or it becomes overwhelmingly ego-dystonic, coupled with mobilization of the flight mechanism.

The therapeutic task within such a model is in some ways an obvious but daunting one. Here is an individual whose development has been aborted—the most profound and regressed of all possible morbid reactions to puberty, except perhaps suicide. In some cases, it can be argued that the regression is not only to a subpubertal but to a prenatal level. Do the resources for development exist in the individual? Can they be mobilized and nurtured? Is the avoidant stance now so chronic that the gulf between it and maturity has become too great to bridge (since growth has already provoked a massive defensive flight at a time when the individual was more in touch with her peers)? And yet it is clear that some individuals can re-cover spontaneously, perhaps having effectively put a temporary brake on what would otherwise have been precocious or unacceptable development at the time. However, so-called "spontaneous remissions" are just as likely to be triggered by meaning-laden life events as the original illnesses were.

The theory holds that the precise biological mechanism involved is the depletion of energy, which then selectively reverses the pubertal process—a relatively expendable development in the face of such a threat to personal survival. This energy, in the form of identifiable calorie-laden food, becomes progressively restricted in the diet. Moderate and often relatively unsuccessful dieting is, of course, a commonplace attempt at self-regulation among teenage females, as noted above. Anorexia nervosa seems most often to arise within this more general setting. High-calorie food can readily come to be experienced as potentially "alive" by the anorexic, should she ever succumb to the temptation to eat it. Within the fully avoidant stance, resting metabolic rate is reduced. Body temperature falls accordingly (thermally protective hair grows); the cardiovascular system is appropriately muted; peripheral circulation closes down. Heat and the pubertal impulse are taken out of the system as pubertally related behavior and its fearful experiential aspects wither. In this sense, anorexia nervosa is a refuge, a foxhole, and a "back-to-the-wall" stance, with nowhere else for the individual to go.

The individual is sadly reduced to a unique form of the biology of starvation—that is, profound calorie depletion, restlessness and sleeplessness, total preoccupation with food, and the impulse to forage. In the presence of plentiful food, this impulse to ingest calories must be kept at bay at all costs. Defensive ritual, social avoidance patterns, and manipulative and tyrannical behavior may erupt, with such strategies being perhaps the only surviving and residual aspects of the individual's previously developing and often maladaptive coping styles. Anorexia nervosa arises in lieu of any attempt at normal personality development. The label "hysterical" may be pejoratively applied as others experience the power of the individual's resistance to intervention. Within this diminished state, many male and female differences are lost. Given the biologically unstable nature of the avoidant stance, and the necessary constant vigilance and exercise of control of the impulse to ingest, some residual sense of security, achievement, and competence can arise when the line is held. This sense is akin to the sense of triumph experienced by the severe ascetic who successfully quells the passions of the body through starvation and exercise, who seeks purity and unity projected to a cosmic level, and who usually escapes the label of "avoidant."

The model can be conveniently construed within the framework of panic disorders, with the attempted solution being the profound avoidant stance. The underlying "dyslipophobia" merges with that experienced by others (again, most often female)—for example, those with bulimia nervosa or with obesity that distresses them. It is also one end of the spectrum of the anxieties that are experienced by many teenage females, and that can prompt a variety of other, less self-destructive defensive strategies than the so-called "eating disorders." The term "eating disorder" no more describes anorexia nervosa than the label "cough" does justice to tuberculosis or lung cancer.

If the original maturational strain has also invoked disgust, then this too will survive to become attached, along with the panic, to any small lapse of dietary control and attendant weight gain. Such disgust (and anger), either conscious or driving the panic, may relate to the "last straw" impact of puberty on a previous childhood experience of sexual abuse; alternatively, it may derive less concretely from family attitudes to sex as fearful or destructive, for instance. Pure panic is more likely to be the response if simple separation or rejection is the challenge that puberty has brought.

The original potential depression (which I have claimed earlier to be the ultimate necessary pathway for recovery from anorexia nervosa, once weight has been restored) will not now be present. Nor will the maturational problem itself; this is the one thing the disorder has solved. Secondary depression is common enough, underlying the brave and defiant but brittle social facade that some anorexics can sustain. This is the depression of exhaustion, of an underlying awareness of wretchedness and hopelessness, and of eventually being abandoned by deskilled aging parents and by battle-weary, deskilled, and angry health care workers. The similarity to substance dependence in such respects is again apparent.

Sooner or later, if dietary restraint gives way to bingeing, then vomiting (and/or laxative abuse, etc.) is the last line of brittle defense. Under these circumstances, the metabolic status changes profoundly, and the whole adjustment becomes still more precarious. The neurotransmitter chemistry of anorexia nervosa, according to such a model as this, could hardly be more distorted. The principal impulses, especially with weight restored to normal, will be flight coupled with anger if the anorexic finds herself at bay. The undoubtedly disturbing and fear-laden impulse to ingest, experienced as potentially uncontrollable, will also still be present.

What then are the social context and other predisposing and precipitating factors for this condition, and how do they fit the model? Apart from being female and subject to the kind of relevant social constraints on adolescence that a middle-class upbringing most often generates, other factors can be a propensity for conflict avoidance behavior within the individual and the family. The sufferer will most often have been compliant as a child, but, if wayward, will have experienced puberty as additionally destructive and found that the anorexic stance is now necessary for belated compliance. The family, eloquently defending its openness, may nevertheless have always skillfully avoided confrontation over really divisive issues. However, the sufferer may still be in no doubt that love and support are conditional upon the control of impulses. Other morbid avoidant behaviors in the family at large, such as obesity, undue nurturing, excessive involvement in husbandry, family enmeshment, substance abuse or dependence, and depression itself may be well to the fore. Denial is the hallmark of the disorder, operating as it does both biologically and psychologically; the individual denies that she is ill and conceals relevant information, including her fear of weight gain. The original maturational problem no longer exists and may never have been articulated, or, if it was, will have been experienced as having an overwhelmingly destructive outcome.

My own thinking about the genetic and constitutional factors at work within anorexia nervosa includes the notion that they may contain the propensity for flight in the presence of strain; for a nurturant diathesis involving high growth rate; and for a unidimensional cognitive organization that concretely links sexual behavior with food and growth. Such possible biological factors, accounting for about half the variation underlying the expression of the condition, may still be susceptible to social modification through psychotherapy. However, the remaining developmental influences are also obvious factors in consideration of relationship-based psychotherapy. What may they be? The present family conflicts, centered on the food table, are the product of deskilled carers/parents who cannot get the individual to eat, and are secondary to the disorder and potentially universal under such circumstances. Little will be learned by focusing on them alone.

The integrity of some parental marriages depends on the continued presence of a child in their midst. Puberty can therefore have a destabilizing impact on some family systems. A given child—say, the youngest, or perhaps the one who is most overtly and potentially identifiable biologically with a restless father—may be left with anorexia nervosa as the only solution to survival of the parental marriage and a sustained but conditional loving bond with the potentially depressed mother. Perhaps the actual existence of the individual, now anorexic, is a symptom reflecting a manipulation 20 years previously to secure a failing marriage; subsequent development, with its conditional love and feared outcome, will hardly have been a seedbed for the emergence of a robust sense of self.

The perceived biological identifications and preferred affiliations of the offspring, ambivalences and all, will be aspects of the family development requiring careful analysis. The assumption that a person is better off putting to one side the relationship with one or the other scapegoated parent fails to acknowledge that a child remains a biological expression of that parent. The anorexic's resolution of this problem through her profound avoidant posture is clearly not a good situation for her.

Childhood sexual abuse, to which about 30% of female anorexics seem to have been subjected, is another experience that can inflame and be inflamed by puberty, rendering the latter intolerable. The origins of such abuse in the family will reflect wider sources of insecurity (lack of healthy and caring communication within the family and between the parents, related substance abuse or dependence, etc.) and will overdetermine the impact of sexual development upon such earlier abusive experience. Therapy may need to define and reframe the abuse in terms of its wider transgenerational and relationship aspects, in order to protect against its potential for possible splitting or other negative effects.

Some children, perhaps as many as 10%, do not have the fathers they think they have! Adolescence may then threaten to express the reality of this circumstance as a child's physical and personality features crystallize out. Or a child's conception may have generated a shotgun marriage, and the child's adolescence may be the key to its breakdown. Adoption brings special strains for an adoptee in adolescence, especially if, for instance, the adopting parents' problems in dealing with sexual issues have contributed to their infertility and to their unease about their daughter's illegitimacy. The continuation of the love and devotion that characterized her childhood may appear conditional on her suppression of adolescent behavior.

Still another scenario I have encountered is one in which growth into adult life brings the threat of hypertrophic cardiomyopathy, Huntingdon's chorea, cystic fibrosis, or other apparent genetic vulnerabilities; in such cases, anorexia nervosa may be experienced as the only potentially effective defensive strategy. Why anorexia nervosa in relation to, say, hypertrophic cardiomyopathy? Well, growth is associated with aging and precipitation of the condition, and brings with it, for instance, the specific risk of cardiac decompensation in pregnancy. If sexuality is perceived as a source of panic or badness anyway, and if the potential for defensive avoidance is there and other, better coping strategies are undeveloped, then the scene can surely be set. I have also seen anorexia nervosa develop as a defense against the teenage eruption of ulcerative colitis and subarachnoid hemorrhage as potentially life-threatening conditions; as always, it is wrapped up in a larger family psychopathology, and puberty is experienced as the destabilizing factor.

Alternatively, if physical development or an aspect of development of temperament in adolescence serves to identify the child physically and temperamentally with an unloved mother, who is rejected by the father to whom the girl has been especially bonded in childhood, then the development of anorexia nervosa may also be experienced as the only solution.

Clearly, the range of maturational problems that can give rise to the condition is endless. Personal and family psychological resources available to deal with such strains will be another major determining factor. The eruption of anorexia nervosa as the defense, rather than some other maladaptive adolescent response or even the capacity to survive and work through such problems, is the specific and necessary mechanism according to the model and has already been touched on.

The greater risk for females of developing eating disorders has been attributed to social pressure in a male-dominated world. I believe the link to be powerfully related to the nature of female puberty. As I have noted earlier, male maladaptive reactions to puberty most often take a different form, and anorexia nervosa in males is very rare.

Background cultural factors are often implicated, especially "fashion." Given the astute marketing philosophies of industry, "fashion" may be more a symptom of a given generation's need than a prompt to its sartorial destiny, though the process is clearly interactive. More relevant may be the broader background structure and social norms of society and its evolution. Anorexia nervosa has often been common in the past and may yield a more stable incidence over time than is claimed. There is evidence that it was common even in the 1870s, let alone the 1920s. Social forces that loosen the structural supports within society may render it a less secure environment for more vulnerable adolescents, who adopt flight responses when under strain. In recent decades, potentially protective customs such as courting and engagement have faded; the spectrum of maternalistic and paternalistic control, from the church through to the family, has lessened; and behavioral ground rules have become uncertain and complicated by new freedoms, such as those invited by the availability of female contraception. The adolescent rebellions of the late 1960s were perhaps recent symptoms of and watersheds for inevitable changes in the limits that could thereafter be set upon behavior. Perhaps anorexics and bulimics are among the casualties of these changes. Equally stifling can be an oppressive culture, which for some may provoke anorexia nervosa as the means of continued bonding when, otherwise, rebellion and rejection would have resulted. This can be seen at the interface and potential clash between permissive cultures and those (e.g., Islam and certain evangelical sects) demanding strict codes of conduct, including culturally restricted marriage.

THE ASSESSMENT

It is the model described above that determines the pattern of assessment my colleagues and I have adopted over the years, as well as our subsequent interventions when sufferers and their families present with the condition already established (Figure 13.1). Anorexia nervosa is ego-syntonic (synchronous with the sense of self); the prospect of intervention is alien and resisted at all costs by the typical anorexic. Occasionally, of course, an individual seeks help. This may be a search for institutional control of a bulimic episode that is threatening the anorexic's capacity to control her weight, though it may be presented as a wish for more fundamental help. Rarely, a request for help may reflect an anorexic's genuine wish to give up the exhausting struggle of sustaining the illness and to escape its grip; such a wish may arise as threshold chronological ages (e.g., 30) are approached, parents die, or the like.

More usually, the anorexic comes to the consultation only because she is trapped by circumstances. She is trying to work out what the price of disengagement from this particular situation will have to be: Will she have to gain a few pounds, show some willingness to relate to you, and so on? It is the same position, for instance, as that confronting the cornered alcoholic.

The purposes of the assessment must include the goal of enabling the anorexic to seriously consider the possibility of real change, with the distant prospect of recovery. She starts in a profoundly avoidant position. She is avoidant in biopsychological terms, because her long-standing anorexia nervosa has completely disconnected her from the precipitating problem; she is also avoidant in terms of her minute-to-minute strategies for sustaining the condition. She has no sense of ever being anything other than anorexic; the task of allowing her to see some light at the end of the tunnel, some prospect of further life rather than the possibility of early death (which she currently accepts with indifference), is formidable. In my view, this is the pivotal intervention in any case of anorexia nervosa.

We normally expect to complete a face-to-face assessment in 3 hours, buttressed by several further hours of planning and production of a report, which thereafter serves as the basic statement concerning the psychopathology behind the case.

I would not normally expect to meet with an anorexic without also meeting with her family. It is this encounter that most often has the immediate potential to reveal the essential under-

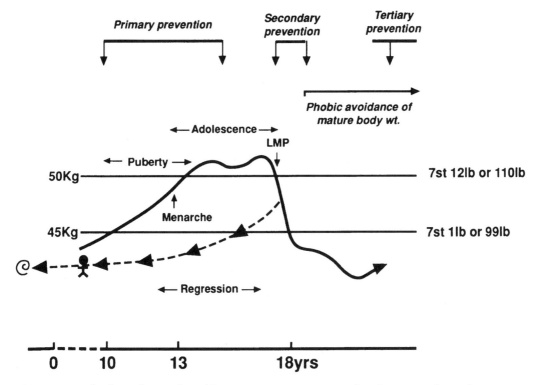

FIGURE 13.1. The three phases of possible preventive intervention within the course of typical anorexia nervosa.

lying maturational pathology. For an understanding of the case and also for treatment purposes, this remains important, whatever the chronological age of the anorexic may be. For example, a 34-year-old anorexic who has been ill since she was 17 has, in my view, been psychologically 9 years old at the most since that time, however well qualified she may be otherwise. Her adolescent developmental psychopathology, which overwhelmed her at the time has since been aborted. Her family, in its own right and also genetically and introjectedly within herself, is as vital an element as ever. You will be reassuring this particular individual that the very most she needs to fear is the picking up of her emotional development again at the age of 17. If this is lost sight of, and if her target weight is not matched accordingly, then a precious building block in the attempt at recovery will have been discarded. Also noteworthy is the fact that she has already failed once at the task of development; now her peers have grown away, her parents aged, and so on. Nevertheless, if the parents cannot help to liberate her (and themselves) now, then the task will be all

the greater and will fall exclusively upon the therapist, with all its transferential demands and reality elements.

It is axiomatic that the more resistant the anorexic or one or both of her parents are to attending, the more important it is that they do attend, or else at the least understand how important you see it as being. This applies whatever the circumstances (e.g., the parents have divorced and remarried). How far therapy will be able to go with involvement of the family will be a judgment to be made later.

It is my custom to see the parents first. Such an arrangement has familiar potential pitfalls (e.g., the perceived collusion with the parents in terms of misguided efforts to achieve weight gain; the smothering of any history of sexual abuse). These need to be attended to forthwith, obviously with the parents themselves, and also subsequently with the anorexic. This is a matter of professional attitude, explanation, and proper handling of initial transferences.

The parents, often long deskilled, may be impatient or desperate to hand over the "case" and often feel that they are being blamed for the illness. It is important to begin by reassuring the parents that "blame" is not going to be a useful concept, but also by emphasizing that their central and overriding importance is not to be doubted. To cite an extreme instance, a biological father who has played no part in the anorexic's upbringing has nevertheless contributed an inescapable half of her genetic makeup. It may be just this factor that has presented as an overwhelming temperamental challenge within the emergence of the offspring's puberty. I reiterate my view that people cannot effectively forge their individuality without first acknowledging their biological inheritance of both body and mind.

The parents are invited initially to report on the history of the illness, before embarking on systematic reviews of themselves, their background, and their relationship. Most parents of anorexics accept the relevance of all this without question by this stage. You will seek, nonjudgmentally, to build up a picture of them both—their temperaments, their childhood backgrounds (often so relevant to the present issue), their belief systems, and their relationship. (A statement such as "Tell me something about your relationship—doubtless you will have had your 'ups and downs'" conveys an invitation to them to disclose. This can be followed later by "Tell me about a time when your relationship was at a low ebb," etc.) With such inquiries, accounts may begin to emerge that clearly link these events with illness onset. Moreover, you can enable them to, and expect that they will, describe aspects of their personal lives and relationship that have never before been shared with others or even with each other. Under such circumstances, therapy will already have begun; this requires the relevant skills from the outset.

You should search for likenesses between the anorexic and her parents. Often parents see their children as like one or the other of them or like someone else in the family, physically and/or behaviorally. Their expectations regarding the child's destiny, and in particular her emerging adolescence, are shaped accordingly. Other possibilities to explore include favoritism and possibilities of nonpaternity. Ask, "If Lucy didn't have anorexia nervosa, what would things be like today, as far as both she and you are concerned?" For example, would the parents have split up? Would the child be estranged because of her behavior?

This initial systematic approach to the parental relationship has been described in greater detail elsewhere (Crisp, 1980/1995). It usually provides the basis for enabling the parents to become involved in subsequent treatment—that is, to become "patients" themselves. This may have been far from their thoughts, but it can be a greatly reempowering process, provided that they can accept the need for personal change—even, for instance (though not often), the ultimate rupture of their own relationship. Other family members (siblings, stepparents, etc.) may also need to be met at this stage and with the same purposes in mind. These systematic assessments, of parents and of other family members, will take 1 to 2 hours.

Next, whoever is undertaking the assessment meets with the individual. The anorexic's overriding fears and wish to flee are likely to have intensified as she has waited within the context described above, trapped by circumstances. Initial reassurance will clearly be in order. By this time, you should have in mind a first working model of the psychopathology of this case, and can begin with an initial judicious sharing of its outline, avoiding premature closure. You should be reassuring about the need for others (e.g., parents, the consultant himself or herself) also to become involved in a new attempt at the growth process. An empathic comment concerning the therapist's awareness of the anorexic's very high levels of panic should be provided. So should reassurance (if possible) that compulsory detention and treatment are not the intention. (First, anorexia nervosa is already a state of "compulsory detention," and such treatment will now compound transferential problems and the psychopathology; second, anorexics close to death can still usually become voluntarily engaged in treatment aimed at helping them recover through this alternative, reempowering approach; third, as we all know, an anorexic's ultimate decision to die is hard to deflect with or without compulsory treatment, and the individual's best chance under such circumstances may be to be offered the package described here.) Finally, the anorexic should be enabled to conclude here and now that you are truly not in collusion with her parents.

Thereafter, the consultation proceeds systematically with conventional history taking. You should use recognized facilitatory skills to maximize the chances of revelation of taboo subjects (e.g., sexual abuse) across the current three generations of the family.

This initial interview with a potential "patient" (a "patient" is defined as someone who has decided that she has a condition she would rather not have, and that there may be someone around to help her get rid of it) will end with a more conclusive sharing of the problem as now identified by the consultant. The offer of help will be made; on average, treatment will need to last for about 6 years,[2] and will usually include the task of gaining weight sooner or later to fully normal adult levels. The outline of the psychotherapeutic help on offer will be shared. The conditions (e.g., regarding weight gain, and hence diet and eating patterns) attached to continuity of treatment along these lines will be stated. This approach is similar to that usually adopted when treating, say, an alcoholic (no drinking) or an acting-out personality-disordered individual (no violence). The treatment is clearly going to stand or fall on the quality of these factors: psychotherapeutic input; the individual's and family's innate and developing capacity to respond; and the structure and support that accompany the behavior constraints concerning weight gain as the necessary condition for the continuing relationship-based psychotherapies. Under certain circumstances, of course (e.g., in some patients who have been ill for 20 years or more), full recovery from the condition will not be the stated goal. Instead, the aim will be the optimal stabilization of the anorexia nervosa for the foreseeable future.

Immediately thereafter, we normally meet with the family as a whole. The understanding so far concerning diagnosis and prognosis is shared, as is the offer of intervention. The diagnostic formulation itself is normally made at four levels:

1. The manifestly abnormal behavior—a function of starvation, the attendant impulse to ingest food, and the battery of defenses against this (i.e., to avoid weight gain above 82% mean matched population weight).
2. Recognition, directly or indirectly, of the underlying phobia about normal body weight and shape (often denied by the patient).
3. Identification of the preceding maturational problem (no longer existing, rarely self-evident, or readily disclosed and now superseded by a nonspecific conflict over eating).
4. Identification of the psychological resources potentially available within the individual and family for the former's growth.

The anorexic is likely at this stage to be in a state of intense panic, despite the approach described above. A few anorexics will be eager to engage with the help being offered, but it is wise to ask that the individual and the family go home, think about the matter carefully, read some relevant literature, and write to the consultant indicating their decisions by the end of the following week. The recommendation given may have been for inpatient or outpatient care, and each will have had its own psychological impact. The prospect of inpatient care invariably brings with it the prospect of tighter immediate control by others over the patient's body weight. In order for this to be perceived in other than negative transferential terms (e.g., as further evidence of control and conditions being imposed over the whole of the anorexic's destiny), an immediate explanation needs to be made along these lines: "Our treatment is aimed to help to liberate you from the trap of your illness, and to help you begin to experience the freedom of being yourself in terms that transcend your body. At the moment, you perceive yourself as only existing in terms of your body size. Although this is important, it does not need to dominate your life. Reactivation of your biological maturity through weight gain will be an essential step towards personal growth." This approach secures the initial engagement of virtually all patients.

It is crucial not to offer the alternative of outpatient care if you believe that inpatient care is necessary. The anorexic will almost always opt for outpatient care if she perceives that option to exist. It is in her makeup to be powerfully avoidant, and she often needs to be protected against this, which will still be there even if you have begun to win her over. On the other hand, many severely ill anorexics can be helped from the start in the much less costly outpatient setting.

TREATMENT

This section of the chapter briefly addresses the form and consent of our treatment package. This package was first created in 1960 and has thus been in development for over 35 years.

The notion that treatment needs to last for about 6 years sound daunting to some patients and their families, as well as to most managers and insurance companies. It is important to clarify the concepts and practices involved.

Treatment must provide a significant new learning experience for the individual concerned, and preferably one that does not create a division between her and her family. The anorexic needs protection from her propensity for psychological splitting and other primitive psychological defenses, which will block any such learning. Movement toward a mature state, increased awareness of feelings, improved capacity to tolerate depression, greater problem-solving skills—these are the goals from the outset.

It is better if parents can be involved, but the alternative must not be to dismiss them. They and their relationship live within their offspring, and no amount of geographical or emotional distancing can change that fact. To deny it is to introduce another serious block to change. One sees it often enough with angry, helpless anorexics, bereft and avoidant of professional help, who are insisting on so-called "self-help" as the only remaining and viable fallback position. Our own self-help book, *Anorexia Nervosa: The Wish to Change* (Crisp, Joughin, Halek, & Bowyer, 1996), begins by examining the concept of self-help, which it presents as the cornerstone of effective professional help. The main aim of our assessment procedure as described above—apart from identifying as much of the psychopathology as possible—is to engage the individual and to involve her in the processes of change, rather than allowing her to continue to feel that everything is being done *to* her.

The treatment alliance, keeping patient and family on board, can be meaningfully sustained over a 6-year period with no more than about 50 outpatient psychotherapy sessions lasting 1 hour each, coupled with 12 or so sessions of expert dietary advice. Other health care professionals in the team may need to become involved from time to time (e.g., a social worker). If an initial inpatient package is needed (and sometimes a second and even third such package), then we still follow it with the basic outpatient package of 50 or so sessions (see Appendix 13.1). The intensive input that goes with inpatient care demands that psychotherapeutic contact not be too quickly diluted thereafter. Continuity, in the sense of there being just one therapist throughout this time, is a most important aim. If it is impossible, then the transition to a second therapist must be planned and worked through psychologically. It is usually also important for the second therapist to carry the same working model of the psychopathology within his or her mind (this model is of course always undergoing updates and revisions as appropriate), and to be part of the team in that and all other senses. The anorexic's potential for psychological splitting will remain powerful; the team members need to protect her against this by working together and by providing continuous supervision of the case in general and the therapy in particular. To this end, the therapist must be able to set aside a further 25 hours for such supervision during the 6-year period. Supervision time can, however, include other cases in appropriately organized teams. Importantly, no member of the team should have anorexia nervosa or any other dyslipophobia!

From the outset, the patient and normally also the parents will have been asked to sign a logbook (Crisp, 1995, p. 3). The relevant passages within it are reproduced below.

1. A statement from us:

You and your family may all experience the psychotherapy that you become involved in as quite challenging and invasive. We believe you know this because we will have told you so but we would like you and any family members involved to commit yourselves here to this aspect of the treatment. You may all find that doing this now in this formal way will help you in the months to come when you are under strain and can look back to this point.

2. Endorsement by the patient and family:

We all understand that we are engaging in psychotherapy and not only consent to this but agree to participate actively with the aim of solving the problems that are currently causing the anorexia nervosa.

Signed

_____

(person with anorexia nervosa)

Signed

_____

_____

(family members)

The logbook provides a basis for self-reflection by the patient in respect of her psychological state and changes within it. The book is structured accordingly, addressing such matters as the following (Crisp, 1995, pp. 14–31):

The meaning of my shape to me
The triggers of my illness and their meaning(s)
My family relationships before and since anorexia
My sense of self—social
My sense of self—sexual
The origins of my anxiety
My use of avoidance to deal with conflict
My family's use of avoidance to deal with conflict
My other moods
Why I approach others in the way that I do
My present or future career; why I have chosen it
My relationships with authority
My impulses and the way I manage them
Difficulties with my choice of food
New things/situations I would like to try
My difficulty gaining/maintaining weight
Any other problems (please specify)

Within the inpatient program, there is a separate "logbook partner"—a member of the team who will share the work being done within the logbook sessions with the key members of the team when the case is periodically reviewed. Of course, the patient must be aware of all such communications and must feel that she is in a position to determine how much is shared and how much within individual therapy is not shared. In the outpatient setting, this role of "logbook partner" will often need to be collapsed into that already occupied by the designated psychotherapist. The same applies to the family work. In the inpatient setting, there are separate family therapists working more intensively with the parents and other family members, but also sharing relevant and agreed elements of this work with the full team. In the outpatient setting, this work will again usually fall on the one psychotherapist and will be discharged through occasional and predictable sessions with the parents alone or together with the patient, still all as part of the 50 or so overall sessions.

The concept of 50 sessions is held as a minimum viable number, lending real credibility to the task in hand. It may need to be extended, but it is the case that the basic package often suffices. Outlines both for free-standing outpatient care and for outpatient care following inpatient treatment are provided in Appendix 13.1. If even this level of therapeutic commitment is impossible, then a scaled-down version still spanning 6 years or so is worth trying and is described in our book of guidelines (Crisp & McClelland, 1996).

The conditions surrounding the program include the patient's and parents' right to contact the therapist or other known and trusted members of the team if there is a problem that cannot otherwise be solved. In a well-run program this rarely happens, but it is a much-valued element; many of our patients have subsequently indicated how supportive they found the knowledge that they could make such contact if necessary. In the United Kingdom, collaboration with the general practitioner/family doctor team will also often be helpful as well as a professionally appropriate measure.

Dietary Advice

If dietary advice is to be given by a dietitian, then that person needs to be a full member of the team, to accept the model, and to have a full understanding of the program. With appropriate psychotherapeutic training, such a person can also become an occasional psychotherapist. This sort of experience, properly supervised, is invaluable in strengthening the team in its identity and goals. These patterns reflect the medical leadership that characterizes our own team.

In our team the selected medical personnel also possess the relevant psychotherapy skills, through the background residency training programs we have; however, these skills are clearly not restricted to medical personnel in principle, and are also sometimes very expertly exercised by some clinical psychologist and social worker colleagues. These attributes include basic competence in individual, family, and group psychotherapy, as well as in cognitive-behavioral approaches. But, to revert to the dietetic dimension, the anorexic for whom full recovery is the aim will have a target weight set, according to general population weight/height tables that relate to her age of illness onset. (These are not actuarial tables; they are reproduced in two of our books [Crisp, 1980/1995; Crisp et al., 1996] and accommodate the effects of advancing age on weight.) Under such circumstances, many anorexics become keen to identify an earlier than actual age of onset! This must be dealt with on a reality basis. The mean target weight for 1,000 anorexics who have come through our service is thus a fraction under 54 kg. In anorexia nervosa, there is a world of difference between 54 and 45 kg. The latter is usually an anorexic and often a fully subpubertal weight, and very far indeed from the normal adult weight, which provides a necessary index of approaching normality. Eventually, the best way to identify full recovery is to wait for the anorexic to report genuinely that such a weight is her "preferred" weight.

Weight gain to target levels, though accepted as essential for treatment, is itself dependent upon the anorexic's continued trust in the prospect of ultimate recovery within the present treatment. This weight will still be associated with mounting panic and (one almost hopes) with mounting depression as she contemplates the real tasks of growth and individuation, which have previously proved overwhelming. This time they require a proper solution; meanwhile, depression—a sense of helplessness but of sustained recognition of the real problem—is appropriate. Also appropriate will be renewed psychotherapeutic effort at this stage.

Ideally, this weight gain will be secured not through counterphobic attitudes, but through a prescribed diet and a conviction that you will be able to protect the patient from overweight and has no secret ambition to promote such overweight. Moreover, the patient must be convinced that you will not lose sight of her mounting distress because of the euphoria of others who either tell her that she looks recovered or else destructively tell her that she is "too fat." Not surprisingly, one parent or the other can sometimes be the culprit under such circumstances.

Dietary advice depends upon the treatment setting and the level of exercise (itself obviously the subject of psychopathological analysis in assessment and of subsequent therapeutic scrutiny). In the inpatient program, with bed rest being the arrangement, a prescription of 3,000 calories per day invites a predictable weight gain of 1 kg/3 pounds per week. Within the assessment style and treatment approach described here, the majority of anorexics can enter the hospital and immediately begin to eat in this way. The notion that the gut needs to adapt is not borne out by the fact that over many years our patients have settled down either immediately or within a few days and begun to eat in

the way described above. Initial resistances reflect ambivalence about the process and then will be expressed in terms of "feeling full" and the like. Figure 13.2 illustrates the rate of weight gain and the steady weight immediately thereafter of a large number of successive patients treated in this way about 15 years ago and reported later (Crisp, Mayer, & Bhat, 1986).

Deviations from such weight gain indicate noncompliance and can act as prompts for psychological exploration (e.g., plateauing of weight significantly often occurs around the 45-kg mark, when the pubertal process is being reactivated). Most of our patients gain weight steadily, as Figure 13.2a shows. Thereafter in the inpatient program, increased mobilization occurs and diet is modified accordingly so as to ensure a leveling off of weight. As the figure also reveals, 21% of the patients we studied did not achieve full target weight (Figure 13.2b), but many of these came close to it and certainly broke through the "82% of mean matched population weight" (see Crisp et al., 1991).

The inpatient program is intensive and also involves twice-weekly group therapy (the goals of this are outlined in Appendix 13.2); body image classes; communication and assertion skills training (the real problem here is to help the anorexic to generalize such developing skills to other settings [the groups, family therapy, the ward routine, etc.] in a constructive way); sex education (it is vital to remember that puberty and full reproductive potential are being reactivated in someone who is socially unskilled and has a very poor sense of boundaries—I have known conception to occur without return of menses); and drama therapy. Most of these and other related treatments have also been part of the basic inpatient package since 1960 and undoubtedly contribute to the overall psychotherapeutic effects. However, it is the core psychotherapy that is the most powerful tool, as research into our treatments shows (see "Outcome" below).

After discharge from the hospital, many patients initially lose some weight. It is essential for them to know that continued psychotherapy may be contingent on their maintaining their discharge weight, or at least embarking now upon a course of regaining it. They may now feel more confident about this task; indeed, they may wish to undertake it, with the conscious expression that it now seems to be under their control and therefore that much more acceptable. During the inpatient program, they

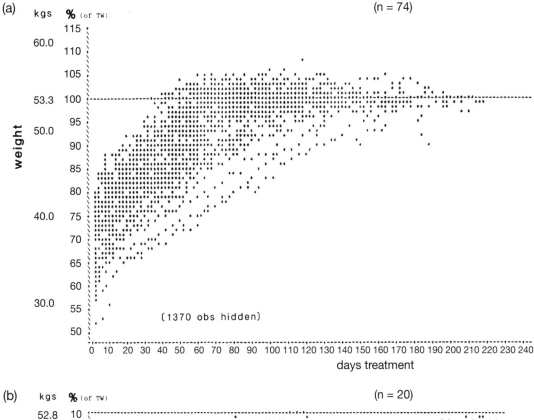

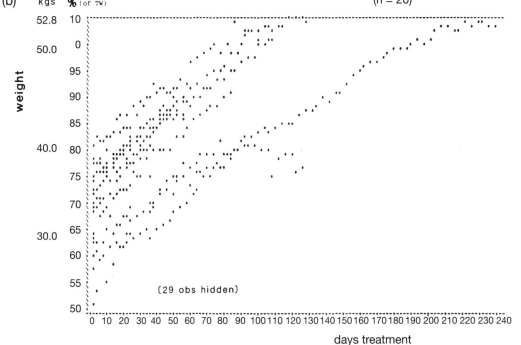

FIGURE 13.2. (a) Composite weight chart of patients reaching target weight. (b) Composite weight chart of those who did not reach target weight. From Crisp, Mayer, and Bhat (1986, pp. 1009 and 1012). Copyright 1986 by the *International Journal of Eating Disorders*. Reprinted by permission.

not infrequently feel that this important aspect of themselves has been taken over by the team, despite our efforts to reempower them in all other respects. The separate *de novo* outpatient program has a less rigid approach to weight gain (the team can afford for this to be so). However, in the 10-bed inpatient program, all the patients gain some small comfort from the fact that they are being treated similarly in respect to their weight, and this takes the weight issue out of the arena as much as can ever be possible with anorexics. Ultimately, the therapeutic task is to render puberty ego-syntonic for them, that is, to make it a process and state they feel in charge of, and one that does not leave them feeling disgusted, worthless, rejected, in danger, and so forth.

The details of the dietary advice for the outpatient package are spelled out in our self-help book (Crisp et al., 1996) and appear here as Appendix 13.3. They were generated by Carol Bowyer, the senior dietitian/nutritionist who worked with me for many years. The three diets, A, B, and C, are intended to (A) prevent further weight loss as an essential first step if treatment is to start, (B) to secure an intermediate weight gain to about 45 kg if recovery is not the goal, and (C) to aim for full recovery.

In all instances, sustained vegetarianism is allowed if the stance predates the onset of the illness. Otherwise, it is treated as a symptom and addressed psychologically, and it is surrendered as part of a pathological weight control strategy. Bingeing (which the inpatient is protected against by the strict dietary program and the explicit instruction that visitors will not bring food in), vomiting, and laxative abuse are subject to the same constraints. Again, within the inpatient program vomiting is not possible because of the conditions of bed rest, and laxative abuse is usually rapidly detected if it is continuing to occur. Appropriate advice and support are given in regard to normal bowel movements.

Psychotherapy

The broad aims of psychotherapy are (1) to support the patient in moving out of the avoidant psychobiological position; (2) to contain her consequent panic, which for her is reality-based (it was previously panic about the possibility of weight gain and has now become displaced onto food); (3) to contain her subsequent depression; (4) to explore and facilitate her potential for a greater sense of competence and own-

ership of her body; (5) to explore and facilitate her potential for an expanding multidimensional perception of the self in ways that are no longer totally dependent upon physical appearance and that promote sufficient self-esteem; and (6) to address her related rekindled psychosocial problems. These broad aims are not qualitatively different from those confronting *all* human beings developmentally as they face the human task of growth toward consciousness and a sense of personal identity—a process requiring the "sadder but wiser" outcome.

As noted earlier, the anorexic has already failed once in the task of growth. Lack of adventurous exploratory childhood behavior; concrete, undifferentiated association of sexual development and impulses with the ingestion of food; and the subsequent failure to recognize or incorporate sexuality as an emerging separate currency for peer relationships frequently represent some flawed developmental building blocks. Such characteristics, rooted in both the biogenetic and personal experiential childhood backgrounds as described earlier, will need to be addressed within the family system—ideally, both as it now exists and also in its incorporated biological (genetic) and introjected (developmental) forms.

The individual, although now technically a patient, starts from a profoundly regressed position that I have suggested is at the least prepubertal, but that in many senses appears psychologically to be more like a prenatal fusion with a "nonnourishing" placenta. In the previous pubertal or postpubertal state, unbridled or even modest expression of impulsivity may have precipitated panic or disapproval in an enmeshed family system, or else shattered the bonds of conditional love. Sometimes, of course, the emergence of anorexia nervosa has reflected a less damaged development, being no more than a temporary break needed within the context, say, of an otherwise unduly rapid and precipitate growth into early puberty and its associated puppy fat, which almost understandably threatened other developing areas of competence (e.g., academic achievement and social exploration). Even so, it invites the question as to why such a radical defense has arisen, instead of any attempt at a less destructive solution. For instance, under such circumstances there may well have been secret panic in the first instance, but no obvious distress/depression or search for help.

The psychotherapeutic tasks of enabling such individuals to develop and thereby to significantly alter the long-term outcome of the condition can appear formidable, and, as previously stated, usually require a long-term dedication to therapy. Apparently major short-term shifts may reflect a more benign natural history in a particular case, but are more likely to prove spurious in the longer term. The ingredients of the psychotherapy mirror many of those that are also key to the overall team approach and have been previously mentioned within that context. They include the following:

1. *Trust.* This will be a product of such factors as the competence of the assessment, the skill of the individual and family psychotherapy, and the quality of the teamwork.

2. *"Conditional" aspects of treatment.* These address the matter of the patient's weight and reflect the "behavioral" elements of the program. They are rooted in the original contract, wherein the individual has agreed (however reluctantly or ambivalently) to the target weight, having understood the reasons for it—that is, reengagement with the biological reality of puberty, and ultimate restoration of the psychobiological position to the chronological age at which the disorder developed and further emotional development was no longer possible. Within this context, the patient will be (a) either fully complying with the dietary plan or, at least, striving to do this; and (b) curbing any vomiting, laxative abuse, excessive exercise, or the like. These behaviors will be subject to scrutiny within the logbook, within the psychological therapies, in day-to-day observation (for inpatients) or within the home setting (for outpatients), and finally through regular weighing and charting of weight.

The hazards of this element of treatment have already been alluded to. For instance, it can only work if the patient has come to trust and believe in the importance of the umbrella psychotherapy. It also runs the risk of being perceived as another form of conditional love, and requires clarification, explanation, and interpretation in that respect. It requires the team to take a unified view of the goal, with everyone fully understanding the processes that are underway, and with no one nursing hidden opinions that, say, the target weight is unreasonable. This aspect of treatment will also come under strain if parental anxieties begin to rise as weight increases, and especially if (as previously described) such anxieties then become focused on the target weight and on a secret wish for it to be less.

3. *Transference.* The limited experience, concrete thinking, and primitive psychological defenses of the average anorexic invite the immediate attribution of powerful superficial transferences toward key members of the team from the outset. From the moment of first contact, control of related countertransferences, diffusion of belief systems rooted in blame, and prompt explanations and interpretations will usually be in order. And yet the patient's concern to differentiate herself from her parents, within either a potentially very primitive or negative early projection onto the therapist, must not be secured at the expense of polarizing oneself in relation to the parents or of splitting the patient's perceptions of the parents into good and bad, respectively.

Such issues, if handled adequately, do not initially depend much on the sex of the therapist, although this may still govern such processes as the ready disclosure of sexual abuse. The possibility of sexual abuse must obviously always be borne in mind, as must that of mistaken parentage. These issues provide obvious further complications to the immediate transferences. They therefore need to be approached nonjudgmentally, and the therapist must be ready and able to address them if and when he or she feels that they are becoming powerfully relevant. However, an interpretation—for instance, "I sense that you are expecting me to feel disgusted about [or, alternatively, to be identified with] your sexual abuse, and I want you to suspend judgment while you get to know me better and to test me out"—will not hold water if it is not true.

As treatment proceeds and deeper attachments between therapist and patient develop, they will come increasingly to contain the elements of reality within the relationship—the mutual dependence. Within this context lies the potential for exposing, containing, and helping with the patient's emerging depression. Solutions will begin to be needed. Under these circumstances, the continued involvement of the "real" parents—that is, the minimization of further splitting and attempts at further reempowering the parents—can become crucial.

Sight must never be lost of the concept behind the target weight. For example, a 30-year-old patient who is a postdoctoral fellow at a university is emotionally 15 years old (or whatever age she was at the onset of illness) when she achieves her 54 kg. This, of course, takes no account of the original fragile emotional development up to that point and prior to the illness, and the patient's current natural regression on this account and in relation to the therapy. These powerful forces can best be contained (involvement of the parents, etc., apart) by the predictable sessional contact that has been prescribed (see Appendix 13.1), of which the patient is fully aware, and also by the teamwork approach, whereby the patient can witness the team functioning healthily as an extended family.

Within the packages described here, the frequency of therapy is substantially reduced as time goes on. The program is structured so as to protect against undue prescribed dependence, while at the same time allowing contact between sessions if necessary. Its strength lies in its promise of at least 6 full years of contact if weight is gained and held. To most patients with anorexia nervosa, such concepts (i.e., 6 years of treatment, target weight related to age of onset) make good sense and invite trust. However, powerful countertransferences arise. The therapist needs to be able to let go, as does any parent. Letting go does not mean total loss of contact, however. We encourage our patients to let us know how they are doing; we follow groups of them up systematically (sometimes after as long as 20 years).

It is the transference issues that benefit most from supervision, since these demand that the therapist look at himself or herself. Such a process not only is important for therapy, but also provides a special opportunity for the personal growth of the therapist—a process that can occur to some extent in healthy parenting, as initially suggested, and that can become a telling factor in sustaining interest in this condition. Because the strains of working with anorexia nervosa are formidable (as we know, it is not possible to help all anorexics), we have to be able to live with failure in regard to patients to whom we have inevitably become attached.

Explanation, clarification, and interpretation are essential aspects of the psychotherapy and provide a basis for improving the patient's communication skills and lateral thinking. Her propensity for avoidance behavior will have affected her capacity to communicate verbally, because she fears verbal expression as a source of conflict. Coaching in related communication skills and assertiveness needs to be provided within the psychotherapy. Examples of explanation and interpretation have been given above.

As always, they must be deployed judicially as processes and must address the whole panoply of the personal and family psychopathology described earlier. They also need to be complemented by listening; it is crucial to continue to talk the patient's own language. By this, I mean that the patient will still be perceiving her destiny in terms of her weight and shape, and attempts to help her develop from this position will need to start from it. One such effort, for instance, will involve examining the precise location of her sense of fatness (a logbook item); its relationship to her female siblings, her mother, and other female relatives; its relevance for sexuality; and her and her parents' concerns about sexuality.

The psychotherapy package also includes the giving of advice. This may include reminding the 30-year-old postdoctoral patient described above that she is currently approaching the emotional age of 15 and should not rush into far-reaching decisions about her career and personal life. This will require that the consultant treat her appropriately and bear the full awareness of her immaturity in mind, without her perceiving this as patronizing. Areas covered will include sex, developing relationships, the need to avoid pregnancy, and so forth. It may even include advice about leaving home, but such decisions are best left primarily to the patient to make within the psychotherapy, being judiciously examined and supported or not as the case may be. Our 30-year-old patient might well be better off living back at home with her parents in the first instance. Moving away, to the other side of the world even, might simply serve to freeze any potential development; she would simply take the conflict (and her parents, genetically and introjectively) with her. After all, it would not be usual for a middle-class girl aged 15 (the emotional age of this hypothetical patient) to leave home.

Work with the Family

Work with the family has been described in some detail in *Anorexia Nervosa: Let Me Be* (Crisp, 1980/1995). Throughout this chapter, I have emphasized the importance of family involvement. Not all parents can respond, but many who start unpromisingly can come to grapple with the tasks in hand. The parents' basic task must be to liberate their daughter. This may go back to lifelong indifference/rejection or may reflect more active panic about growth, impulsivity, and separation. Such backgrounds may require at least some further scrutiny of where the parents "come from," what has secured their relationship, and so on. It may occasionally require examination of what has ruptured their relationship and some reattribution of related blame. It is after all especially difficult for a child to integrate her parents' make-ups within herself, both biogenetically and through developmental identifications and attachments, if their relationship is powerfully and primitively ruptured. Anorexia nervosa will have been the only solution for a patient, who has thereby banished the destructive and bad part of herself—the part identified with the bad parent.

The emergence of sexual abuse as a factor is especially fraught with danger, but such abuse has often been perpetrated by a brother or other male relative rather than by the father. If the perpetrator is the father, then the abuse may already be a background feature of a disrupted marriage; if it has occurred secretly within an enmeshed, noncommunicative, and heavily defended family, then the prospects are not promising. Unexpected rupture of the parental marriage may be the outcome, but beneficial therapeutic outcome for the patient is rare. A period of intensive work may need to be done with the patient first, to help her decide whether to share sexual abuse information with her parents. Any such sharing often best occurs thereafter within a family session.

The emergence of nonpaternity will need to be dealt with on an individual-case basis. We have at times clarified the matter medically, with good therapeutic effects. In one case, the clarification of paternity doubt in favor of the mother's husband not only resecured the marriage in a fruitful way: It reduced the father's depression and high alcohol consumption, and, more pertinently, it liberated the patient to get on with her life through a clearer view of herself and the consequent tasks ahead. She had not been aware of the real uncertainty concerning her paternity until after treatment had started. However, her childhood emotional insecurity, inflamed by the onset of puberty, had always been fueled by the unspoken possibilities that characterized her parents' marriage.

Some sessions with the parents together and apart from the patient (all part of the 50 overall sessions whenever possible) can be very helpful. Suitably orchestrated, such sessions allow the parents to continue to share things about themselves with each other that have previously been taboo (e.g., aspects of their own adolescences). Previous avoidance of such issues may have blocked any capacity for the mother, for instance, to talk with her daughter about sexual matters in the past. Now she may more readily be supported in doing this within future family meetings, which will usually also involve the father.

Parents also run the risk of becoming depressed. Whereas previously the mother was depressed, now the father may be, or vice versa. Other reactions may erupt (e.g., heavy drinking, major weight change). I have witnessed a myocardial infarction in a mother at the point of her daughter's achieving her target weight—a development probably precipitated by the related strains. Such events can be guarded against, once one becomes aware of the major stress endured by some parents who are genuinely trying to help by engaging in their daughter's treatment.

To summarize:

- Parents, through accompanying treatment, can sometimes play an important role in helping their daughter escape the grip of anorexia nervosa.

- In doing so they run the risk of personal upheaval and strains in their relationship, though the therapy also aims to address these problems and to help them achieve as good an outcome for them as possible.

- Such involvement can be helpful at any chronological age so far as the patient is concerned, though it may be somewhat less relevant or necessary if the illness onset is exceptionally late and has occurred within the context of another relationship. However, a late onset will have arisen within the context of a reactivated adolescent conflict, which can usually still be examined fruitfully in relation to the earlier nuclear family.

- At the least, involvement of the patients' parents, spouse/partner, or other family members should aim to minimize the potential block on change and recovery in the patient, which may otherwise operate powerfully—for example, if the illness is cementing the parental marriage on behalf of one or the other parent (usually the mother), or if the patient is married and the illness is cementing the marriage for the husband.

Areas of Therapist Competence

The necessary areas of therapist competence have already been briefly touched on. In case they may be helpful, the minimum training requirements (followed by several further years of "in-service" supervised experience) for the spectrum of relevant skills are outlined in Appendix 13.4.

OUTCOME

The natural history of core cases of anorexia nervosa is often one of chronicity and, significantly often, early death. "Spontaneous" recovery can also occur, but such recovery will be as importantly related to life events as was the onset. The impact of treatment on this natural history (as distinct from the effect of brief life-saving interventions) can only be usefully judged in the long term—if possible, within internally controlled studies, and always with careful follow-up. Comparisons of outcome between different clinical populations receiving different treatments are not defensible unless the populations concerned can be shown to have been very similar in their initial makeup.

Our own outcome studies have been reported over the years, but more recently we have described two further studies. The first of these (Crisp et al., 1991) involved random allocation of 90 patients to one of four treatment conditions, including "no further treatment by us." The other three conditions were the inpatient package briefly described above, the outpatient package described above, and an outpatient group approach involving separate group therapy for patients and for parents. Within these conditions we deployed the same principles of treatment as described above. However, a major and inevitable departure was the ability to provide only 12 follow-up outpatient sessions, all concentrated within the first year after assessment, for patients receiving the inpatient package. This constraint was a function of impoverished psychotherapeutic resources, which were insufficient to allow us to take on any additional commitments over and above those being routinely undertaken. Inevitably, the inpatient package offered much more intensive initial treatment. The recruitment to the study spanned the period 1982–1987.

The methodological problems within the study have been reported on elsewhere (Gowers et al., 1988). They included the following:

1. The impossibility of retaining contact with a control group that had not even been assessed in the first instance.

2. The use of the "no further treatment by us" group for control purposes under these circumstances, despite the therapeutic impact that we are convinced stems from the initial assessment procedure, one purpose of which is to engage the individual and family as "patients." This effect would have been complicated in the "no further treatment" group by the impact of the subsequent random allocation and rejection of those patients and families for treatment (this was the hardest aspect of the study).

3. The problem of having to allocate any one case to the randomly chosen setting when we judged that either inpatient or outpatient care would have been more beneficial in that instance.

4. The inability to deliver more than the 12 follow-up outpatient psychotherapy sessions spread over only 1 year, when our firm belief, as stated, is that the need and the promise should be for a 6-year contract. Thus many of the inpatients did well until this enforced point of discharge loomed.

The total follow-up extended over a 5-year period. Figure 13.3 shows the outcomes in weight terms by the 1-year follow-up. It can be seen that the patients who accepted the inpatient package reached, at their maximum point, almost 100% of mean matched population weight (on average, almost 55 kg). The enforced allocation to inpatient care when outpatient care would have been better ensured greater rejection of such treatment than usual; however, as the figure shows, all patients were included in the outcome analysis, regardless of whether they accepted treatment. It can also be seen how the weight of the "no further treatment by us" population (in the figure, the "one-off" group) only rose to the lower limit of puberty and then retreated from it. Many of these had received active treatment, including extensive hospitalization elsewhere (inevitable because of the severity of their illnesses). Our two outpatient populations also did very well, and actually ended the first year better than the inpatient population—not surprisingly, since the

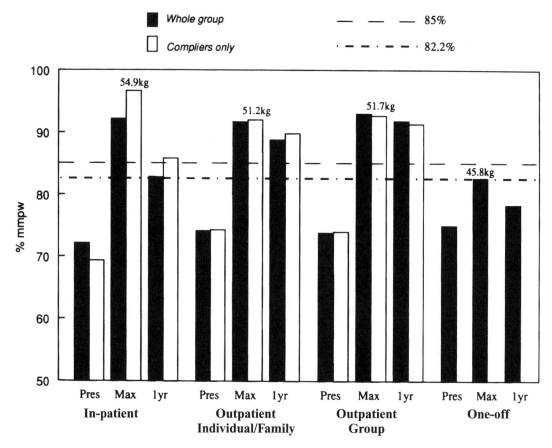

FIGURE 13.3. Mean body weight (without clothes), expressed as percentage of mean matched population weight (mmpw) at presentation, at maximum, and at 1-year follow-up, for the three treatment groups and the control ("one-off") group. The figure shows percentage of mmpw for current age; treatment was aimed at mmpw for age of onset (i.e., very slightly lower weights). From Crisp et al. (1991, p. 331). Copyright 1991 by the Royal College of Psychiatrists. Reprinted by permission.

latter, exposed to the intensive inpatient package in the first instance, suddenly felt almost abandoned on discharge with only the prospect of 12 attenuated sessions of follow-up. Nevertheless, at the 2-year follow-up, the individually treated outpatient population was still doing especially well (Gowers, Norton, Halek, & Crisp, 1994). In retrospect, it was a weakness of the study to concentrate these few follow-up sessions within the first 12 months and not to spread some of them over the later period.

These weight improvements in the first and subsequent years of follow-up were mirrored in other measures (e.g., dietary, menstrual, social, sexual), as compared with these measures for the control group. The differences between the populations at the 2-year follow-up are illustrated by weight comparisons between the outpa-

tient group involved in individual/family therapy and the control group; these are presented in Table 13.1. There have been just two deaths—one on the waiting list for treatment and one within the inpatient group. Together, these findings indicate that, in the short term, our treatments are significantly beneficial. The project based follow-up after the 2-year period unfortunately became contaminated and impractical because some of the "no further treatment by us" cohort had to be taken into our treatment programs. These patients had become desperately ill; their need for care could not be met elsewhere in our region, and the obligation to treat and our wish to do so supervened.

The second study involved a 22-year follow-up of 104 female patients originally assessed

TABLE 13.1. Outcomes at 1 and 2 Years: Weight and Body Mass Index (±/*SD*s)

	Outpatient psychotherapy (n = 20)	One-off assessment (n = 20)
Weight		
Presentation	40.31 kg (± 3.8)	41.02 kg (± 6.1)
One year	48.76 kg (± 6.2)°	43.92 kg (± 8.0)
Two years	52.51 kg (± 8.5)°	46.24 kg (± 8.6)
Change at 2 years	12.05 kg (± 8.4)	5.21 kg (± 6.3)
Weight as % of mean matched population weight		
Presentation	74.5% (± 6.9)	75.0% (± 8.5)
One year	88.9% (± 11.7)°	79.5% (± 14.1)
Two years	94.5% (± 14.0)°	83.0% (± 15.4)
Body mass index (wt/ht^2)		
Presentation	15.52 (± 1.4)	15.84 (± 1.7)
One year	18.97 (± 2.0)°	16.93 (± 2.8)
Two years	20.09 (± 2.8)°°	17.83 (± 3.2)
Change at 2 years	4.54 (± 3.0)°	1.99 (± 2.5)

Note. The data are from Gowers et al. (1994). Adapted by permission from John Wiley & Sons.
° $p < .05$ (*t* test across groups).
°° $p < .01$ (*t* test across groups).

and treated according to need between 1968 and 1972 (Crisp, Callender, Halek, & Hsu, 1992). These patients were earlier followed up at between 4 and 7 years (Crisp, Kalucy, Lacey, & Harding, 1977; Hsu, Crisp, & Harding, 1979). In particular, only four of these patients have so far died. The patient population was chronically and severely ill at the outset, comparable in such respects with those reported elsewhere. Table 13.2 shows differences in mortality among several such populations at 20-year follow-up. Our own 4% mortality rate is not different from that expected within the comparable general population, though the causes of death were in some instances obviously related to anorexia nervosa. In particular, if these differences can be attributed to the impact of our treatments, then the numbers dying from suicide can be claimed to be reduced from around 5 or so per 100 to 1 per 100 over a 20-year period.

It is extremely difficult to be categorical about the impact of treatment on such a disorder as anorexia nervosa, but we view our data as supporting the effectiveness of our treatment for a significant number of individuals and families. We also view the data as showing that our treatment is not capable of curing everyone with anorexia nervosa. In this chapter, on behalf of my team over the years, I have tried to share some of our methods in the hope that they may be of interest. The references cited in the text amplify various aspects of the model and related interventions. I have now retired from this work at St. George's Hospital Medical School; I wish my readers good luck with their own.

TABLE 13.2. Mortality in Anorexia Nervosa at 20-Year Follow-Up

	Causes of death			
	Anorexia nervosa	Suicide	Other	Total deaths
St. George's[a] (n = 108)	2 (2%)	1 (1%)	1 (1%)	4 (4%)
Aberdeen[a] (n = 63)	3 (5%)	4 (6%)	1 (2%)	8 (13%)
Maudsley[b] (n = 41)	3 (7%)	3 (7%)	1 (2%)	7 (17%)
Sweden[c] (n = 94)	12 (13%)	5 (5%)	2 (2%)	19 (20%)

[a]The data are from Crisp, Callender, Halek, and Hsu (1992).
[b]The data are from Ratnasurya, Eisler, Szmukler, and Russell (1991).
[c]The data are from Theander (1985).

NOTES

1. Because most individuals with anorexia nervosa are female, I use feminine nouns and pronouns throughout the chapter to refer to such individuals. (An exception is Appendix 13.4, where masculine pronouns are used for general psychiatric patients and therapists for the reason noted there.)

2. As we know, everyone is different. Some patients will not need such a lengthy program. They may already be on the road to recovery when they come to the consultation; others may need longer if therapeutic resources can be stretched that far; obviously some may never recover despite one's best long-term efforts, although the anorexia may survive because of them. The program described here is therefore put forward as a realistic model that is applicable in round terms to the majority of cases, producing the kind of results described later.

REFERENCES

Crisp, A. H., Burns, T., Drummond, L., Heavey, A., Lieberman, S., Norton, K., & Powell, A. S. (1993). *The learning of communication skills and psychotherapy: Educational goals, content and processes.* London: Department of Mental Health Sciences, St. George's Hospital Medical School.

Crisp, A. H., Callender, J. S., Halek, C., & Hsu, L. K. G. (1992). Long-term mortality in anorexia nervosa: A 20-year follow-up of the St. George's and Aberdeen cohorts. *British Journal of Psychiatry, 161,* 104–107.

Crisp, A. H., Kalucy, R. S., Lacey, J. H., & Harding, B. (1977). The long-term prognosis in anorexia nervosa: Some factors predictive of outcome. In R. A. Vigersky (Ed.), *Anorexia nervosa* (pp. 55–65). New York: Raven Press.

Crisp, A. H., Mayer, C. N., & Bhat, A. V. (1986). Patterns of weight gain in a group of patients treated for anorexia nervosa. *International Journal of Eating Disorders, 5,* 1007–1024.

Crisp, A. H., Norton, K., Gowers, S., Halek, C., Bowyer, C., Yeldham, D., Levett, G., & Bhat, A. (1991). A controlled study of the effect of therapies aimed at adolescent and family psychopathology in anorexia nervosa. *British Journal of Psychiatry, 159,* 325–333.

Gowers, S., Norton, K., Halek, C., & Crisp, A. H. (1994). Outcome of outpatient psychotherapy in a random allocation treatment study of anorexia nervosa. *International Journal of Eating Disorders, 15,* 165–177.

Gowers, S., Norton, K., Yeldham, D., Bowyer, C., Levett, G., Heavey, A., Bhat, A., & Crisp, A. H. (1988). The St. George's prospective treatment study of anorexia nervosa: A discussion of methodological problems. In D. Hardoff & E. Chigier (Eds.), *Eating disorders in adolescents and young women* (pp. 301–311). London: Freund.

Hsu, L. K. G., Crisp, A. H., & Harding, B. (1979). Outcome of anorexia nervosa. *Lancet, i,* 62–65.

Lieberman, S., Hafner, R. J., & Crisp, A. H. (1978). Teaching psychotherapy in mental hospitals. *British Journal of Psychiatry, 111,* 398–402.

Ratnasurya, R. H., Eisler, J., Szmukler, G. J., & Russell, G. F. M. (1991). Anorexia nervosa: Outcome and prognostic factors after 20 years. *British Journal of Psychiatry, 158,* 495–503.

Seidensticker, J. F., & Tzagournis, M. (1968). Anorexia nervosa: Clinical features and long term follow-up. *Journal of Chronic Diseases, 21,* 361–367.

Theander, S. (1985). Outcome and prognosis in anorexia nervosa and bulimia: Some results of previous investigations compared with those of a Swedish long term study. *Journal of Psychiatric Research, 19,* 493–508.

The following books can all be obtained through the Psychology Press, c/o Afterhurst, 27 Church Road, Hove, BN3 2FA, England:

Crisp, A. H. (1995). *Anorexia nervosa: Let me be.* Hove, England: Erlbaum. (Original work published 1980)

Crisp, A. H. (1995). *Anorexia nervosa: Patient's log book.* Hove, England: Erlbaum.

Crisp, A. H., Joughin, N., Halek, C., & Bowyer, C. (1996). *Anorexia nervosa: The wish to change* (2nd ed.). Hove, England: Psychology Press.

Crisp, A. H., & McClelland, L. (1996). *Anorexia nervosa: Guidelines for assessment and treatment in primary and secondary care* (2nd ed.). Hove, England: Psychology Press.

The last three titles are available as the "Anorexia Nervosa Clinician's Pack" from the Psychology Press as above.

APPENDIX 13.1
Outpatient Treatment Plans

FREE-STANDING OUTPATIENT TREATMENT PLAN FOR ANOREXIA NERVOSA (INFORMATION FOR PATIENTS AND STAFF)

The free-standing plan involves 6 years of contact with the specialist team. Following the initial assessment and identification of developmental psychopathology, the greatest density of psychotherapy sessions (sometimes also involving other family members) is within the first year. Thereafter, the frequency of sessions diminishes within the overall framework of expected discharge from care at the end of the sixth year.

Year 1	Weekly for 6 weeks	6	
	Every 2 weeks for 20 weeks	10	24
	Every 3 weeks for 24 weeks	8	
Year 2	Monthly	12	
Year 3	Every 2 months	6	
Year 4	Every 3 months	4	
Year 5	Every 4 months	3	
Year 6	Concluding session	1	
	Total sessions	50	

In addition, sessions with the team dietitian will be as follows:

Year 1	Every 2 months	6
Year 2	Every 4 months	3
Year 3	Every 6 months	2
Years 4–6	Annually	3
	Total sessions	14

This program is dependent upon the patient's capacity to gain weight in an agreed-upon way within it and to maintain it thereafter. Often the expectation will be that normal adult body weight is achieved in this way. Deviations from, suspension followed by review of, or curtailment of the program may arise if it becomes evident that this specialized treatment is not helpful in altering the course of the anorexia nervosa for the better.

TREATMENT PLAN FOLLOWING INPATIENT TREATMENT FOR ANOREXIA NERVOSA (INFORMATION FOR PATIENTS AND STAFF)

Year 1	Following the assessment and identification of the developmental psychopathology, *the first 4–5 months will be taken up with inpatient treatment.* Thereafter, there will be an extended period of further core psychotherapy and dietetic support as a basic arrangement. These psychotherapy sessions should usually unfold as follows:	

	Weekly for 14 weeks	14	23
	Every 2 weeks for 4 months	9	
Year 2	Every 3 weeks	17	
Year 3	Every 3 months	4	
Year 4	Every 4 months	3	
Year 5	Every 6 months	2	
Year 6	Concluding session	1	
	Total sessions	50	

Usually there will also be some further separate family therapy sessions, providing continuity with the prior separate inpatient family therapy, and now aiming at conclusion within 2 years. Six to nine sessions during this period is the norm.

In addition, follow-up sessions with the team dietitian will usually be as follows:

Year 1	Every 3 months	4
Year 2	Every 4 months	3
Year 3	Every 6 months	2
Years 4–6	Annually	3
	Total sessions	12

Deviations from, suspension followed by review of, or curtailment of this program may arise if body weight cannot be maintained or if other crises occur and there is a question about the suitability of continued specialist treatment.

APPENDIX 13.2
Operational Policy for Small-Group Psychotherapy for People with Anorexia Nervosa as Part of an Intensive Hospital Care Program

CHARACTERISTICS OF THE PATIENTS

There are currently 10 inpatient places and several day patient places for people with anorexia nervosa. This unit is situated in a larger 43-bed unit providing care for people with a variety of psychiatric problems.

GOALS OF THE TREATMENT

The goals of treatment are to enhance symptom relief and personal growth in the patients whenever possible, and always to avoid damaging the patients.

THE PSYCHOPATHOLOGY AND ITS TREATMENT

Free-ranging anorexia nervosa has a psychopathology that allows little or no conventional social access. It is a conflict avoidance stance that has harnessed the mechanism of psychobiological regression through the banishment of pubertal processes. It is sustained at the price of constant vigilance within the context of the need to maintain an inherently unstable subpubertal body weight. The individual's identity is substantially reduced to the psychobiology of starvation—incessant thoughts of food, impulses to forage and to eat, and the necessary battery of defenses against this. The ego boundary becomes limited and subject to the same forces (e.g., "badness" is collapsed into weight gain; foraging and hoarding, within the context of loss of greater sense of self, lead to "stealing").

Ideally, acceptance of the treatment program reflects a degree of trust that has developed as a result of the initial assessment and exploration of the underlying maturational problem. It includes motivation to explore change and to accept weight gain and its confrontational consequences. It needs to be fostered. It, and the associated weight gain, render the patient slightly more accessible to social interventions (including those within group psychotherapy). However, the patient remains defensive and with only a slowly increasing sense of personal boundaries and social competence. Even therapeutically intended social interventions run the risk of being perceived as invasive, persecutory, and destructive. The habitual family and personal defenses include splitting mechanisms (e.g., splitting of the staff within the primitive transferences), avoidance mechanisms (e.g., noncommunication and denial), and excessive manipulation and control of others. At the same time, the patient has difficulty in differentiating herself from what is happening in the people around her (e.g., other anorexics, nonanorexic but impulse-ridden patients on the unit), and she will be affected by this. The overall psychotherapy approaches to anorexia nervosa are aimed at enabling the patient to gain insight into the adaptive nature of the condition (i.e., how it has provided a solution to maturational problems) and to learn to cope with reemerging maturational conflict as weight is gained. This is done through the following means:

1. Meeting primitive transferences by control of countertransference and interpretation.
2. Thereby improving communication and enabling patients and their families to share thoughts and feelings more safely.
3. Helping the patients and families to solve the problems that arise as a result of these interventions (e.g., coping with the task of separation–individuation); this in its turn will require patients and their families to tolerate more dysphoria (through such newly found nonjudgmental but genuine and professional support as is available). Also, helping patients to develop self-esteem and new areas of competence through such processes as self-revelation, learning, and practice.

THE ROLE OF GROUP PSYCHOTHERAPY

The group probably requires to be oriented to the needs of the anorexic patients, but must also address the needs of any occasional nonanorexic patients in the group. However, addressing the psychopathology of adolescence is usually relevant to all patients in one way or another.

This group is inevitably characterized by special boundary problems. First, there is the influence on it of the other inpatients, including those with problems that the anorexics are heavily defended against and have limited resources to handle. Second, the patients typically have very limited healthy ego structure, individually and as a group (note the apparent inactivity and noninvolvement of anorexics in the ward milieu). Third, there are the psychological consequences of hospital admission, which involves acceptance of psychiatric patient status and the consequent risks of dependence and impaired self-esteem (however, the profound regression of free-ranging anorexia nervosa is surrendered by anorexics who accept admission, and this militates against sustained hostile dependence within treatment). Fourth, the contractual obligation to be in the group brings with it transference problems of a special kind for patients with anorexia nervosa, which essentially itself has been a state of "compulsory detention." Fifth, the therapist must play a dual role in requiring "good" compliance with the weight gain program, while at the same time adopting a nonjudgmental approach to the consequent maturational psychopathology. Sixth, the turnover of group membership can be rapid. Finally, a variety of therapists must sometimes be used.

The potential therapeutic factors in group psychotherapy have been identified as follows:

1. Catharsis.
2. Self-disclosure.
3. Learning from interpersonal action (e.g., learning how to relate adaptively).
4. Universality (i.e., learning that one's own problems are not unique).
5. Acceptance (i.e., being valued and belonging).
6. Altruism (i.e., having something to contribute to solving other people's problems).
7. Guidance (i.e., learning how to tackle one's own problems).
8. Self-understanding (i.e., learning something important about oneself that is liberating).
9. Vicarious learning (i.e., learning through identification and through watching other people solve their problems).
10. Instillation of hope (i.e., gaining of a sense of optimism through the achievement of others in the group).

Other commentators, discussing inpatient groups with the characteristics identified in this document, have emphasized the relative importance of the less invasive factors such as catharsis, universality, altruism, and instillation of hope. Patients themselves believe such factors to be important. However, the boundaries among the 10 factors listed above are overlapping. Moreover, despite the particular defensiveness of anorexics, they are concurrently being intensely involved elsewhere in individual/family/marital psychotherapy, communications skills training, psychodrama, and the ward milieu, and should therefore be potentially more open to self-disclosure and exploration within the group, provided that the context is right. Indeed, the group can be potentially fruitful in this sense, in that such processes within it can facilitate a sense of universality and vicarious learning throughout the group (including the nonanorexic patients). Because of the patients' low self-esteem, therapists can often helpfully reveal any positive regard they have, being careful to avoid transference traps. They can also often usefully actively encourage communication, including the invitation of comments. Moreover, the therapists can carefully point out areas of conflict, discriminatingly "raising the temperature" in a session, in order to encourage working through conflict rather than avoiding it. Active but also sensitive interventions of this kind can help anorexics to feel safe, whereas prolonged silences may reinforce their habitual avoidance mechanisms and leave them feeling as incompetent as ever. Such silences can also become intolerable when they are incompatible with patients' helpless perceptions of expectations that they should be communicating.

Such therapy three times weekly requires expertise in the conductors. Given the boundary problems and the particular defensive strategies of anorexics, there are also obvious advantages in having as much continuity of therapist involvement as possible. The group is then more likely to complement usefully the many other facilitatory relationships that spring up between various members of the team and the patients. The tasks within the group should transcend these processes and be more focused.

The group is open to outside observation by invited staff, students, and visitors, with the permission of the group members, and on the basis that professional confidentiality is maintained.

SUPERVISION

1. Weekly, of the Tuesday group behind the one-way screen.
2. Once monthly, based on (a) reports from the conductors, and (b) video film excerpts of a sample group.

APPENDIX 13.3
Eating Plans

	A No. of portions	B No. of portions	C No. of portions
Breakfast			
Cereal	1	1	1
Bread	1	2	2
Fat	1	2	2
Jam/marmalade	—	—	2 teaspoons
Midmorning			
Fruit	—	1	1
Lunch			
Bread	1	2	2
Protein	1	1	2
Fat	1	2	2
Salad/vegetables	√	√	√
Fruit	1	1	1
Chocolate cookie or biscuit	—	—	1
Midafternoon			
Fruit	1	—	1
Cookie or biscuit	—	1	2
Evening meal			
Starch	1½	1½	2
Protein	1	2	2
Fat	1	1	2
Salad/vegetables	√	√	√
Fruit	1	—	—
Dessert	—	1	1
Bedtime			
Cookie or biscuit	—	1	2
Milk throughout the day	1	1	1

Note. See below for details of what constitutes a "portion."

CONVERSION FACTORS

1 fluid ounce = 25 ml
1 ounce = 25 g

WHAT CONSTITUTES 1 PORTION?

Starch

Bread: 1 slice from a large medium-sliced loaf (whole wheat or white)
Potato (baked or boiled): 100 g
Potato (mashed): 1 rounded tablespoon
Rice (boiled): 2 rounded tablespoons (weight before cooking 25 g)
Pasta (boiled): 2 rounded tablespoons (weight before cooking 25 g)

Breakfast Cereal

Bran flakes or cornflakes: 25 g
Shredded wheat: 2 biscuits
Muesli: 25 g

Protein

For lunch:
  Eggs: 1 large
  Cheese (cheddar type): 25 g
  Cottage cheese: 100 g
  Baked beans: 2 tablespoons
  Tuna fish: 50 g
For evening meal:
  Red meat: 50 g cooked weight
  Chicken: 50 g cooked weight
  White fish: 100 g cooked weight
  Beans (e.g., kidney): 100 g (after soaking)
  Lentils: 25 g (dried)

Fat

Butter/margarine: 1 teaspoon
Vegetable oils: 1 teaspoon
Low-fat spreads: 2 teaspoons
Mayonnaise: 1 teaspoon
Oily salad dressing: 1 teaspoon

Milk

Whole: 300 ml
Semiskimmed (2%): 450 ml

Fruit

Apple or orange or pear: 1 medium
Banana: 1 small
Fruit juice: 150 ml
Soft fruit (e.g., raspberries, strawberries): 150 g

Dessert

Yogurt, pudding, etc. (not diet varieties): 1 individual pot (135–150 calories)
Vanilla ice cream: 2 scoops

Chocolate Cookie or Biscuit

Individually wrapped biscuit: 1
Two-finger Kit-Kat: 1
Small chocolate chip cookies: 3

PREPACKAGED MEALS

Calorie content of ready-prepared meals for the evening meal: Diet A, 250–300 calories; Diet B, 350–400 calories; Diet C, 450–500 calories.

Note. This appendix is adapted from Crisp, Joughlin, Halek, and Bowyer (1996, pp. 69–71). Copyright 1996 by the Psychology Press. Adapted by permission.

APPENDIX 13.4
The Learning of Communication Skills and Psychotherapy

This appendix is condensed and adapted from a booklet describing the requirements for learning communication skills; also psychodynamic and cognitive-behavioral psychotherapy, in our educational programs for trainee doctors (residents) in psychiatry. They are reproduced here because they serve to identify the minimal skill levels I consider necessary to provide effective psychotherapy for individuals with anorexia nervosa. Professionals other than psychiatrists may also find them helpful for this purpose. (*Note.* The use of masculine pronouns reflects usage in the original booklet and is not intended to be sexist.)

EDUCATIONAL GOALS

Basic Clinical Communication Skills (not detailed here)

Dynamic Psychotherapies

General Goal

To produce a general psychiatrist who has a critical appreciation of psychodynamic theories and can apply that understanding to himself, to his colleagues, and in the treatment of his patients.

Specific Objectives

(1) A degree of self-awareness that permits the therapist to understand more about his reactions to patients and his own range of psychological defense mechanisms. He should have some heightened awareness of his own temperament and prejudices. He should understand something about his motivation to be a psychiatrist. He should be able to recognize and acknowledge his feelings as they arise within his work, in regard to both the frustrations and the rewards.

(2) The ability to contain or harness his self-awareness for the purpose of helping the patient.

(3) The ability to assess and formulate the patient's presenting psychopathology (and that of significant others and their relationship[s] with the identified patient) in psychodynamic terms, and to hypothesize concerning its origins, both developmentally and as a product of the patient's current relationships and experiences.

(4) The ability to assess the patient's (associated) personality structure and resources in psychodynamic terms.

(5) An associated elementary ability to identify conscious and unconscious strategies that the patient uses for modifying anxiety or conflict (such as avoidance, denial, projection, projective identification, and reaction formation), and that influence the patient's ability to change.

(6) Elementary ability to determine whether the dynamic psychopathology is amenable to psychotherapy of any kind, taking into account other factors such as age and present relationships.

(7) Elementary ability to determine the type (e.g., individual, family, group) and depth (e.g., supportive, reeducative, interpretative, reconstructive) of intervention, and also the timing (e.g., crisis intervention, suitability for waiting list) that such intervention should take.

(8) A basic understanding of the knowledge and theory underlying psychotherapeutic interventions, combined with the ability to link theory and practice.

(9) An associated elementary ability personally to conduct individual psychotherapy.

(10) An associated elementary ability, with or without a cotherapist, to conduct couple or family psychotherapy.

(11) An associated elementary ability, with or without a cotherapist, to conduct psychotherapies in small groups and in a large (milieu) group.

(12) An associated elementary ability to undertake crisis intervention therapy.

(13) An associated elementary ability to conduct supportive psychotherapy.

(14) An associated ability to make effective use of the supervisory provisions that need to be available.

(15) An ability to deploy the techniques necessary to assess, as far as possible, the nature and effectiveness of such dynamic psychotherapies.

Cognitive-Behavioral Psychotherapy (not detailed here)

CONTENTS OF TEACHING

Basic Clinical Skills (not detailed here)

Dynamic Psychotherapies

To avoid too much overlap or repetition in this section, the knowledge, skills, and attitudes required to carry out basic individual dynamic psychotherapy are first described. Following this, the contents of teaching referring to family therapy, to small- and large-group therapies, to crisis intervention techniques, and to supportive psychotherapy are outlined only insofar as they differ from that of individual dynamic psychotherapy.

1.0 Individual Dynamic Psychotherapy

1.1 Knowledge

The trainee should learn about:

(a) Psychodynamic formulations of mental illness and health.
(b) Concepts of body–mind relationships.
(c) Developmental theories of personality.
(d) Concepts of causality.
(e) Concepts of meaning (including the significance of metaphor, dream, fantasy, etc.).
(f) Historical development of concepts in dynamic psychotherapy.
(g) The currently clinically useful psychodynamic concepts.
(h) (United Kingdom only:) The practice of individual psychotherapies in the National Health Service and other settings.
(i) Importance and difficulties of research into assessment of outcome and process of dynamic psychotherapeutic treatment.

1.2 Skills

The trainee should practice:

(a) Observation of his inner self in relation to patients in treatment.
(b) Therapeutic use of self-awareness (see (1) under "Specific Objectives," above).
(c) Psychodynamic formulation of a case.
(d) Identification in a patient of the preferential use of particular defenses and other unconscious communications.
(e) Judgment as to whether a patient might benefit from dynamic psychotherapy (of whatever type).
(f) Writing appropriate letters of referral for dynamic psychotherapy.
(g) Undertaking individual dynamic psychotherapy with selected neurotic patients without regular supervision.
(h) Using a supervisor to further the trainee's therapeutic effectiveness.
(i) Recognizing transference and other defensive phenomena that may arise during psychotherapy (such as regression) and dealing appropriately with them.

(j) Offering interpretations.
(k) Tolerating emotional material.
(l) Ending psychotherapy sessions appropriately.
(m) Evaluating the difference between the patient's psychodynamic status at the end of treatment and the initial assessment findings.

1.3 Attitudes

The trainee should sustain:

(a) Genuine interest in the patient.
(b) A reflective attitude.
(c) Readiness to tolerate uncertainty.
(d) Readiness to listen to the patient.

And the trainee should practice:

(e) Readiness to learn from the patient about how the patient sees himself, and his perception and experience of the trainee in relation to himself.
(f) Recognition of the importance of attending to process as well as content of psychotherapy.

2.0 Couple/Family Therapy

2.1 Knowledge

The trainee should learn about:

(a) The family life cycle and its effects on family members.
(b) Varieties of normal structure and functioning.
(c) Characteristics of abnormal families.
(d) Family phenomena (e.g., defensive identification, projection, role distortion, enmeshment, family myth).
(e) Different schools of family therapy.
(f) Different family therapeutic techniques.

2.2 Skills

The trainee should practice:

(a) Engaging family members in the context of the family interview.
(b) Determining the level and quality of family functioning; determining suitability for family therapy.
(c) Identifying family phenomena.
(d) Making therapeutic use of information related to the family's past.
(e) Deploying a range of family therapeutic techniques.
(f) Accepting and making use of supervision (including live supervision).

2.3 Attitudes

The trainee should learn to:

(a) Conceive of the family as the unit for treatment.
(b) Attend to process as opposed to content of psychotherapy transactions.

3.0 Small-and Large-Group Psychotherapies

3.1 Knowledge

The trainee should learn about:

(a) The concept of social nature of the individual.
(b) The effect of leadership style on group members.
(c) The concept of the therapeutic community and its variants.
(d) Specific group phenomena (including therapeutic and adverse factors).
(e) The concept of demoralization in groups (e.g., staff burnout).
(f) The concept of group boundaries and open and closed systems.
(g) Intergroup relationships and related problems.
(h) The potential detrimental effects of the "institution."
(i) Different schools of group psychotherapy.
(j) Aspects of group psychotherapy technique.
(k) The range of group treatments.

3.2 Skills

The trainee should practice:

(a) Identifying group phenomena displayed by the group.
(b) Attempting to understand psychological disturbances arising within the group system.
(c) Treating psychological disturbances arising within the group system.
(d) Leading a ward small group.
(e) Leading a ward or unit community meeting.

3.3 Attitudes

The trainee should practice:

(a) Oscillating between "figure" and "ground"—individual and group.

4.0 Supportive Psychotherapy

4.1 Knowledge

The trainee should learn about:

(a) The "sick role" and secondary gain.
(b) The values and dangers of dependence.

(c) Aspects of institutional transference.
(d) Splitting and projection (in relation to negotiating with multiple agencies).
(e) Reinforcement and shaping techniques.

4.2 Skills

The trainee should practice:

(a) Making an assessment of the patient's capacity to sustain his present functioning or even improve it.
(b) Maintaining an awareness of the transference and countertransference even when there is no intention of interpreting them; also, learning to recognize when transference interpretations *can* be useful.
(c) Exploring the anxieties surrounding prognosis, in order to give specific and effective reassurance.
(d) Enhancing treatment compliance by exploring the significance of treatment for the patient.
(e) Shifting styles (e.g., directive, nonjudgmental, confrontational) and activities (e.g., exploration, reeducation, ventilation) more rapidly than in other therapeutic modes.
(f) Identifying and delineating meaningful goals and tasks.
(g) Focusing on and rewarding adaptive behavior, and at times minimizing symptomatology.
(h) Finding honest means of encouragement.
(i) Writing succinct but meaningful notes so that other staff members can, if needed, replace the trainee.

4.3 Attitudes

The trainee should develop a capacity for:

(a) Greater acceptance of individual variation.
(b) Respect for the patient's need to make sense of his experience, despite the process's being "noninterpretive."
(c) A genuinely collaborative relationship with the patient, despite the process's being "supportive."
(d) A willingness to deal with practical and dynamic issues concurrently.

5.0 Crisis Intervention

5.1 Knowledge

The trainee should learn about:

(a) The concept of "emotional homeostasis" and the creative potential for crises.

(b) The differences between accidental, external hazards and emotional crises; the Eriksonian "eight stages of man" (Erikson, 1963).

(c) The various vulnerability factors (developmental phases, coexistent physical or social stress, absence of adequate family support, social or cultural isolation, intrapsychic residues).

(d) The protective factors (the patient's strengths—emotional, social, intrapsychic).

(e) The natural history and characteristics of crisis (time course, expression of dependence needs, reactivation of old conflicts).

(f) The phases of a crisis (habitual problem-solving behavior, increasing arousal, novel problem solving, resolution).

5.2 Skills

The trainee should practice:

(a) Making an assessment incorporating the degree of decompensation, nature of hazards, intensity of crisis, patient's ego strengths, and family strengths.

(b) Selecting an appropriate level of crisis intervention (symptom suppression, crisis support, crisis intervention).

(c) Carrying out basic crisis intervention procedures (clarification and redefining, encouragement of expression of emotions, mobilization of individual and family resources, challenging maladaptive coping, rehearsing healthy coping, anticipation and use of early termination).

5.3 Attitudes

The trainee should adopt a positive attitude toward:

(a) The potential value of a crisis to the patient.

(b) The possibility of lasting psychological change's occurring in the course of short interventions.

(c) The importance of manipulating social networks to ensure healthy psychological functioning of patients.

PROCESS

The "Grammar of Psychotherapy" course (run by the peripatetic associate professor in dynamic psy-

chotherapy) provides teaching on the topic of the psychiatrist–patient relationship and represents three 2-hour seminars and three 2-hour follow-up sessions. This course should be attended by all trainees.

Over the first 3 years of training, there should be supervised experience in individual dynamic psychotherapy with at least two patients, one of which should be for a period of not less than 18 months. Supervision should be weekly and should be provided by a consultant psychotherapist. The residency educational program provides formal teaching of the knowledge base underpinning the various dynamic psychotherapies and should be attended by all trainees. The training should be augmented locally by seminars on the dynamic psychotherapies. This should be done by making dynamic psychotherapeutic topics approximately 25% of the local teaching program.

All trainees should have a supervised experience of leading (or coleading) an outpatient or inpatient group. For the former this should be a continuous period, and for the latter it should be a cumulative period of at least 1 year. Supervision should be available via local consultant group psychotherapists or other suitably qualified personnel (Lieberman, Hafner, & Crisp, 1978).

Training in group psychotherapy should ideally be augmented by attendance at sensitivity groups or other group training with an experiential element. At least at one point in their rotational scheme, trainees should have the opportunity of working in a therapeutic milieu (or in a ward environment where there are regular small- and large-group meetings of patients and staff, together with review meetings following these).

All trainees should have the opportunity of attending at least three family therapy workshop days. These should be arranged locally by consultant psychotherapists. Trainees should treat at least two families, this work being supervised by the use of a one-way screen by a suitably qualified therapist or in a family therapy clinic.

Supportive psychotherapy is conventionally the domain of the general adult psychiatrist. All trainees should have supervised experience of this with at least three patients (each of at least 6 months' duration). Supervision should be by a consultant psychiatrist and/or senior resident.

Training in crisis intervention should be experiential and gained in on-call and liaison assessment of crises. Teaching will be by trainees' senior colleagues in the team.

Note. This appendix is condensed and adapted from Crisp et al. (1993). Copyright 1993 by the Department of Mental Health Sciences, St. George's Hospital Medical School. Adapted by permission.

CHAPTER 14

Interpersonal Psychotherapy for Bulimia Nervosa

CHRISTOPHER G. FAIRBURN

Interpersonal psychotherapy (IPT) is a short-term focal psychotherapy in which the goal is to help patients identify and modify current interpersonal problems. It was developed in the late 1960s as a treatment for clinical depression, the premise being that since interpersonal difficulties contribute to the onset and maintenance of depression, their resolution is likely to hasten recovery.

More recently IPT has been applied to other problems, including recurrent depression, bipolar disorder, substance abuse, marital problems, and eating disorders (Klerman & Weissman, 1993; Weissman & Markowitz, 1994). In addition, adaptations have been devised for adolescents (Mufson, Moreau, Weissman, & Klerman, 1993) and the elderly (Frank et al., 1993). The focus of this chapter is on its application to bulimia nervosa.

THE STATUS OF INTERPERSONAL PSYCHOTHERAPY FOR BULIMIA NERVOSA

Two studies, both conducted by my group at Oxford, provide empirical support for the use of IPT to treat bulimia nervosa. In the first (Fairburn, Kirk, O'Connor, & Cooper, 1986), a form of cognitive-behavioral therapy (CBT) designed specifically for treating bulimia nervosa (Fairburn, 1981; Fairburn, Marcus, & Wilson, 1993) was compared with a short-term focal psychotherapy in which the emphasis was on iden-

tifying and modifying interpersonal problems accompanying the eating disorder, rather than on the eating disorder itself. This treatment was nondirective and noninterpretive in character. In its first stage, each patient's current interpersonal problems were identified from a detailed assessment of the patient's past and from an examination of the circumstances under which episodes of overeating tended to occur. In the second stage, these problems became the focus of treatment, with patients being encouraged to think about them in depth and consider possible ways of changing. In the final few sessions, the focus shifted toward reviewing what had been learned in treatment and applying it to the future.

The results were striking (see Figure 14.1). Patients in both treatment conditions improved substantially, with the changes being maintained over a 12-month treatment-free follow-up period. Although some findings favored CBT, it was nevertheless clear that the short-term focal psychotherapy had a major and sustained impact on the disorder.

The second Oxford study (Fairburn et al., 1991; Fairburn, Jones, Peveler, Hope, & O'-Connor, 1993) was designed to replicate and extend the findings of the first study with a larger sample size. Seventy-five patients were randomly assigned to three treatments, CBT, behavior therapy (BT), and IPT. CBT was essentially the same treatment as that used in the first trial. BT was a dismantled version of CBT, consisting solely of those behavioral procedures

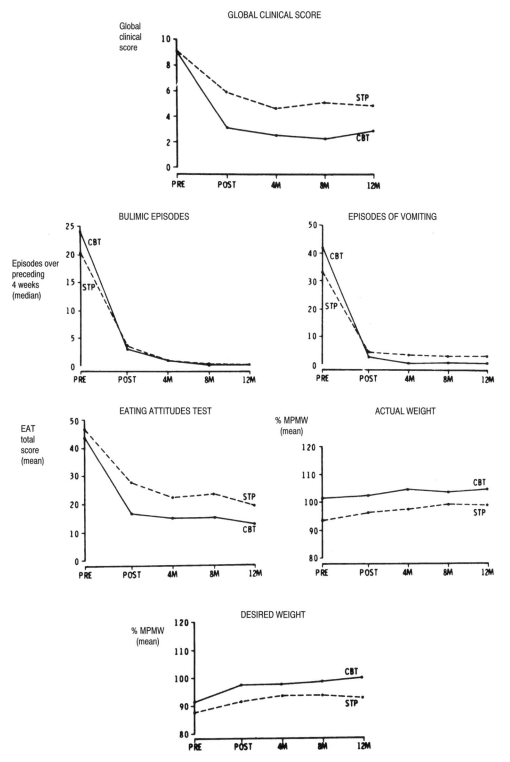

FIGURE 14.1. Changes in eating disorder psychopathology and weight following treatment with cognitive-behavioral therapy (CBT) or short-term focal psychotherapy (STP). From Fairburn, Kirk, O'Connor, and Cooper (1986). Copyright 1986 by Pergamon Press, Ltd. Reprinted by permission.

directed at normalized eating. IPT was chosen in place of the original interpersonal treatment, since it was similar to it in style and focus, but had the advantages of being better known and having a treatment manual available.

The findings at the end of treatment indicated that all three treatments had a substantial effect, with the results favoring CBT (Fairburn et al., 1991). However, the effects of the three treatments differed over time. Patients who received BT did not do well; indeed, over the 12-month treatment-free follow-up period, almost half the patients either dropped out or had to be withdrawn on clinical grounds. The poor maintenance of change with BT is illustrated by the rapid decline in the proportion who met strict criteria for a good outcome (see Figure 14.2). This course of events contrasted sharply with that following CBT and IPT, where there

was no tendency for the patients' state to deteriorate (Fairburn, Jones, et al., 1993). As can be seen in Figure 14.2, CBT was rapid in achieving its effects, with almost all the changes occurring during treatment itself; with IPT, the changes were slower to develop but continued during follow-up.

A longer-term follow-up has been conducted on the patients in these two trials; the average length of follow-up being 6 years (Fairburn et al., 1995). Perhaps surprisingly, given the length of follow-up and the fact that over a third had received subsequent treatment (the proportions were the same across the three treatments), differential treatment effects were observed even after this long interval. Those subjects who had received BT fared the worst: At follow-up 86% had an eating disorder as defined in the *Diagnostic and Statistical Manual*

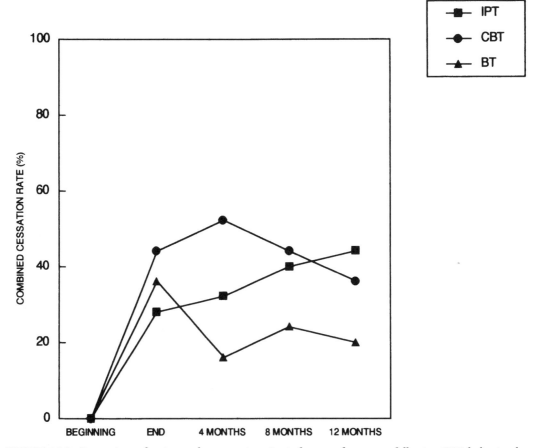

FIGURE 14.2. Proportions of patients who met strict criteria for a good outcome following CBT, behavior therapy (BT), or interpersonal psychotherapy (IPT). From Fairburn, Jones, Peveler, Hope, and O'Connor (1993). Copyright 1993 by the American Medical Association. Reprinted by permission.

of Mental Disorders, fourth edition (DSM-IV), compared to 37% of those who had received CBT and 28% of those who had received one of the two forms of focal interpersonal psychotherapy. These findings are similar to those at 12-month follow-up. They indicate that BT had an immediate but short-lived effect, with patients subsequently tending to relapse. In contrast, the majority of patients who received CBT or a focal interpersonal psychotherapy did well, with the treatment effects observed at 12-month follow-up being still present on average 6 years later.

Taken together, the findings of these two trials provide strong evidence that bulimia nervosa responds to psychological treatments that are not cognitive-behavioral in character. However, this is not to imply that bulimia nervosa responds to any psychological intervention—far from it. The relative ineffectiveness of BT is testimony to this fact. Furthermore, it is common clinical experience that many patients with bulimia nervosa have received psychotherapy in the past with limited or only transitory benefit. What the findings of the two Oxford trials do suggest is that short-term psychotherapies that focus on modifying current interpersonal problems are a promising alternative to CBT. IPT is the leading treatment of this kind.

THE PRACTICE OF INTERPERSONAL PSYCHOTHERAPY FOR BULIMIA NERVOSA (IPT-BN)

IPT for bulimia nervosa (IPT-BN), as developed by our group at Oxford, closely resembles IPT for depression. Thus it is a noninterpretive, nondirective form of individual psychotherapy involving 15 to 20 sessions, which last 50 minutes each and extend over 4–5 months. The treatment has three stages, each of which will be described in turn. For further details about the practice of IPT in general, readers should consult the IPT manual (Klerman, Weissman, Rounsaville, & Chevron, 1984).

Stage 1

Stage 1 usually occupies three to four sessions. The goals are threefold:

1. To describe the rationale and nature of IPT.

2. To identify current interpersonal problems.

3. To choose which of the interpersonal problems should become the focus of the remainder of treatment.

Describing the Rationale and Nature of IPT

It is explained that to help people break out of a self-perpetuating problem such as bulimia nervosa, it is necessary to find out what is keeping it going and then address the maintaining factors in treatment. It is explained that interpersonal difficulties are common in bulimia nervosa although many patients have limited awareness of them because of the distracting influence of their preoccupation with thoughts about eating, shape, and weight. The interpersonal difficulties play an important role in maintaining the eating disorder through a number of mechanisms; for example, many binges are precipitated by interpersonal events and circumstances, such as having an argument or feeling lonely. The therapist may say something along the following lines:

> The relevance of relationships to bulimia nervosa has been highlighted by the results of two recent treatment studies, which have shown that treatments that modify current interpersonal problems have a major beneficial effect which appears to be well maintained. IPT is the best substantiated of these treatments.

It is further explained that in IPT there is little emphasis on the patient's eating problem as such, except during the assessment stage (Stage 1). Instead, the focus is on the patient's interpersonal difficulties. This is because focusing on the eating disorder would tend to distract the patient and therapist from dealing with the interpersonal difficulties.

Patients are also forewarned that IPT has two distinct phases, which are quite different in character. In the first, which occupies the first three or four sessions, the goal is to identify those interpersonal difficulties that would be best to focus on. The therapist may say:

> This will involve a detailed review of your past and present relationships, and I will take the lead in asking you questions. This phase of treatment will end with our agreeing upon the problem or problems that should be the

focus of the remainder of treatment. There-after, our sessions will change in style. You will become largely responsible for the content of the sessions, and I will take more of a back-seat role. Gradually we will learn more about your interpersonal difficulties and ways of changing them. Your role will be not only to explore these difficulties in our treatment sessions but you must also experiment with ways of changing. Doing so will shed further light on the nature of your problems, and it may lead to change.

It is important to stress the time-limited nature of the treatment. As performed in Oxford, IPT has a fixed number of sessions (usually 16), and these are held at weekly intervals until near the end of treatment, when they are held every 2 weeks. Therefore, even at the outset, it is possible to give the patient a good idea of when treatment is likely to end. The fact that the treatment has a fixed number of sessions helps the therapist stress the importance of working hard at treatment:

> This is an opportunity to change—an opportunity to break out of what has been a long-standing problem. It is essential that you make the most of the opportunity by giving the treatment priority in your life. Not doing so is likely to limit the progress that we can make.

Other ground rules also need to be explained. For example, in Oxford we say that sessions will always end on time (50 minutes after they are due to start), and it is the responsibility of both the therapist and patient to ensure that they start promptly. Exchanging telephone numbers in case of unforeseen problems is a good idea.

Identifying Current Interpersonal Problems

Three sources of information are used to identify current interpersonal problems.

1. *A history is taken of the interpersonal context in which the eating problem developed and has been maintained.* This helps identify current interpersonal problems. It also highlights links between changes in the eating problem and the occurrence of interpersonal events, thereby stressing the importance of interpersonal factors to the eating problem. This helps

the patient see the relevance of this form of treatment.

Four separate histories are taken, starting from the patient's birth. The first is a history of the eating problem and how it has evolved. Key events and dates are recorded—for example, the ages at which the patient first began to diet, binge, and purge. The timing of major changes in weight are noted, as is prior experience of treatment. The second history is of the patient's interpersonal functioning prior to and since the development of the eating problem. Relationships with family and peers are especially relevant here. The third history is of significant life events, many of which will already have been identified. The fourth history is of problems with self-esteem and depression. The history taking should culminate in the creation of a "life chart" in which separate columns are allocated to each domain. A typical life chart is shown later in the chapter (see Figure 14.3).

The patient should be encouraged to play an active role in the history-taking and the creation of the life chart. Looking though old diaries and photographs can be helpful, as can discussions with relatives and friends. The whole process usually takes two to three sessions.

2. *An assessment is made of the quality of the patient's current interpersonal functioning.* This involves asking about the patient's social network. Inquiries should be made about family members, the patient's spouse or partner, confidants, work contacts, and friends and acquaintances. The topics to be addressed include frequency of contact, positive and negative aspects of each relationship, mutual expectations, intimacy, and reciprocity.

3. *The precipitants of bulimic episodes are identified.* In each of the assessment sessions, the therapist asks whether there have been any binges (objective or subjective), and, if so, inquires about the circumstances preceding them. Since it is common for bulimic episodes to be precipitated by interpersonal events, they serve as "markers" of current interpersonal problems.

Choosing Which Problem Areas Should Become the Focus of Treatment

By the third or fourth session, the nature of the patient's interpersonal difficulties should be clear. Usually they belong to one of the four standard "problem areas" described in the IPT manual (Klerman et al., 1984)—namely, grief, interpersonal role disputes, role transitions, or interpersonal deficits. (These problem areas are discussed later in the chapter.) The next step is to decide which of the problem areas should become the focus of the remainder of treatment. This decision should be a mutual one. When more than one problem is identified, progress will be facilitated if the therapist suggests the order in which they should be tackled. In the main, it is best if the simplest and most readily soluble of the problems is addressed first; for example, unresolved grief can often be tackled relatively quickly, in part because it does not generally require others to change. Tackling the most soluble problem first also has the advantage that progress on one front often leads to progress on others. Not only are the patient's morale and overall sense of competence enhanced when progress is made on a problem, but barriers to progress in other areas may be eroded or removed.

In some cases, the interpersonal problems identified have no clear connection to the eating disorder. IPT appears to be just as useful in these cases; this observation suggests that it operates at least in part through general mechanisms, rather than simply by tackling the immediate precipitants of binges.

Stage 2

The second and third stages of the treatment are virtually identical to IPT for depression, as described in the IPT manual, although in IPT-BN for bulimia nervosa the patient is perhaps placed under greater pressure to change. Stage 2 generally involves about eight weekly sessions.

At the end of Stage 1, the therapist reminds the patient that the treatment will now change in character:

As we discussed at the outset, from this point on the nature of our sessions will change. Instead of me asking you questions, you will take the lead. Your task will be to focus on the problems we have identified and consider them in depth and from all possible angles. In this way, you will come to a better understanding of them. A key part of this process is thinking what changes are possible and how you could bring them about. You will need to consider all the possible alternatives, together with their pros and cons. And it is important for you to experiment with

ways of changing. By doing so, not only will you get a better idea of the nature of the problems, but you may well be able to influence them.

The sessions from this point on are largely patient-led. The therapist's job is to ensure that the patient remains focused on the identified problem areas, gains a better understanding of them, and attempts to change. After reminding the patient of the session number and of how many sessions remain, the therapist opens each session with a general inquiry such as "Where shall we start today?" Thereafter, the patient takes the lead.

The therapist is active but not directive. The patient is encouraged to explore the problem areas and to consider ways of changing; the attempts to change then become the focus of subsequent sessions. The therapist helps the patient remain focused by ensuring that the subject matter is relevant and by providing clarification when needed. For example, one patient described helping her father adapt his house. This was relevant, since their relationship was one of the agreed-upon problem areas. However, she then went on to discuss the nature of the adaptation; the therapist had to intervene at this point, since the interpersonal focus had been lost. Clarification takes the form of pointing out themes and inconsistencies, highlighting points that the patient might miss. For example, another patient had three problem areas that appeared quite distinct. The therapist made an important clarifying intervention by pointing out that a factor contributing to each problem was the patient's desire to avoid conflict at all cost. Clarification does not extend to making "interpretations," in which reference is made to a theoretical view on the disorder and its treatment. Throughout, the focus remains on the present.

The therapist should ensure that the patient remains aware of the task at hand. At the end of each session, the therapist should provide a brief resumé in which he or she summarizes what has been covered. In addition, at intervals during Stage 2, the therapist reviews progress by considering each of the problem areas and assessing what has been achieved and what remains to be done.

The need to change is stressed at regular intervals. It is important to note that this constitutes general encouragement to change, rather than pressure to take a specific course of action.

As illustrated later, the therapist is active in supporting and reinforcing attempts to change, but is not directive in the sense of making specific recommendations. Formal problem solving as employed in CBT is not used, although the therapist helps patients consider the various options available to them. There is little use of behavioral procedures. Exceptions include the reenacting of key exchanges to get a clearer idea of what was said, as well as the role playing of important future exchanges. For example, a patient was about to face a job interview after she had been off work for over a year. Having encouraged her to consider how she would account for the period of unemployment, the therapist helped her rehearse her response at interview through the use of role play.

Rarely is reference made to the therapist–patient relationship, since doing so can complicate and undermine IPT. An exception is when treating those patients with interpersonal deficits whose social network is so impoverished that one of the few relationships available for examination is that between the therapist and patient. Reference to the therapist–patient relationship can also be useful when patients would be helped by feedback about how they come across to others. This is illustrated later in the chapter.

Interestingly, most patients make few, if any, references to their eating disorder. If they do, the therapist should shift the focus away from the eating problem and onto its interpersonal context. Detailed discussion of the eating disorder and its symptomatic management are not part of IPT-BN for bulimia nervosa as currently practiced (see "Indications and Future Directions").

Stage 3

The third stage of treatment comprises the final three or four sessions. These may be held at 2-week intervals. There are two related goals: The first is to ensure that the changes that have been made during treatment continue following discharge, and the second is to minimize the risk of relapse.

Unlike the transition between Stages 1 and 2, there is no sharp change in style between Stages 2 and 3. Instead, the sessions continue much as before, except that there needs to be a review of treatment in which what has been achieved and what has not are considered. When progress on a particular problem area is being discussed, the therapist should help the patient look toward the future:

> As you know, we only have three more sessions to go. What do you envisage happening regarding _____ over the coming months? How can you make sure that you build upon what you have achieved so far?

By this point, it should be clear what changes are likely to be made and what changes may not take place. The therapist should ensure that the patient has realistic expectations. For example, the therapist might say:

> Given what has emerged during treatment, it seems unlikely that _____ will start to behave differently in the foreseeable future. If this is the case, what do you think *you* should do?

The therapist should also help the patient predict areas of future difficulty.

It is not uncommon for patients at this stage in treatment to make reference to their eating problem. Unless their eating problem is so troublesome as to make the ending of treatment impossible, our practice in Oxford is to remind patients that the evidence suggests that it often takes months for the full benefits of IPT to be felt (as illustrated in Figure 14.2; Fairburn, Jones, et al., 1993). We point out to those patients tempted to start further treatment that in our opinion they might be wiser to delay doing so, since in this way they will be able to see whether there is continuing improvement, and, if so, attribute it to the changes that they have already set in motion—something that they would be unable to do were they to have further treatment. However, the patients are also told that their eating problem is likely to remain an "Achilles heel," in the sense that it may recur at future times of difficulty. We encourage patients to view any deterioration as a useful "early warning signal." It is a sign that they need to review what is happening in their lives and perhaps take some action.

It is unusual for patients receiving IPT to have difficulty accepting the ending of treatment. This is because it is made clear at the outset that treatment is time-limited, and patients are reminded at the beginning of each session of the number of sessions remaining. Nevertheless, therapists should always ask patients how they feel about the ending of treatment—not least because this provides an opportunity to emphasize what has been achieved and to stress the patient's probable competence at dealing with future areas of difficulty.

The Four Problem Areas

Grief

Our experience suggests that problems with grief are not common among patients with bulimia nervosa. They were judged to be present among 12% of the patients in our second trial (Fairburn, Jones, et al., 1991, 1993). As mentioned earlier, they can often be resolved comparatively quickly, and it is therefore worth addressing them first. The goal is to help patients face the loss, assess exactly what has been lost, and start to move on. Facing the loss requires them to think in detail about the events surrounding the loss and express their feelings about it. Patients need to be educated about the grief process and variations on it. Profound feelings of sadness are common, but so are feelings of anger and guilt. Reconstructing the relationship—both its positive and its negative aspects—is central to the assessment of exactly what has been lost and is needed to counter the idealization that so commonly occurs. As patients become less focused on the past, they should be helped to think about the future and the establishment of new interests and relationships.

Interpersonal Role Disputes

Interpersonal role disputes were present in 64% of the patients in our second trial. Such disputes may be with any figures of importance in the patients' lives, including spouses or partners, parents, children, friends, and employers. The aim of treatment is to help clarify the nature of the dispute, consider the possibilities for change on both sides, and then actively explore them. The outcome may be a renegotiation of the relationship or its dissolution.

Since the standard form of IPT is conducted on a one-to-one basis, the other party in any dispute is not directly involved. In most cases, this seems fine and the results are good; however, in the case of marital disputes, we have encountered a few instances in which it might have been preferable to involve a patient's spouse/partner. For example, it may be worth arranging supplementary conjoint sessions in those cases in which a marital dispute is the primary problem and progress is limited. Weissman and Klerman (1993) have described an adaptation of IPT specifically for patients with marital disputes.

Role Transitions

Problems with role transitions are common in this patient group. Not surprisingly, given their age, these often involve establishing independence from their parents. The goal of treatment is to help the patient abandon the old role and adopt a new one. This involves exploring exactly what the new role involves and how it can be mastered. Often there are associated role disputes which need to be addressed at the same time.

Problems with role transitions are not confined to the difficulties of late adolescence and early adulthood. They include problems coping with other life changes, such as leaving college, changing jobs, getting married, and becoming a parent. They were judged to be present among 36% of the patients in our second trial.

Interpersonal Deficits

Interpersonal deficits are present when the patient gives a long history of difficulty in initiating or maintaining intimate relationships. Some degree of social isolation is common in bulimia nervosa and needs to be addressed, but longstanding interpersonal deficits are much less common. They were present in just 16% of the patients in our second trial. This is fortunate, since such patients are difficult to help. Many have an avoidant or schizoid personality disorder, as defined in DSM-IV.

To help these patients, it is necessary to determine why they have this difficulty in forming or maintaining relationships. As mentioned earlier, it may be appropriate to examine the nature of the patient–therapist relationship, since this may be such a patient's only close relationship and it is present to be observed. Solving the identified problems is often difficult, however, although for those with social skills deficits role playing can be helpful.

AN ILLUSTRATIVE CASE HISTORY

The patient was a 22-year-old college student who was studying physics. She was referred by her primary care physician for the treatment of an "intractable eating problem." Assessment indicated that she had the purging type of bulimia nervosa. In addition, she met criteria for major depressive disorder. Both disorders had been present since she was aged 16.

The patient complained of being "unable to stop eating." She denied having any other problems. She had recurrent objective bulimic episodes, many of which involved the consumption of very large amounts of food. These episodes, which occurred at least daily, were followed by compensatory self-induced vomiting. She also took large quantities of laxatives several times a week. Between the bulimic episodes she dieted to an extreme degree, her goal being to eat less than 1,200 calories daily. She was vigilant about her appearance and weighed herself at least twice daily. She was 5'7" tall and 137 pounds in weight (body mass index = 21.5).

Stage 1

The therapist, who had not been involved in the patient's assessment, introduced himself. He asked about the processes that had led to her referral. She explained that 2 months earlier she had sought help from her primary care physician. The physician had provided simple counseling and advice, but this had proved unhelpful. The doctor had therefore suggested that specialist help was needed, especially since the problem was long-standing and the patient had not benefited from treatment in the past.

The therapist described the nature and rationale of IPT (as outlined earlier). It was agreed that treatment would involve 16 weekly sessions. The likely date of the final session was identified.

The remainder of the first session and the next three sessions were devoted to the identification of current interpersonal problems.

Identifying Current Interpersonal Problems

1. *The interpersonal history.* The patient's problems with eating had begun when she was aged 14, shortly after she changed to a new school. She started to diet and lost more than 20 pounds over 6 months. Although the diagnosis was not made at the time, she would have met diagnostic criteria for anorexia nervosa. At the age of 15, her control over eating began to break down and her weight started to increase.

At first her binges were small, but once she started to vomit as well, they increased in size to become true DSM-IV binges (Fairburn & Wilson, 1993). By the time she was 16 (the timing was relatively easy to establish, since it could be related specifically to her progress through school), her current eating pattern was established and her weight had increased to its present level.

In her last year of secondary school, when she was aged 18, she was referred to a local psychiatrist for the treatment of depression. The psychiatrist detected the eating disorder, and the patient was treated with antidepressant drugs and a form of dynamic psychotherapy. This resulted in a slight improvement in her mood and eating habits, but the benefits were short-lived.

Over the subsequent 4 years, the patient's bingeing and vomiting continued unchanged. There was a slight improvement after she started college, but she continued to eat little outside her binges and for a while lost weight.

From her personal history, it emerged that she was an only child. Her father was a lawyer and her mother a teacher. Both were very involved with their work. The family had liberal values although there was a clearly stated expectation that she would "do well." Neither parent showed her much affection during her childhood, but for different reasons. Her father seemed uncomfortable expressing his feelings, but she felt sure that he was fond of her. In contrast, she found her mother "distant," "cold," and rivalrous. Her relationship with her parents had deteriorated over the previous summer, when they had a protracted argument over how she was to spend the vacation. She wanted to travel abroad with a girlfriend, but her parents forbade this; they insisted that she was too young, it was not safe, and she ought to be using the time more productively.

The first event of note in her history was the change in schools, which took place when she was aged 13. Having been at an ordinary local school, she was transferred to an *avant garde* school favored by her parents. This school had little structure or discipline, and a casual attitude to work was *de rigueur* among the pupils. She did not fit in, since she enjoyed schoolwork—something that was strongly reinforced by her parents. She was rejected by the other children, who accused her of being a snob, possibly because of her parents' professional backgrounds and her accent. She had no friends or confidants. It was at this time that she began to diet. She spent an unhappy 5 years at this school. Matters improved slightly in the last 2 years, when she was taught with others planning to go on to a university.

She came to college with one other person from her school. During their first 2 years they spent a great deal of time together. However, her friend became become cooler at the beginning of the third year, and in the second term they had a major argument in which her friend described her as "dependent," "aloof," and "arrogant." Since then they had seen little of each other.

Her problems with depression and low self-esteem tracked the state of her eating problem. They had begun shortly after she entered the *avant garde* school and had persisted ever since. They had been particularly bad since the breakup of the relationship with her girlfriend. She thought that her feelings of depression and loneliness were what had led her to seek help.

2. *Current relationships.* The loss of the relationship with her girlfriend was a great blow, since the girlfriend was the patient's only confidant. She had a boyfriend, but they were not close. They had been going out for almost 2 years, but this simply involved seeing each other at weekends and going to parties. The relationship had an aggressive side to it, in that her boyfriend was offensive and offhand. On the other hand, she said that the relationship suited her, since it was "not too bothersome."

She had no other friends, but she did have a circle of people with whom she played cards. She knew their names and what subjects they were studying, but little else.

3. *Precipitants of bulimic episodes.* Most of the patient's binges seemed to be habitual rather than triggered by specific events. She invariably overate in the afternoon and sometimes did so in the morning. Unusually for patients with bulimia nervosa, she rarely overate in the evening. No specific triggers emerged, other than unstructured time and the feelings of loneliness that characterized her afternoons.

Choosing Which Problem Areas Should Become the Focus of Treatment

Between the third and fourth sessions, the therapist asked the patient to create a life chart summarizing her interpersonal history. An adaptation of this life chart is shown in Figure 14.3. Clear links between her eating problem

and the occurrence of interpersonal events were evident. On the basis of this information, and that gathered from the assessment of her social network and the precipitants of her binges, the therapist proposed that the following three areas would be worth focusing on:

1. *The difficulty with her parents.* This was presented as a role transition problem rather than as an interpersonal dispute: The patient was being treated as a child.

2. *The difficulties with her boyfriend.* The therapist suggested that there was an interpersonal dispute between the patient and her boyfriend, since, contrary to her claims, it was likely that they had differing expectations of each other.

3. *Social isolation.* The therapist pointed out that the patient's social network did not include any friends or confidants. The therapist did not class the problem as an interpersonal deficit (as defined earlier), since it appeared that she had the ability to form intimate relationships. Instead, he wondered whether a social skills problem might be acting as a barrier to the forming of relationships. The accusations of her being a "snob" and "arrogant" seemed relevant and worth exploring.

The patient accepted that the first and third problem areas would be worth exploring. It was obvious that something had to be done in regard to her parents, and over the previous few months she had become increasingly aware of her social isolation. However, she did not regard the relationship with her boyfriend as a problem, and so it was decided to put it aside.

The fifth session ended with the therapist reminding the patient that the sessions would now change in style.

Stage 2

The sixth session coincided with the end of the term and the start of the summer vacation. After the previous summer's argument with her parents, the patient had no specific plans about how to spend the 8 weeks of vacation, other than that she expected to be based at home. The therapist suggested that she ought to give treatment priority, since this would maximize the chances of success. He also suggested that her being at home might make it easier to deal with the first of the agreed-upon problem areas—her relationship with her parents.

Age	Eating problem	Relationships	Events/ circumstances	Depression/ low self-esteem
13			Change in school	
		No friends, called a "snob"		
14	Begins to diet, rapid weight loss			
15	Meets criteria for anorexia nervosa			
	Starts to binge, weight begins to rise			Depressive symptoms develop
16	Starts to vomit, weight now back to previous level			Pronounced depressive symptoms
	Regular binge eating and vomiting (meets criteria for bulimia nervosa)			
17				
18			Referred to psychiatrist for treatment of depression	
	Eating disorder detected by psychiatrist		Receives antidepressants and psychotherapy	
	Short-lived improvement in eating habits			Short-lived improvement in depression
19			Starts at college	
	Transitory decrease in frequency of binge eating and vomiting, some weight loss	Spends much time with V. (girlfriend from school)		
20		Starts seeing R. (boyfriend)		
21		Major argument with parents over vacation plans		
22		Breakup of friendship with V. Accused of being "aloof," "arrogant," and "dependent"		
				Worsening of depressive symptoms
			Seeks help from college doctor	

FIGURE 14.3. A "life chart" of a patient with bulimia nervosa.

The patient talked about her concern that treatment was becoming too intrusive. She did not like dwelling on herself: "Life is bad enough without having to think about it the whole time." The therapist commented that one has to face up to problems in order to overcome them, and that some degree of introspection is necessary to bring about change.

One topic dominated the seventh session. On arriving home, the patient decided to tell her parents about the eating problem. This was the first time that she had mentioned it to them.

Her parents reacted differently. Her father seemed genuinely shocked and at a loss as to what to say. Her mother said that she had known all along. Neither parent raised the subject again during the entire week. The patient was angry and upset at their lack of reaction: She had divulged a major problem, and her parents had barely responded. The patient then went on to describe her need to be perfect. She felt that she had been "infected" by her parents' drive to succeed, and that this had made her "obsessed with performance." She had to succeed at everything she did. It was therefore highly significant for her to admit to her parents that she had an eating problem. Their lack of response was very hurtful. The therapist suggested that her parents' behavior reinforced the need for treatment to focus on her relationship with them. The patient agreed.

The patient was somewhat hostile in the next session. She said that she felt worse than when she had started treatment, and that she disliked the lack of guidance. The therapist restated the rationale behind IPT and the reason for not focusing on her eating. The patient then went on to discuss her parents' response to her admission that she had an eating problem. She said that her father seemed to be avoiding her. He was spending even more time than usual away at work and her mother was busying herself with preparations for the end of the school term. She felt angry and rejected.

Between the eighth and ninth sessions, the patient raised with her parents their apparent indifference to her revelation. Both said that they wanted to help but were unsure how to do so. At mealtimes, her father started to make awkward and inappropriate comments about what she ate. Her mother bought a number of self-help books on eating problems and left them on her bed, saying, "These should help." The patient started to feel more angry than rejected. She also reported that her eating was "awful." The therapist said that this was understandable, given the tension at home.

The 10th session opened with the patient's saying that she had been thinking about her relationship with her parents and felt it was worth distinguishing between her parents' rights and their expectations. She thought that they had a right to expect her to make the most of her time at college. It was also reasonable for them to expect her to fit into the home routine when she was with them during the vacation. On the other hand, given her age and circumstances, she thought it was not appropriate for them to expect her to be an outstanding academic, and not reasonable for them to dictate what she did during the vacation. The therapist said that he thought the distinction between rights and expectations seemed useful. He stressed the need to change, since attempts to change might yield useful information.

At the 11th session, the patient was more cheerful than she had been up to this point. She reported that the previous evening she had confronted her parents with their controlling be-

havior, their inappropriate expectations, and their apparent need for her to be perfect and trouble-free. She told them that they needed to forge a new relationship, since she was no longer going to accept the old one. She said that she would continue to work hard at college and would obey reasonable house rules when at home, but in other respects she planned to follow her own priorities. Her parents responded by saying that they would think about what she had said. The therapist was strongly supportive of the patient.

Between the 11th and 12th sessions, the patient returned to college. The aftermath of the confrontation with her parents had been disappointing. They had simply carried on with their busy lives, not mentioning the subject at all. She had therefore decided to spend the remaining week or so of the vacation back at college. The therapist reinforced this decision, saying that it demonstrated to her parents her determination to redefine her relationship with them. It also fitted in well with the stage that she had reached in treatment: Although she had made considerable progress with respect to her parents, her social isolation had not been addressed. The therapist also suggested that it might be worth reconsidering her relationship with her boyfriend. The patient said that before the next session she would set time aside to think about these matters.

The 13th session opened with the patient's saying that she had decided to break off her relationship with her boyfriend, since it was basically unhealthy. Indeed, she announced that she had telephoned him to say that she did not intend to see him again. The therapist expressed concern at this abrupt termination of the relationship. The patient retorted that just as her relationship with her parents had needed attention, so did her relationship with her boyfriend, but in this case there was little to be gained by continuing it. She thought that his aggression and offhand behavior were probably his ways of coping with the fact that he felt threatened by her. She said that she wanted to establish a relationship with someone who was sufficiently secure not to be intimidated by her.

The therapist suggested that perhaps many people found her intimidating and that this could lie behind the accusations of her being "arrogant" and a "snob." Since the patient seemed skeptical at this proposal, the therapist took the unusual step for IPT (as described earlier) of commenting on his own experience of the patient, saying that he could see how people might find her threatening. He said that certain aspects of her behavior contributed to this impression. For example, her gait was striking in that she walked very fast and upright, rather like a model on a catwalk, and her speech was unusually rapid and fluent. As a result, she had a self-confident air that might keep people at a distance. The therapist said that he suspected there was a marked contrast between how he knew she felt about herself and her circumstances, and how she appeared to others.

The patient was taken aback by this intervention and started to cry. She began to talk about her loneliness. She also said that she had recently realized that she never admitted to having any problems. While acquaintances at college would talk about their difficulties with work, boyfriends, and so on, all she talked about were her achievements. She felt that she had learned this style of communicating from her parents, who only wanted to know about her accomplishments. She thought it kept people at a distance and meant that she did not receive support from others. The therapist encouraged her to think more about this matter, since he thought it was likely to be contributing to her social isolation—the one problem that had not been addressed so far. He asked her to think about ways that she might be able to change.

Stage 3

The 14th session was dominated by further discussion of how the patient appeared to others. She was now convinced that this was a fundamental problem and had to be addressed. She had decided to make two changes. First, she planned to be more open with others and to discuss any difficulties that she was having. Second, she thought that she would take up a sport. At school she had been dismissive of peers who were interested in sports (a view shared by her parents), but recently her attitude had changed and she felt envious of them. She thought that taking up a new sport would be a good way of getting to know a new circle of people. She said that she had decided to learn to play squash. The therapist supported these changes. Near the end of the session, the therapist reminded her that there were just two more sessions to go. She said that she was aware of the impending end of treatment and was worried, since she felt that she was only just beginning to change.

The therapist said that he thought she had turned a corner, and that he was confident she would be able to build upon what had been achieved.

The 15th session was much like the 14th. The patient reported that she was now spending more time with her fellow students. She was making a point of listening to their problems with work and discussing her own. She had told two students of her difficulties with eating, and both of them had seemed amazed. She had also played squash on three occasions and was enjoying it.

The therapist used the last third of this session to review what had been achieved in treatment. The therapist and patient agreed that the difficulty with her parents had been addressed, although the extent to which her parents had changed was not clear. Fortuitously, her parents had contacted her earlier in the week, saying that they would like to visit. This provided an opportunity for her to reassess her relationship with them. The second area of difficulty, the relationship with her boyfriend, had also been addressed—although only by eliminating the relationship. Once again, the therapist expressed misgivings over the appropriateness of this solution, but the patient insisted that she had followed the right course of action. The therapist asked about future relationships with boyfriends and any problems she envisaged forming or maintaining them. The patient simply said that she would prefer having no relationship to having one with the wrong person. Finally, the therapist mentioned the third problem area, social isolation. It was agreed that definite progress was being made on this front.

At the final session, the patient reported that the visit of her parents had gone well. They appeared eager to see her and had expressed interest in her overall well-being. She had enjoyed their visit and was looking forward to the Christmas vacation. She thought that they seemed relieved that she was now doing things her way; it was as if a burden had been taken from them. In other respects, there was little to report. She felt that she now had several friends in college and she was seeing them regularly. Her work was going well.

The therapist asked about her eating and mood. The patient seemed almost surprised at the question. She said that her eating had been "awful" over the summer, but that since her return to college it had improved greatly. She had not binged or vomited for 3 weeks; indeed, she had not given the problem much thought. She said that she also felt much better about herself and was no longer depressed in mood. The therapist told her that continuing improvement was likely. He also reminded her that binge eating serves as a marker of other difficulties, and that it might recur at times of stress. Therefore, should there be a resurgence of the eating problem, she should take stock.

Further Progress

Although no formal plans were made to follow up the patient, she was contacted approximately 6 and 12 months after she completed treatment. As predicted, her eating problem had continued to improve. At the 12-month follow-up, she had no residual eating disorder psychopathology: She was not binge-eating, vomiting, or misusing laxatives, and her scores on the Eating Disorder Examination subscales (Fairburn & Cooper, 1993) were in the normal range. Socially, she had also made great strides. She had several close girlfriends, two of whom she had vacationed with in the summer. She also felt that she was more popular in college. Her relationship with her parents was much better than it had been; indeed, they now enjoyed each other's company. She had no boyfriend.

HOW DOES INTERPERSONAL PSYCHOTHERAPY (IPT-BN) WORK?

Neither of the Oxford studies was designed to investigate how focal interpersonal psychotherapies work. The fact that IPT and CBT are so different in practice makes it likely that, at least to some extent, they have their own particular modes of action. Our finding that IPT took longer than CBT to achieve its full effect supports this view (Fairburn, Jones, et al., 1993), although another possibility is that it operates though the same mechanisms as CBT but not so efficiently. (See Frank & Spanier, 1995, for further discussion of the mechanism of action of IPT.)

Our clinical observations as therapists during our studies may shed light on the mechanisms of action of IPT. We observed repeated instances of patients' making major positive changes in their relationships, particularly with respect to parents, spouses/partners, peers, and employers. Often these changes set in train oth-

er positive events, many of which were still evolving at the end of treatment. It seems as if successful IPT may operate by bringing about "fresh-start" events (Brown, Adler, & Bifulco, 1988). Although the precise relationship between interpersonal changes and alterations in eating disorder features has not been addressed in our research, and could not be assessed by the therapists since they were not aware of the state of the patients' eating problems, it is possible to see how improved interpersonal functioning could have a beneficial effect. At least four processes may be operating:

1. The patients' realization that they are able to bring about changes in what have often been entrenched interpersonal problems may lead them to feel more capable of changing other aspects of their lives, including their eating problem.
2. The improvement in mood and self-esteem may result in a decrease in the severity of the patients' concerns about appearance and weight; this development may decrease their tendency to diet, which in turn may lessen their vulnerability to bingeing.
3. The increase in the patients' social activity may decrease the amount of unstructured time they have, thereby further reducing their vulnerability to binge eating.
4. The reduction in the frequency and severity of interpersonal stressors may lead directly to a decrease in the frequency of binge eating.

Through the operation of processes of this type, it is not difficult to see how the eating disorder may be progressively eroded. It is also easy to see how the full effects of IPT may take longer to be expressed than those of CBT, since CBT probably operates directly on the disturbed eating habits and attitudes, whereas with IPT these changes may be secondary. However, the effects of IPT cannot be exclusively the product of changes in interpersonal functioning, since some change occurs almost immediately (see Figure 14.4).

INDICATIONS AND FUTURE DIRECTIONS

In contrast to the substantial body of evidence supporting CBT as a treatment for bulimia nervosa (Wilson & Fairburn, in press), the evidence supporting IPT is much more modest. It

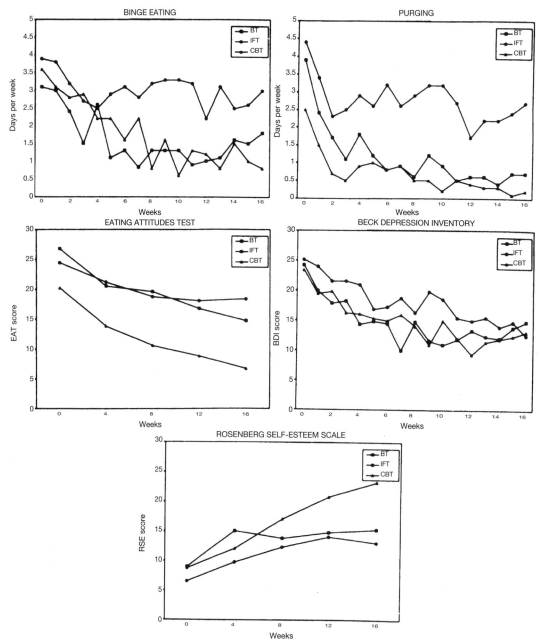

FIGURE 14.4. Symptomatic change during the treatment of bulimia nervosa. From Jones, Peveler, Hope, and Fairburn (1993). Copyright 1993 by Pergamon Press, Ltd. Reprinted by permission.

cannot therefore be recommended as a first-line treatment. In my opinion, it is best viewed as a promising alternative to CBT. IPT should probably be reserved for those patients who either fail to respond to CBT or will not accept it. For example, we have had some success using IPT with patients who have both bulimia nervosa and insulin-dependent diabetes mellitus—

a patient group that can be difficult to engage in CBT (Peveler & Fairburn, 1992).

There is a clear need for more research on the use of IPT to treat bulimia nervosa. In progress is a two-center trial in which the Oxford comparison of CBT and IPT is being repeated. This study is designed to see whether the original findings can be replicated. In addition, its large sample size will allow other important questions to be addressed. For example, an issue of considerable interest is whether the same types of patients benefit from the two treatments or whether there are "mode-specific" predictors of response. If different patient characteristics are found to predict response to CBT and IPT, this might allow the matching of patients to treatments, thereby improving overall outcome.

In addition to the need to substantiate the effectiveness of IPT, there is a need to improve the treatment. Its cost-effectiveness might be enhanced by administering it in a group format. Work by Wilfley et al. (1993) with obese patients who binge-eat suggests that this might be possible. The effectiveness of the treatment might be enhanced by adding techniques from CBT directed at the disturbed eating habits and attitudes. Indeed, it would seem logical to amalgamate IPT and CBT, so that both the eating disorder and the accompanying interpersonal problems could be directly addressed in a single treatment. Unfortunately, this is not possible, since the styles of the two treatments are so different as to make them immiscible. Instead, our group is experimenting with combining IPT with the use of a self-help program based directly on CBT (Fairburn, 1995). Patients receive IPT exactly as described in this chapter; at the same time, they follow the self-help program with the encouragement of the therapist. This combination seems to work well.

ACKNOWLEDGMENTS

I am most grateful to G. Terence Wilson, PhD, for his thoughtful comments on an earlier version of this chapter.

The research described in the chapter was supported by grants from the U.K. Medical Research Council (8008656 and 8921076) and the Wellcome Trust (13961). I hold a Wellcome Principal Research Fellowship (046386).

REFERENCES

Brown, G. W., Adler, Z., & Bifulco, A. (1988). Life events, difficulties and recovery from chronic depression. *British Journal of Psychiatry, 152,* 487–498.

Fairburn, C. G. (1981). A cognitive behavioral approach to the management of bulimia. *Psychological Medicine, 11,* 707–711.

Fairburn, C. G. (1995). *Overcoming binge eating.* New York: Guilford Press.

Fairburn, C. G., & Cooper, Z. (1993). The Eating Disorder Examination (12th edition). In C. G. Fairburn & G. T. Wilson (Eds.), *Binge eating: Nature, assessment and treatment* (pp. 317–360). New York: Guilford Press.

Fairburn, C. G., Jones, R., Peveler, R. C., Carr, S. J., Solomon, R. A., O'Connor, M. E., Burton, J., & Hope, R. A. (1991). Three psychological treatments for bulimia nervosa: A comparative trial. *Archives of General Psychiatry, 48,* 463–469.

Fairburn, C. G., Jones, R., Peveler, R. C., Hope, R. A., & O'Connor, M. (1993). Psychotherapy and bulimia nervosa: The longer-term effects of interpersonal psychotherapy, behavior therapy and cognitive behavior therapy. *Archives of General Psychiatry, 50,* 419–428.

Fairburn, C. G., Kirk, J., O'Connor, M., & Cooper, P. J. (1986). A comparison of two psychological treatments for bulimia nervosa. *Behaviour Research and Therapy, 24,* 629–643.

Fairburn, C. G., Marcus, M. D., & Wilson, G. T. (1993). Cognitive-behavioral therapy for binge eating and bulimia nervosa: A comprehensive treatment manual. In C. G. Fairburn & G. T. Wilson (Eds.), *Binge eating: Nature, assessment, and treatment* (pp. 361–404). New York: Guilford Press.

Fairburn, C. G., Norman, P. A., Welch, S. L., O'Connor, M. E., Doll, H. A., & Peveler, R. C. (1995). A prospective study of outcome in bulimia nervosa and the long-term effects of three psychological treatments. *Archives of General Psychiatry, 52,* 304–312.

Fairburn, C. G., & Wilson, G. T. (1993). Binge eating: definition and classification. In C. G. Fairburn & G. T. Wilson (Eds.), *Binge eating: Nature, assessment, and treatment* (pp. 3–14). New York: Guilford Press.

Frank, E., & Spanier, C. (1995). Interpersonal psychotherapy for depression: Overview, clinical efficacy, and future directions. *Clinical Psychology: Science and Practice, 2,* 349–369.

Frank, E., Frank, N., Cornes, C., Imber, S. D., Miller, M. D., & Morris, S. M. (1993). Interpersonal psychotherapy in the treatment of late-life depression. In G. L. Klerman & M. M. Weissman (Eds.), *New applications of interpersonal psychotherapy* (pp. 167–198). Washington, DC: American Psychiatric Press.

Jones, R., Peveler, R. C., Hope, R. A., & Fairburn, C. G. (1993). Changes during treatment for bulimia nervosa: A comparison of three psychological treatments. *Behaviour Research and Therapy, 31,* 479–485.

Klerman, G. L., & Weissman, M. M. (Eds.). (1993). *New applications of interpersonal psychotherapy.* Washington, DC: American Psychiatric Press.

Klerman, G. L., Weissman, M. M., Rounsaville, B. J., & Chevron, E. S. (1984). *Interpersonal psychotherapy of depression.* New York: Basic Books.

Mufson, L., Moreau, D., Weissman, M. M., & Klerman, G. L. (1993). *Interpersonal psychotherapy for depressed adolescents.* New York: Guilford Press.

Peveler, R. C., & Fairburn, C. G. (1992). The treatment of bulimia nervosa in patients with diabetes mellitus. *International Journal of Eating Disorders, 11,* 45–53.

Weissman, M. M., & Klerman, G. L. (1993). Conjoint Interpersonal psychotherapy for depressed patients with marital disputes. In G. L. Klerman & M. M. Weissman (Eds.), *New applications of interpersonal psychotherapy* (pp. 103–128). Washington: American Psychiatric Press.

Weissman, M. M., & Markowitz, J. C. (1994). Interpersonal psychotherapy: Current status. *Archives of General Psychiatry, 51,* 599–606.

Wilfley, D. E., Agras, W. S., Telch, C. F., Rossiter, E. M., Schneider, J. A., Cole, A. G., Sifford, L., & Raeburn, S. D. (1993). Group cognitive-behavioral therapy and group interpersonal psychotherapy for the nonpurging bulimic individual: A controlled comparison. *Journal of Consulting and Clinical Psychology, 61,* 296–305.

Wilson, G. T., & Fairburn, C. G. (in press). Treatment of eating disorders. In P. E. Nathan & J. M. Gorman (Eds.), *Psychotherapies and drugs that work: A review of the outcome studies.* New York: Oxford University Press.

CHAPTER 15

The Etiology and Treatment of Body Image Disturbance

ANN KEARNEY-COOKE
RUTH STRIEGEL-MOORE

Slade (1988) describes body image as "the picture we have in our minds of the size, shape, and form of our bodies" and the feelings we have concerning these characteristics and our constituent body parts. Disturbed body image is a well-known feature of both anorexia nervosa and bulimia nervosa (Bruch, 1962, p. 20). Body image disturbance in eating disorders is a multidimensional phenomenon that involves perceptual, attitudinal, and behavioral features (Cash & Brown, 1987; Garfinkel & Garner, 1982; Kearney-Cooke, 1989; Rosen, Saltzberg, & Srebnik, 1989; Slade, 1994; Thompson, 1990; Williamson, 1990). Body image disturbance in women with eating disorders has been attributed to cultural standards for beauty, learning within the family, disturbances in development of self-identity and effectiveness, disturbances in psychosexual development, and deficits in self-esteem (Rosen, 1990). Compared to other variables, body image appears to be among the important prognostic factors for anorexia nervosa (Button, 1986) and bulimia nervosa (Freeman, Beach, Davis, & Solyom, 1985).

Recently, clinical researchers of eating disorders have begun to extend their focus from body image distortion and body image dissatisfaction to the ways in which cognitions about the body affect body image and self-image. For example, overvaluation of weight and shape is now recognized as a major symptom of anorexia nervosa and bulimia nervosa (American Psychi-

atric Association, 1994). We have found it useful to apply the construct of "schemas" to our work with women who experience body image disturbance. As described in the work of cognitive therapists such as Aaron Beck and his colleagues (Beck, 1967; Beck, Freeman, & Associates, 1990; Beck, Rush, Shaw, & Emery, 1979), schemas are central cognitive structures within the system of the self. Schemas have been defined as "stable, cognitive patterns that provide a basis for screening out, differentiating, and coding stimuli that confront the individual" (Beck et al., 1979, pp. 12–13), and as "specific rules that govern information processing and behavior" (Beck et al., 1990, p. 8).

Once a negative body schema is formed, it serves a powerful maintenance function for body image problems because the schema determines what is noticed, attended to, and remembered about experiences (Padesky, 1994). A woman who believes "I am not attractive; thus, I am not lovable" will notice and remember negative comments about her body more readily than positive reactions. She will focus on bodily defects, flaws, and errors, noticing these more than strengths. She will attribute her successes and failures to her appearance. She will tend to surround herself with others who are obsessed with their appearance. She will tolerate negative comments about her appearance because they fit her view of her body. Once formed, a negative body schema is maintained in the face of contradictory evidence through processes of not noticing, distorting, and discounting contradictory information (Beck et al., 1990; Hastie, 1981). Thus a woman whose body schema for many years has been "My body is defective—I am too fat" will look at a list of data supporting "My body is fine" and say to the therapist, "Yes, I see the evidence, but I am still too fat. I feel embarrassed about how I look. My boyfriend only said I look good because he felt sorry for me." Padesky (1994) describes this process as the "Swiss cheese phenomenon." Using this concept with eating disorders, we listen as clients describe letting experiences or comments that would improve their body image slip through the "holes," but holding on to negative statements.

From such phenomena as phantom limb syndrome, eating disorders, body dysmorphic disorder, and depression, we know that body image is based on the physical self but is not synonymous with it. We know that the translation from the physical body to the mental representation of the body, and then to attitudes and behavior toward the body, is a complex and emotionally charged developmental process. The results of this process, such as body image distortion, body hatred, or other negative body experiences, have puzzled researchers and clinicians for years. We are still left with unanswered questions like the following: What happens in development that causes the mental picture of the body to be quite different from the actual physical appearance of the body? Why do some individuals become obsessed with their bodies, feel intensely dissatisfied with them, and structure their lives around changing them, while others with a similar body type experience dissatisfaction, feel that they would like to lose 20 pounds, but forget it and get on with their day? Why do some individuals experience shifts in their images of their bodies, while others tend to have a stable body image?

In this chapter, we first introduce two major pathways to body image disturbance. We realize that there may be additional pathways, but we focus on those pathways we have encountered in a majority of our clients. Subsequent sections of this chapter illustrate therapeutic techniques we have developed to help clients construct more positive body images and to change their body schemas. We describe ways to assist clients in adopting attitudes that facilitate change, as well as techniques to replace negative images with more positive ones.

PATHWAYS TO THE DEVELOPMENT OF BODY IMAGE DISTURBANCE

After listening to the stories of many clients with body image disturbance and following the literature on eating disorders, we would like to describe two possible pathways to the development of body image disturbance among eating-disordered clients. Regardless of the pathway, these clients are left with negative body images and schemas about their bodies, which serve a powerful maintenance function for their eating disorders. Later, we describe how guided imagery and cognitive-behavioral techniques can be used to help clients develop alternative, positive schemas for their bodies.

Pathway 1: Internalization as the Key Process

Moore and Fine (1968) define "internalization" as a progressive process by which external interactions between the organism and outer world are replaced by inner representations of these interactions and their end result. We believe that for one group of clients, a combination of key events (e.g., sexual abuse, multiple surgeries) and/or significant relationships (e.g., interactions with a mother who is obsessed with her body or a father who is overly focused on appearance) leaves them with a tremendous "charge" around their bodies and with internalized negative representations of their physical selves.

For example, Alice, a 28-year-old bulimic client, described growing up with a mother and aunts who were obsessed with their own appearance and constantly talked about the shape and weight of other women. She described almost feeling paranoid when she left a family gathering, because she knew they would be talking about her hair, clothes, and weight. Her father, a successful businessman, was as concerned about her weight gain as she was during the first 6 months of treatment. She remembered that although her father rarely hugged her or affectionately touched her, he often commented about how she looked. She also described an image of her body as repulsive and dirty, which she attributed to a long-term incestuous relationship with an older brother, who told her that her genital area smelled bad. To overcome the shame, she developed elaborate rituals to keep her body and clothes clean. Hers was a family in which joy was derived primarily from achievement (including the achievement of "looking good"), rather than from the security and warmth of human connection. This led to an obsession with her shape and weight, to the point that almost all feedback was filtered through the lens of the body. The attainment of the perfect body was a way to gain prestige and admiration within her family. Her ability to attain the ideal shape and weight brought her a feeling of accomplishment, which temporarily rescued her from the emptiness and isolation of her world. Sculpting herself into a "statue to be admired" felt safer than having to be vulnerable and enter into close relationships with others. But this way of relating left her "hungry" and addicted to the notion that if she could only lose 2 more pounds or wear a smaller dress size, she would feel better.

For clients in this group, the first goal of body image treatment is to assist them in reconstructing the key relationships and events that have left them with negative body representations. Techniques to help clients understand the role of parents, peers, culture, sexual experiences, and so forth have been described in other publications (Kearney-Cooke, 1989; Kearney-Cooke & Striegel-Moore, 1994; Wooley & Kearney-Cooke, 1986) and do not constitute the focus of this chapter. The second goal of treatment is to help clients develop alternative schemas for their bodies; treatment techniques related to this goal are described later in the chapter.

Pathway 2: Projection as the Key Process

Human identity cannot be separated from the house it lives in—the body (Fisher, 1990). Body schemas are crucial to early personality development, especially to the differentiation of the self from the world as the sense of body boundaries is formed. Because the body is the only object in a person's perceptual world that simultaneously is perceived and is part of the self, theorists have proposed an equation between body feelings and personality patterns (Fisher, 1966; Schilder, 1935). The unique closeness of the body to the individual's identity maximizes the likelihood that the body reflects and shares in the person's most important preoccupations.

Fisher (1966) writes that the body, like all significant objects, can become a "screen" on which one projects one's most intense concerns.

Some clients project onto their bodies their experiences of overwhelming internal states and/or interpersonal struggles that they feel inadequately equipped to deal with. They perceive their bodies as changeable; hence, projecting their feelings of being out of control onto their bodies permits these clients the illusion that they have a means of restoring control.

Because most of the clients' time is spent changing their bodies, they do not develop the skills to handle the overwhelming feelings or interpersonal deficits that lead to profound feelings of inadequacy. These clients believe that "If I change my body, I will change myself and feel more competent in the world." The efforts they expend to change their bodies offer temporary relief from the aversive emotional states by offering distraction and by permitting the clients to narrow their cognitive focus to a highly structured task that appears manageable (see also Heatherton & Baumeister, 1991). Moreover, the clients may hold on to the "myth of transformation" commonly associated with efforts to change appearance—namely, that by changing one's body one may change one's life.

Unfortunately, Western culture reinforces this myth of transformation. In our image-conscious society, developing an image seems to have become more important than developing an authentic self (Gergen, 1991). This is especially true for women. From early childhood, girls in our society learn from many socialization agents that appearance is extremely important, that beauty is an essential part of their worth, and that acceptance or rejection by others depends to a large extent on how they look (Rodin, Silberstein, & Striegel-Moore, 1985; Striegel-Moore, 1993; Striegel-Moore, Silberstein, & Rodin, 1993). As a result, most women experience a tremendous "charge" around their bodies. The following is an example of this process.

Amy, a 28-year-old anorexic who had struggled with an eating disorder for 10 years, entered group therapy and was beginning to connect with other members of the group. Group members encouraged her to eat meals with others, and she planned to eat with her sister and brother-in-law on a Friday night. The sister and her husband were golfing and got delayed; Amy began to feel physically hungry and yearned to be out with them rather than being home alone. She then reported feeling fat, flabby, and afraid that she was gaining too much weight. She got on her treadmill. As she exercised, she began to discount her yearnings to be with her sister, and began to feel better. She was sweating, burning calories, and feeling that she had regained control. The process is illustrated in Figure 15.1.

For this group of clients, the initial goal of therapy is to help them decode their negative talk about their bodies and understand the function it serves. Clients are asked to keep track of the times each day that they feel negative about their bodies, and of the people and events connected with those times. They are told that the body is the house a person lives in, and that whenever they talk negatively about their bodies they are talking negatively about themselves. They are asked to consider the possibility that at these times when they tend to feel fatter, they might be distracting themselves from feelings or interpersonal struggles that are too difficult to handle.

For example, Amy realized that whenever she felt "hungry" for people or food, she felt out of control and hopeless about getting her needs met. She would look in the mirror, see herself as fat, believe that fatness was the cause of her hopelessness and depression, and experience a distortion of her body image. Her focus would then switch to changing her body, which played an important role in maintaining her eating disorder. In an attempt to seek active mastery, she focused on something concrete (her body) that she could effectively control. She converted helplessness to action. A transient sense of mastery occurred, and the action (exercise) regulated the self-state. As she wrote about times she felt negative about her body, she began to see the negative body talk as a signal that an internal experience needed to be understood.

Writing it down helped Amy organize the series of interactions and internal experiences and their significance. Writing thus increased her understanding and mastery by giving active form to an otherwise unknowable internal experience (Krueger, 1989).

Facilitating the Development of Alternative Body Images and Body Schemas

Whether the central factor in the development of body image disturbance is internalization or projection, both groups of clients are left with maladaptive body schemas (Figure 15.2). Therefore, we believe that treatment of body image disturbance involves not only working through historical material related to body hatred and understanding projections onto the body, but also developing and strengthening alternative, more adaptive body schemas. Such schemas must be developed in order for the clients to be able to take in more positive feedback about their bodies. Hence, the second goal of treatment is to help both groups of clients develop alternative schemas for themselves and their bodies.

It is difficult for eating-disordered clients to change their body image. Body image is a complicated phenomenon, closely connected to the earliest experience of the self and of the self in relation to others. The cultural focus on women's bodies as an object (on billboard, TV, etc.), together with the use of the female body to sell and to seduce, further complicates efforts to change a negative body image. Women are exposed on a daily basis to information that confirms their self-critical views of their bodies (Bordo, 1993). Once a negative body image is formed, one sees the world through a negative body schema, making it difficult to change one's body image. We share with our clients that we believe it is difficult but possible to develop an alternative image of the body.

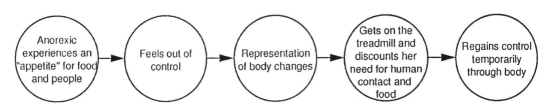

FIGURE 15.1. The role of body in self regulation.

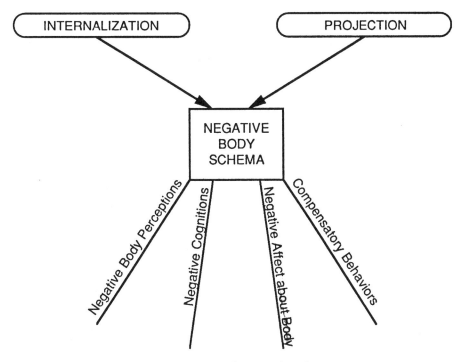

FIGURE 15.2. Body image disturbance.

DEVELOPMENT OF ATTITUDES OF CHANGE

Before we describe techniques to help clients create alternative body images, we discuss our efforts to encourage clients to develop attitudes which will help enhance the process of change.

An Attitude of Deliberateness

We share with clients the research of Wolin and Wolin (1993), summarized in a book entitled *The Resilient Self.* These researchers set out to study the effects of alcoholic parents on their children's adjustment. The initial assumption was that a high percentage of children of alcoholic parents would become alcoholics themselves; contrary to this assumption, only 25% of children of alcoholic parents became alcoholics. Wolin and Wolin (1993) then continued their research by studying the 75% of children who did well. In their book, they describe how these children practiced "deliberateness." These children improved deliberately and methodically upon their parents' lifestyle. They married into strong and healthy families and developed meaningful family rituals. They also engaged in a self-repair process, whereby they actively did things to keep themselves strong for battling the adversity within. For example, instead of coming home and drinking beers at night as their alcoholic parents did, they scheduled leisure activities or coached their children's sport teams.

The point in sharing this with clients is to illustrate that it is difficult to change such a basic aspect of the self as body image. Change involves understanding and working through the past and decoding projections onto the body, but at some point the clients must focus their energy on the hard work of changing. This involves their being deliberate about being in situations where body acceptance is more important than body perfection. It involves their cultivating relationships with individuals who are capable of extending unconditional regard to others (Rogers, 1951). It involves the clients' practicing guided imagery, repetitively keeping data logs, and teaching others new ways of talking about and touching their bodies. Without such sustained efforts, clients may spend their lives complaining about and mistreating their bodies/selves. They may solidify a helpless and victimized stance in life. We emphasize with clients that they are not responsible for their body image struggles, but that they are responsible for taking on the challenge of developing a solution.

A New Definition of Power

The message in Western culture is that power for a woman equals the ability to make her body look like the present beauty ideal. Women are encouraged to look outside themselves and to adopt a lifestyle that enables them to reach the beauty ideal at any cost. As women look outside themselves at the current ideals for their age, it is like looking into a funhouse mirror; the images that come back via magazines or TV are not realistic. Nevertheless, women are told that they can meet these ideals if only they try hard enough. Many women internalize these standards, become profoundly dissatisfied with themselves (Davis, 1985), and spend countless hours and dollars attempting to achieve an impossible look (Freedman, 1986).

Eating-disordered clients often report feeling the most empowered when they are losing weight. They often attain an illusory/grandiose feeling of power through controlling their bodies and being thinner than others. This illusory sense of power is a protection against a terrifying awareness of the fragility or helplessness that goes with a poorly defined identity. Therapists must challenge female clients to develop a new kind of power—intrinsic power. According to Horner (1989), "intrinsic power" refers to a sense of mastery, of competence, of potency in one's dealings with the world of things and with the world of people.

We believe that intrinsic power can be strengthened by helping women to focus on themselves and to define their own visions—in other words, to take themselves seriously enough to articulate what they value in life. This includes developing a new relationship with their bodies. Women might begin by tuning out what is politically correct or the present fashion "craze," and, with their own metabolism and bone structure in mind, defining what would be a realistic weight and shape. It then involves developing a lifestyle that supports their own goals. It means honoring the many seasons of a woman's body, such as menstruation, childbearing years, and menopause, and the physical changes associated with different life stages. It involves women's experiencing themselves as the writers and rewriters of the story about their bodies. This involves a shift from a reactive stance of trying to sculpt their bodies (and often themselves) into the current ideal to a more proactive, life-affirming focus on acceptance of their bodies and a commitment to take care of them.

Much energy is generated as women develop intrinsic power rather than the illusory power of body perfection. Therapy then needs to address how each client can deal with the uncomfortableness others may feel with a woman's new approach to her body. For example, one client shared an effective, simple response she gave when people commented on her body. When others would comment on her weight, she would say, "You are saying this because . . ." She thus shifted the burden of explanation back to the critical person, where it belonged. She found that fewer comments were made about her body after this new response, and she felt empowered in a new way.

A New Approach to Pace of Change

We have found that it is important to discuss with clients that they are not going to make the shift from body hatred to body acceptance overnight. But through the repetitive practicing of the techniques described in treatment, women will find themselves spending more of their time accepting their bodies and less time loathing their bodies. They will find that when they do feel bad about their bodies, they can employ the new strategies they have learned, and as a result can shift back more quickly to a greater level of body acceptance. We emphasize that a little bit of change each day leads to a marked shift in body image over time. We stress that women do not need to reach complete body acceptance; even women without eating disorders are not accepting of their bodies 100% of the time. But the goal is to develop a realistic body image—to listen to the body and to take care of it. The therapist must function as the container of hope and as the record keeper of progress. For example, we remind clients of shifts that have already occurred in their body images; of the times when they have rebounded from body loathing; and of the shifts taking place within when they are able to feel better about their bodies through other activities besides losing weight.

DEVELOPMENT OF ALTERNATIVE BODY SCHEMAS THROUGH GUIDED IMAGERY

The past three decades have seen a proliferation of research and reports about the clinical application of guided imagery in the treatment of a wide range of disorders (Crits-Cristoph & Singer, 1981; Schultz, 1978; Singer & Pope, 1978). Guided imagery has been a powerful tool in treatment approaches ranging from psychosomatic psychotherapy (Reyker, 1977) to behavior therapy (Wolpe, 1958). Hutchinson (1983) wrote that the most important features of imagery as a transformational tool include efficiency and economy in affective arousal; access to preverbal, primary-process material; circumvention of defensiveness and resistance; and creation of new mental patterns. We now describe how guided imagery can be used to help clients develop alternative body schemas.

Guided Imagery I: Rewriting the Script

The first type of guided imagery helps clients develop more adaptive schemas by reevaluating their body schemas in the developmental contexts in which they originated. Furthermore, it provides clients with a powerful first experience of what it would be like to hold different schemas and to respond to their bodies/selves and others in new ways. The steps of this technique can be summarized as follows:

1. Imagining an early life scene that evoked the schema of the current body image distortion.
2. Focusing on the emotions experienced, beliefs activated, and behaviors elicited or suppressed.
3. Exploring the image of body/self that the client extracted from the experience.
4. Developing an alternative schema.
5. Writing a new script.

We illustrate these steps through the story of Janet, a 24-year-old bulimic woman who was no longer binge-eating, but was still struggling with an unstable body image and body hatred. She described feeling disgusted with her body during the week. the therapist asked her when she felt the most disgusted. She described being in a meeting at the hospital where she worked, when she felt her body looked shorter and fatter, her cheeks were beginning to widen, and she looked less feminine. She felt self-conscious and was afraid that everyone was looking at her. The therapist asked her to recall exactly what was happening to her at that moment. She reported that she was asked to defend her position on a case. She felt inadequate and insecure, and thought she could never be articulate with these doctors. She then began to feel hatred toward herself.

1. *Imagining an early life scene that evoked the schema of the current body image distortion.* In using this technique, the therapist begins by asking the client to recreate the original setting in which the negative body image arose. For example, Janet's therapist instructed her to imagine a magic carpet or rope permitting her to go back through time, back to a scene where she had experienced similar feelings of inadequacy. The therapist told Janet to begin to see herself getting younger—to see the house or apartment she grew up in, and playgrounds or schools she went to—until she "found" the scene where she felt inadequate and self-conscious.

The client recalled the following: "I am sitting at the dinner table, and my mother and stepfather begin to fight. My stepfather is a lawyer and he loves to debate. He starts putting my mother down, and I jump in to defend her. he yells and makes fun of me; I keep yelling back, but begin to cry. I sink. I am acting like a baby. I run into my room, look in the mirror, and see my round cheeks, freckles, and fat body."

2. *Focusing on the emotions experienced, beliefs activated, and behavior elicited or suppressed.* Upon evoking the earlier schema, the therapist's task now is to explore the affective, cognitive, and behavioral components of this experience. This is illustrated in the following dialogue between Janet and her therapist:

THERAPIST. What are you experiencing?

CLIENT. Sadness, hopelessness.

THERAPIST. What did you learn about yourself in this scene?

CLIENT. I learned that I was not good enough, I was stupid, and my face is found and ugly.

THERAPIST. What was silenced in you during this experience?

CLIENT. My fighter self, my effective self.

3. *Exploring the image of body/self that the client extracted from the experience.* The therapist then explores fully the conclusions the client has drawn about her body, and examines the logic behind these conclusions. For example, Janet concluded, "I am not good enough, fat, and a baby."

4. *Developing an alternative schema.* In this step, the client is asked to create a new role from which to reexperience the original event. In Janet's care, she first imagined going back and having the mental capacities of her adult self and the power of speaking up to her stepfather. She imagined feeling good about her body and her ability to speak up. She also imagined a discussion with her mother about how she was no longer going to fight the mother's battles for her.

5. *Writing a new script.* As a final step, the therapist and client join efforts to create a new script. The new script may be difficult and complex to create, and may require the client and therapist to brainstorm together to find the right script. This script provides a powerful first experience of what it would be like for the client to hold a different schema and respond in a more empowered way. The new script then needs to be applied to other, similar experiences.

Janet created a script in which she imagined stronger roots from her feet going into the floor to a rich soil to support her. She thought out how to speak up to her stepfather in the words of an adult self—for example, by not allowing herself to get humiliated, but instead sticking to the issues at hand. She wrote out this script, role-played it in the session, and then practiced it outside the session. Each time a similar situation occurred at work, she would practice responding with a new image of self and write it in her data log. The therapist encouraged her to teach and discuss in the session each time how she handled difficult situations to strengthen the new schema. She began to report a more positive, consistent image of her body as she learned to handle interpersonal situations more effectively.

In summary, this imagery technique of rewriting the script helps clients develop more adaptive schemas of their bodies/selves. Clients reevaluate their original schemas in the developmental contexts in which they originally occurred, and learn to respond to people and events on the basis of alternative images and sets of beliefs about the self. They are then encouraged to be deliberate about practicing these new ways with people in the present. They become the teachers in the session, where the therapist asks many questions about how they were able to speak up, what they said to themselves, and what their bodies were saying. This serves to empower clients further, because they are largely responsible for creating the revised scripts.

Guided Imagery II: Letting Go of the Old Schema and Creating a New One

The second type of imagery helps clients develop and strengthen alternative, more adaptive schemas of their bodies/selves. The steps in this technique can be summarized as follows:

1. Relaxing and tuning in to the body.
2. Creating a wise and compassionate figure.
3. Letting go of negative images.
4. Creating an alternative body schema.

For this type of imagery, we illustrate the steps by giving the words a therapist might actually say to a client.

1. *Relaxing and tuning in to the body.* The therapist begins as follows:

Close your eyes and begin to take some deep breaths. Gently focus on your breathing. Do not do anything with your breath except watch it. Let your body breathe at its own pace. Watch it go in and watch it go out. Remember, there is nothing you need to hold onto, nothing you have to do. Just experience your breath. Experience the life force moving in and out of you. (*The therapist waits 2–3 minutes.*) You are now beginning to see yourself walking along a beach. You hear the crashing waves, the sounds of the sea gulls, children playing. You see cliffs in the distance.

2. *Creating a wise, compassionate figure.* The therapist goes on:

You begin to see a figure on the cliffs. You realize the figure is wise and compassionate, knows your body's story, and is behind you 100% in the change process. This could be a spiritual figure, a person you've known or read about, or one you create. Look at his or her face. Sense the kindness, gentleness. Feel the love and acceptance.

3. *Letting go of negative images.* The therapist continues:

> You begin to see negative images of your body; you hear yourself saying negative things to yourself about your body; you hear others talking in negative ways about your body. Imagine that the wise figure turns to you and reaches out his or her hand, and this hand is like a magnet. Those negative images and thoughts begin to leave you.

This step is repeated as often as necessary, and examples from the past week or negative reactions to the body described in the session are used to assist the client in letting go of negative feelings.

4. *Creating an alternative body image.* The therapist says:

> Now look to the sky and realize there is a screen in the sky where you can see new images of yourself. You are aware that this is your body, your life. You hear yourself talking to yourself in a more positive way. What are you saying? . . . You experience yourself listening to the information your body is teaching you about hunger, about fullness, about tiredness. Instead of ignoring your needs, you see yourself stopping eating when you are full . . . resting when you are tired . . . feeding yourself when you are hungry. You have the courage to accept and express yourself as a _____ year-old woman, and you are no longer looking outside yourself to try to reach an external standard. You feel empowered as you attain a realistic shape and weight. You see yourself teaching others how to treat your body. What are you telling them? . . . Who do you see yourself telling this to? . . . You see yourself buying fabrics and colors that feel good on your body. Feel these fabrics. What do they feel like? . . . You feel a shift taking place within and feel the support of the figure behind you. Just allow the images to unfold . . . A new way of experiencing yourself and your body . . . You feel more whole, more solid . . . When I count to three I want you to open your eyes, still feeling relaxed and calm. With each number, feel the new image of yourself strengthening within. One, two, three.

We feel it is useful to repeat this imagery with clients for 10–15 minutes every other session. The clients should be encouraged to teach the therapist about the images developing on the screen, and also to teach family members and friends, so they can assist in developing these alternative images.

We believe that guided imagery is an especially powerful tool, because body image is an image that clients have the potential to change. It is a powerful technique for psychic reconstruction, as well as for the creation of alternative images of the body.

DEVELOPMENT OF ALTERNATIVE SCHEMAS THROUGH COGNITIVE-BEHAVIORAL METHODS

In the preceding section, we have described how guided imagery can be used to develop alternative schemas. We now discuss how a "positive continuum" and "positive data logs" can be used to strengthen an alternative schema that has been developed through guided imagery.

Use of a Positive Continuum

To further the adoption of alternative, adaptive body schemas, we ask clients to chart the presence of their new schemas on a continuum ranging from 0% to 100%. Most clients with eating disorders have a highly detailed but negative view of their bodies. They can enumerate countless ways in which their bodies are inadequate, and they collapse these negative views into a global category that does not permit any gradation of degrees of attractiveness–unattractiveness. A major purpose of emphasizing a continuum is to shift dichotomous, absolute beliefs to more balanced, differentiated beliefs. In addition, at this stage in the treatment, it is important to focus only on positive aspects of body image, rather than focusing on aspects that are disliked.

> For example, Andrea, a bulimic client, was trying to develop the new belief "I am developing a healthy body image." On the initial continuum, she rated herself at 0%; this is not unusual for a client struggling with an eating disorder. The therapist asked her to place other people she knew on this continuum. She placed friends and people she liked in the 40–80% range. In helping Andrea and other

clients construct criteria for the continuum, the therapist explained that body image is not just shape and weight, but body functioning, health, capacity to bear a child, and so forth. The therapist then asked Andrea what it was about her friend Mary that made her rate her at 80% on the continuum. Andrea responded, "Mary is thin, dresses nice, walks around in a confident way; she reaches her hands out when she meets you; she is comfortable getting on the floor and playing with children." The therapist asked Andrea whether she could use those same "eyes" and evaluate herself on the continuum. Andrea then spoke about "messing up in many areas," but feeling good about her two pregnancies and being proud of how she ate, went through labor, and so on. She did feel proud of her body for that. She then rated herself at 15% on the continuum. This small shift on the continuum was in the direction of endorsing the new schema. Andrea had to consider her body as a bit more likable and capable to move from 0% to 15%.

Every few weeks, it is important to ask clients to rate their new schemas. The therapist asks the clients to talk about times they felt more accepting of their bodies. The schema range can be used to identify experiences and moods during the week that support either the old or new schemas. Continuum ratings allow the clients to subjectively quantify the schema change process.

Use of Positive Data Logs

To help clients begin to rate themselves more positively, it is necessary to teach them on a daily basis how to look for observations that are consistent with their new, more adaptive schemas. This is a difficult task, because the assignment asks them to look for or perceive things they tend to ignore or normally let go. The therapist must encourage clients' persistence in recording positive data about their bodies even when they do not quite believe these data. The therapist must be vigilant in the session about possible data for the log. Initially, the therapist can assume that clients will discount, distort, or simply not notice any positive data. The following dialogue demonstrates this process.

THERAPIST. Did you notice anything this week to write in our data log to support the belief "My body is fine"?

CLIENT. No, I tried. But there is nothing to support it. I still feel fat, heavy.

THERAPIST. OK, tell me about your week.

CLIENT. [The client talks about work and family, then describes the following:] I went dancing with my friends and felt great. My husband does not like to dance, so I have not been out dancing for 5 years. I forgot how much rhythm I have. I am a fairly good dancer. Also, it was fun to be out with the nurses I work with.

THERAPIST. Tell me more about how you like to dance. What was that experience like? What kind of music do you like?

CLIENT. I love music [from the 1970s and 1980s]. It brought back memories of myself in college. I felt somewhat attractive, light on my feet. Some of the male nurses danced with me too.

THERAPIST. Do you think it is possible that your experience out with your friends, moving through space, dancing, could quality on the positive data log as your body's being more likable because you have a body full of rhythm? Remember, the data we are looking for to write in your log include tiny experiences like the [dancing]. Why don't you write this in your log?

The therapist must teach clients to be vigilant, to record small amounts of evidence, and to pay attention to moments when they feel accepting of their bodies. Clients with eating disorders often have a tendency to pay attention only to evidence based on body weight and shape. It is important to teach clients that body image is affected by other aspects of behavior. Categories that are useful for clients to consider include the following:

Comforting things they do for their bodies (wearing comfortable clothing, calling a friend when sad, crying, taking a bubble bath).

Times their bodies feel good (dancing, wearing a favorite fabric or color).

Times they listen to their bodies (eating when hungry, stopping eating when full, resting when fatigued).

Teaching others how they want their bodies treated ("You're saying this because . . . ," "You eat what you want, but I am eating this . . . ").

Thoughts indicating new attitudes about their bodies ("I am energetic and feel great").

For example, a 45-year-old binge eater named Teri described the following change in body image occurring as a result of widening her conception of body image. She described waking up feeling depressed, looking in the mirror, and feeling disgusted at how fat she was. She wanted to stay in bed all day and order pizza to be delivered. However, she had been working on her data log the night before and remembered other things she could do to feel better. She got up, took a walk, put on a dress in her favorite color and fabric, scheduled a facial for after work, and came to the group. She felt better about her body as the day went on. She spent time in the group discussing the reasons why she was depressed and action strategies to fight depression. She began to see that when she treated her body well and faced the truth behind a difficult feeling state, she had a better body image.

SUMMARY

We have described two pathways we believe can lead to body image disturbance among eating-disordered clients. The first pathway is one in which a child's repeated actual experiences and interactions with important adults become internalized for the child as a working model of body image. The second pathway involves the projection onto the body of uncomfortable internal states; in this case, changing the body serves an important role in self-regulation. Regardless of the pathway, these clients are left with a negative body image that plays a powerful role in the maintenance of their eating disorders. We have then described how guided imagery and cognitive-behavioral techniques can be used to help clients develop alternative, more positive schemas of their bodies.

As we wrote this chapter, it became clear to us that this is definitely a work in progress. Many questions arose in the writing. Are there two distinct pathways? Are there more than two pathways? Are these pathways associated with different personality structures? If so, what are the implications of these for the treatment? Are there other treatment methods available to create alternative body schemas? As we listen

more seriously to eating-disordered women as they talk about their bodies, can we learn at a deeper level the function of the body obsession in these clients' lives and techniques to treat it effectively?

Our hope is that this chapter will assist in further understanding of the body image construct. Such advancement is important, because the body image construct is widely considered to play a central role in the etiology and maintenance of eating disorders. We are also aware of the need to evaluate empirically the various techniques we have described here. Despite considerable interest in body image, and despite an increasing number of controlled treatment outcome studies (for a review, see Fairburn, Agras, & Wilson, 1992), few researchers have concentrated on the specific aspects of treating body image disturbances (Cash & Brown, 1987; Garner & Bemis, 1982; Rosen et al., 1989). Clearly, more research is needed on the etiology and treatment of body image. Further research will lay the groundwork for the development of a comprehensive theory of eating disorders—a theory in which the construct of body image occupies a prominent position.

REFERENCES

American Psychiatric Association. (1994). *Diagnostic and statistical manual of mental disorders* (4th ed.). Washington, DC: Author.

Beck, A. T. (1967). *Depression: Clinical, experimental, and theoretical aspects.* New York: Harper & Row.

Beck, A. T., Freeman, A., Pretzer, J., Davis, D. D., Fleming, B., Ottavani, R., Beck, J., Simon, K. M., Padesky, C., Meyer, J., & Trexler, L. (1990). *Cognitive therapy of personality disorders.* New York: Guilford Press.

Beck, A. T., Rush, A. J., Shaw, B., & Emery, G. (1979). *Cognitive therapy of depression.* New York: Guilford Press.

Bordo, S. (1993). *Unbearable weight: Feminism, western culture, and the body.* Berkeley: University of California Press.

Bruch, H. (1962). Perceptual and conceptual disturbances in anorexia nervosa. *Psychosomatic Medicine, 24,* 187–194.

Button, E. (1986). Body size perception and response to outpatient treatment in anorexia nervosa. *International Journal of Eating Disorders, 5,* 617–629.

Cash, T. F., & Brown, T. A. (1987). Body image in anorexia nervosa and bulimia nervosa: A review of the literature. *Behavior Modification, 11,* 487–521.

Crits-Cristoph, P., & Singer, J. (1981). Imagery in cognitive behavior therapy: Research and application. *Clinical Psychology Review, 1*(1), 19–32.

Davis, L. L. (1985). Perceived somatotype, body cathexis, and attitudes towards clothing among college females. *Perceptual and Motor Skills, 61*(3), 1199–1205.

Fairburn, C. G., Agras, W. S., & Wilson, G. T. (1992). The research on the treatment of bulimia nervosa: Practical and theoretical implications. In G. H. Anderson & S. H. Kennedy (Eds.), *The biology of feast and famine* (pp. 317–339). San Diego: Academic Press.

Fisher, S. (1966). Body attention patterns and personality defenses. *Psychological Monographs: General and Applied, 80*(9), 1–29.

Fisher, S. (1990). The evolution of psychological concepts about the body. In T. Cash & T. Pruzinsky (Eds.), *Body images: Development, deviance, and change* (pp. 3–20). New York: Guilford Press.

Freedman, R. (1986). *Beauty bound: Why we pursue the myth in the mirror.* Lexington, MA: Lexington Books.

Freeman, R. J., Beach, B., Davis, R., & Solyom, L. (1985). The prediction of relapse in bulimia nervosa. *Journal of Psychiatric Research, 19,* 349–353.

Garfinkel, P. E., & Garner, D. M. (1982). *Anorexia nervosa: A multidimensional perspective.* New York: Brunner /Mazel.

Garner, D. M., & Bemis, K. M. (1982). A cognitive behavioral approach to anorexia nervosa. *Cognitive Therapy and Research, 6*(2), 123–150.

Gergen, K. J. (1991). *The saturated self: Dilemmas of identity in contemporary life.* New York: Basic Books.

Hastie, R. (1981). Schematic principles in human memory. In E. T. Higgins, C. P. Herman, & M. P. Zanna (Eds.), *Social cognition: The Ontario symposium* (Vol. 1, pp. 39–88). Hillsdale, NJ: Erlbaum.

Heatherton, T. F., & Baumeister, R. F. (1991). Binge eating as escape from self-awareness. *Psychological Bulletin, 110,* 86–108.

Horner, A. (1989). *The wish for power and the fear of having it.* Northvale, NJ: Jason Aronson.

Hutchinson, M. G. (1983). Transforming body image: Your body or foe? *Women and Therapy, 1,* 59–67.

Kearney-Cooke, A. M. (1989). Reclaiming the body: Using guided imagery in the treatment of body image disturbance among bulimic women. In L. M. Hornyak & E. K. Baker (Eds.), *Experiential therapies for eating disorders* (pp. 11–33). New York: Guilford Press.

Kearney-Cooke, A. M., & Striegel-Moore, R. H. (1994). Treatment of childhood sexual abuse in anorexia nervosa and bulimia nervosa. A feminist psychodynamic approach. *International Journal of Eating Disorders, 15*(4), 305–319.

Krueger, D. W. (1989). *Body self and psychological self: A developmental and clinical integration of disorders of the self.* New York: Brunner/Mazel.

Moore, E. B., & Fine, D. (1968). *A glossary of psychoanalytic terms and concepts.* New York: American Psychoanalytic Association.

Padesky, C. A. (1994, December). *Schema change processes in cognitive therapy of personality disorders.* Paper presented at the Milton H. Erickson Annual Conference, Los Angeles.

Padesky, C. A. (1994). Schema change processes in cognitive therapy. *Clinical Psychology and Psychotherapy: An International Journal of Theory and Practice, 1*(5), 267–278.

Reyker, J. (1977). Spontaneous visual imagery: Implications for psychoanalysis, psychopathology, and psychotherapy. *Journal of Mental Imagery, 2,* 253–274.

Rodin, J., Silberstein, L. R., & Striegel-Moore, R. H. (1985). Women and weight: A normative discontent. In T. B. Sonderegger (Ed.), *Nebraska symposium on motivation* (pp. 267–308). Lincoln: University of Nebraska Press.

Rogers, C. (1951). *Client-centered therapy.* Boston: Houghton Mifflin.

Rosen, J. C. (1990). Body image disturbances in eating disorders. In T. Cash & T. Pruzinsky (Eds.), *Body images: Development, deviance, and change* (pp. 3–20). New York: Guilford Press.

Rosen, J. C., Saltzberg, E., & Srebnik, D. (1989). Cognitive behavior therapy for negative body image. *Behavior Therapy, 20,* 393–404.

Schilder, P. (1935). *The image and appearance of the human body.* New York: International Universities Press.

Schultz, D. (1978). Imagery and the control of depression. In J. L. Singer & K. S. Pope (Eds.), *The power of human imagination.* New York: Plenum Press.

Singer, J. L., & Pope, K. S. (Eds.). (1978). *The power of human imagination.* New York: Plenum press.

Slade, P. D. (1988). Body image in anorexia nervosa. *British Journal of Psychiatry, 153*(Suppl. 2), 20–22.

Slade, P. D. (1994). What is body image? *Behavior Research and Therapy, 32,* 497–502.

Striegel-Moore, R. H. (1993). Etiology of binge eating: A developmental perspective. In C. G. Fairburn & G. T. Wilson (Eds.), *Binge eating: Nature, assessment, and treatment* (pp. 144–172). New York: Guilford Press.

Striegel-Moore, R. H., Silberstein, L. R., & Rodin, J. (1993). The social self in bulimia nervosa: Public self-consciousness, social anxiety, and perceived fraudulence. *Journal of Abnormal Psychology, 102,* 297–303.

Thompson, J. K. (1990). *Body image disturbance: Assessment and treatment.* Elmsford, NY: Pergamon Press.

Williamson, D. A. (1990). *Assessment of eating disorders: Obesity, anorexia, and bulimia nervosa.* Elmsford, NY: Pergamon Press.

Wolin, S. J., & Wolin, S. (1993). *The resilient self.* New York: Villard Books.

Wolpe, J. (1958). *Psychotherapy by reciprocal inhibition.* Stanford, CA: Stanford University Press.

Wooley, S. C., & Kearney-Cooke, A. M. (1986). Intensive treatment of bulimia and body image disturbance. In K. D. Brownell & J. P. Foreyt (Eds.), *Physiology, psychology and treatment of eating disorders* (pp. 477–501). New York: Basic Books.

CHAPTER 16

Family Therapy for Anorexia Nervosa

CHRISTOPHER DARE
IVAN EISLER

> Psychotherapy is the totality of therapeutic . . . procedures
> determined by the consideration of psychological phenomena
> which have previously been studied, and above all by the
> consideration of the laws which regulate the development of these
> psychological phenomena. . . . In a word, psychotherapy is the
> application of psychological science to the treatment of disease.
> —*Janet (1925, p. 1208)*

> All who drink this remedy recover in a short time except those
> whom it does not help, who all die. Therefore, it is obvious that it
> only fails in incurable cases.
> —*Attributed to Galen (2nd century A.D.)*

In writing this chapter, our aim is to bring together three perspectives on the family therapy of anorexia nervosa: (1) the theoretical models that provide the general framework for family interventions; (2) the growing empirical evidence for the efficacy of family therapy in anorexia nervosa; and (3) the clinical conceptualizations that guide the clinician in the moment-to-moment interactions with families. We recognize that however strongly a practice is committed to empirically investigated therapies, a great deal of clinical activity must be determined by clinical experience rather than detailed empirical data. This is inevitable, as there will always be considerable limitations on the proportion of the therapist's business with anorexic patients that can be justified by recourse to formal scientific work. At all stages in any one clinical encounter, a therapist has to make choices of possible behaviors. Some behaviors, such as the demonstration of warmth, sympathy, and consistent, flexible attention, are applicable to all patients. An overall decision as to a general strategy may have been shown to be valid by a control trial. But for much of what the therapist does, empirical support is absent, minimal, or contradictory.

This is true for all therapies, but in family therapy the potential determining variables are greatly increased—partly through the simple increase in the number of people the therapist has to relate to, and partly because of the complexity of the issues of family structure, family relationships, and family beliefs. Even if only a small proportion of these variables are relevant to the specific conduct of therapy, the range of determinants is potentially enormous.

The theoretical models and the conceptual

understanding of how change is brought about are therefore crucial in guiding clinical practice. Theoretical models, however, also run the risk of becoming enclosed self-justifying entities, and it is therefore important that they remain open to systematic evaluation. Our own practice in the family therapy of anorexia nervosa has changed considerably under the impact of our empirical studies. In this chapter we provide a structure for identifying the theoretical origins of the many different suggestions for the conduct of family therapy in anorexia nervosa. We then indicate how these suggestions are incorporated into our practice, and how that practice is justified by the evidence from research.

THE DEVELOPMENT OF FAMILY THERAPY FOR ANOREXIA NERVOSA

The field of family therapy for anorexia nervosa is vast, and any new publication under this title can only be commenced with a feeling of hubris. Family therapists have discussed work with anorexic patients for many years (e.g., Selvini Palazzoli, 1974; Minuchin, Rosman, & Baker, 1978; Wynne, 1980). In the field of eating disorders, there has likewise long been an acceptance of a problem in relation to the families of the patients, and hence an acknowledgment of a possible place for family interventions in the management of anorexia nervosa (Gull, 1874; Bliss & Branch, 1960; Bruch, 1973; Morgan & Russell, 1975). There is a gradual accumulation of empirical evidence indicating the circumstances in which the use of family therapy is most clearly indicated. We are also beginning to acquire information about the manner in which family interventions need to be modified to be successful, depending on the age of the patient at the time of therapy, the patient's age at onset of the illness, and the family characteristics. As would be expected, writers from within the field of eating disorders are more likely to specify the patient characteristics (age, duration of illness, etc.), whereas within the family therapy field, family factors (patterns of interaction, family structure, family life cycle stages, etc.) are much more thoroughly considered.

Anorexia nervosa has a special place in the development of family therapy, for it has played an important role in the work of a number of influential figures in family therapy (Minuchin, Selvini Palazzoli, Stierlin, Whitaker, White, Liebman, etc.). For this reason, anorexia nervosa can be seen as having become a paradigm for the therapy, in much the same way that hysteria served as a paradigm for psychoanalysis and phobias served for behavior therapy. The first conjectures as to the usefulness of family therapy in the treatment of anorexia nervosa came from Salvador Minuchin and his colleagues at the Philadelphia Child Guidance Clinic, and from Mara Selvini Palazzoli at the Milan Center. They believed that they had observed quite specific characteristics of the families within which anorexia nervosa arose. Their ideas were couched in quite a different language, referencing contrasting conceptual fields, and so it is difficult to compare the formulations of the two schools of thought. Nevertheless, there is clear overlap between these accounts. Both emphasize the closeness of the relationships within the family, the blurring of boundaries between generations, and a tendency to avoid open disagreement or conflict. The Philadelphia and Milan groups each evolved therapeutic strategies directed toward changing those qualities of the family that, in turn, were believed to offer the possibility of helping the patient.

Family therapy is far from being a unified conceptual system. There are a number of different models in the field; though these exhibit considerable overlap, they also constitute quite distinctive views of the nature of family therapy and the mechanisms that bring about change. All the major models of family therapy have had proponents who have applied them to the treatment of eating disorders. We have structured our presentation around a discussion of the main models of family therapy that have been used in the treatment of patients with anorexia nervosa (structural, strategic, Milan systemic, post-Milan, and feminist[1]), and that provide elements for our own practice, which we have immodestly called "the Maudsley approach." We have evidence for the extent of the efficacy of our model, as well as some evidence for the factors that contribute to its successful execution. Our model contains a theory about the development and treatment of anorexia nervosa, and its therapeutic procedures have clear connections with the other models we describe.

ETIOLOGICAL SCHEMES AND THE NATURE OF FAMILY THERAPY

The Traditional Model

Figure 16.1 is a simplistic illustration of the traditional view as to the relationship among the illness, the patient, and the origin of the disorder (see also Dare, 1993). The illness is labeled the "symptom" and is represented as a rectangle within the diagram. The psychology of the person is illustrated as the "personality" upon which biological, social, familial, and peer pressures have influence. Personality characteristics have a central position in most theories of the nature and development of anorexia nervosa:

> The remarkable consistency of clinical observations about anorexic personality features is matched by an unusual cross-theoretical convergence in the interpretation of their etiological significance. Dominant conceptual models assign such a central causal role in the emergence and maintenance of anorexic symptomatology, maintaining that the profoundly maladaptive behavior

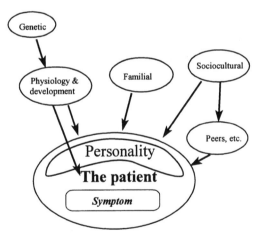

FIGURE 16.1. The traditional medical view of single or additive etiological factors. Genetic, sociocultural, familial, and peer group influences are seen as impinging in isolated and unidirectional ways on the psychobiological constitution of the individual. Genetic, social, and familial influences are seen as impinging similarly on the personality of the individual. Treatment, whether pharmacological, cognitive, psychodynamic, or family-therapeutic, is directed at correcting the problem in the individual. Psychoeducation is directed toward minimizing peer group or cultural pressures, given the patient's vulnerability.

of self-starvation acquires functional value only in the context of specific dispositional traits. (Vitousek & Manke, 1994, p. 137)

In Figure 16.1 the symptoms are portrayed as though they exist as a property of the individual; hence they are placed within the ellipse labeled "The patient." The various factors that have been postulated as giving rise to anorexia nervosa are portrayed as existing outside the patient, but as impinging upon her in a unidirectional way and as unrelated to one another.[2] Most of the literature on the topic suggests similar views as to the cluster of "ingredients" in a causal explanation for anorexia nervosa. Genetic factors have their impact upon the developing psychobiological systems of the individual. At a given, developmentally determined stage, illness processes evolve and symptoms become manifest. Likewise, sociocultural, familial, and other environmental factors influence the individual, increasing or decreasing her vulnerability to developing the eating disorder and having some potential to modify the symptomatic presentation.

In this model, treatment is also hypothesized as operating within the individual, countering the effects of the etiological vulnerability by inducing or enhancing protective factors. A variety of therapies can be categorized according to their relationship to the theoretical model. Psychological treatments are seen as comparable to pharmacological agents, operating within the individual to alter the psychobiological state. The diagram points to the possibility of psychoeducational treatments' being directed to reduce the effects of sociocultural and peer pressures. Within this model, a family intervention is conceived either as modifying the dysfunctional nature of the family or as leading to a "parentectomy" (Harper, 1983)—that is, leading to the removal of the child from the negative influence of the family.

Limitations of this traditional medical model, based as it is upon concepts of linear causality, have been described by many people in the field of eating disorders, but the critiques evolved by a variety of schools of family therapy are highlighted in the next few sections. The headings denote schools of family therapy as applied to anorexia nervosa. Some of the so-called "schools" are self-proclaimed entities, whereas others (e.g., the strategic therapies) represent a relatively diverse collection of ideas and techniques from a number of different centers.

Structural Family Therapy

Minuchin and his coworkers at the Philadelphia Child Guidance Clinic (Minuchin et al., 1975, 1978; Liebman, Minuchin, & Baker, 1974) developed a model for the treatment of anorexia nervosa, while at the same time evolving a persuasive and significant school whose general principles have been subject to considerable theoretical challenge but continue in practice to be widely influential in the conduct of family therapy. The basis for their approach to the treatment of anorexia nervosa is the "psychosomatic family model" which is best illustrated by the following quotation:

> This model holds that three factors in conjunction are necessary for the development of severe psychosomatic illness in children. First, the child is physiologically vulnerable; second, the child's family has the four following transactional characteristics: enmeshment, overprotectiveness, rigidity, and lack of conflict resolution. Third, the sick child plays an important role in the family's pattern of conflict avoidance; and this role is an important reinforcement for his symptoms. (Minuchin et al., 1975, p. 1032)

We do not discuss the model here in any detail, except to indicate its implications for the conduct of therapy and to evaluate the evidence for the specificity of the theory. The style of therapy has been clearly elaborated by a number of writers—for example, by Sargent, Liebman, and Silver (1985).

Figure 16.2 summarizes the theory of the symptom and the process of structural family therapy. A nuclear family is portrayed, although it is clear that there are examples of patients with anorexia nervosa in all types of family organizations. Two children are shown, one of whom (the patient) is enclosed within an ellipse connecting her to her mother, while the other child (the patient's sibling) is shown on the boundary of the family—that is, on the point of leaving home. The symptom is shown as placed amidst the family, but mostly as laid *upon* the patient. Minuchin (see the diagram of an "open systems model of psychosomatic disease" in Minuchin et al., 1978, p. 22) makes it clear that he sees physiological and extrafamilial stressors as contributing to the development of anorexia

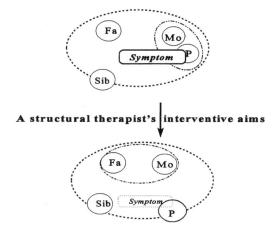

A family with an anorexic patient

A structural therapist's interventive aims

FIGURE 16.2. A model of structural family therapy intervention. The symptom is shown as though it were only a property of the family and the individual. It is wholly contained within a dysfunctional family structure; the correction of this structure through appropriate interventions contributes to a resolution of the symptom.

nervosa, so that Figure 16.2 is not a wholly accurate account of Minuchin's understanding of the origins of the disorder. The emphasis in his accounts of therapy, however, is upon the alteration of a dysfunctional family as the focus of treatment.

Structural interventions are shaped by the perceived dysfunctional state of the family: "The goal is to alter the family organization through limiting some patterns of family interaction while encouraging others" (Sargent et al., 1985, p. 261). If the therapist perceives the family as having difficulties in resolving conflicts, then that is what the therapist works upon. If the family shows a tendency to accept alliances between the child and the parent, then directive interventions are made to encourage a stronger coalition between the two parents, while placing the children in a stronger sibling subsystem. The family members are encouraged to have a more open style of communication among themselves and with the outside world. All these things are addressed because, as they are dealt with, the functional improvement within the family is believed to diminish the processes that give rise to the symptom:

> In structural family therapy the techniques are used within the structural goals of the therapy

thereby taking into full account the purposes of the symptoms . . . such techniques are carried out within a comprehensive process that not only removes symptoms, but also opens and firms up new structural channels for responding to the motivations that were sustaining the symptoms in the first place. (Aponte & VanDeusen, 1981, p. 334)

To facilitate the structural change, therapy sessions with the parental couple, with the patient, or with any other combination of family members may be needed.

To enable direct observation of the way the family's apparent dysfunction is manifested in the eating problem, the Philadelphia Child Guidance Clinic team has used participant observation of a family meal as a therapeutic occasion (Rosman, Minuchin, & Liebman, 1975). The interventions can be understood as clearly deriving from the "psychosomatic family" model. The parents are encouraged to decide jointly what they want their daughter to eat. The family is prevented from avoiding the conflict that the meal situation is likely to engender, thereby breaking the habitual pattern of interaction. In taking control of their daughter's eating, the parents must distance themselves from her fears of being engulfed by them, and thus, paradoxically, must increase the distance in their relationship with her. At the same time, the need to work together as parents will often bring the parents closer together and increase their belief in themselves (see also Dare, Eisler, Russell, & Szmukler, 1990; Eisler, 1993). Such structural interventions are often very powerful and have a visible and immediate effect on the way the family is organized around the symptom.

The empirical evidence for the efficacy of the approach, particularly with adolescent anorexia nervosa, is compelling. Minuchin et al. (1978) reported a good outcome in 80% of cases in their follow-up study of 52 adolescent anorexics. Martin (1985), using a comparable treatment approach, reported very similar findings from her Toronto study. In our own approach (which we discuss in more detail later in the chapter), there is a strong structural component in working specifically with adolescents; the results of our controlled treatment studies (Russell, Szmukler, Dare, & Eisler, 1987; Dare et al., 1990; Eisler, Hodes, Dare, Russell, & Dodge, 1996) showing the efficacy of family therapy for adolescent anorexia nervosa provide further evidence in support of this approach.

Strategic Family Therapy

Some of the activities described as structural family therapy directly attack the role of the symptom, and in this sense are strategic interventions. Some of Minuchin's associates are or have been advocates of strategic family therapy. For example, Jay Haley was director of research at the Philadelphia Child Guidance Clinic, and M. Duncan Stanton developed his research in the family therapy of substance abuse and dependence while at the clinic (Stanton, Todd, & Associates, 1982). Stanton's integration of structural and strategic approaches in the treatment of patients with substance use disorders has some resemblance to our own work with anorexic families. However, specific aspects of strategic therapy diverge from those of structural therapy, and the two approaches differ in some conceptual respects as well.

Haley (1973), in particular, takes a strongly "agnostic" view of the causes of psychological disorders. This is illustrated in Figure 16.3, where the symptom is placed outside the individual and the family—not to suggest an external origin or location, but to express the lack of interest in and speculation about etiology that characterizes both Haley's work and the discussion by Madanes (1981, pp. 39–48) of the treatment of eating disorder patients. In this figure, the family configuration is the same as in Figure 16.2, with a sibling on the point of leaving home and the patient involved with the mother. The symptoms of the illness are shown outside the family ellipse, but as having effects upon the individual, the patient, and the family. The uni-directional arrows are intended to portray the illness as a burden on the family; it puts limits on the normal process of life cycle development, but no specific function is postulated for it. The interventions are shown as being directed toward limiting the impact of the symptom on the individual and the family.

Most of the technical writings of the strategic therapists in this model have been concerned with developing powerful, focused techniques for inducing change. Prescribing behaviors with paradoxical intentions is the form of intervention most closely identified with this group. Examples are the prescription of "no change for the time being"; advising the performance of behaviors that challenge the symptom (e.g., advising an anorexic patient to eat a little more, to get up her strength to oppose her parents' insistence that she eat; recommending areas in which the patient might be more stubborn and obstinate other than through starvation). Haley's (1984) concept of "therapeutic ordeals," although not specifically devised for anorexia nervosa, is relevant because they can be congruent with the asceticism of the patient.

Strategic interventions have been criticized as being "tricky," manipulative, and disrespectful (Treacher & Carpenter, 1984). Particularly when the patient is so ill and her parents so understandably distressed, the therapist must be extremely careful to be responsible and sympathetic. Proponents of strategic models of therapy would also argue that it is crucial for the therapist to have a good theoretical grasp of the possible impact of the intervention (thus a "no change" prescription implies that the symptom can be controlled, and also puts the responsibility for the continued existence of the symptom on the therapist, reducing feelings of guilt and blame). The change that strategic therapy intends is illustrated in the lower part of Figure 16.3. The symptom is shown as still existing, but in a less intense form; this implies that the illness is not necessarily eliminated, but rather that its influence on the family and individual is weakened. The alterations in family functioning are expected to be less dramatic than those to which the structural family therapist aspires.

Milan Systems Therapy and the Post-Milan Developments

In discussing strategic therapy, a distinction has to be made among those such as Haley, who have kept to a relatively atheoretical stance; the Palo Alto Mental Research Institute group (e.g., Watzlawick, Beavin, & Jackson, 1967; Watzlawick, Weakland, & Fisch, 1974), whose members have been concerned with a specific theory of change; and the Milan systems group of therapists, whose early work fits into the strategic model, but whose innovations have become the basis of a separate school (see Tomm, 1984a; MacKinnon, 1983).

In the original formulations of the Milan approach (Selvini Palazzoli, 1974; Selvini Palazzoli, Boscolo, Cecchin, & Prata, 1978), the central idea was that the family has become a rigidly organized interactional system in which the symptoms of the illness play an important role as a powerful homeostatic mechanism. The Milan group developed a very specific style of interviewing (Selvini Palazzoli, Boscolo, Cecchin, & Prata, 1980; Tomm, 1984b), which aims to

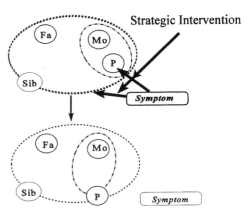

FIGURE 16.3. A model of straegic family therapy intervention. The family is the same one as in the model of structural family therapy (see Figure 16.2). However, the symptom is placed, "atheoretically," outside the family, although it is seen as having strong influences on the individual and the family. After treatment (in the lower half of diagram), the family is seen as showing some reorganization, but less than intended within structural therapy; the symptom is shown as persisting in a more shadowy form. Although the patient may be seen to be closely tied to the mother, no "dysfunction" is implied in this model. The strategic interventions are derived from Haley's formulations (Haley, 1973; Madanes, 1981). They aspire to be powerful in disconnecting the symptom from its role in dominating the relationship between the patient and the family. This disarticulation is intended to provide an opportunity for the patient and the family members to reenter age-appropriate lives.

elicit information about the family system, and at the same time introduces a new perspective that emphasizes the interconnectedness of different aspects of family life. This allows the therapist to develop a hypothesis about the nature of the family organization and the "function" of the symptom in this organization. End-of-session interventions, usually in the form of a "message to the family," are used to reframe the observed pattern in a way that gives it a new, positively connoted meaning. Some interventions also include a prescription of a task that challenges the perceived pattern.

The main departure from the strategic model developed by the Milan group was the notion that the therapist needs to maintain a neutral stance not only in relation to the family (i.e., not taking sides), but also as to whether change should occur (and, if so, what direction it should take). This should not be understood as therapeutic nihilism. Rather, it is an expression of a view of the family as a homeostatic system, in which direct pressure for change is likely to be met by a counterpressure to maintain the system in an unchanged, balanced state. Instead of making direct interventions, the therapist therefore interviews the family in a way that elicits differences; these become new information in the family system and encourage the family members to become observers of their own family process, challenging their beliefs about themselves and about their relationships.

In the early 1980s, the original Milan group split up and moved in different directions. Mara Selvini Palazzoli, together with Giuliana Prata, moved back closer to the strategic origins of the model and in some respects also closer to the structural model (Jones, 1988). This is perhaps best exemplified by the strategic intervention most often associated with Selvini Palazzoli's later work—the "invariable prescription" or "secret couple task:"[3]

> We invited the parents to attend the following session without the daughters. In this session we gave them this prescription: "Keep everything about this session absolutely secret at home. Every now and then, start going out in the evenings before dinner. Nobody must be forewarned. Just have a written note saying, 'We'll not be home tonight.' If when you come back, one of your daughters inquires where you have been, just answer calmly, 'These things concern only the two of us.'" (Selvini Palazzoli, 1986, pp. 341–342)

Selvini Palazzoli stresses the strategic nature of the intervention, highlighting the importance of the secrecy of the task and the authority that this gives the therapist. However, the use of this task for the parents, which requires them to establish and proclaim a separate private life as a couple, can be seen to have implications for the structure of the family in terms of its hierarchical organization and internal intergenerational boundaries. In this respect, there is a clear convergence between the approaches of Selvini Palazzoli and the Philadelphia group.

The theoretical ideas that were pursued by the other half of the Milan group (Luigi Boscolo and Gianfranco Cecchin) and later developed by many others (e.g., Boscolo, Cecchin, Hoffman, & Penn, 1987; Hoffman, 1985; Penn, 1982; Campbell, Draper, & Huffington, 1991; White, 1987), increasingly challenged the conceptual and ideological basis of existing family therapy practice. The initial shift from concepts of individual dysfunction to ones of family dysfunction gave way to the realization that assumptions about family "normality" are also questionable, for any such beliefs must be strongly socially, geographically, and historically determined. An important influence on the field has been the work of the theoretical biologists (e.g., Maturana & Varela, 1988), who have argued that reality is always a constructed reality—that is, known only through the psychological and social process of making sense of perceptual data. Therapy is seen as being concerned more with the beliefs and meanings attached to behaviors than with the behaviors per se. The assumption is that the family members develop an understanding (a "story") that describes their beliefs and attitudes. The illness is embedded and in some ways "cocreated" by these stories.

Therapy is shown in Figure 16.4 as a process of the therapist's engaging the family members in discussions about themselves. The expertise of the therapist is in facilitating the evolution of

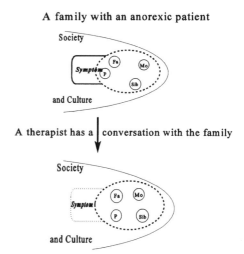

FIGURE 16.4. A post-Milan family therapy intervention. Contemporary family therapy is absorbing a combination of postmodern and feminist ideas; these are resulting in styles of family therapy which ascribe more power to the family and patient. The symptom is seen as arising from socially constructed views as to the nature of feminity, of body shape, and of the adolescent developmental process. The therapist is seen not as an expert in the illness who helps the family or patient change, but as someone who can facilitate the evolution of a different story for the family.

different meanings (different beliefs, explanations about cause, interpretations of their own histories and relationships, etc.) The therapist has no special rights or privileges concerning "truer" or "more healthy" stories, since "truth" and "health" are only social conventions shaped by linguistic practice. The therapist's "insights" are as suspect or as accurate as the family's own, but no more likely to be helpful, because they are no less likely to be bounded and controlled by the pressure of social process. The therapist helps the family members think about their own views, leads them to question and explore their own understanding, and encourages them to take charge of their own beliefs.

Obviously, many of these "new" clinical propositions are uncontentious aspects of good therapy, representing sensible modesty and a respectfulness of the family. They can be taken to arise out of a belief that the individual and the family have to take charge of their own lives (this is discussed further in the section on feminist family therapy). There is also, however, an important theoretical shift in this understanding of the role of the therapist in the process of change. The therapist is seen no longer as a detached observer of the family system, who has the power to intervene from outside to change the system, but rather as someone who offers for the time being to *join* the family system, enabling it to observe and modify itself (Hoffman, 1985; Tomm, 1987a, 1987b). An example may help to illustrate this: A structural therapist identifying an extremely close relationship between mother and daughter may intervene directly by interrupting the mother when she is speaking for her daughter and encouraging the daughter to speak for herself. The Milan (or post-Milan) therapist is more likely to adopt a stance of curiosity (Cecchin, 1987) and ask the daughter, "What would happen if you did not wait for your mother to speak for you? Is it more likely to strengthen her wish to help you find the right solutions for you, or her wish to see you grow up and become independent?"

The Milan systems model has been widely used; next to the structural approach of Minuchin, it has probably had the greatest influence on the family therapy of eating disorders. Although there are no published control studies comparing it with different approaches, Stierlin and his colleagues in Heidelberg (Stierlin & Weber, 1989) have published a detailed follow-up study of 42 families using this approach. The sample was heterogeneous, including both anorexics and some bulimics, approximately two-thirds of whom were 18 years or younger when therapy started. Even though fewer than a quarter of the patients had been ill for more than 3 years, all but two had had one or more previous attempts at treatment (64% outpatient and 56% inpatient). The treatments were generally quite brief, commonly lasting no more than 6 months, and continuing for more than a year in only 25% of cases. The intensity of the treatments was also low, with an average number of six sessions per family. The length of follow-up varied between 2 and 9 years. The most interesting aspect of the results is the fact that at the time that treatment ended, the improvements were generally quite modest (particularly in terms of symptomatic change); by the time of the follow-up, however, approximately two-thirds of the patients had achieved a relatively normal weight and were menstruating. A similar pattern of change was also observed in the patients' social functioning, both in relation to their families and in relation to their peers.

Feminist Family Therapy

Feminist family therapy is not, strictly speaking, a "school of therapy" with which one can associate a particular theoretical model and a set of therapeutic techniques. Rather, it provides a stance toward therapy that is a basis for a critique of some of the approaches developed in other models. In discussing the techniques of family therapy, Luepnitz (1988) suggests: "Feminism is not a set of therapeutic techniques but a sensibility, a political and aesthetic center that informs a work pervasively. One does not merely make clinical interventions in the family as a feminist; one also greets and sets the fee as a feminist" (p. 231). She also states: "In feminist therapy, patients come to have compassion for their own dilemmas, to see their desires for nurturance as wholesome and self-preserving, and to learn to meet their needs with open requests" (p. 228). Likewise, in their discussions of family therapy techniques, Schwartz and colleagues (Schwartz, Barrett, & Saba, 1985; Schwartz & Barrett, 1988) acknowledge and elaborate on the importance of the ideas, but they do not argue for defined feminist methods. In their approach to treatment, they suggest the application of structural and strategic techniques.

Feminist perspectives have provided two important contributions to the family therapy of anorexia nervosa (and bulimia nervosa). The first arises out of the general feminist critique of the inequitable position of women in society. This inequality includes (1) the expectation that women will be nurturers and caretakers, and (2) the demand for conformity to the culturally defined norms of physical attraction. This combination forms the matrix within which eating disorders develop (Orbach, 1979; Chernin, 1985; Schwartz & Barrett, 1988; Luepnitz, 1988). Schwartz and Barrett (1988), for instance, explore the internalization of family and sociocultural elements from a feminist perspective to specify the context within which an eating disorder develops: "We now see anorexia nervosa and bulimia not simply as aberrant sets of eating habits but as rigid and extreme patterns of thinking, feeling, and interacting with others. These patterns, we have found, are established within the individual's familial and sociocultural contexts" (p. 131). They continue:

> Consequently, eating disorders maintain both the position of the dependent person in need of constant care and attention and the position of being powerful and overcontrolling demagogue. This indirect method of gaining power and control, while remaining subordinate is congruent with the societal message that women are taught. . . . A woman can perform overresponsible and sacrificial tasks and only reward herself sparingly. The physical numbing effects that result from both self-starvation and purging creates a denial system that helps a person deny hunger, feelings, and needs. Consequently, she can take care of others' needs and deny her own. (Schwartz & Barrett, 1988, pp. 132–133)

The sociocultural expectations placed upon women are particularly important during the adolescent passage. As Ussher (1989) remarks of the woman in adolescence, "As she looks at her changing body and compares it to the internalized norm of beauty, she is at a distance from it. In the most extreme case this sense of splitting, the loss of control, can result in anorexia" (p. 39). The general critique also raises questions about the idea that the anorexic family is pathological or dysfunctional (as suggested by Minuchin and Selvini Palazzoli). The notion that there is something wrong with such a family invites the question as to what style of family organization is "right" and how "rightness" can be defined (see Jones, 1990). This line of inquiry stems from questions about the "normal"

relationship between men and women and the "normal" form of marriage.

The feminist account of the sociocultural context that gives rise to the development of eating disorders is relevant to the practice of family therapy, but, of course, is not specific to it. The second contribution from feminist theory is more focused; it concerns the nature of therapy, and, in particular, the role that the therapist has in the therapeutic process. Feminist therapists argue for the importance of reducing the differences in power between therapist and client, and of viewing therapy as a partnership (see Burck & Daniel, 1990). They have therefore been particularly critical of structural and strategic approaches, which emphasize issues of hierarchy and control within families and address them by interventions that require the therapist to be the "powerful expert." As Jones (1990) states, "I am therefore unlikely to believe in, or to urge families to practice, the exercise of power in intimate relationships which so easily shades over into the abuse of power—by men over women, and by parents over children" (p. 64). Although we do not entirely concur with this view, and would generally encourage parents of anorexic adolescents to take charge of their daughters' eating, we recognize the importance of helping parents to do this in a way that is firm but not abusive. We have found (see Squire-Dehouck, 1993) that particularly in families where there is a high level of criticism or hostility, highly challenging and confrontational techniques may be counterproductive, unnecessarily raising feelings of guilt and blame.

In Figure 16.5, the feminist view of the societal influences that pervade the lives of the individual and the family is illustrated by the numerous arrows emanating from the ellipse representing sociocultural influences, "irradiating" the permeable ellipse containing the family. The symptom is shown as existing outside and in the family and as overlying the patient. The interventions contained in the attitudinal stance that Luepnitz (1988) describes are directed toward directly addressing the ways in which that the culture is being expressed. In our own practice, we often talk directly about the advertising pressures that prescribe a specific shape for women. We describe the shape as being like a woman early in puberty, and contrast it with the ideal of the "hunky" male, whose secondary sexual characteristics are by no means unaccented in advertising images. We also point to the eco-

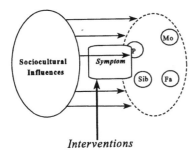

Interventions

FIGURE 16.5. A model for feminist family therapy interventions (and ways to counteract sociocultural influence). Sociocultural influences (definitions of gender roles and of what constitutes acceptable body shape) are shown as creating the disorder (a "culture-bound syndrome") by their influenes on the individual and family. Interventions can be devised to reduce the putative pathogenic effects (i.e., psychoeducation, consciousness enhancement).

nomic advantages that food and fashion industries gain from promoting an image of femininity that is difficult for a woman of average size and shape to attain, and then selling products that appear to offer hope of achieving the fostered vision. On the whole, however, we agree that the impact of feminism is not in the definition of specific techniques, but rather in the development of therapeutic attitudes. These attitudes include an expectation of equality, a strong opposition to any use of male power against women, and a special respect for the emerging individuality and femininity of an anorexic woman.

A SYSTEMIC VIEW OF A MULTIFACTORIAL MODEL: THE MAUDSLEY MODEL

Our own approach to the family therapy of anorexia nervosa is based on the proposition that an interactional systems model can best account for the multifactorial etiological influences leading to the illness. This mode is shown in Figure 16.6. Interventions are deployed to systematically address the multiple sites at which it is possible to intervene in the putative mechanisms creating and maintaining the disorder. These factors operate within a specific cultural and family context. An important aspect of our model is that there is a relatively predictable developmental/life cycle process

created by and interacting with the biosocial context.

In Figure 16.6, the illness is shown as existing outside the individual, as though the manifest, externally perceived symptomatology constitutes the whole of the illness. This is a simplification used not only to make a contrast with the medical model, but also to emphasize the plasticity and interpersonal qualities of the presentation of psychological disorders (see Shorter, 1992, for an account of the historical progress of one variety of psychosomatic disorder, seemingly in response to prevailing medical beliefs). By placing the symptoms outside the individual and the family, we are stressing the importance of external sources (e.g., sociocultural) for the

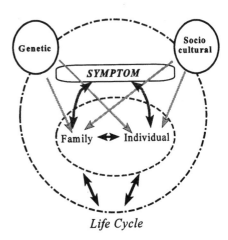

Life Cycle

FIGURE 16.6. The Maudsley systemic model of etiology. This figure illustrates the elements we believe to be therapeutically relevant in the multifactorial etiology of anorexia nervosa. Social and genetic (and physiological) influences affect the family and (through the biological parents) the individual. These influences are unidirectional. The outer circle represents the encompassing, organizing effect of the life cycle, which is in turn formally ordered by genetic and social influences. These interactions are two way because the psychological state of the individual and the family also influences their movement through and experience of the life cycle. The individual and the family are in interaction throughout life, either through direct processes or through internalized processes in the individual. This is indicated both by the inner ellipse and by the double-ended arrow between the family and individual. The symptom, having arisen as an outcome of the complex interaction of the etiological factors, in turn has an influence on the individual and family psychology; while the symptom persists, it structures, in a powerful way, the trajectory of the life cycle (see Dare, 1993).

illness. In addition, we are emphasizing the major impact of the symptoms on the functioning of the individual and the family, once the symptoms have established their grip on the patient. The most obvious are the well-known effects of starvation on an individual's mood, behavior, and social functioning (Keys, Brozek, Henschel, Mickelsen, & Taylor, 1950; Vitousek & Manke, 1994). Comparable studies of the effects of starvation in an individual on the whole family have not been reported, and are improbable. However, it is highly likely that some of the apparent "dysfunction" reported in families of an anorexic patients is not an antecedent of the eating disorder, but is the result of the development of a life-threatening illness in a previously well child, of the above-mentioned changes in the child's mood and behavior, of the possible experience of covert blaming by professionals, and of the common failure of initial therapeutic endeavors. The power of the feedback interactions of the symptoms is indicated by the bidirectional arrows in Figure 16.6.

In the model, genetic influences are seen as assailing both the individual and the family. Although genetic transmission takes place through the parents, the individual has a unique genetic constitution. The nature of this genetic influence is quite unclear: it is mediated through physiological qualities (e.g., the ability to endure the pangs of hunger by means of specificities of endorphin metabolism; see Huebner, 1993) or via specific personality traits (see Strober, 1992)? In our form of family therapy, we advocate the view that the genetic aspects of the development of anorexia nervosa can be seen in two ways: *either* as a disadvantage (a tendency to develop anorexia if a course of slimming is undertaken), *or* as a quality with a potential for good (the capacity to put up with hardship and to persevere). The task for family therapy is to potentiate the good possibilities of the genetic endowment and to minimize the negative effects.

In Figure 16.6, genetic inputs are portrayed as shaping the symptomatic presentation. For example, it is possible to argue that the specific genetic context makes it more likely that an anorexic than a bulimic form of eating disorder will occur. Likewise, sociocultural inputs (specifically, the "slimming culture" and the complexities of gender-based attitudes toward the nature of adult individuation) are portrayed as impinging on the individuals of the family and clearly have a strong effect on the nature of

family organization. The family is shown as bounded by an elliptical dashed line, in order to suggest the relative openness of the family—a quality that can be called "semipermeable," to indicate both the consistency of the structure but also the fact that influences and people can move across the boundary. The structure of the diagram also shows a link between the family (as a transmitter of sociocultural values, attitudes, and expectations) and the individual. The symptom is structurally connected to sociocultural impacts in accordance with the notion of eating disorders as "culture bound" syndromes (Gordon, 1990), which suggests modifications in the incidence as well as the actual symptoms as outcomes of social changes. For example, Russell (1979) pointed out that a hitherto undescribed variant of anorexia nervosa, "bulimia nervosa," had become apparent. Subsequently, Russell (1993, 1995) suggested that the appearance of bulimia nervosa was associated with a more general phenomenon—namely, that eating disorders were subject to change in their forms, psychological contents, and incidence. The change over time in the contents of eating disorders—for example, the apparent evolution of a fear of fatness as part of these disorders—is paralleled by cross-cultural differences. It seems that in some cultures (e.g., the ethnic Chinese of Hong Kong), fear of fatness is not a feature of these conditions (Hsu & Lee, 1993).

An important element of Figure 16.6 is the presence of the life cycle as an organizing principle. The life cycle is considered to be an extension of the concept of development. That is, though the biological, physiological substrate for psychological maturation creates what Erikson termed a "ground plan" (Erikson, 1968), the cultural specifics have an effect on how the ground plan shows itself. How the individual and the family have adapted to and assimilated the cultural impingements in turn alters progress through the current phase and has an effect on the entry to and hence the passage through the subsequent phase.

Figure 16.7 elaborates the links between the Maudsley model and the models of therapy described earlier. It extends Figure 16.6 by including the theoretical sites for intervention that are associated with the Maudsley model. Many authors have commented upon the multifactorial origins of anorexia nervosa and have proposed the need to change a number of the patient's psychological structures. For example, Andersen (1987) comments: "In summary, the ap-

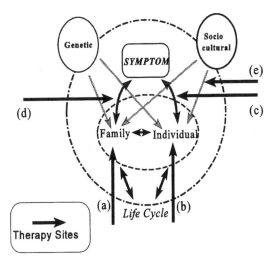

FIGURE 16.7. Theoretical sites for therapy. The figure repeats Figure 16.6, except that lettered arrows have been added to show the possible sites for therapeutic interventions. Thus therapies may seek to change (a) the individual, (b) the family, (c) the role of the symptom in the life of the individual, and the symptom. All treatments have to accept the genetic organization of the individual and the currently unchangeable aspects of society as given.

proach to self-induced starvation requires a simultaneous or sequential attention to the actual behavior of starvation, to the irrational thoughts prompting this behavior, to the meaning of the behavior in the patient's life, and to any aspect of mood disorder that is present" (p. 529). We suggest that family systems theory and family therapy techniques can go far beyond an approach based on the individual alone. Not only have they opened up the possibility of discerning new modes of intervention to change the family; they have created a way of thinking that permits the incorporation of a much wider range of interventive possibilities. The labeling (a) through (e), in the next paragraph refers to the lettered sites for intervention in Figure 16.7.

Powerful interventions directed toward the individual or the family may, through creating marked change in (a) individual or (b) family functioning, alter the balance of forces within the whole system. More modest intentions may direct therapy toward reducing the feedback actions whereby the illness (the "symptoms") controls (c) the individual and her trajectory through the life cycle, or (d) the relationship between the individual and the family. Lastly,

interventions can be directed toward minimizing the impact of (e) sociocultural qualities— that is, the ideals of body shape and the gender values that contribute to self-formation (identity) in adolescence and young adulthood. In all our interventions, we hold in mind the powerful consequences of starvation for the functioning of the individual, as well as their profound impact upon the family. Whenever a patient is in a malnourished state, we remind the patient and her family that they are all suffering as much from the consequences of the starvation (whatever its origins) as from whatever gave rise to the problem in the first place. Most families are highly alarmed by the onset of the illness. This leads them to reevaluate their preceding relationships and often to come up with highly self-critical and negative views as to their mutual influences. The parents often fear that their daughter is suffering from the consequences of their own failings, and believe that treatment should consist of helping the patient get over those ill consequences. Reiteration by the therapist of the likely effects of starvation on the person and their reversal on recovery of proper levels of nutrition should accompany many interventions, whatever their additional focus may be.

EMPIRICAL VALIDATION OF THE THEORETICAL MODELS OF FAMILY THERAPY

Our treatment approach has been shaped by a series of controlled trials, in which family therapy has been compared with different forms of control therapies in an effort to identify the specific indications for family therapy (see Dare et al., 1995, for an overview of the Maudsley studies of family therapy). A crucial feature of the studies has been the careful delineation of different subgroups (defined by prognostic criteria) of patients with anorexia nervosa. This subdivision has enabled the specificity of family therapy to be assessed. In our clinical work, we have also been influenced by the different theoretical conceptualizations described earlier in the chapter, and many of the interventions that we use can clearly be seen to derive from these models. Although we have not attempted to test the different models directly, a number of our research findings provide support or in some instances, contraindication to different aspects of these models.

Our most robust finding is that adolescents with a relatively short duration of anorexia nervosa respond extremely well to family therapy interventions both in the short term (Russell et al., 1987; Dare et al., 1990) and at long-term follow-up (Eisler, Hodes, et al., 1996). (We have some evidence that adolescents suffering from bulimia nervosa may respond equally well to family therapy; see Dodge, Hodes, Eisler, & Dare, 1995.) The model of therapy utilized with adolescent anorexic patients in many ways most closely resembles the structural model (though it also contains strategic and psychoanalytic elements—see Dare, 1988, and Dare & Eisler, 1992), but with a number of important modifications. Like the Philadelphia group, we commonly support the parents in taking control of their daughter's eating. With an acutely ill adolescent, this is usually an effective intervention: It prevents the need for admission to a hospital, raises the parents' morale, and is also an important step in engaging the family in further therapeutic work. However, in engaging the family around this task, we make no assumption that the observed pattern of family functioning is dysfunctional or that the aim of therapy is to reverse such dysfunction.

For instance, a structural therapist observing what might be thought of as the stereotypical pattern of a "peripheral" father and an "overinvolved" mother may seek to increase the father's involvement, with the aim of freeing the mother to move to a less involved position (an intervention that can be easily seen to imply that the "real" problem is the mother's overinvolvement). Although we recognize the complementarity of such parental positions, we believe it is presumptuous for us to assume that we know what kind of organization is going to work best in a given family. We also know how easy it is for some interventions to become covertly blaming of the family, and perhaps in particular of the mother. We will therefore focus on exploring the advantages of being very close, as well as of being able to take a more detached position. We will stress that in order to help their daughter, the parents will need to make use of both positions. We may also point out that we see evidence that in fact both parents appear to be pulled in opposite directions—both fearing for their daughter's life and therefore wanting to intervene, and at the same time worrying that if they do too much they will become intrusive and overbearing. We will then explore the way in which the anorexia locks them into the seemingly rigid opposing positions in which one parent speaks for "caring closeness" and the other for "respectful distance."

Some of the techniques derived from the "psychosomatic family model"—namely, those aimed at helping the family to break a habitual pattern of conflict avoidance—are in our experience unnecessary and in some cases are contraindicated. In a study in which we compared conjoint family therapy with a family intervention in which parents were seen separately from their adolescent daughters (Le Grange, Eisler, Dare, & Russell, 1992; Eisler, Dare, et al., 1996), we found that the latter treatment (which by its very nature made it impossible to use some of the more challenging and confrontational interventions characteristic of the Philadelphia group) was just as effective as our customary conjoint therapy; in families where there were high levels of criticism or hostility, it was, if anything, more effective. A 2-year follow-up of the original pilot study (Squire-Dehouk, 1993) found that in this group of families the occurrence of conflicts was associated with feelings of guilt and blame. It is our view that interventions for conflict avoidance can be counterproductive with such families, particularly in the early stages of treatment, and should therefore be used with extreme caution.

Because of our findings that higher levels of criticism have a detrimental effect on the engagement and outcome of therapy with anorexic patients (Szmukler, Eisler, Russell, & Dare, 1985; Le Grange, Eisler, Dare, & Hodes, 1992), we have made particular efforts to understand both the individual psychological mechanisms and the family processes involved in criticism. We view criticism as being strongly linked to feelings of guilt and blame (Dare et al., 1990), and we always find it useful to spend some time discussing the nature of the illness, stressing in particular that we do not see the family as the origin of the problem. We concur with White's account of a message to help a family's burden of guilt: "I told them that I had even come across mothers who wholly and secretly blamed themselves for their daughters problems, swallowing the distorted view that has so often appeared in popular and professional literature that anorexia nervosa is caused by intrusive and overbearing mothers" (White, 1987, p. 118). Although some of our interventions have the appearance of psychoeducational input, we also explore with the family difficulties in separating anger and blame or anxiety and guilt, as well as the interactional patterns that may be maintaining such difficulties.

The only other controlled trial of family therapy in adolescent anorexia nervosa has been that of Robin, Siegel, Koepke, Moye, and Tice (1994). Their findings confirmed the effectiveness of family interventions, but their control treatment (an "ego-oriented individual therapy") was reported as being equally effective. However, in the individual therapy group, the parents were also seen bimonthly for 54 minutes a session throughout the 16 months of therapy. This study therefore contributes to the overall compelling evidence that in adolescent anorexia nervosa, parents need to be part of the treatment program. Although there is no evidence that there is any specific advantage in seeing the parents with the patient in the same session, it is usually more convenient to see the family conjointly. Whether the patient is seen on her own or together with the family, our experience shows that the therapist must pay close attention to the inner experience of the patient and of other family members, and must use this understanding to make contact with each family member. In this way, the therapist demonstrates an interest in, knowledge of, and respect for the differing as well as the shared experiences within the family.

With adult anorexic patients, the empirical evidence supporting particular treatment approaches is less clear. This is partly because the adult patients that we see tend to be quite chronically ill, and it is unlikely that any one treatment approach is going to turn out to be a panacea. Nevertheless, findings from our recent studies indicate that family therapy is more effective than either individual psychodynamic or individual supportive therapy even for adult patients, particularly if the illness started during adolescence (Russell, Dare, Eisler, & LeGrange, 1992). The style of therapy that we have evolved with this group of patients is different, as one would expect, from the one we have described in relation to adolescent anorexia nervosa patients. This is only partly attributable to the differences in age and family organization. With an adult patient there is also usually a different level of anxiety, as well as less pressure to find a rapid resolution of the crisis. As often as not, the patient is at a low but relatively stable weight; even if she is losing weight, it is often possible to engage her in treatment on the understanding that she will prevent further weight loss. In contrast with our work with adolescent patients, we would not expect parents (or partners, in the case of married patients) to become involved in the issue of weight control. We spend much more time trying to demote dietary preoccupation as a medium of family communication and to promote age-appropriate relationships. Even though the relationship issues that are addressed in treatment may be very similar to those that come up in the work with adolescents, the way that we address them tends to be different. Although we do not adopt a consistently neutral position in the way that is advocated by the Milan group, we usually explore the beliefs and perceptions within the family in a way that resembles the Milan style. Our interventions are most likely to take the form of a question (e.g., "When your mother comments like this, are you more aware of her worry about you or her irritation?") or an observation ("I've noticed how difficult it is to talk about the relationship between you and your daughter, as if you believed that you were being criticized for being too close"). Consistent warmth and a positive, supportive attitude are used to counter the family members' tendencies to self-blame and self-justification.

In practice, we have also been influenced by psychodynamic considerations concerning the development of the self, particularly in those patients with anorexia nervosa who have marked features of borderline personality disorder. In exploring the transference–countertransference issues within individual therapy with such a patient, the therapist has to find a way to work with the patient's coexisting longing for and terror of personal closeness (see Dare & Crowther, 1995a, 1995b; Dare, 1995). Too much display of intimate understanding and emotional closeness causes the patient to withdraw into her symptomatic preoccupations, and yet too aloof a therapeutic relationship is felt as cold and rejecting. Interpretation of this transference pattern can be helpful, although the therapist must also be careful to maintain an accurate balance of closeness and distance. The experience of working in intensive individual therapy has been very usefully transferred to the style of making contact with the patient in our forms of family therapy, whether or not we also see the patient on her own (see below).

Adult patients are often reluctant at first to involve other family members in therapy. This is usually attributable to a mixture of feeling that they have already been too much of a burden on their families, a fear that other family members will take center stage, and a fear that they may say or do things that other family members may find upsetting. Discussing the advantages of inviting other family members to sessions, and how, when, and in what combination it would be best to ask them to come, is often in itself a powerful intervention. One patient, who had agonized over a number of sessions about the difficult relationship with her parents and how she would manage if they came to some sessions with her, reported the following:

I thought carefully about our last discussion. I decided to try it out on my own first. I asked my dad to come for a walk with me and just listen to what I had to say. I told him the things I have never been able to say to him, and to my surprise he just listened. He got quite upset, and I nearly gave up halfway through. But I was determined not to give up. He gave me a hug just before we got home. It made me feel really guilty about saying all those things to him. But I am still glad I did it.

We continued to discuss the possibility of her parents' coming for a number of sessions, thinking about the kind of issues that might come up and who would say what. Although the parents never actually came, it often felt as if they were present in the room.

COMBINING INDIVIDUAL THERAPY WITH FAMILY INTERVENTION IN ANOREXIA NERVOSA

Enthrallment with the technical and conceptual innovations of the many family therapists who have created such a transformation in the psychotherapy of anorexia nervosa may lead some clinicians to conclude that family therapy is always a sufficient treatment. Clearly, we do not take this view, but agree with the Louven group from Belgium:

Many family therapists have a strong belief that once they have changed the family structure, strengthened the coalition between the parents, and made clear intergenerational boundaries, or once the anorectic [sic] daughter starts to live on her own, improvement in all levels (including the symptoms) will follow automatically. Therapists

who focus only on the interactions in the family neglect sometimes considerable developmental retardation which exists in anorexic patients. Many patients, once they gave up their anorectic [sic] symptoms, go through a period of a "loss of identity." They often feel empty or insecure and have to make a completely new start. Therefore, they will need the support and guidance of the therapist over a long time. (Vanderlinden & Vandereycken, 1984, p. 278)

In our own practice, we often combine individual and family therapy (see Eisler, 1995, for a detailed case description). As we see it, there are tasks for family therapy and tasks for individual work. In keeping with our systemic multifactorial model, we seek therapeutic leverage at a sufficient number of sites to provide sustained change. By this we do not mean that individual psychological change is necessarily always best achieved by individual therapy, or that changes in family relations always require conjoint family interventions. On the contrary, it is our experience that within family therapy it is possible to address many different issues, such as the difficulties of affect management and identity formation, as well as more direct relationship issues. Similarly, as we have described earlier, individual sessions can often be used effectively as a means of input into the family. We also find that a combination of individual and family therapy (usually by the same therapist), whether they are delivered in parallel or in sequence, can have a mutually facilitating effect on both forms of treatment.

CONCLUSIONS

We have advocated that family therapy for anorexia nervosa be based on a theoretical model in which multiple sites for therapy are identified. We have argued that the clinician needs to draw both on empirical findings and on a conceptual framework to determine the specific forms of interventions to be used. It is important, at this point, to urge caution and a critical self-evaluation. It is all too easy to devise plausible theoretical explanations of our activities, which may ignore factors that are just as salient in determining what we do. For instance, it is worth noting that the different styles of therapy that have evolved in different centers (e.g., Philadelphia and Milan) have been developed with quite different groups of patients. Although this is seldom acknowledged, it has undoubtedly been an important (though not the only) factor shaping the theoretical models. The work described by Minuchin and colleagues was conducted to a large extent with adolescents with a relatively short duration of illness, and was carried out in close collaboration with a pediatric team. In contrast, the Milan group tended to work with rather chronically ill patients, many of whom traveled a long distance to obtain the specialist treatment. The differences in treatment approaches between the two centers clearly reflects these differences in patient populations.

Similarly, we have often been struck by the way in which theoretical explanations are often put forward for different models of inpatient treatment programs in different countries (e.g., a psychodynamic explanation for using a slow rather than a rapid refeeding program), without taking into account that probably the most powerful determining factor is likely to be the nature of the health service provisions in each country (e.g., availability of beds). Much of the advice given on the inpatient treatment of anorexia nervosa suggests that the management of the dietary restriction is "behavioral." In practice, however, much of the activity often appears to be punitive: The patient is kept on a strict regimen of bed rest and restriction of visitors and occupation, with "privileges" being allowed as a result of weight increase. This does not always accord closely with principles of modern learning theory; indeed, it often seems more to be an acting out of the patients' own asceticism and self-punishment. We would advise similar caution and self-observation when accounts of individual or family therapy are being considered. We say this on the basis of our experience as therapists, as well as of our work as teachers and supervisors in a number of different treatment projects. Family systems approaches offer a number of new and important insights and have led to many important treatment innovations. However, the many clinical accounts of the family and anorexia nervosa also have to be seen as resembling an elaboration of the families' own self-blaming—their self-accusations of somehow having caused the problem. Such observations make us view all aspects of our own clinical practice with benign skepticism, and they encourage us to continue to confront our clinical and theoretical conceptualizations with empirical research evidence.

NOTES

1. We have not included behavioral family therapy in our discussion because, somewhat surprisingly, it has not figured much in the literature on eating disorders, in spite of the fact that behavioral and cognitive-behavioral approaches have had such an impact on individual treatments of bulimia nervosa.

2. Because most patients with anorexia nervosa are female, we use feminine nouns and pronouns in this chapter to refer to such patients.

3. This task was first used in 1979 (in the treatment of a family with a 16-year-old anorexic) before the Milan group split up, but was later developed as a standard "invariable" intervention by Selvini Palazzoli as a way of breaking up what she describes as "psychotic family games" (Selvini Palazzoli, 1986; Selvini Palazzoli & Viaro, 1988).

REFERENCES

Andersen, A. E. (1987). Contrast and comparison of behavioral, cognitive-behavioral and comprehensive treatment methods for anorexia nervosa and bulimia nervosa. *Behavior Modification, 11,* 522–543.

Aponte, H. J., & VanDeusen, J. M. (1981). Structural family therapy. In A. S. Gurman & D. P. Kniskern (Eds.), *Handbook of family therapy.* New York: Brunner/Mazel.

Bliss, E. L., & Branch, C. H. (1960). *Anorexia nervosa: Its psychology and biology.* New York: Hoeber.

Boscolo, L., Cecchin, G., Hoffman, L., & Penn, P. (1987). *Milan systemic family therapy.* New York: Basic Books.

Bruch, H. (1973). *Eating disorders: Obesity, anorexia nervosa and the person within.* New York: Basic Books.

Burck, C., & Daniel, G. (1990). Feminism and strategic therapy: Contradiction or complementarity? In R. J. Perelberg & A. C. Miller (Eds.), *Gender and power in families.* London: Tavistock/Routledge.

Campbell, D., Draper, R., & Huffington, C. (1991). *Second thoughts on the theory and practice of the Milan approach to family therapy.* London: Draper Campbell.

Cecchin, G. (1987). Hypothesizing, circularity, and neutrality revisited: An invitation to curiosity. *Family Process, 26,* 405–413.

Chernin, K. (1985). *The hungry self: Women, eating and identity.* New York: Times Books.

Dare, C. (1988). Psychoanalytic family therapy. In E. Street & W. Dryden (Eds.), *Family therapy in Britain.* Milton Keynes, England: Open University Press.

Dare, C. (1993). Aetiological models and the psychotherapy of psychosomatic disorders. In M. Hodes & S. Morey (Eds.), *Psychological treatments in disease and illness.* London: Gaskell.

Dare, C. (1995). Psychoanalytic psychotherapy for eating disorders. In G. O. Gabbard (Ed.), *Treatments of psychiatric disorders.* Washington, DC: American Psychiatric Press.

Dare, C., & Crowther, C. (1995a). Psychodynamic models of the eating disorders. In G. I. Szmukler, C. Dare, & J. Treasure (Eds.), *Eating disorders: Handbook of theory, treatment and research.* Chichester, England: Wiley.

Dare, C., & Crowther, C. (1995b). Living dangerously: Psychoanalytic psychotherapy for anorexia nervosa. In G. I.

Szmukler, C. Dare, & J. Treasure (Eds.), *Eating disorders: Handbook of theory, treatment and research.* Chichester, England: Wiley.

Dare, C., & Eisler, I. (1992). Family therapy for anorexia nervosa. In P. Cooper & A. Stein (Eds.), *The nature and management of feeding problems in young people.* New York: Harwood Academics.

Dare, C., Eisler, I., Colahan, M., Crowther, C., Senior, R., & Asen, E. (1995). The listening heart and the chi square: Clinical and empirical perceptions in the family therapy of anorexia nervosa. *Journal of Family Therapy, 17,* 31–58.

Dare, C., Eisler, I., Russell, G. F. M., & Szmukler, G. I. (1990). Family therapy for anorexia nervosa: Implications from the results of a controlled trial of family and individual therapy. *Journal of Marital and Family Therapy, 16,* 39–57.

Dodge, E., Hodes, M., Eisler, I., & Dare, C. (1995). Family therapy for bulimia nervosa in adolescents: An exploratory study. *Journal of Family Therapy, 17,* 59–78.

Eisler, I. (1993). Families, family therapy and psychosomatic illness. In S. Moorey & M. Hodes (Eds.), *Psychological treatments in human disease and illness.* London: Gaskell.

Eisler, I. (1995). Combining individual and family therapy in adolescent anorexia nervosa: A family systems approach. In J. Werne (Ed.), *Treating eating disorders.* San Francisco: Jossey-Bass.

Eisler, I., Dare, C., Russell, G. F. M., Szmukler, G. I., Le Grange, D., & Dodge, E. (1996). *A controlled trial of two forms of family intervention in adolescent eating disorder.* Manuscript in preparation.

Eisler, I., Hodes, M., Dare, C., Russell, G. F. M., & Dodge, E. (1996). *A five year follow-up of a controlled trial of family therapy in severe eating disorder.* Manuscript submitted for publication.

Erikson, E. H. (1968). *Identity: Youth and crisis.* New York: Norton.

Gordon, R. A. (1990). *Anorexia and bulimia: Anatomy of a social epidemic.* Oxford: Blackwell.

Gull, W. W. (1874). Anorexia nervosa (apepsia hysterica, anorexia hysterica). *Transactions of the Clinical Society of London, 7,* 222–228.

Haley, J. (1973). *Uncommon therapy: The psychiatric techniques of Milton H. Erickson.* New York: Norton.

Haley, J. (1984). *Ordeal therapy.* San Francisco: Jossey-Bass.

Harper, G. (1983). Varieties of parenting failure in anorexia nervosa: Protection and parentectomy revisited. *Journal of the American Academy of Child Psychiatry, 22,* 134–139.

Hoffman, L. (1985). Beyond power and control: Toward a 'second order' family systems therapy. *Family Systems Medicine, 3,* 381–396.

Hsu, L. K. G., & Lee, S. (1993). Is weight phobia always necessary for a diagnosis of anorexia nervosa? *American Journal of Psychiatry, 150,* 1466–1471.

Huebner, H. E. (1993). *Endorphins, eating disorders and other addictive behaviors.* New York: Norton.

Janet, P. (1925). *Psychological healing: A historical and clinical study* (Vol. 2). London: George Allen & Unwin.

Jones, E. (1988). The Milan method—*quo vadis? Journal of Family Therapy, 10,* 325–338.

Jones, E. (1990). Feminism and family therapy: Can mixed marriages work? In R. J. Perelberg & A. C. Miller (Eds.), *Gender and power in families.* London: Routledge.

Keys, A., Brozek, J., Henschel, A., Mickelsen, O., & Taylor, H. L. (1950). *The biology of human starvation* (2 vols.). Minneapolis: University of Minnesota Press.

Le Grange, D., Eisler, I., Dare, C., & Hodes, M. (1992). Family criticism and self starvation: A study of expressed emotion. *Journal of Family Therapy, 14,* 177–192.

Le Grange, D., Eisler, I., Dare, C., & Russell, G. F. M. (1992). Evaluation of family therapy in anorexia nervosa: A pilot study. *International Journal of Eating Disorders, 12,* 347–357.

Liebman, R., Minuchin, S., & Baker, L. (1974). An integrated treatment program for anorexia nervosa. *American Journal of Psychiatry, 131,* 432–436.

Luepnitz, D. A. (1988). *The family interpreted: Psychoanalysis, feminism, and family therapy.* New York: Basic Books.

Madanes, C. (1981). *Strategic family therapy.* San Francisco: Jossey-Bass.

MacKinnon, L. (1983). Contrasting strategic and Milan therapies. *Family Process, 22,* 425–440.

Martin, F. E. (1985). The treatment and outcome of anorexia nervosa in adolescence: Prospective study and 5 year follow-up. *Journal of Psychiatric Research, 19,* 509–514.

Maturana, H. R., & Varela, F. J. (1988). *The tree of knowledge: The biological roots of human understanding.* Boston: Shambala.

Minuchin, S., Baker, L., Rosman, B. L., Liebman, R., Milman, L., & Todd, T. C. (1975). A conceptual model of psychosomatic illness in children. *Archives of General Psychiatry, 32,* 1031–1038.

Minuchin, S., Rosman, B. L., & Baker, L. (1978). *Psychosomatic families: Anorexia nervosa in context.* Cambridge, MA: Harvard University Press.

Morgan, H. G., & Russell, G. F. M. (1975). Value of family background and clinical features as predictors of long-term outcome in anorexia nervosa: A four year follow-up study of 41 patients. *Psychological Medicine, 5,* 355–371.

Orbach, S. (1979). *Fat is a feminist issue.* London: Paddington Press.

Penn, P. (1982). Circular questioning. *Family Process, 21,* 267–280.

Robin, A. L., Siegel, P. T., Koepke, T., Moye, A. W., & Tice, S. (1994). Family therapy versus individual therapy for adolescent females with anorexia nervosa. *Journal of Developmental and Behavioral Pediatrics, 15,* 111–116.

Rosman, B. L., Minuchin, S., & Liebman, R. (1975). Family lunch session: An introduction to family therapy in anorexia nervosa. *American Journal of Orthopsychiatry, 45,* 846–853.

Russell, G. F. M. (1979). Bulimia nervosa: An ominous variant of anorexia nervosa. *Psychological Medicine, 9,* 429–448.

Russell, G. F. M. (1993). The social psychiatry of eating disorders. In D. Bhugra & J. Leff (Eds.), *Social psychiatry.* Oxford: Blackwell.

Russell, G. F. M. (1995). Anorexia nervosa through time. In G. I. Szmukler, C. Dare, & J. Treasure (Eds.), *Eating disorders: Handbook of theory, treatment and research.* Chichester, England: Wiley.

Russell, G. F. M., Dare, C., Eisler, I., & Le Grange, P. D. F. (1992). Controlled trials of family treatments in anorexia nervosa. In K. A. Halmi (Ed.), *Psychobiology and treatment of anorexia nervosa and bulimia nervosa.* Washington, DC: American Psychiatric Press.

Russell, G. F. M., Szmukler, G. I., Dare, C., & Eisler, I. (1987). An evaluation of family therapy in anorexia nervosa and bulimia nervosa. *Archives of General Psychiatry, 44,* 1047–1056.

Sargent, J., Liebman, R., & Silver, M. (1985). Family therapy for anorexia nervosa. In D. M. Garner & P. E. Garfinkel (Eds.), *Handbook of psychotherapy for anorexia nervosa and bulimia*. New York: Guilford Press.

Schwartz, R. C., & Barrett, M. J. (1988). Women and eating disorders. *Journal of Psychotherapy and the Family, 3*, 131–144.

Schwartz, R. C., Barrett, M. J., & Saba, G. (1985). Family therapy for bulimia. In D. M. Garner & P. E. Garfinkel (Eds.), *Handbook of psychotherapy for anorexia nervosa and bulimia*. New York: Guilford Press.

Selvini Palazzoli, M. (1974). *Self starvation: From the intrapsychic to the transpersonal approach*. London: Chaucer.

Selvini Palazzoli, M. (1986). Towards a general model of psychotic family games. *Journal of Marital and Family Therapy, 12*, 339–349.

Selvini Palazzoli, M., Boscolo, L., Cecchin, G., & Prata, G. (1978). *Paradox and counterparadox*. New York: Jason Aronson.

Selvini Palazzoli, M., Boscolo, L., Cecchin, G., & Prata, G. (1980). Hypothesizing–circularity–neutrality: Three guidelines for the conductor of the session. *Family Process, 19*, 3–12.

Selvini Palazzoli, M., & Viaro, M. (1988). The anorectic process in the family: A six-stage model as a guide for individual therapy. *Family Process, 27*, 129–148.

Shorter, E. (1992). *From paralysis to fatigue: A history of psychosomatic illness in the modern era*. New York: Free Press.

Squire-Dehouk, B. (1993). *Evaluation of conjoint family therapy versus family counselling in adolescent anorexia nervosa patients: A two year follow-up study*. Unpublished dissertation submitted in partial fulfillment of BPS Statement of Equivalence for MSc in Clinical Psychology, Institute of Psychiatry, University of London/Surrey University.

Stanton, M. D., Todd, T. C., & Associates. (1982). *The family therapy of drug abuse and addiction*. New York: Guilford Press.

Stierlin, H., & Weber, G. (1989). *Unlocking the family door*. New York: Brunner/Mazel.

Strober, M. (1992). Family–genetic studies. In K. A. Halmi (Ed.), *Psychobiology and treatment of anorexia nervosa and bulimia nervosa*. Washington, DC: American Psychiatric Press.

Szmukler, G. I., Eisler, I., Russell, G. F. M., & Dare, C. (1985). Anorexia nervosa, parental "expressed emotion" and dropping out of treatment. *British Journal of Psychiatry, 147*, 265–271.

Tomm, K. (1984a). One perspective on the Milan systemic approach: Part I. Overview of development, theory and practice. *Journal of Marital and Family Therapy, 10*, 113–125.

Tomm, K. (1984b). One perspective on the Milan systemic approach: Part II. Description of session format, interviewing style and interventions. *Journal of Marital and Family Therapy, 10*, 253–271.

Tomm, K. (1987a). Interventive interviewing: Part I. Strategizing as a fourth guideline for the therapist. *Family Process, 26*, 3–13.

Tomm, K. (1987b). Interventive interviewing: Part II. Reflexive questioning as a means to enable self-healing. *Family Process, 27*, 167–183.

Treacher, A., & Carpenter, J. (1984). *Using family therapy*. Oxford: Blackwell.

Ussher, J. M. (1989). *The psychology of the female body*. London: Routledge.

Vanderlinden, J., & Vandereycken, W. (1984). Directive family therapy in adult patients with severe or chronic anorexia nervosa. *International Journal of Family Psychiatry, 5*, 267–280.

Vitousek, K., & Manke, F. (1994). Personality variables and disorders in anorexia nervosa and bulimia nervosa. *Journal of Abnormal Psychology, 103*, 137–147.

Watzlawick, P., Beavin, J. H., & Jackson, D. D. (1967). *Pragmatics of human communication*. New York: Norton.

Watzlawick, P., Weakland, J., & Fisch, R. (1974). *Change: Principles of problem formation and problem resolution*. New York: Norton.

White, M. (1987). Anorexia nervosa: A cybernetic perspective. *Family Therapy Collections, 20*, 117–129.

Wynne, L. C. (1980). Paradoxical interventions: Leverage for therapeutic change in individual and family systems. In M. Strauss, T. Bowers, S. Downey, S. Fleck, & I. Levin (Eds.), *The psychotherapy of schizophrenia*. New York: Plenum Press.

IV

HOSPITAL AND DRUG TREATMENTS

CHAPTER 17

Inpatient Treatment of Anorexia Nervosa

ARNOLD E. ANDERSEN
WAYNE BOWERS
KAY EVANS

The comprehensive treatment of eating disorders (EDs), especially anorexia nervosa, often requires inpatient care as part of a long-term program to restore healthy mental, physical, and social functioning. Sir William Gull (1874) suggested more than a century ago that many patients suffering from anorexia nervosa improve only after care in a hospital, temporarily separated from family and friends. He prescribed treatment with nutritional rehabilitation and "moral" (psychological) counseling.

Third-party payers are relentlessly cutting funding for inpatient care of psychiatric disorders in general and EDs in particular. The best defense against imprudent, economically driven, but scientifically unwise decreases in necessary inpatient care for ED patients is to demonstrate empirically the capacity of a treatment program to bring about symptom resolution and long-term relapse prevention. This type of program must achieve safe, prompt, and effective short-term hospital-based improvement; it must also prepare patients for transition to a less intense, stepped-down, partial hospital treatment, followed by long-term continued outpatient care emphasizing relapse prevention and health promotion. Our goal in this chapter is to describe a proven, up-to-date, integrative, multidisciplinary program for the comprehensive inpatient treatment of anorexia nervosa (and, to a lesser extent, other EDs); we

note changes in treatments since the last description (Andersen, Morse, & Santmyer, 1985), and provide suggestions for future research.

Anorexia nervosa is generally diagnosed by the criteria of the *Diagnostic and Statistical Manual of Mental Disorders,* fourth edition (DSM-IV; American Psychiatric Association [APA], 1994; see Walsh & Garner, Chapter 3, this volume). This widely used, committee-based product represents a reasonable and useful compromise on the diagnosis of EDs, rather than enduring truth, since the fundamental etiology and mechanism of EDs remain incompletely understood. The more time-tested general principles of Russell (1970) for diagnosis of anorexia nervosa continue to be sound. Anorexia nervosa is diagnosed when an individual suffers from (1) substantial self-induced starvation; (2) the presence of a morbid fear of fatness and relentless pursuit of thinness; and (3) abnormality of reproductive hormone activity secondary to weight loss, but also possibly as a result of independent hypothalamic abnormality.

An outdated, pessimistic view of the effectiveness of treatment for anorexia nervosa still prevails at times in some treatment centers. The opposite mistake of considering EDs as minor, voluntary, or self-indulgent disorders of spoiled or worried young people leads to underestimation of the clinical significance of anorexia nervosa. This fascinating, serious, but highly treatable disorder generally begins in teens and young adults with the endorsement of sociocultural norms promoting weight loss during the crucial identity-forming years; this leads to serious weight loss or lack of adequate gain, overriding the body's physiological regulation of hunger and satiety. The result is an imprisonment or entrainment of normal eating behavior into the service of dealing with age-old issues of identity, self-esteem, mood regulation, and family functioning, rather than in the maintenance of a normal "set point" of weight. This disorder is not only a common source of chronic adolescent morbidity, but occasionally a fatal disorder, with a documented rate of up to 19% earlier-than-expected death compared to controls in one long-term follow-up (Theander, 1985). More recent studies support a lower but still distressing long-term death rate.

The conceptual model most appropriate for guiding the treatment of anorexia nervosa is that of a multifactorial etiology. The infectious-disease model of the 19th century (a model based on finding the single cause of a disease) led to effective treatment of such diseases with antibiotics, or prevention by inoculation and sanitation. EDs, however, have never been adequately explained by single etiologies; they require a more complex, multifactorial understanding of both origin and treatment. Since treatments logically grow out of assumptions about the nature of a disorder, with etiological beliefs leading *pari passu* to treatment strategies, the clearest possible description of known contributing factors is important for guiding effective treatment of anorexia nervosa.

Some advances in the field of inpatient treatment of anorexia nervosa and other EDs in the last decade include the following:

- The formal division of anorexia nervosa in DSM-IV into diagnostic subtypes: the restricting and the binge-eating/purging subtypes (APA, 1994; see Walsh & Garner, Chapter 3, this volume).
- Development of the first guidelines by the APA (1993) for a specific set of psychiatric disorders, the EDs.
- Increased awareness of the multiple symptomatic as well as occult medical complications associated with anorexia nervosa, with evidence for significant differences in medical complications be-

tween subtypes (see Mitchell, Pomeroy, & Adson, Chapter 21, this volume).
- Demonstration of the equal effectiveness of treatment for males.
- Demonstration that the rate of nutritional restoration in anorexia nervosa can be increased to approximately 3 pounds per week, instead of a previous standard of 2.2 pounds (1.4 vs. 1 kg/week).
- Increased utilization of the body mass index (BMI) in place of population-based reference norms for weight calculations, and recognition of the limitations of BMI as well.
- Recognition of the effect of EDs on the physiological regulation of eating behavior, hunger, and satiety.
- Increased recognition of the comorbid psychiatric conditions associated with anorexia nervosa, with a recent emphasis on co-occurrence of obsessive–compulsive disorder.
- Demonstration of the effectiveness of family therapy for long-term maintenance and relapse prevention after inpatient treatment, especially for patients under age 18 (Russell, Szmukler, Dare, & Eisler, 1987).
- Development of patient "care maps" utilizing a logic tree (algorithm), examples of which are provided later in this chapter.
- Relentless attempts by third-party payers in the United States to decrease inpatient length of stay for EDs on a financially driven basis, despite the demonstration of effectiveness of inpatient psychiatric care. Arbitrary decreases in insurance benefits for the care of EDs are greater than decreases in funding of less treatable medical disorders.
- The increasing availability in many areas of a full spectrum of care for EDs, with stepwise transitions between full inpatient care, partial hospitalization, outpatient treatment, community residential programs, and support groups.
- Increased awareness of the broad spectrum of severity of EDs. This has led to a "stepped-care" approach to treatment, with simple but effective psychoeducation in some early cases as the only treatment, and months of inpatient care and years or decades of aftercare in very complex cases (see Garner & Needleman, Chapter 5, this volume).

- Cautious reintroduction of hyperalimentation in selected severe cases of anorexia nervosa.
- Replacement of single concepts of etiology or treatment (e.g., theories of hypothalamic origin, feminist theories, strict behavioral paradigms, pharmacological treatment alone) by increasingly uniform adoption of a multidimensional concept of origin leading to multidisciplinary team treatment. Empirically demonstrated vulnerability factors differentially predisposing individuals to EDs include specific personality traits or disorders (e.g., the Cluster B and C personality disorders in DSM-IV); family mood disorder; family obesity; participation in interest groups or sports requiring thinness; possible past sexual abuse; female gender; young age; and living in a society or subgroup promoting weight loss and dieting behavior.
- Attempts to develop a predictive equation for a single individual's risk of developing an ED.

This chapter begins with a description of criteria for inpatient admission, initial evaluation methods, and medical stabilization, and then focuses on three relatively distinct but related areas of interest: unit management and structure; psychological testing and psychotherapy; and nutritional and medical aspects of treatment. Finally, the chapter concludes with comments on the discharge process and on research issues. A practical protocol (see Appendix 17.1) summarizes our safe, effective, and proven approach to weight adjustment and maintenance. The emphasis in the chapter is on our experience over 25 years of treatment and research, rather than on a broad review of the literature (Bowers & Andersen, 1994; Andersen, 1995), but references are made to research applicable to clinical care.

CONCEPTUAL FRAMEWORK FOR EATING DISORDERS

EDs are dynamic disorders. They evolve and progress from the personal endorsement of slimness as a highly valued sociocultural norm. The roots of anorexia nervosa begin in the preschool and early grade school years rather than in the adolescent and early adult years, when cases are formally diagnosed. The multi-

ple factors *predisposing* to illness, *precipitating* the illness, *promulgating* the illness, and *ameliorating* the illness may be different. An understanding of origin does not necessarily lead to understanding of perpetuating factors. Medical factors play a significant role in sustaining the established illness, even if not in the origin of the illness, although this point is still debated. EDs differ from many other medical and psychiatric disorders by being as much "friends" as "foes." Frequently appearing to offer Faustian solutions to important crises in development, to mood regulation, or to distressed family dynamics, in actuality they offer only partial, temporally effective solutions, with a high cost in arresting maturational development and in producing physical danger.

ADMISSION, EVALUATION, AND MEDICAL STABILIZATION

Admission to a hospital for treatment of a complex disorder such as anorexia nervosa (or bulimia nervosa) remains a clinical decision based on multiple factors. (See Figure 17.1 for our "care map" concerning the level of treatment intensity required for a given patient; this logic-tree approach guides decision making from initial assessment through aftercare.) Some of the most common clinically significant reasons for admission are as follows:

1. Severe or rapid self-induced weight loss (or lack of normal gain), usually to less than 85% of normal weight or with significant medical, psychological, and social abnormality.
2. Lack of response to a reasonable trial of outpatient treatment, with lack of improvement in weight or binge–purge symptoms.
3. Significant psychiatric comorbidity, including major depressive disorder; severe obsessive–compulsive disorder; borderline personality disorder with impulsive behaviors; substance abuse or dependence; and/or self-harm plans or behaviors.
4. Significant medical complications, including hypokalemia, cardiac abnormalities, comorbid diabetes mellitus, and so on.
5. Lack of outpatient facilities, or a toxic/barren family or psychosocial environment.
6. Diagnosis and treatment of weight

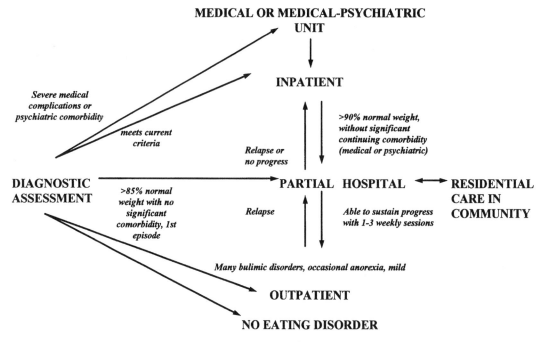

FIGURE 17.1. Care Map 1: Level of treatment intensity.

loss/low weight or binge–purge behavior in atypical cases, from medical or psychiatric referrals where diagnosis is uncertain but significant problems exist in eating behavior or weight.

Many of these factors interact with or potentiate each other. For example, a very rapid weight loss of 25 pounds may be medically more dangerous than a slower weight loss of 40 pounds. Hypokalemia with an irregular but nonbradycardic heartbeat may be more medically serious than a very slow, regular heartbeat of 40, gradually attained.

For a patient to be admitted to an inpatient unit for EDs, a physician or other health professional must initiate a request for placement. Unless there is a necessity for emergency admission, a process of thorough preparation is beneficial for patient care. The following steps are involved in the preparation for admission:

1. Diagnostic confirmation.
2. Description of program to patient and family (parents, spouse).
3. Ventilation of fears and fantasies.
4. Visit to program site if possible.
5. Receipt of previous diagnostic and treatment records.

6. Consideration of contract regarding specific features of program if commitment is weak.
7. Discussion of treatment goals with all participants—patient, family, treatment team, referral source.
8. Initial psychoeducation regarding the origin and treatment of EDs.

Because of the inherent ambivalence of many patients (and sometimes their families) toward treatment, admission for EDs differs from admission for other complex but strictly medical or surgical conditions. Patients may have fears that they will be made to become overweight, or may entertain fantasies that they will have a time of recreation and leisure instead of intensive and rigorous treatment.

Prior to admission, members of the treatment team are available to patients, their families, and their health professionals to provide information and to answer any questions about treatment. Contact with the treatment team before coming to the hospital reassures patients and families. The availability of tours of the unit may decrease anticipatory anxiety. When a patient is admitted, the patient and family are oriented to unit functioning and daily routines; this enables the treatment team to enlist the family's help and collaboration in the treatment process and to observe the family's interactional patterns, as well as to explain each discipline's role in treatment.

After admission, treatment is guided by clear, specific, achievable goals. The emphasis in some programs on simple weight restoration as the only goal for treatment of anorexia nervosa goes against Hilde Bruch's sage warning to avoid letting these patients "eat their way out of [the] hospital" (Bruch, 1974). The opposite and overly ambitious extreme in treatment goals—complete reorganization of family structure, resolution of all dynamic conflicts, complete normalization of personality, and the like—represents an exercise in unreality. An illustrative sample of significant but achievable goals for the inpatient care of anorexia nervosa is as follows:

1. Restoration of a healthy body weight (adequate and stable) and a healthy body composition.
2. Development of eating behavior that is normal in time, manner, and content.
3. Development of social comfort, personal confidence, and knowledge of balanced nutrition, with practice in eating meals in a wide variety of situations.
4. Treatment of comorbid psychiatric disorders.
5. Moderate, appropriate exercise behavior.
6. Resolution of major distorted cognitions regarding body weight, body image, fear of fatness, pursuit of thinness, and so on.
7. Resolution or initiation of treatment of significant medical complications.
8. Improved family/interpersonal interaction.
9. Formulation and resolution of central dynamic conflict.
10. Development of age-appropriate identity.
11. Aftercare plans for treatment.
12. Relapse prevention plans and readmission criteria.

Weight restoration (a vital if not exclusive goal) means restoration of a fully healthy body weight, with rebuilding of body and organ tissue—not excessive fluid weight, as may occur with hyperalimentation. Restoration of a healthy body weight is best seen as a means, not an end, to comprehensive treatment. The conclusive work of treatment involves a fundamental and enduring change of thinking concerning body weight and shape, in order to decrease the patient's overinvestment in thinness as a means of dealing with crucial central issues in life (e.g., mood regulation, identity, or family stability) that are best attained by other more healthy, developmentally appropriate means. To deal with patients' existential guilt about having an ED or self-criticism for the burden of the ED on their families, we often say: "There are no bad reasons for developing EDs. The ED is simply not an effective or lasting way of dealing with these issues, and the price you pay is too high. Let's find other ways to achieve your goals, whatever they are."

Administrative preparation of a patient for admission and financial approval for continuation of inpatient care usually requires interaction with third-party payers. As noted earlier, this is becoming increasingly difficult with managed-care programs, which frequently deny inpatient care on a fiscal instead of a scientific basis. Interaction with third-party payers requires thorough preparation regarding the facts of the case and relentless advocacy for truly adequate care. Unless approval for admission is rapidly granted by the first "gatekeeper," it is generally more effective to speak only with board-certified psychiatrists. Tape recording of conversations for possible future reference to these important decisions may be useful, if the other party is notified that such taping is occurring. All decisions should be confirmed by fax or mail. It is easy for a clinician to be put on the defensive in seeking approval for treatment when the only questions asked by managed-care reviewers are whether the patient is suicidal or has severe medical abnormalities. Anorexia nervosa patients frequently die with normal laboratory values. The primary reason for admission is usually not acute suicide risk or severe medical abnormality alone, but the need to reverse the course of a potentially deadly, serious, progressive illness through a structured, multidisciplinary inpatient program that integrates nutritional rehabilitation, psychotherapy, and behavioral relearning, in a manner that is not practicable on an outpatient basis. Since contracts for health care are set up with the advice of expert legal counsel, it is only prudent for patients or family members who believe that the patients have been denied reasonable benefits to obtain their own legal counsel regarding interpretation of contract benefits, and to use litigation as needed to secure contract benefits.

Whenever possible, collaboration with managed care is highly desirable, but unfortunately it is not always possible. It is logical that anorexia nervosa patients should receive combined medical and psychiatric benefits for care based on their physical and psychiatric symptoms in the initial starved state, until >90% of a healthy weight is achieved. By analogy, a person with a depressive illness and a broken leg following a suicide attempt by jumping from a ledge requires both orthopedic and psychiatric care. Truly adequate funding for EOs requires legislative mandate.

THE EVALUATION PROCESS

Admission to an ED unit is followed by a biopsychosocial evaluation as summarized in Table 17.1. (A more detailed discussion of psychological testing is provided later in the chapter.) The general recommendations in the table, of course, may be individualized for patients according to their needs.

A comprehensive psychiatric evaluation utilizes a detailed interview for all psychiatric symptoms, with special focus on features pertinent to the EDs. The clinical exam will ideally be supplemented by standardized assessment instruments, such as the Eating Disorders Examination (EDE; Fairburn & Cooper, 1993), the most comprehensive instrument available. A part of the psychiatric evaluation that is too often neglected is the integrative formulation of the case, including the summary of pertinent features, diagnosis and differential diagnosis, etiological factors, treatment plans, prognosis, and central dynamic formulation.

The medical evaluation includes a physical examination and appropriate laboratory studies to document the presence and severity of the medical component, as well as those variables that may be markers of the treatment process. Thyroid hormones (especially T_3), luteinizing hormone (LH) and estrogen in women, or testosterone in men are laboratory parameters correlated with adequacy of weight restoration.

Social and family histories are best obtained by an experienced social worker, in the context of giving support and education to the family during the evaluation process.

Evidence of the severity of anorexia nervosa

TABLE 17.1. Comprehensive Admission Evaluation

1. *Comprehensive psychiatric evaluation:* History, mental state examination, and formulation.

2. *Physical examination:* Note emaciation, vital signs (including orthostasis), lanugo hair, acrocyanosis, height, weight, edema, parotid gland tenderness, hair loss, nail softening, jaundice, scars on dorsum of hand, abdominal tenderness, etc.

3. *Laboratory studies:*

	Admission	Discharge
	Heme-7 with differential	D°
	Urinalysis with microscopic exam	D°
	Electrolytes	D°
	General screen (glucose, calcium, phosphate, TP, albumin, AST, LDH, AlkPtase, total bilirubin, uric acid)	D°
	Lipid profile	D°
	Thyroid: free T_4, thyroid-stimulating hormone, T_3	D°
	Chest X-ray	D
	Electrocardiogram	D°
	Bone mineral density	D
	Bone age (if growth retardation present)	D
	Serum estradiol (in females)	D°
	Testosterone (in males)	D°
	Consider Zn, Mg blood levels	D°

4. *Social work:* Family evaluation (semistructured interview).

5. *Other:*

	Patient photograph	D°
	Imaging for atypical neurological features (MRI)	D

Note. Studies to be repeated routinely at discharge are indicated by D. Studies to be performed at discharge if results are abnormal on admission or for other specific indications are indicated by D°. Some initial studies, if abnormal, may be repeated more often (e.g., heme-7).

and a patient's overall condition may be provided by a photograph of the patient at the time of admission, in shorts and sleeveless top. Toward the end of treatment in the context of individual or group psychotherapy, a review of the pretreatment photograph may allow the patient to gain a healthy perspective on the former degree of illness, often denied prior to treatment.

MEDICAL STABILIZATION

The initial goal of medical stabilization in anorexia nervosa is to differentiate slowly produced symptoms of starvation that are part of the body's adaptive response to decreased energy intake and that will generally respond to simple nutritional rehabilitation from those medical signs and symptoms that are either life-threatening or atypical. This distinction requires the clinician to acquire a thorough understanding of the body's adaptive responses to starvation—a process often best begun by reading the monumental and fascinating work of Keys, Brozek, Henschel, Mickelsen, and Taylor (1950) on experimental starvation. Many of the social behaviors and psychological symptoms attributed to anorexia nervosa are in fact results of starvation, and will normalize with restoration of a healthy body weight. The rapidity of weight loss, methods of weight loss, physical examination results, and laboratory tests are some of the factors that need to be understood in the acute medical stabilization of the patient. Many patients with the restricting subtype of anorexia nervosa are dehydrated on admission because of voluntary fluid restriction practiced to lower the scale weight or due to laxatives/diuretics.

Rehydration may produce an apparently rapid decrease in hematocrit and hemoglobin, but usually simply represents normalization of the intravascular fluid. Sometimes unequilibrated body fluid extravasates into the extravascular space, producing edema (usually peripheral, rarely central). Irregular heartbeats, signs of a significantly thinned or soft myocardial wall, and low core temperature are all danger signs. Patients are seldom altered in their state of consciousness, and may in fact appear to have more energy than the staff, despite their extreme emaciation. Studies have not yet concluded whether supplementation of low serum mineral micronutrients such as zinc is necessary or helpful, but hypophosphatemia often requires replacement treatment and may only emerge during early refeeding. If atypical mental features are present, or there are indications of pituitary microadenoma or other central nervous system lesion, an imaging study of the brain by computed tomography or magnetic resonance imaging (MRI) may be useful. MRI usually shows a decrease in brain size and ventricular dilatation.

MANAGEMENT AND STRUCTURE OF THE INPATIENT UNIT

The Therapeutic Milieu

We employ the concept of a therapeutic milieu as an invaluable context for inpatient treatment of EDs. The therapeutic milieu gives patients the opportunity to recreate in the hospital environment the same dynamics that governed their lives outside the hospital, and affords the treatment staff and patients everyday situations in which to change these dynamics. The unit environment becomes a microcosm of the patients' previous everyday world. The patients are no longer passive recipients of treatment, but become active participants and co-creators in health improvement.

The skilled management of an inpatient unit for patients with EDs is of paramount importance to the outcome of treatment. Consistency of goals and methods is required to keep the focus of treatment on the true issues. This consistency is provided by a protocol that deals with all the routine specifics related to the restoration of weight, exercise, level of observation, and privileges (see Appendix 17.1). Following these practices in the protocol leaves the patient and treatment team free to focus on the underlying relational dynamics, cognitive distortions, and abnormal behaviors that sustain EDs, instead of engaging in endless skirmishes about predictable recurring situations such as the number of calories prescribed or body weight. The unit's therapeutic milieu and psychological principles of treatment derive from the general features of cognitive–behavioral therapy (CBT), as developed by Aaron T. Beck (see Wright, Thase, Beck, & Ludgate, 1993, for applications of CBT to inpatients). Psychoeducation and psychodynamic treatment provide the "shoulders" supporting the main therapeutic emphasis on CBT. All treatment staff members involved in caring for ED patients on our unit have been trained in the CBT model.

Multidisciplinary Team Approach

A multidisciplinary team approach to treatment grows logically from the concept of EDs as involving a multifactorial etiology and a wide variety of individual needs. The team focuses on the goal of changing illness behavior and thinking patterns not only in the protected environment of the inpatient unit, but in practical, "real-life situations; the latter are prepared for both through role play and *in vivo,* so that changes will endure after discharge. Patients receive consistent supportive information regarding diminution of illness behavior and thinking, as well as support, praise, and guidance on the process of attaining appropriate maturity in behavior, thinking patterns, and defense mechanisms.

Transforming a general psychiatric unit into a uniform, effective specialty unit for treating EDs can be accomplished effectively and at low cost. CBT, which is manual-based and achievable in a short time of training, provides a pragmatic treatment model that fits with the simultaneous use of psychopharmacology and psychodynamics. This model has psychoeducational materials that can be used to create a collaborative relationship with the patient. A specialty unit based on CBT enhances staff morale and improves the specificity of treatment.

Treatment Team Functioning

Upon admission to the unit, a patient is assigned to a treatment team consisting of a staff psychiatrist, a psychiatric resident, a psychologist, a primary nurse, a social worker, an occupational therapist, a dietitian, and an activities therapist. Some patients will also need a vocational rehabilitation therapist, or, if they are students, an educational consultant. We focus on helping patients to develop coping skills for good stress management, to decrease compulsive exercise, to utilize leisure time constructively, to learn nutrition and cooking skills, to practice assertiveness and relaxation, to stabilize mood, to prevent weight loss, and to diminish perfectionism. The treatment modalities include group, individual, and family methods. Team members work closely together on these issues to provide the patients with the structure and support they will need in treatment, to avoid "splitting," to balance support with healthy limits, and to balance supervised with independent work.

Program Scheduling

Patients are actively involved in some form of treatment much of the day. They begin with a psychoeducational group, in which they learn about the effects of starvation, as well as principles of healthy social and psychological functioning. They then participate in an activities therapy group to allow for leisure-time skill building. Occupational therapy focuses on meal planning and purchasing. Twice a week, the patients participate in a coping skills group that emphasizes role playing. On two other days, patients participate in a CBT group, led jointly by a clinical psychologist and a clinical nurse specialist. Three times a week, a body perception group is led by a clinical nurse specialist followed by snack and discussion. Dinner is followed by a group discussion. Social recreational activity is offered from 7:00 P.M. until 8:30 P.M. The program is summarized in Table 17.2.

Complex Patients

Besides the challenges presented by typical cases of EDs serious enough to be admitted to inpatient care, some patients present additional complexities. Male patients occur in a 1:10 ratio to female patients; the presence of male patients on a unit adds a dimension of gender divergence, with male issues of etiology, sexuality, and social roles needing to be addressed. It is valuable for female patients to learn to relate to male patients in a therapeutic context, especially if gender relations were troubled prior to admission.

Adolescents are often in the midst of the psychosocial task of identity formation described by Erikson (1968) as central to the teen years. Many anorexic adolescents are caretakers of their parents (reversed parenting), to the detriment of their own development; such adolescents need to learn to nurture themselves and play appropriately. Perfectionistic, extremely sensitive adolescents need to learn to relax and have fun, while impulsive adolescents need to internalize reasonable limits.

Patients with diabetes or other comorbid medical conditions have many issues that usually fall between the interface of medicine and psychiatry. The medical care is addressed as needed, but is not allowed to become the central focus of the treatment (see Powers, Chapter 24, this volume).

Patients with substance dependence are best

TABLE 17.2. Program Schedule

Time	Sunday	Monday	Tuesday	Wednesday	Thursday	Friday	Saturday
8:00–9:00 A.M.		Breakfast	Breakfast	Breakfast	Breakfast	Breakfast	Breakfast
8:15–9:00 A.M.	Breakfast						
9:00–9:30 A.M.		Psychoeducation group	Psychoeducation group	Psychoeducation group	Psychoeducation group	Psychoeducation group	
9:30–10:30 A.M.	Activity if no school or tutor	°Activity if no school or tutor	Activity if no school or tutor	Activity if no school or tutor	Activity if no school or tutor	Activity if no school or tutor	
10:30–11:00 A.M.				Leisure education group			
11:00–1:00 A.M.				OT cooking group			
11:45–12:30 P.M.	Lunch	Lunch	Lunch	Lunch	Lunch	Lunch	Lunch
12:30–1:30 P.M.				Coping skills group		Coping skills group	
1:00–2:00 P.M.		Tutor		Body perception group		Body perception group	
1:30–3:00 P.M.			CBT group		CBT group		
1:30–2:30 P.M.			Activity if no group	Activity if no group	Activity if no group	Activity if no group	Activity if no group
2:00–3:00 P.M.		Body perception group					
2:30–3:00 P.M.	Snack if ordered	Snack if ordered	Snack if ordered	Snack if ordered	Snack if ordered	Snack if ordered	Snack if ordered
3:45–4:45 P.M.		Activity	Activity	Activity	Activity	Activity	Activity
5:00–5:45 P.M.	Dinner	Dinner	Dinner	Dinner	Dinner	Dinner	Dinner
6:00–7:00 P.M.	Study hall	Study hall	Study hall	Study hall	Study hall	Study hall	
7:00–8:30 P.M.		°Activity	Activity	Activity	Activity	Activity	Activity
8:30–9:00 P.M.	Snack if ordered	Snack if ordered	Snack if ordered	Snack if ordered	Snack if ordered	Snack if ordered	Snack if ordered
11:00 P.M.	Bedtime	Bedtime	Bedtime	Bedtime	Bedtime	Bedtime	Bedtime

°Varied daily by recreational therapy and unit staff to include social and leisure activities.

withdrawn from their dependence before admission, if possible. It is essential for this population to deal with both their ED and their substance dependence, or they may switch back and forth between their illnesses rather than achieve true recovery from their dual disorders. They often benefit from referral for additional treatment upon completion of the ED program. (See Mitchell, Specker, & Edmonson, Chapter 23, this volume.)

Patients who are parents are provided with parenting classes while in treatment. Children are included in family therapy sessions if they are old enough to participate. Teaching is aimed at helping the patients avoid fostering an ED in their children, as often occurs. Many of the young mothers on our unit entered treatment only after they noticed their young children were imitating their own self-starving or purging behaviors.

The diagnosis of one or more comorbid psychiatric disorders (mood disorders, anxiety disorders, OCD, and personality disorders, etc.) often accompanies the diagnosis of an ED. Indeed, EDs seldom occur without two to four additional psychiatric diagnoses. It is helpful to assess whether these diagnoses are truly independently comorbid disorders or are the secondary results of starvation and/or binge–purge behaviors. Secondary comorbid psychiatric conditions often improve with weight restoration alone. Reevaluation of comorbid weight restoration then allows the clinician to treat enduring conditions.

Program Self-Evaluation and Patient Evaluation

It is essential to review the treatment program periodically and make changes as needed—for example, when impasses are reached in patient care or new data are published. In these days of health care reform and managed health care, clinicians must continue to focus on delivering truly comprehensive care with the most cost-effective methods possible, but never at the expense of sound treatment.

PSYCHOLOGICAL TESTING AND TREATMENT

Psychological Testing

Psychological assessment during inpatient treatment contributes vital quantitative and qualitative information about ED symptomatology, as well as about personality factors, general psychiatric symptomatology, and intellectual/neuropsychological functioning. Pretreatment assessment can be completed at any stage during inpatient treatment, but offers the greatest amount of information if finished within the first 3 to 5 days of hospitalization. A list of generally useful psychological tests is provided in Table 17.3.

ED psychopathology can be assessed with valid and reliable tests that target this area. Brief self-report measures such as the Eating Disorder Inventory (EDI; Garner, 1991), the Eating Attitudes Test (EAT; Garner & Garfinkel, 1979), and the Eating Inventory (Stunkard & Messick, 1987) identify specific aspects of the disorder, including desire for thinness, binge–purge behavior, and restraint in eating. The EAT and the first three subscales of the EDI (Drive for Thinness, Bulimia, and

TABLE 17.3. Useful Tests for Psychological Evaluation upon Admission

Admission	Discharge
Personality	
_____ MMPI-2	_____ D°
_____ SNAP	_____ D
_____ SIDP-IV	_____ D
_____ NEO-PI-R	_____ D
Intellectual/neuropsychological functioning	
_____ WAIS-R (Adults/Adolescents)	_____ D
_____ WISC-III (Children)	_____ D
_____ Trail Making Test, Category Test, Wisconsin Card Sorting Test (if indicated)	_____ D°
Mood/anxiety disorders	
_____ Beck Depression Inventory	_____ D°
_____ Hamilton Depression Rating Scale	_____ D°
_____ Beck Anxiety Inventory	_____ D°
_____ Yale–Brown Obsessive Compulsive Scale	_____ D°
Eating disorders	
_____ EAT	_____ D°
_____ EDI	_____ D°
_____ Eating Inventory	_____ D°
_____ EDE	_____ D°

Note. See text for full titles of abbreviated tests. As in Table 17.1, tests to be repeated routinely at discharge are indicated by D; tests to be repeated at discharge if results are abnormal on admission or for other specific indications are indicated by D°.

Body Dissatisfaction) are additionally useful for documenting change during treatment. A valuable assessment tool, mentioned earlier, is the EDE (Fairburn & Cooper, 1993); this test is designed to assess broad clinical features of an ED, especially attitudes and behaviors related to the illness over the preceding 4 weeks.

Because the EAT and EDI are valid, reliable, and easily administered instruments, these tests are useful both to document severity of illness at admission and to record improvement during treatment. They can also indicate areas for emphasis in treatment. Finally, they may offer prognostic information and guidance for outpatient follow-up, establishing baseline scores at the time of transition from inpatient care to partial hospital or outpatient care.

It is vital to assess personality functioning and the presence of Axis I comorbid disorders, such as depression and anxiety disorders (Margolis, Spencer, DePaulo, Simpson, & Andersen, 1994). Paper-and-pencil inventories such as the Minnesota Multiphasic Personality Inventory—2 (MMPI-2; Hathaway & McKinley, 1989) and the Schedule of Nonadaptive and Adaptive Personality (SNAP; Clark, 1993) help to identify patients with these vulnerabilities. Other tools such as the Structured Interview for DSM-IV Personality (SIDP-IV; Pfohl, Blum, & Zimmerman, 1995), an interview-based measure, may identify additional DSM-IV Axis II traits or disorders. Along with instruments that evaluate state personality features (e.g., the MMPI-2), the assessment of trait aspects of personality can aid the psychotherapeutic process; for example, the Five-Factor Model of Personality (NEO-PI-R; Costa & McCrae, 1985) can be used to assess dimensional rather than categorical features.

Mood disorders are the Axis I comorbidity most commonly associated with EDs. Tests that evaluate for depression include the Beck Depression Inventory (Beck, Ward, Mendelson, Mock, & Erbaugh, 1961) and the Hamilton Rating Scale for Depression (Hamilton, 1960), though evaluators should be aware that some skewing will be found on weight-related questions. Instruments that assess anxiety disorders, such as the Beck Anxiety Inventory (Beck, 1990) or the Yale–Brown Obsessive Compulsive Scale (Goodman, et al., 1989), should also be used as indicated. Often treatment of comorbid conditions presents as serious a challenge as treatment of the primary ED.

Intellectual functioning warrants assessment for a number of reasons. Many patients or their parents have expectations for the patients' academic or vocational performance that are based more on their persevering traits than on their inherent giftedness. Evidence of actual level of intellectual functioning may be sympathetically used to change these expectations. The Wechsler Adult Intelligence Scale—Revised (WAIS-R; Wechsler, 1981) or the Wechsler Intelligence Scale for Children, third edition (WISC-III; Wechsler, 1991) can assess such functioning efficiently.

Use of standard intelligence tests can also alert the treatment team to ED-induced alteration in brain function. There is growing evidence of neuropsychological dysfunction among low-weight patients with EDs (Bowers, 1994; Hamsher, Halmi, & Benton, 1981). The use of a short battery of neuropsychological tests can inform the treatment team about deficits in a patient's cognitive functioning. For example, neuropsychological testing can recognize problems with abstract thinking and reasoning, which are particularly important for patients involved in psychotherapy. Abstract reasoning can be assessed with the Wisconsin Card Sorting Test (Berg, 1948), the Category Test (DeFillippis, McCampbell, & Rogers, 1979), and the Trail Making Test (Spreen & Strauss, 1991). When cognitive dysfunction is found, it is important to repeat the testing after weight restoration to determine whether these neuropsychological changes have been reversed.

General Comments on Psychotherapy

Individual psychotherapy represents the most common psychotherapeutic intervention during inpatient treatment of anorexia nervosa (Garner, 1985). It constitutes a primary treatment for this and other EDs because of the significant psychosocial impairment that these patients experience (Bruch, 1973), particularly a global sense of ineffectiveness and dysphoria. Such problems impede social, occupational, familial, and educational development. Individual psychotherapy is used most often as a therapeutic agent to change distorted attitudes, beliefs, and behaviors. Only a limited amount of psychotherapy can be carried out during hospitalization, but this component may be extremely helpful for good long-term outcome. Inpatient psychotherapy creates a smooth transition to vital long-term outpatient psychotherapy. Most inpatient programs integrate individual therapy with family and group methods.

These patients often view psychotherapy as threatening. They are being asked to give up behaviors, beliefs, and an approach to life that may have provided a comparatively simple and partially effective solution to complex problems. Thinness and weight control offer concrete and easily measured markers of self-control and self-esteem. Without these simple but illness-based measures, life is seen as more complicated and ambiguous. An anorexic patient's anxiety may become high if an adequate replacement for self-starvation is not forthcoming. Medical recovery from the disorder (a positive goal to many physicians) may be perceived by the patient as a loss of specialness, and thus as a negative event, if accompanying psychotherapy to change attitudes toward weight is not integrated into the weight restoration. Often a patient will go through the motions of listening to educational information and attending treatment activities while attempting to defeat the treatment team at every turn. Acceptance of treatment depends upon building a trust that a satisfactory substitute for the disorder will emerge as the psychotherapeutic process continues.

Increasing a patient's desire for treatment can be accomplished by commending the patient's willingness to consider treatment as a sign of health. This sets a positive tone from the beginning. Defining the need for treatment as a failure of coping strategies, rather than as a personal failure of the patient, helps to reduce the sense of stigma that so often demoralizes patients. The following typical statement by a therapist captures this tone:

> There are no bad reasons for developing an ED. This illness usually represents an attempt to deal with challenges in personal development, self-esteem, mood regulation, or family functioning. It works to some extent, but in the end it is not successful, as well as being dangerous. Our goal is never to criticize you for the disorder, but to ask you to work with us to understand how it came about, and then to "trade in and trade up" so that whatever the purposes behind the disorder are, you can accomplish them in a healthy and effective way.

Individual therapy thus conveys to the patient that treatment involves a joint and cooperative effort in developing new and successful tactics to deal directly and effectively with the personal and developmental issues involved in the disorder.

Behavioral therapy and psychological interventions vary among inpatient programs, according to the type of program, patient features, and the training of the treatment team. Most programs emphasize some form of unspoken or explicit behavior therapy and contingency management. Healthy behaviors are systematically reinforced through positive and negative consequences. Programs that do not claim to use explicit contingencies usually employ more subtle positive and negative reinforcement principles; they are just not defined formally. It is important to make the contingencies within a program as clear as possible to both patients and staff members, in order to create a consistent and effective program.

In a review of ED treatment programs comparing medication versus psychotherapy, Agras (1987) reported that treatment results were poorer in strictly medication-oriented programs than in programs employing psychotherapy and behavior therapy. In addition, programs that used some features of behavior therapy resulted in fewer days of hospitalization. It should be noted that weight normalization achieved by way of behavior therapy, though helpful, is not equivalent to comprehensive treatment of EDs. Behavior therapy may best be seen as one aspect of a total treatment program that includes psychosocial and medical interventions.

CBT as a Central Theme for All Unit Psychotherapies

CBT has been shown to be effective in the treatment of bulimia nervosa (Wilson & Fairburn, 1993; see Wilson, Fairburn, & Agras, Chapter 6, this volume). CBT for the treatment of bulimia nervosa employs many strategies that can be applied to the treatment of anorexia nervosa, although its effectiveness in anorexia nervosa has not yet been definitively demonstrated. Shared goals in treatment of the two disorders include decreased illness-driven eating and social patterns, and their replacement by healthy behaviors. Because anorexia nervosa and bulimia nervosa share symptoms (overemphasis on body shape and weight, rigid dietary habits), CBT seems well suited for the treatment of a heterogeneous mix of EDs during inpatient treatment (Eckert & Mitchell, 1989; Wilson & Fairburn, 1993; Bowers, 1993; Fairburn & Cooper, 1989). CBT can be learned in a short time by all members of the treatment team, is logical and testable, and is based on clear manuals for training.

Individual psychotherapy utilizing a cognitive perspective during inpatient treatment has been advocated to deal with the crucial developmental issues of EDs (Bowers, 1993). Although supportive psychotherapy and psychoeducation are often used during the early phases of inpatient care, it is reasonable to start concomitantly with a more aggressive, well-defined cognitive-behavioral approach from the earliest days of treatment—an approach that becomes increasingly effective as a stable, adequate weight is achieved.

The cognitive-behavioral model of anorexia nervosa (many aspects of which are also applicable to bulimia nervosa) represents a developmental theory that emphasizes primacy of the cognitions as mediating factors for distressed emotions, resulting in abnormal behavior (Garfinkel & Garner, 1982; Garner, 1985; Garner & Bemis, 1982; see Garner, Vitousek, & Pike, Chapter 7, this volume). Cognitive-behavioral theory also accommodates factors from psychodynamic and biological paradigms. Through various life experiences (called "schemas"), specific distorted ideas regarding the self, the world, and the future are learned, which then create vulnerability to the disorder. A cognitive model views anorexia nervosa as a final common pathway of multiple events or experiences (Garfinkel & Garner, 1982). Adolescents affected are most often introverted, sensitive, persevering, and isolative youngsters, who develop the idea that weight loss will somehow alleviate psychological distress and dysphoria (Garfinkel & Garner, 1982; Garner & Bemis, 1982, 1985). Dieting and attaining thinness become the common ways for these individuals to exercise control over their internal and external environments (Garner & Bemis, 1982, 1985). At the same time, the patient decreases food intake, and is reinforced by social praise for achievement of weight loss. Weight loss next leads to increased social isolation and reinforces the distorted cognitions and maladaptive behaviors of anorexia nervosa.

CBT also places a high value on the expression and understanding of emotions. Increased awareness of emotions is gradually achieved through the therapist's observation of inconsistencies, incongruities, and inappropriate emotional reactions to the patient's everyday events. Confirmation and reinforcement of emotions that are a genuine part of the patient's past and present experiences are essential. Analogies, hypothetical situations, and Socratic questioning may all be used to help the patient see that reactions in specific situations are distorted. The patient can initially recognize that in a hypothetical sense emotion is acceptable, but only for other people, not for him or her. The patient is encouraged to identify accurately and to express all emotions, especially "unacceptable" emotions. With the therapist serving as a model for expression of emotion, the patient can then learn that open expression of emotions does not lead to rejection (Garfinkel & Garner, 1982) or out-of-control behavior. For emotionally immature but intellectualized younger patients, indirect methods such as poetry reading and writing may be helpful (Woodall & Andersen, 1989).

CBT attempts to help the patient recognize and change the rigid standards employed to determine self-worth. Setting reasonable standards for competence (emphasizing adequacy, not perfection), and learning to accept "in-betweens," are very important. Self-acceptance, despite normal personal shortcomings and failures to meet unrealistic standards, is a fundamental goal for the psychotherapist working with an anorexic (or a bulimic) patient. Helplessness and incompetence can be decreased by encouraging efforts at mastery in areas that have been avoided because of fear of failure (Garfinkel & Garner, 1982).

Dynamic Principles

As noted above, CBT accommodates a concomitant psychodynamic paradigm, especially the formulation of Hilde Bruch (1973, 1974). Bruch postulated a central psychodynamic role in the etiology of EDs, proposing that EDs represent a struggle for self-respect and the development of a secure identity. According to Bruch, a major factor in the development of ED psychopathology is the failure of parents to regard an adolescent child as an autonomous individual; the child is treated instead as a means of meeting the parents' needs. Although psychotherapy can use ideas from several models, its foundation needs to be a relationship based on mutual trust.

Group Therapy

Individual psychotherapy during inpatient treatment is generally combined with family and group therapy. Group therapy in the treatment of EDs is increasingly recognized as an important, effective, economical psychotherapeutic tool (Hall, 1985). A blend of process orientation (Yalom, 1995) and cognitive-behavioral principles (Lee & Rush, 1986; Bowers & Andersen, 1994) appears to be most effective; it gives the group latitude to deal with personal and interpersonal issues, with a focus on the cognitive and developmental factors involved with EDs. The group can also influence the perceptions of the patients and permit the patients to assist in one another's recovery through self-disclosure and confrontation of symptomatic behavior, ideas, and attitudes. A difference from outpatient group therapy is that the pool of inpatients is limited by the inpatient census, reducing the ability to screen patients for an ideal mix. An inpatient group may be more heterogeneous diagnostically (including patients with anorexia nervosa and bulimia nervosa), but the common themes of both EDs unite the otherwise diverse population into a psychologically homogeneous group.

A process orientation schema capitalizes on a group's curative factors (Yalom, 1995)—elements of the group process that become primary tools to promote change. These include an instillation of hope, feelings of universality, an opportunity for altruism and interpersonal learning, the imparting of information, the development of socializing techniques, and the corrective recapitulation of the primary family unit. Group therapy with others suffering from similar symptoms allows isolative individuals to overcome feelings of shame and secrecy. A central factor for instilling a sense of hope is to show that it is possible to confront and change the seemingly unresolvable issues surrounding food and weight (Lee & Rush, 1986; Yalom, 1995).

Body Perception Group

The body perception group helps patients come to terms with their body distortions. It first shows them how these distortions affect their lives and sustain EDs, and then assists them in adopting a healthier perspective. The patients are alternately supportive and confrontive with one another, helping each other in ways not possible in individual therapy. Often the distortion of body size and shape is not completely resolved, but patients learn to diminish the impact of these thoughts and begin to put them into a healthier perspective.

Family Therapy

Scientific evidence (Hall, 1987; Russell, Szmukler, Dare, & Eisler, 1987; Dare, Eisler, Russell, & Szmukler, 1990; Crisp et al., 1991) and clinical experience strongly suggest that some form of family therapy (or at least family meetings) is mandatory during inpatient treatment. This is especially true for patients who are under the age of 18, live at home, and have a stable family environment (Russell et al., 1987; Dare et al., 1990; Crisp et al., 1991). Inpatient treatment often offers the family an opportunity to become an effective unit. The family members are not blamed for their past problems; rather, they receive concern and support, along with the message that family change needs to occur together with the patient's improvement.

An approach to family therapy that will encompass all ages and family units is one that is pragmatic, eclectic, and flexible, using elements of structural, strategic, and cognitive-behavioral interventions (Vanderlinden & Vandereycken, 1991). The focus of therapy is on here-and-now issues that facilitate change in the family. The treatment team requests the family's help, support, and cooperation during the process of therapy. The family therapist must develop and communicate nonblaming, constructive hypotheses regarding the meaning of the ED for the family as well as the patient.

Family therapy may have multiple goals. These include redesigning family boundaries, decreasing the patient's role in parental or family disputes, and educating the family about the etiology and symptoms of the disorder. In addition, family therapy can ward off blame, help the family members communicate more effectively, and help the patient become a more independent individual (Hall, 1987). Family therapy also endeavors to increase development of an age-appropriate style of individual and family functioning, to diminish enmeshed or disengaged styles, and to assist children to make age-appropriate changes as they mature. A major goal is to promote or prepare the way for a transition to adult-to-adult relationships instead of entirely parent–child interactions.

Vandereycken, Kog, and Vanderlinden (1989) provide a cogent discussion of whether families are "architects or victims" of EDs. When family members are not able to modify their behaviors, especially if these behaviors are destructive to healing, separation of the patient from the family may be warranted during treatment (Hall, 1987) and occasionally afterwards. It may be equally important for family members to begin psychotherapy themselves. Individual or marital therapy can be important, particularly when family members have unresolved problems with substance use or depression (Vandereycken et al., 1989; Andersen et al., 1985). Continued outpatient family therapy is strongly recommended after the patient has been discharged, especially when the patient is under the age of 18.

NUTRITIONAL REHABILITATION

Setting the Goal Weight Range

There are several approaches to setting the goal for desired weight. In general, we strive for a healthy normal weight. The two sets of standards we generally use are (1) the Metropolitan Life tables (Metropolitan Life Insurance Company, 1959, 1983) for patients 18 and over, and (2) the nomograms devised by Frisch and McArthur (1974) for achieving the weight necessary for return of menstrual periods in anorexic females. A reasonable goal is the midrange of the weight on the Metropolitan Life chart for a given height (with appropriate age correction and occasionally frame correction). In general, patients being restored from anorexia without past obesity have initial target weight derived from 1959 MetLife table, while patients with a personal history of overweight, are initially targeted for 1983 weight, about 10 pounds higher than 1959. Individualization of weight goal additionally considers normal T_3, normal LH, normal estrogen/testosterone, and normal core temperature. For female patients under age 18, with amenorrhea secondary to anorexia nervosa, we use the weight identified by Frisch and McArthur for a 50% chance of return of menstrual periods. It should be noted that the weight for return of periods is about 10 pounds higher than the weight required to begin cycles during normal development. For patients below age 14, weights may be chosen from pediatric development charts.

Picking a number from a chart is not the whole answer, however. Some attention should be given to the weight at which a patient functioned well if he or she had a time of stable weight and height before the onset of illness. The average anorexic patient often begins dieting at 5–10% above the "ideal" weight. There is a rationale for setting the goal weight of these patients at 5–15% above the "ideal" weight, since many of these patients may in fact be biologically normal only when they are above the "ideal" in weight. Few patients accept this reasoning in practice, however.

Where practical considerations dictate a short treatment period, moderate weight gain (to 90% of normal) may have to be accepted as the next best goal for an anorexic patient, with close follow-up required in a partial hospitalization program or the outpatient clinic. A goal weight range, rather than a single point, should be set so that patients can fluctuate comfortably within a 4-pound (1.4-kg) range.

The weight goal is not firmly set when a patient comes into the hospital, but only after treatment has been underway for several days or weeks. The weight range is made as a decision among the team members if variation from protocol is needed. Since it is our practice not to tell patients their goal weight range until they are in the middle of it, changes can be made by staff members without incurring the wrath or fear of patients that we are breaking promises about a given weight range.

Concepts in Achieving Weight Restoration

The essential concepts of this phase of our program are as follows: Food is prescribed as medication and is eaten in normal form. Milkshake-type products are used only on rare occasions and for energy intakes above 3,500 calories per day or in a special medical situations. Within 24 hours of admission, virtually all of our patients begin to eat regular prescribed meals. The following summary talk is given to all of our incoming patients:

> You have an illness that has changed your perception about your body's size and your body's need for food. We are going to ask you to trust us to prescribe your food like medication. This may be difficult for you because of your fear that you may lose control, eat too much, and become overweight. Our goal, however, is never to make anyone overweight, and we will not let you gain too

much. But we will ask you to accept our judgment about your nutritional needs and to eat everything that we prescribe for you. You may be anxious during part of the program, but we will have nurses with you much of the time to give you support and encouragement.

We do not know where this illness comes from. It seems to come from many factors, including some features of your personality, such as perfectionism; some family stresses; perhaps some biochemical changes in your body; and going on a diet. Whatever the cause, we do not blame anybody. We think people are often blamed for this problem, but we do not feel your parents are to blame or you are to blame.

Please be honest with us and trust us. We know that there is a great temptation to dispose of your food secretly or to vomit to avoid the effects of eating. We want to concentrate not on your gaining weight, but on your losing your disorder and building a healthy body. If you are anorexic, we think that your hands and feet will be less cold; you will have more energy and less restlessness; your thinking will be clearer. Our goal is to make you a happier and healthier person. You may experience some discomfort as you go through the nutritional rehabilitation, but we will try to make you as comfortable as possible. We want you to regain control of your life and to continue your growth and development in a healthy manner, free from the eating disorder.

Nurses and nursing assistants initially remain with a patient for 24-hour support and supervision, until a normal eating pattern has been established and comprehensive assessment of the patient's psychological and physical state have been obtained. Nurses sit with patients at all meals and encourage them to eat. A nasogastric tube is rarely required. No cases (out of more than 700) have required hyperalimentation. The emphasis is on empathizing with the patients' fear of fatness, giving psychological support, and using the milieu for group encouragement. The promise that patients will not be allowed to become overweight is kept. No discussion of weight or calories is permitted; rather, the emphasis is on patients' achieving self-understanding of their feelings and thoughts. Fears of fatness are interpreted as symptoms of illness. The combination of an empathic nursing-supervised weight restoration program, using normal food in a milieu setting and group support, results in patients' beginning to eat three meals a day with only moderate anxiety. Occasionally, very anxious patients receive a small amount of an antianxiety agent (lorazepam, 0.5 mg 1 hour before meals) for a week or two. Rarely, small doses of phenothiazines may be used.

A number of methods are unacceptable, including forcing patients to eat; using a passive interpretive psychotherapy alone, with no attention to altering eating patterns; and using appetite-stimulating medications alone, without psychological support.

Food Prescribed

For an anorexic patient, the initial food prescribed begins with 1,200 to 1,500 calories per day, according to the patient's admission weight; this food is low in fat, salt, and lactose. The enzymes for digesting fat and milk products take time to be restored after starvation, and the body should not be challenged with these products until these inducible enzymes have been regenerated. No diet foods of any kind are allowed. (See Appendix 17.1.)

The dietitian plays an essential role in relating to both patients and staff, taking a complete nutritional history from the patients upon admission, and after that not discussing treatment directly with the patients until their weight is in the maintenance range. Every day, however, the dietitian is present at staff rounds to help make decisions about changes in dietary programs. If the dietitian and the patients are allowed to interact directly during nutritional rehabilitation, the patients may requires endless changes in their menus. We allow patients to name three specific foods to delete from their menus, but other than these three specific choices (e.g., artichokes, pork chops, and scrambled eggs), they do not determine the foods prescribed. During the maintenance phase, the nutritionist becomes active again in direct conferences with patients, teaching them to choose balanced meals (first, types of food, and then, quantities). Vegetarianism is permitted only if it was part of an established religious or philosophical practice preceding the onset of the disorder (e.g., a patient was a Seventh-Day Adventist).

Calories are increased by 500 every 4 to 5 days until a maximum of between 3,500 and 4,500 calories per day is achieved. The exact number will depend on the individual rate of weight gain, the height of the patient, and the presence of gastrointestinal discomfort. If too many low-energy foods are allowed in the diet, then the physical quantity occupied by 3,500 to 4,500 calories a day becomes enormous. Once nutritional rehabilitation has been underway for several weeks, most calories can be prescribed in fairly dense form, including a moderate amount of fats and sweets. A detailed program for nutritional rehabilitation is described in Appendix 17.1, with specific suggestions for food items.

General Comments

The person supervising an anorexic patient at a given meal makes the final decisions. Endless discussions about the contents of the meal are not allowed. Signs of staff splitting are watched for carefully, and comments about what other staff members have "allowed" are politely ignored. The key is consistent, empathic, insightful supervision, with encouragement of the development of normal eating patterns. Two additional points need to be emphasized.

First, an increase in weight does not automatically produce a normal eating pattern in an anorexic patient. Specific teaching about balanced patterns of nutrition, role modeling, and working out the patient's fears of fatness in psychotherapy are all important in achieving normal eating patterns as well as normal weight.

Second, weight gain is a means to an end and not an end in itself. The reasons for prompt weight restoration in anorexia nervosa are to eliminate the physical and mental symptoms of starvation and to help establish normal, healthy behavior. Many confusing psychological symptoms are produced by starvation. Intensive psychotherapy is only partially effective at best in the starved patient. Weight gain by itself is only the beginning of the process of healing, but it is a necessary first step.

Specific Problems and Suggestions

If a patient refuses to eat, a confident, supportive approach by the nursing staff almost always overcomes this refusal. Group encouragement from other patients is helpful. At times the staff members worry about whether their own weight influences patients. We try to avoid hiring either grossly overweight or severely emaciated nurses. We also try not to hire nurses who have active EDs themselves.

If patients induce vomiting so quickly that it cannot be prevented, we ask them to help the staff clean it up. The approximate volume vomited is replaced by an equal volume of a nutritious milkshake. Most of the time, the patients express relief that they are not allowed to vomit. Nurses accompany them to the bathroom and stand outside the stall. They stand to the side of the shower while a shower is taking place. Occasionally a patient is very behaviorally disordered and attempts to strike out at a staff member. This is discouraged by time in the "quiet room" and, again, by a supportive and empathic but firm approach. Frequent staff meetings are necessary to deal with the staff's feelings (both reality-based and countertransferential) about the patients' attitudes and behaviors.

Most medical consequences of nutritional rehabilitation are transient and generally mild to moderate. The commonly occurring peripheral edema is treated by having patients elevate their feet, limiting salt in the diet, and at times by holding calories constant for a week without increases. Diuretics are not needed. Rarely, patients develop gastric dilatation, a potentially fatal problem.

MEDICAL AND PHARMACOLOGICAL TREATMENT

Exercise Program

A graduated exercise program is introduced after admission as clinically permitted, and is adjusted to the physical status of the patient (especially bone density and cardiac status). It is a major source of encouragement for patients to begin stretching and walking soon after admission. Weight restoration will be better distributed if there is ongoing, moderate, appropriate exercise. Compulsive, driven exercise is discouraged; strenuous forms of exercise such as aerobics are not introduced until a patient is in the maintenance weight range, and only then if such exercise is consistent with medical parameters.

Role of Medications in Treatment

The use of medicines to stimulate appetite is generally unhelpful and counterproductive, for two reasons. First, appetite mechanisms in the patients' brains are normal. Second, without psychotherapeutic improvement, increased appetite leads to increased anxiety and attempts to vomit or exercise.

Antidepressants have been advocated for both anorexia nervosa and bulimia nervosa, and may well have a role in treatment of comorbid depression in both disorders (Needleman & Weber, 1977; Hudson, Pope, Jonas, & Yurgelun-Todd, 1985). Our practice, however, has been to prescribe antidepressants only after patients' weights are normal, their eating patterns are normal, and they have had experience with intensive psychotherapy. After these three approaches have been employed, if a patient still meets criteria for major depressive disorder, then antidepressants are prescribed. (See Figure 17.2 for our "care map" concerning the treatment of anorexia nervosa with comorbid depression.) The current reports in the literature are not yet sufficiently convincing in our view to suggest that antidepressants have a routine role during the low-weight phase of illness. Fluoxetine is approved for treatment of bulimia nervosa. We use selective serotonin reuptake inhibitors (SSRIs) for treatment of the binge-eating/purging subtype of anorexia nervosa in selected cases only, since CBT alone is often effective.

Obsessive–compulsive symptoms may also be improved with weight restoration, and should be reevaluated after weight restoration before medications are used to treat them. Exceptions may of course occur. Occasionally patients benefit from prokinetic agents (cisapride) to decrease bloating, or H_2 blockers (ranitidine) where reflux esophagitis is present.

RETROSPECTIVE COMMENTS

Using the nursing-supervised management of nutritional rehabilitation as described above, we have had an average weight restoration of 9–12 kg (20–26 pounds) per anorexic patient. There have been no deaths. There has been one case of congestive heart failure in a patient with prior valvular disease. Transient pedal edema and nonspecific gastrointestinal symptoms occur fairly often (Waldholtz & Andersen, 1990), but generally respond quickly to conservative treatment. Patients are told about these symptoms in advance and generally have anticipated them when they have occurred.

Male anorexic patients show a dramatic indeed, often a fivefold increase in their testosterone levels (Andersen, Wirth, & Strahlman,

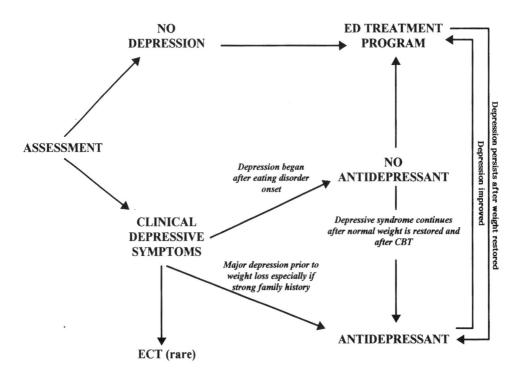

FIGURE 17.2. Care Map 2: Treatment of anorexia nervosa with depression symptoms.

1982). This increase is accompanied by a return of sexual fantasies, erections, and sexual drive. A modest percentage of female anorexic patients achieve return to menstrual cycles while in treatment; most of the time this does not occur until after discharge, if it occurs at all (Andersen, Hedblom, & Hubbard, 1983).

Patients interviewed after treatment generally state that the close nursing supervision during the first week or two of treatment was emotionally difficult because of the lack of privacy. They believe, however, that it was an essential part of the program for them and that they would have found ways to avoid weight restoration if other methods had been used. Most agree that leaving the hospital and getting back to everyday life is an even more difficult experience.

THE DISCHARGE PROCESS

Aftercare planning begins as close as possible to the time of admission. EDs severe enough to require inpatient treatment will require experienced long-term follow-up, usually from 1 year to several years. The characteristics of satisfactory aftercare include making a predischarge decision about whether a patient should step down to partial hospitalization or outpatient treatment alone. We involve the aftercare team in the discharge process, transmitting information about the course of treatment, and sharing both the philosophy and practice of treatment. Patients returning to rural areas or to areas without experienced professionals may soon worsen in their symptomatology. This is particularly true in view of the increasingly frequent problem of managed-care-driven discharge of patients before they have had a chance to establish adequate weight or healthy patterns of behavior. Data do not support the frequently practiced discharge of anorexic patients at very low weight, immediately after medical danger or self-harm danger has passed, but while they are still far short of a healthy body weight.

After inpatient care, the next challenge becomes relapse prevention. Relapse after discharge is more probable in cases where patients at the time of discharge were still low in weight, continued to experience severe distortion of body image, practiced vomiting, or experienced a continued severe drive for thinness and/or morbid fear of fatness. Relapse is more probable when patients have unresolved comorbid psychiatric problems, do not have experienced follow-up outpatient facilities for continued treatment, or return to seriously disturbed family situations. During the immediate posthospital course, emphasis on maintaining a normal weight through normal patterns of eating behavior is the cornerstone for future psychological work. A central goal of inpatient treatment is to have the patient internalize the structure of the program. Upon discharge, the patient is then able to self-regulate eating behavior according to nutritional needs, rather than in the service of psychological conflicts or deficits.

Readmission to the hospital for treatment of relapse will generally be more effective and shorter if it occurs sooner rather than later. Prompt readmission should occur when a patient falls below 85% of target weight, but a higher threshold may be appropriate. In addition, maintenance of body weight in the metastable weight range of 85–90% of target, without improvement after 6 months, should also warrant readmission. Other proven reasons for readmission to the hospital include return of severe depressive illness or serious medical complications of an ED. Because EDs are spectrum disorders with a variable course and severity, a subgroup of patients may require repeated admissions. There is a tendency to blame patients for a return to illness, as if EDs were entirely voluntary, and to take a negative or punitive view toward ED patients requiring readmission. For the minority of patients who do have chronic, severe, and relapsing EDs, readmission is necessary whenever indicated by clinical symptomatology and should not be a source of stigma or rejection.

RESEARCH ISSUES

Elsewhere (Bowers & Andersen, 1994), we have described the relative lack of progress in research in anorexia nervosa in the last decade, compared to the vigorous research on bulimia nervosa. No effective pharmacological treatment has been found for treatment of the central psychopathology of anorexia nervosa, and it is possible that none will be found, but the search certainly should continue for adjunctive pharmacological therapies.

Patients with EDs present us with a rare chance to understand the effect of extremes in weight and eating behavior on human physiology, psychology, and social behavior. Every patient can teach us something new about these disorders. A research-oriented way of thinking by a clinical staff does not require high-technology methodology, but rather a mental set of questions about the nature of the EDs and their treatment. Investigation into a new ED category, binge ED, continues to grow. Other syndromes not yet described undoubtedly exist. Additional understanding of EDs will come from research into all aspects of the disorders, whether this research consists of reports on highly technical biomedical features, studies of new treatment strategies, or clinical observations of the history of these disorders and contributing factors. As patients are effectively brought to a healthy weight during inpatient treatment, the next therapeutic challenge of relapse prevention becomes increasingly crucial. Investigations of psychotherapeutic strategies (especially CBT) versus pharmacological strategies (especially the SSRIs) for relapse prevention are underway.

Whether prevention of anorexia nervosa is at all possible remains a highly controversial issue. At a minimum, early identification (secondary prevention) is improving. The Scandinavian countries have taken a more vigorous approach toward primary prevention, whereas the United States and Great Britain have tended to emphasize early diagnosis followed by therapeutic intervention. We believe that prevention strategies will be more successful if they are focused on higher-risk children with several known predisposing factors, rather than on unrealistic efforts to change the broader sociocultural norms promoting slimness.

SUMMARY

This chapter has attempted to describe a pragmatic, thoroughly tested inpatient program for EDs, with an emphasis on the treatment of anorexia nervosa; however, we acknowledge that other methods (described elsewhere) may also be effective. Our method emphasizes a multidisciplinary approach whose goals are to reestablish healthy weight, to improve patterns of eating, to teach healthy social behavior, to decrease core psychopathology, to promote healthy age-appropriate patterns of conflict resolution, and to promote healthy living in a weight-preoccupied society. The indispensable requirements for treatment success include an intimate knowledge of the longitudinal biopsychosocial process of development of EDs; utilization of a multidisciplinary team approach; possession of a genuine interest in treatment; realistic optimism about lasting improvement in these patients; and continued staff education and program review.

REFERENCES

American Psychiatric Association (APA). (1993). Practice guidelines for eating disorders. *American Journal of Psychiatry, 150,* 212–228.

American Psychiatric Association (APA). (1994). *Diagnostic and statistical manual of mental disorders* (4th ed.). Washington, DC: Author.

Andersen, A. E. (1995). Sequencing treatment decisions: Cooperation or conflict between therapist and patient. In G. Szmuckler, C. Dare, & J. Treasure (Eds.), *Handbook of eating disorders* (pp. 363–377). New York: Wiley.

Andersen, A. E., Hedblom, J. E., & Hubbard, F. A. (1983). A multidisciplinary team treatment for patients with anorexia nervosa and their families: Preliminary report for long-term outcome. *International Journal of Eating Disorders, 2,* 181–192.

Andersen, A. E., Morse, C., & Santmyer, K. (1985). Inpatient treatment of anorexia nervosa. In D. M. Garner & P. E. Garfinkel (Eds.), *Handbook of psychotherapy for anorexia nervosa and bulimia* (pp. 311–343). New York: Guilford Press.

Andersen, A., Wirth, J., & Strahlman, E. (1982). Reversible weight related increase in plasma testosterone during treatment of male and female patients with anorexia nervosa. *International Journal of Eating Disorders, 1,* 74–83.

Agras, W. S. (1987). *Eating disorders: Management of obesity, bulimia, and anorexia nervosa.* Elmsford, NY: Pergamon Press.

Beck, A. T. (1990). *Beck Anxiety Inventory.* San Antonio, TX: Psychological Corporation.

Beck, A. T., Ward, C. H., Mendelson, M., Mock, J., & Erbaugh, J. (1961). An inventory for measuring depression. *Archives of General Psychiatry, 4,* 561–571.

Berg, E. A. (1948). *The Wisconsin Card Sorting Test.* Madison, WI: Wells.

Bowers, W. A. (1993). Cognitive therapy for eating disorders. In J. H. Wright, M. E. Thase, A. T. Beck, & J. W. Ludgate (Eds.), *Cognitive therapy with inpatients: Developing a cognitive milieu* (pp. 337–356). New York: Guilford Press.

Bowers, W. A. (1994). Neuropsychological impairment among anorexia nervosa and bulimia patients. *Eating Disorders: Journal of Treatment and Prevention, 2,* 42–46.

Bowers, W. A., & Andersen, A. E. (1994). Inpatient treatment of anorexia nervosa: Review and recommendations. *Harvard Review of Psychiatry, 2,* 193–203.

Bruch, H. (1973). *Eating disorders: Obesity, anorexia nervosa and the person within.* New York: Basic Books.

Bruch, H. (1974). Perils of behavior modification in treatment of anorexia nervosa. *Journal of the American Medical Association, 230,* 1419–1422.

Clark, L. A. (1993). *Schedule of Nonadaptive and Adaptive Personality*. Minneapolis: University of Minnesota Press.

Costa, P. T., & McCrae, R. R. (1992). *NEO-PI-R: Professional manual*. Odessa, FL: Psychological Assessment Resources.

Crisp, A. H., Norton, K., Gowers, S., Halek, C., Bowyer, C., Yeldham, D., Levett, G., & Bhat, A. (1991). A controlled study of the effect of therapies aimed at adolescent and family psychopathology in anorexia nervosa. *British Journal of Psychiatry, 159,* 325–333.

Dare, C., Eisler, I., Russell, G. F. M., & Szmukler, G. I. (1990). The clinical and theoretical impact of a controlled trial of family therapy in anorexia nervosa. *Journal of Marriage and Family Therapy, 16,* 39–57.

DeFillippis, N. A., McCampbell, E., & Rogers, P. (1979). Development of a booklet form of the Category Test: Normative and validity data. *Journal of Clinical Neuropsychology, 1,* 339–342.

Eckert, E. D., & Mitchell, J. E. (1989). An overview of the treatment of anorexia nervosa. *Psychiatric Medicine, 7,* 293–315.

Erikson, E. H. (1968). *Identity: Youth and crisis.* New York: Norton.

Fairburn, C. G., & Cooper, P. J. (1989). Eating disorders. In K. Hawton, P. M. Salkovskis, J. Kirk, & D. M. Clark (Eds.), *Cognitive behavior therapy for psychiatric problems* (pp. 277–314). New York: Oxford University Press.

Fairburn, C. G., & Cooper, P. J. (1993). The Eating Disorder Examination (12th Edition). In C. G. Fairburn & G. T. Wilson (Eds.), *Binge eating: Nature, assessment, and treatment* (pp. 317–360). New York: Guilford Press.

Frisch, R. E., & McArthur, J. W. (1974). Menstrual cycles: Fatness as a determinant of minimum weight for height necessary for their maintenance or onset. *Science, 185,* 949–951.

Garfinkel, P. E., & Garner, D. M. (1982). *Anorexia nervosa: A multidimensional perspective.* New York: Brunner/Mazel.

Garner, D. M. (1985). Individual psychotherapy for anorexia nervosa. *Journal of Psychiatric Research, 19,* 423–433.

Garner, D. M. (1991). *Manual for the Eating Disorder Inventory (EDI).* Odessa, FL: Psychological Assessment Resources.

Garner, D. M., & Bemis, K. (1982). A cognitive-behavioral approach to anorexia nervosa. *Cognitive Therapy and Research, 6,* 123–150.

Garner, D. M., & Bemis, K. (1985). Cognitive therapy for anorexia nervosa. In D. M. Garner & P. E. Garfinkel (Eds.), *Handbook of psychotherapy for anorexia nervosa and bulimia* (pp. 107–146). New York: Guilford Press.

Garner, D. M., & Garfinkel, P. E. (1979). The Eating Attitudes Test: An index of the symptoms of anorexia nervosa. *Psychological Medicine, 9,* 273–279.

Goodman, W. K., Price, L. H., Rasmussen, S. A., Mazure, C., Delgado, P., Heninger, G. R., & Charney, D. S. (1989). The Yale–Brown Obsessive Compulsive Scale (Y-BOCS): II: Validity. *Archives of General Psychiatry, 46,* 1012–1016.

Gull, W. W. (1874). Anorexia nervosa (apepsia, hysterica, anorexia hysterica). *Transactions of Clinical Endocrinological Metabolism, 49,* 806–809.

Hall, A. (1985). Group psychotherapy for anorexia nervosa. In D. M. Garner & P. E. Garfinkel (Eds.), *Handbook of psychotherapy for anorexia nervosa and bulimia* (pp. 213–239). New York: Guilford Press.

Hall, A. (1987). The place of family therapy in the treatment of anorexia nervosa. *Australian and New Zealand Journal of Psychiatry, 21,* 568–574.

Hamilton, M. (1960). A rating scale for depression. *Journal of Neurology, Neurosurgery and Psychiatry, 23,* 173–184.

Hamsher, K. S., Halmi, K. A., & Benton, A. L. (1981). Prediction of outcome in anorexia nervosa from neuropsychological status. *Psychiatry Research, 4,* 79–88.

Hathaway, S. R., & McKinley, J. C. (1989). *The Minnesota Multiphasic Personality Inventory—2.* Minneapolis: University of Minnesota Press.

Hudson, J. I., Pope, H. G., Jonas, J. M., & Yurgelun-Todd, D. (1985). Treatment of anorexia nervosa with antidepressants. *Journal of Clinical Psychopharmacology, 5,* 17–23.

Keys, A., Brozek, J., Henschel, A., Mickelsen, O., & Taylor, H. L. (1950). *The biology of human starvation* (2 vols.). Minneapolis: University of Minnesota Press.

Lee, N. F., & Rush, A. J. (1986). Cognitive-behavioral group therapy for bulimia. *International Journal of Eating Disorders, 5,* 599–615.

Margolis, R., Spencer, W., DePaulo, R., Simpson, S. G., & Andersen, A. E. (1994). Psychiatric comorbidity in subgroups of eating disordered inpatients. *Eating Disorders: The Journal of Treatment and Prevention, 2*(3).

Metropolitan Life Insurance Company. (1959). *Metropolitan height and weight tables.* New York: Author.

Metropolitan Life Insurance Company. (1983). *Metropolitan height and weight tables.* New York: Author.

Needleman, H. L., & Weber, D. (1977). The use of amitriptyline for inpatients with anorexia nervosa. In R. A. Vigersky (Ed.), *Anorexia nervosa* (pp. 357–362). New York: Raven Press.

Pfohl, B., Blum, N., & Zimmerman, M. (1995). *Structured Interview for DSM-IV Personality: SIDP-IV.* Iowa City: University of Iowa Press.

Russell, G. F. M. (1970). Anorexia nervosa: Its identity as an illness and its treatment. In J. H. Price (Ed.), *Modern trends in psychological medicine* (vol. 2, pp. 131–164). London: Butterworths.

Russell, G. F. M. (1979). Bulimia nervosa: An ominous variant of anorexia nervosa. *Psychological Medicine, 9,* 429–448.

Russell, G. F. M., Szmukler, G. I., Dare, C., & Eisler, I. (1987). An evaluation of family therapy in anorexia nervosa and bulimia nervosa. *Archives of General Psychiatry, 44,* 1047–1056.

Spreen, O., & Strauss, E. (1991). *A compendium of neuropsychological tests.* New York: Oxford University Press.

Stunkard, A. J., & Messick, S. (1987). *Manual for the Eating Inventory.* San Antonio, TX: Psychological Corporation.

Theander, S. (1985). Outcome and prognosis in anorexia nervosa and bulimia: Some results of previous investigations, compared with those of a Swedish long-term study. *Journal of Psychiatry Research, 19,* 493–508.

Vandereycken, W., Kog, E., & Vanderlinden, J. (1989). *The family approach to eating disorders: Assessment and treatment of anorexia nervosa and bulimia.* New York: PMA.

Vanderlinden, J., & Vandereycken, W. (1991). Guidelines for the family therapeutic approach to eating disorders. *Psychotherapy and Psychosomatic, 56,* 36–42.

Waldholtz, B., & Andersen, A. E. (1990). Gastrointestinal symptoms in anorexia nervosa: A prospective study. *Gastroenterology, 98,* 1415–1419.

Wechsler, D. (1981). *Manual for the Wechsler Adult Intelligence Scale—Revised.* New York: Psychological Corporation.

Wechsler, D. (1991). *Manual for the Wechsler Intelligence Scale for Children* (3rd ed.). San Antonio, TX: Psychological Corporation.

Wilson, G. T., & Fairburn, C. G. (1993). Cognitive treatments for eating disorders. *Journal of Consulting and Clinical Psychology, 61,* 261–269.

Wilson, G. T., & Pike, K. M. (1993). Eating disorders. In D. H. Barlow (Ed.), *Clinical handbook of psychological disorders* (2nd ed., pp. 278–317). New York: Guilford Press.

Woodall, C., & Anderson, A. E. (1989). The use of metaphor and poetry therapy in the treatment of the reticent subgroup of anorexic patients. In E. Baker & L. Hornyak (Eds.), *Experimental therapies for eating disorders* (pp. 191–206). New York: Guilford Press.

Wright, J. H., Thase, M. E., Beck, A. T., & Ludgate, J. W. (Eds.). (1993). *Cognitive therapy with inpatients: Developing a cognitive milieu.* New York: Guilford Press.

Yalom, I. (1995). *The theory and practice of group psychotherapy* (4th ed.). New York: Basic Books.

APPENDIX 17.1
Inpatient Protocols for University of Iowa Health Center Eating Disorders Unit: Weight Adjustment and Maintenance (for Staff Only)

POLICY

Inpatients with EDs are guided to achieve standard, normal weight for height as readily as permitted by their physical status. They are protected from abnormal behaviors, such as inappropriate choice of foods, bingeing, purging, or excessive exercise, as they progress toward normal weight. At normal body weight, they practice maintaining their weight and improving their capacity to eat normally and think in a healthy way about body size and shape. For the sake of (1) agreement among staff members, and (2) improvement of their illness, patients require a treatment regimen that is consistently adhered to, follows simple rules, and is described in considerable detail.

PROCEDURE

A. Determining goal weight
  1. Underweight patients:
     a. Goal weight is defined as a 4-pound range in the desirable weight for a person of medium frame of the same sex and height without shoes and without clothing, according to the 1959 table of the Metropolitan Life Insurance Company. (Copyright 1959 by the Metropolitan Life Insurance Company. Reprinted by permission.)

ft.	in.	Women	Men
4	9	98–102	
4	10	101–105	
4	11	104–108	
5	0	107–111	
5	1	110–114	115–119
5	2	114–118	118–122
5	3	117–121	121–125
5	4	122–126	124–128
5	5	126–130	128–132
5	6	130–134	132–136
5	7	134–138	136–140
5	8	138–142	140–144
5	9	142–146	144–148
5	10	146–150	149–153
5	11		153–157
6	0		158–162
6	1		162–166
6	2		167–171
6	3		172–176

b. Subtract 1 pound from the table above for each year the person is below the age of 25 until age 18.

c. If a female patient is known not to menstruate at the standard goal weight, the goal weight is raised to that of a patient 1 inch taller.

d. Young women below 18 years of age will be brought to a weight at which they have a 50% chance of onset of menses (for primary amenorrhea) or a 50% chance of return of menses (for secondary amenorrhea), according to Frisch and McArthur (1974).

2. Overweight patients: Goal weight is a 4-pound range in the desirable weight for a person of medium frame of the same sex and height without shoes and without clothing, according to the 1983 table of the Metropolitan Life Insurance Company. (Copyright 1983 by the Metropolitan Life Insurance Company. Reprinted by permission.)

ft.	in.	Women	Men
4	9	110–114	
4	10	113–117	
4	11	115–119	
5	0	117–121	
5	1	120–124	130–134
5	2	124–128	131–135
5	3	126–130	1 33–137
5	4	130–134	136–140
5	5	133–137	139–143
5	6	136–140	144–148
5	7	139–143	144–148
5	8	142–146	147–151
5	9	145–149	150–154
5	10	148–152	154–158
5	11		157–161
6	0		161–165
6	1		16 4–168
6	2		168–172
6	3		170–174

3. Patients are weighed on admission, the morning after admission, and then on Mondays, Wednesdays, and Fridays, unless otherwise indicated. They are weighed in the morning after voiding, wearing nightclothes, with back to scale.

4. *No information about weight (goal range, cur-*

rent weight, increases or decreases) is given to patients or families by any staff member. Patients will be told when they are in goal range by their primary nurse, in a systematic, planned manner.

B. Nutritional rehabilitation

Note: No information about energy intake (calorie level) is discussed with patients. They have no access to written information about calories.

1. Meal patterns
   a. Three meals per day.
   b. Zero to two snacks (none after 8:30 P.M.).
   c. One "family-style" meal on the unit per week, staffing permitting.

2. Dietary content
   a. Physiological considerations
      1) Patients with validated, medically documented food allergies or intolerances have diets without these foods.
      2) Low salt, low lactose, low fat for the first 4–7 days.
      3) Low salt until edema resolved.
      4) Two diet sodas/day maximum are permitted for normal-weight or overweight patients. No low-calorie or diet products are permitted with underweight patients. Gum, candy, etc., will be prescribed by treatment team.
      5) If liquid dietary supplements are required above a certain level of energy intake (i.e., 3,500 calories in females), they will be prescribed on an individual basis by the treatment team.
   b. Calorie progression for underweight patients
      1) For first 4 days, 1,500 calories/day; then increments of 500 calories/day every 4 days to 3,500 calories per day on 16th hospital day.
      2) If patient is at less than 70% goal weight on admission, begin with 1200 calories/day for 4 days before progressing to 1,500 calories/day. Will require 20 days to reach 3,500 calories/day.
      3) In goal weight range, treatment team adjusts calories to maintain weight in midrange.
   c. Weight progression on 3,500 calories/day for underweight patients
      1) Expect 3 pounds/week weight gain.
      2) If less than 2.5 pounds/week:
         a) Keep patient close to observer at all times at table.
         b) Observe for mobilization of edema

fluid as possible cause of lesser weight gain.
         c) Increase to standard eating disorders observation (EDO) if abnormal behaviors *appear* to be present.
      3) If after 1 week of standard observation, weight gain is still less than 2.5 pounds/week:
         a) Increase daily calories by 500-calorie/day increments every 4 days until weight gain is at least 2.5 pounds/week.
         b) Increase to 24-hour EDO if *clear indications* of abnormal behaviors are present.
   d. Dislikes: Patients may designate three specific foods they do not want in their diets.
      1) Examples of appropriate designations: okra, tofu, squid. Also, subcultural or familial food exclusions clearly present by report of an independent informant *prior to* the onset of the earliest symptoms of an eating disorder. Examples: pork (for Muslims), all meat (for Seventh-Day Adventists).
      2) Examples of inappropriate designations: meat (in most cases—but see above), starch, fat, baked products, cake.

3. Practice by patients
   a. Selecting food
      1) Selecting *items* of food occurs first and proceeds as follows:
         a) For patients with anorexia nervosa (AN), when weight gain is consistent and weight is at 90% of target level.
         b) For patients with bulimia nervosa (BN), after 2 weeks.
         c) Only when patients are comfortable with protocol; after instruction by dietitian on nutritional balance; and as per protocol unless contraindicated by team.
      2) Selecting *amounts* of food (portions), using exchange list, proceeds as follows:
         a) When patients are selecting items appropriately (after 1 week, for BN patients), and when AN patients are in middle of goal weight range.
         b) Only after instruction by dietitian in the use of exchanges. Staff monitors all selections; no dietetic foods allowed unless BN patients need to lose weight.
   b. Planning, purchasing, preparing meals
      1) Patients participate in occupational

therapy meal preparation group, and also practice eating in a cafeteria or restaurant under nursing staff supervision, as follows:

   a) When they are selecting items appropriately (see above).

   b) Unless contraindicated by team.

   c) At a frequency dependent on adequate staffing.

  2) Patients practice eating in a cafeteria or restaurant alone or with friends/family as follows:

   a) For AN patients, when they are in goal weight range.

   b) When they are selecting portions appropriately (see above).

   c) Unless contraindicated by the primary multidisciplinary team.

C. Exercise

  1. All patients may do mild stretching exercises within their physical limitations for 30 minutes each day, observed by the staff, and may walk during the physical activity group, unless they abuse these privileges.

  2. Patients who are at 80% of their goal weight, are gaining 2.5 or more pounds per week, and have bone densitometry measures in the normal or mildly deficient range may participate in the physical activity group and in the aerobic exercise group as long as they continue with this weekly weight gain and as long as they do not exercise inappropriately.

  3. Patients who are at 80% of their goal weight, are gaining 2.5 or more pounds per week, and have bone densitometry measures in the moderate or severely deficient range may participate in *low-impact* activities in the physical activity group and in the aerobic exercise group as long as they continue with this weekly weight gain and as long as they do not exercise inappropriately.

D. Eating disorders observation (EDO)

  Note: Possible EDO levels are 24 hours, 8 A.M.–10 P.M., meals plus 2 hours, meals plus 1 hour, and meals only. Standard EDO is 8 A.M.–10 P.M..

  1. Standard EDO on admission: 8 A.M. until 10 P.M. for at least 1 week. Patients may go to all prescribed therapeutic activities while on EDO, provided that their physical state and mental state permit, and on condition that staff members directing the activities will be responsible for direct observation of patient at all times (monitoring bathroom visits, etc.).

2. Indications for decreasing EDO to meals plus 2 hours:

  a. After at least 1 week on standard EDO, patient shows the capacity to control urges for abnormal eating behavior.

  b. Patient is gaining 2.5–3 pounds/week with no abnormal behaviors.

  c. The decrease is not contraindicated.

3. Indications for decreasing EDO to meals plus 1 hour:

  a. An AN patient has attained bottom of goal range, or is 1 week from anticipated discharge and not in goal weight range (e.g., insurance limitation).

  b. A BN patient has completed 2 weeks on the unit.

  c. The decrease is not contraindicated.

4. Indications for decreasing EDO to meals only:

  a. Patient has been doing well at meals plus 1 hour for 3 days.

  b. The decrease is not contraindicated.

5. Indications for discontinuation of EDO:

  a. Patient has been doing well at meals only for 3 days.

  b. The decrease is not contraindicated.

6. Indications for increasing EDO at meals:

  a. Unexplained weight fluctuations.

  b. Strong impulses to behave inappropriately.

  c. Staff suspicion that the patient is behaving inappropriately.

  d. Abnormal or increasing amylase.

7. Indications for 24-hour EDO:

  a. A new and unfamiliar patient has a possible or known history of vomiting or exercise abuse.

  b. See "Indications for increasing EDO" (item 6 above).

8. Consequences for inappropriate behavior on EDO: Response by treatment team after discussion.

9. Decisions about level of EDO (initial and subsequent): Per protocol unless contraindicated.

10. Authorization for changes in EDO:

  a. Initiation or increase in hours requires the order of a physician, psychologist, or nurse.

  b. Discontinuation or decrease in hours requires the order of a physician or psychologist.

11. EDO during visits by family or friends:

  a. A family member or friend of a cooperative patient may assume the responsibility of EDO on the unit or on hospital grounds, if agreed upon by the treatment team and ordered by a physician or psychologist.

b. Minors must first have written permission from a parent or guardian to see a particular visitor.

12. EDO when patients go on or off campus with staff for therapeutic activities:

a. The staff member invites only the number of patients that will permit him or her to maintain EDO as if the patients were on the unit.

b. Minors must first have a note in the chart that a parent or guardian has consented before going off campus with a staff member.

E. Therapeutic leave of absence (TLOA)

1. Patients do not have TLOA during the hours of EDO, unless the need for TLOA is an overriding humanitarian concern, such as death of or serious illness in a close family member. In these cases:

a. A nurse teaches the family member or friend accompanying the patient on the emergency TLOA to do EDO, emphasizing the need to keep the patient in direct view at all times. The nurse instructs the family member or friend to return the patient to the observer.

b. Minors must first have written permission from a parent or guardian before going on a TLOA unaccompanied by a parent or guardian.

2. Discussion about TLOA:

a. The patient knows that TLOA does not occur during EDO times.

b. The patient submits to the primary nurse a written request for TLOA, including date, hours, and persons to be accompanying the patient.

c. The patient discusses with the nurse the value and risks of TLOA.

d. To prevent "staff splitting," the nurse does not inform the patient of his or her decision about TLOA; rather, the nurse tells the patient that it will be discussed with the treatment team.

e. The primary nurse writes his or her recommendation on the request for TLOA and places it in the chart rack with morning report materials, for discussion in morning rounds and agreement with the attending physician.

F. Goal weight maintenance plan

1. Weigh Monday, Wednesday, and Friday for first week in goal weight range.

2. Decrease calories after reaching midpoint, until weight is stable within goal weight range.

3. Reduce EDO as rapidly as patient can tolerate without abnormal eating behaviors (See D3–D5.)

4. Increase exercise to patient's satisfaction as long as it is consistent with maintaining goal weight, it lasts no more than 1 hour per day, staffing permits, and exercise is not abused by patient.

5. Have patient do one of the following at least daily to increase confidence and practice in normal eating:

a. Purchase and prepare a meal under staff supervision.

b. Eat in a cafeteria or restaurant.

c. Go on TLOA to test resisting abnormal eating behaviors and to practice healthy behaviors out of the hospital.

6. Arrange appropriate outpatient therapy.

G. Activity levels

Attached is the description provided to patients:

Patient Activity Levels: Adult Units

Restricted to the Unit

You are frequently restricted to the unit for the first few days. This is to assure that you will be available for appointments, and to allow us to become acquainted with you and your needs. For clinical referrals, you must be accompanied by a nurse or nursing assistant. You may make telephone calls on the pay phone at the nurse's discretion. You may have visitors on the unit at the nurse's discretion. You may attend scheduled activities on your unit. No passes will be allowed.

Supervised

After the first week, you may engage in supervised activities at the nurse's discretion unless these are contraindicated by physical or psychological circumstances.

Level I: You may attend activities scheduled for the gymnasium and large classroom. These activities include crafts, gym activities, music, and volleyball. You may be accompanied on a one-to-one basis while on this level. No passes will be allowed. Generally for patients with low weight, patients who are medically unstable, or patients with distressed mood or illness behaviors present.

Level II: In addition to the above, you may also attend scheduled activities in the immediate vicinity of the hospital, including the outside court and grounds, General Hospital, the Quadrangle, the Field House, Carver–Hawkeye Arena, and the Recreation Building. No passes will be allowed.

Level III: In addition to the above, you may attend any scheduled activities therapy events and activities within a 25-mile radius of Iowa City, including such activities as swimming, roller skating, bicycling, and field trips. In general, for patients who are at more than 85% of body weight, and if not contraindicated. *Special events over 25 miles outside of Iowa City will require a special order.*

Routine

On routine activity level, you may participate in all activities therapy events and activities. You may go out alone for 1 hour in the morning and 1 hour in the afternoon. You must sign out at the nurses' station (name, time, destination, and estimated time of return). You may go the coffee shop at University Hospital, the activities therapy gym, the hospital courtyard, or the Quadrangle. Your time off the unit must be spent on hospital grounds. Please sign in at the time of your return. You may have passes, if ordered by the physician. You may be allowed to see visitors off the unit area at the discretion of the nurse manager.

General requirements for routine activity:

AN—patient is at middle of goal range, and demonstrates responsible attitudes and behaviors.

BN—after 3 weeks, and patient demonstrates responsible attitudes and behaviors.

Others—per staff.

CHAPTER 18

Partial Hospitalization

ALLAN S. KAPLAN
MARION P. OLMSTED

The Day Hospital program (DHP) for eating disorders utilizing group treatment was established at The Toronto Hospital in 1985. The initial impetus for this program evolved from the clinical need for intensive treatment of eating disorders, following the closure of the 12-bed inpatient unit at the Clarke Institute of Psychiatry that had previously provided in-hospital care for patients severely ill with anorexia nervosa. Because of financial constraints, the Ontario provincial government at the time was unwilling to open any more inpatient beds at The Toronto Hospital, where the eating disorder treatment team (under the leadership of Dr. Paul Garfinkel) had moved. The idea of treating patients with eating disorders, who would previously have required hospitalization, as outpatients in day treatment was also suggested by increasing evidence that inpatient care was often fraught with difficulties for both staff and patients and was associated with a high rate of recidivism. As a result of these financial and clinical concerns, an alternative model for the treatment of severely ill patients with eating disorders—one that would be both cost-effective and clinically effective—was developed. A day treatment program that would provide intensive treatment and nutritional rehabilitation during daytime hours, but would forgo the "hotel" aspect of treatment, was funded by the Ontario government in 1985.

DESCRIPTION OF THE PROGRAM

The DHP originally conceived and implemented (Piran & Kaplan, 1990) operated 5 days per week (Monday through Friday), 8 hours each day, although in November 1994 it was reduced to 4 days per week. The program treats a maximum of 12 patients at any time. The average length of stay is between 10 and 11 weeks and ranges from 6 to 14 weeks (see page 359, New Directions). The program is staffed by a multidisciplinary treatment team consisting of a full-time psychologist, a psychometrist, an occupational therapist, a nutritionist, two social workers, and a nurse, as well as a part-time psychiatrist. There is one secretary assigned full time to the DHP.

The goals of the program are threefold: (1) the normalization of disturbed eating behavior, and the complete cessation of bingeing–purging and other behaviors aimed at weight control; (2) nutritional rehabilitation through adequate caloric intake and, when necessary, weight gain; and (3) the identification of psychological and familial processes that serve to perpetuate each patient's eating disorder.

The DHP integrates biological, psychological, familial, and sociocultural interventions. Biological interventions focus on the treatment of medical complications that result from starvation, bingeing, and purging. Pharmacotherapy (most commonly selective serotonin reuptake inhibitors) is prescribed to approximately half the patients, in order to stabilize their mood or to facilitate a cessation of binge eating. Nutritional rehabilitation is achieved through the prescription of a balanced meal plan, consistently usually of between 1,800 and 3,000 calories per day, depending on the need for weight maintenance or weight gain; the calories are spread over three meals and two snacks, which incorporate phobic foods and binge foods. Lunch, a snack, and dinner are provided during the treatment hours, and an evening snack is given to each patient to take home at night. Patients are required to provide their own breakfast. Patients are usually prescribed liquid supplements when they require calorie levels beyond maintenance (about 2,200 calories) for weight gain.

The psychological treatment consists of intensive group psychotherapy, which incorporates psychoeducational, cognitive, behavioral, and interpersonal paradigms (Kaplan, Kerr, & Maddocks, 1992). The group experiences are divided between those that deal directly with disturbed attitudes and behaviors centering around eating and weight, and those that deal with more general areas of psychopathology. An emphasis is placed on acquiring skills and insights that will facilitate normalization of eating outside of program hours. All participants in the DHP are encouraged to bring close friends, family members, or significant others for a family therapy assessment. When indicated, subsequent family therapy focuses on symptom separation and establishing appropriate boundaries. Sociocultural interventions in the DHP include providing vocational counseling, arranging supportive housing, and establishing community supports.

INDICATIONS AND CONTRAINDICATIONS FOR ADMISSION

To enter the DHP, all patients must meet *Diagnostic and Statistical Manual of Mental Disorders,* fourth edition (DSM-IV) criteria for an eating disorder—either bulimia nervosa, anorexia nervosa, or eating disorder not otherwise specified. All patients must have had some previous potentially effective outpatient treatment (Kaplan & Garfinkel, 1995) that has failed to have a significant impact on their eating be-

havior. Patients and families have to be motivated to become involved in an intensive treatment program with the agreed-upon expectation of symptomatic change, as opposed to only psychological understanding without behavioral change. Patients also have to demonstrate some capacity, however limited, to relate in a group setting. There are relatively few contraindications for involvement in the DHP. These include (1) acute medical risk that precludes out-of-hospital treatment, such as severe emaciation or cardiovascular or gastrointestinal complications requiring in-hospital care; (2) acute suicide risk; and (3) severe substance abuse or dependence, which clearly interferes with the normalization of weight, appetite, and eating.

ADMINISTRATIVE AND FINANCIAL STRUCTURE

The DHP is part of an integrated ambulatory care program for eating disorders. The other components of this program consist of a transition program and an outpatient clinic. A community outreach program, an information center, a consultation service, and an inpatient program make up the rest of the eating disorders program.

The ambulatory care program is funded by a special grant from the Ministry of Health (MOH) of the province of Ontario. The budget for this grant is approximately $700,000 (Canadian), which covers all expenses except for physicians' fees, which are reimbursed on a fee-for-service basis through the Ontario Health Insurance Plan. Approximately 65% of this budget funds the DHP. The money flows from the MOH to The Toronto Hospital's finance department, which administers it. The majority of the budget is divided between salaries and ongoing capital costs, such as food provisions for the patients in the DHP. The Toronto Hospital does not cover any cost overruns that the ambulatory care program may incur, and the budget must be strictly adhered to. The hospital provides only the physical space for the program; all other costs are paid from the MOH grant. Because the monies flow under a separate MOH grant, the program's budget is protected from budgetary cuts imposed by the hospital, but is subject to other financial constraints that the MOH may impose.

Excluding physicians' fees, the cost of DHP

treatment is approximately 22% that of inpatient care (for residents of Ontario, the cost per patient per week of day treatment is $804, and that of inpatient treatment is $3,722). All health care in Canada is financed by the national government, but providing health care is the responsibility of each province. Residents of the province of Ontario do not pay directly for their health care, although health care is financed primarily through a tax structure that is significantly higher than that of the United States (53% in Canada vs. 30% for the highest U.S. tax bracket). At this time there is no system in Ontario that limits the amount of care that can be provided for any particular patient or illness, as occurs in the United States with managed care (Kaye, Kaplan, & Zucker, 1996). However, the Ontario government has set a ceiling on the total amount of money it will expend for physicians' fees and leaves it up to physicians' organizations to divide the resources. The government has also set ceilings on the earnings of individual physicians. Private billing of patients by physicians is illegal in the Ontario health care system.

The administrative issues that arise in directing the DHP are quite complex. The director is responsible for the hiring, evaluation, and potential firing of staff members who work under her. For example, the nurses working in the DHP report directly to the director of the DHP, not to nursing administration in the hospital. The head of the eating disorders program and the director of the DHP are responsible for developing and maintaining the budget of the DHP. Such responsibility involves periodic meetings with hospital personnel and with personnel from the MOH, the funding body. Justification for capital costs, the hiring of new personnel, shifting of funds from one classification to another, and requests for additional funds all require approval from the MOH and constitute an important part of the director's administrative duties. Finally, specific negotiations with consulting medical and surgical house staff and physicians have had to be undertaken, in order for these staff personnel to agree to do consultations on medically or surgically ill patients in the DHP. These staff members generally consult only in regard to inpatients and not to outpatients in the hospital.

ADVANTAGES OF DAY TREATMENT

The DHP has both clinical and financial advantages. The clinical advantages of treating patients in an outpatient group psychotherapeutic format relate to the outpatient nature of the program, as well as to the group treatment itself. The clinical advantages of outpatient treatment over inpatient care are compelling. The in-hospital treatment of bulimic as well as anorexic patients is difficult and taxing for both the staff and the patients. These patients often have serious underlying character pathology, which manifests itself during hospitalization through the development of regression, hostile dependence, unstable mood, and impulsive behavior (including self-harm). Such patients often perceive external control as punitive and are compelled to oppose therapeutic maneuvers by splitting the staff. They may also comply superficially with treatment, but may continue secretly to adhere to distorted attitudes and beliefs and to engage in illness-related behaviors. Because of these factors, the inpatient treatment of eating disorders requires a high staff-to-patient ratio, and staff members must be specially trained professionals who are required to maintain a significant level of vigilance. This results in expensive and at times inefficient use of highly trained personnel and facilities (Kennedy, Kaplan, & Garfinkel, 1992).

The outpatient aspect of the DHP addresses several of these difficulties. Regression and dependence are minimized, because patients have to maintain themselves in a functioning state outside of the hospital during intensive outpatient treatment. This approach not only promotes autonomy, but provides opportunities for the generalization of newly acquired tools with which to regulate eating behavior. On a daily basis, the patients must actively confront disturbed areas of functioning (e.g., relationships, vocational issues, impulsivity) while simultaneously attempting to normalize their eating and weight. Such an approach therefore facilitates the difficult yet crucial process of internal integration of external controls. Because patients are not totally externally controlled, there is less of a need for them to oppose treatment; thus, there is a greater likelihood that such treatment will be perceived empathically rather than punitively. By its nature, day treatment is less psychosocially disruptive than inpatient care, as patients are able to maintain contact with supportive relationships that facilitate the process of recovery.

The clinical advantages of group treatment have become clearer over time. Group treatment provides an atmosphere of mutual support while increasing the power of therapeutic intervention through group confrontation and pressure. Dependence and regression are controlled, as the intensity of relating is diffused by the nature of the group interaction. The sense of isolation that develops as a result of disturbed eating patterns is alleviated by mutual sharing of what have been previously felt to be humiliating and degrading behaviors. This process of sharing helps patients "own" their illness rather than denying or dissociating it (Kaplan & Spivak, 1996).

Finally, there are obvious financial advantages to treating seriously ill patients, who would otherwise have required in-hospital care, as outpatients. The outpatient component of treatment lessens the need for hospital beds and is cost-effective, in that resources are directed at providing treatment rather than at housing patients. Nurses, who constitute the single costliest expense in running an inpatient unit, spend most of their evening and weekend hours engaged in activities not directly associated with patient care; the costs of such hours, obviously, are eliminated in a day treatment program. Other costs that are not directly aimed at providing care can also be eliminated in a day program. For example, ward clerks often spend much of their time dealing with the paperwork associated with admissions and discharges from the hospital, as well as costs related to housekeeping and laundry.

DISADVANTAGES OF DAY TREATMENT

There are clinical as well as administrative difficulties in utilizing an intensive outpatient group psychotherapeutic format to treat seriously ill patients with eating disorders. For some patients, the day treatment model does not provide as strong a sense of containment as might be found on an inpatient unit. Such containment in the DHP evolves from the holding environment provided by supportive group interaction, as opposed to the physical structure of an inpatient unit. Some patients, because of their underlying character disturbance, do not or cannot supportively engage in the group process; the intensive group interaction can lead to their being scapegoated, with subsequent psychological fragmentation and deterioration. In addition, for patients who are able to engage in the group therapy, there is often a period of emotional instability as their eating and weight normalize. Intense affect, which had been bound by disordered eating behaviors such as caloric restriction, bingeing, and vomiting, becomes freed up and can potentially overwhelm a patient's ability to cope. At such times, patients can act out by attempting self-harm through self-mutilation or overdosing on/abusing drugs or alcohol. At such times, patients may require in-hospital treatment (often in a crisis unit) to allow these intense feelings to pass. Unless there is access to such a unit, treatment in a day hospital setting can become untenable and potentially dangerous for some patients.

For the staff members who work in such a program, its outpatient nature requires continual monitoring of patients' mental status, for the reasons just described. The ability to deal with unstable patients, many of whom are at risk for self-harm, requires considerable clinical skills. Such skills are taxed by the intense and continuous staff–patient interaction required to provide an empathically controlling environment. Staff members can and do feel at times as if they are attempting to fill a bottomless pit, and this can lead directly to staff burnout. Contributing further to this possibility are pathological group processes whereby patients' angry and intolerable feelings are projected onto staff members, who are then devalued and made to feel as if they are sadistically tormenting patients, especially during mealtimes (when a high level of staff vigilance is required). Being unaware of such issues can lead to a sense of therapeutic nihilism. To prevent these and other difficulties from developing, the staff in such a unit has to function as a closely knit, mutually supportive group, with frequent communication, agreed-upon treatment goals, and clearly established models of intervention. In addition, there is a blurring of boundaries in terms of staff identity and responsibilities, as all staff members are required to function as group therapists, as supervisors of meals, and as assessors of mental status. Such responsibilities often do blur discipline-specific identities, and this can create stress for staffers who are not used to such role diffusion.

EFFICACY

From April 1, 1985, to October 31, 1994, the 5-day DHP treated over 500 patients with eating disorders. The number of admissions and the number of patients who completed the 5-day DHP are shown in Table 18.1. The diagnostic

TABLE 18.1. Description of Admissions to the DHP (April 1, 1985, through October 31, 1994)

	n	% of total	% of female first admissions
Total admissions	527	100	—
First admissions	476	90	—
Second admissions	42	8	—
First admissions, females	459	87	100
Program completers (≥ 4 weeks treatment)	408	77	89
Noncompleters (< 4 weeks treatment)	51	10	11

TABLE 18.3. Demographic and Clinical Features

	ANR (n = 51)	ANBN (n = 61)	BN (n = 236)
Age (years)	24.6 (5.7)	25.5 (7.0)	25.4 (6.7)
Duration of illness (years)	6.5 (4.8)	8.3 (7.4)	8.3 (6.4)
Duration in program (weeks)	11.1 (3.1)	11.1 (3.0)	10.2 (2.4)°
% single	78.4	70.5	81.1

Note. In this and subsequent tables, column entries in parentheses are standard deviations.
°$p = .04$ (ANBN > BN).

breakdown of these patients is shown in Table 18.2. Close to 60% of the patients had bulimia nervosa, and a further 30% had anorexia nervosa (either the binge-eating/purging or the restricting subtype, according to DSM-IV). As can be seen in Table 18.3, the patients' mean age was about 25 years, and most had been ill for 6½ to 8½ years. They stayed in the program for an average of 10 to 11 weeks; 80% of the patients stayed for at least 4 weeks, the minimum amount of time required for a "therapeutic dose" of treatment for most patients. Three-quarters of the patients were single. When bulimic patients entered the program, they were bingeing an average of 11 times a week and vomiting an average of 14 times a week. Anorexic patients entered the program with a mean body mass index (BMI) of 16, corresponding to approximately 77% of matched population mean weight (MPMW). (See Tables 18.4 and 18.5.)

The program was highly effective in the short term in alleviating symptoms (Maddocks & Kaplan, 1991). Bulimic patients left the program

on average bingeing and vomiting less than once a week over the last 4 weeks of treatment (see Table 18.5). Slightly over 50% of the patients with bulimia nervosa left the program with no episodes of bingeing or vomiting during the last month of treatment, and a further 32% left the program bingeing and/or vomiting less than DSM-IV threshold frequency criteria (see Table 18.6). Anorexic patients gained approximately 6 kg in weight and left the program with a mean BMI of 21, corresponding to 88% of MMPW; those who binged and purged showed significant decreases in these behaviors (see Tables 18.7 and 18.8). The program was also effective in reducing disturbed attitudes and beliefs about weight and shape (as measured by the Eating Disorder Inventory), as well as in reducing comorbid symptoms such as depression, with patients moving from the severely depressed range on the Beck Depression Invento-

TABLE 18.2. DSM-III-R Eating Disorder Diagnoses (n = 408)

Diagnosis	n	%
Bulimia nervosa (BN)	236	58.0
Anorexia nervosa and bulimia nervosa (ANBN)[a]	65	16.0
Anorexia nervosa, restricting (ANR)	58	14.0
Eating disorder not otherwise specified	49	12.0

[a]The ANBN patients would be diagnosed as having the binge-eating/purging subtype of anorexia nervosa in DSM-IV.

TABLE 18.4. Weight-Related Features

	ANR (n = 51)	ANBN (n = 61)	BN (n = 236)
Admission weight (kg)	45.2 (5.6)	46.6 (3.7)	63.2 (15.5)°
Admission weight as % MPMW	76.2 (7.4)	78.5 (5.0)	105.7 (21.4)°
Maximum weight as % MPMW	104.8 (13.9)	109.2 (14.5)	124.7 (24.0)°
Minimum weight as % MPMW	69.1 (8.9)	72.1 (6.9)	86.2 (12.5)°

°$p = .001$ (BN > ANR, ANBN).

TABLE 18.5. Change in Bingeing and Vomiting Frequency over Treatment in Bulimia Nervosa Patients (n = 224)

	No. of episodes per week		Mean change
	Admission	Discharge	
Bingeing	10.9 (9.8)	0.7 (1.3)	−10.2 (9.6)°
Vomiting	14.0 (12.0)	1.1 (1.9)	−12.9 (11.7)°

Note. Data are presented only for patients with symptoms in the month prior to admission.
°p = .001.

TABLE 18.7. Weight Change over Treatment in Anorexia Nervosa Patients

	Admission	Discharge
ANR (n = 51)		
Weight (kg)	45.2 (5.6)	50.6 (6.4)°
% MPMW	77.2 (7.7)	85.2 (8.5)°
ANBN (n = 61)		
Weight (kg)	46.6 (3.7)	52.2 (4.6)°
% MPMW	78.7 (5.2)	88.0 (6.8)°

°p = .0001.

ry to the nondepressed range over the course of treatment. Over the course of a 2-year follow-up of some of the bulimic patients treated in the DHP, the gains made during intensive treatment were for the most part sustained (Maddocks, Kaplan, Woodside, Langdon, & Piran, 1992). Of the patients in this subgroup who left the program free of symptoms, 80% remained for the most part asymptomatic over the follow-up period (Olmsted, Kaplan, & Rockert, 1994).

NEW DIRECTIONS

In 1994, a review of the eating disorders program led to the decision that a cheaper version of the DHP should be tested, to determine whether efficacy could be maintained while cost-effectiveness was increased. A related directive emphasized the importance of providing more follow-up treatment.

Empirical work conducted in the DHP setting provided a rationale for revising the program. A study of the relationship between treatment dose and response in bulimia nervosa patients treated in the DHP showed that 41% obtained good symptom control immediately on

entering the program. In contrast to slower treatment responders, these rapid responders had better symptom control at the end of DHP treatment and had a significantly lower relapse rate over a 2-year follow-up period (16% vs. 57% relapse rate; Olmsted, Kaplan, Jacobsen, & Rockert, 1996). This suggested that the patients who benefited most from the DHP might respond well to a shorter, less intense program. On the other hand, the patients who struggled, took longer to achieve symptom control, and were more likely to relapse after leaving the DHP might benefit from more intense follow-up treatment. The follow-up study of bulimic patients mentioned above showed that the large majority of relapses occurred within the first 6 months after treatment: At 6 months the relapse rate was 25%, and by 24 months it had increased to only 31% (Olmsted et al., 1994). This suggested that follow-up treatment focused on relapse prevention was critical for the first 6 months following treatment in the DHP.

In November 1994, the DHP was reduced to 4 days weekly (Tuesday through Friday). In the latter part of 1995, a shift toward shorter length of stay for bulimia nervosa patients was initiated. The goal is to move from stays of 10–11 weeks to stays of 6–8 weeks. The basic structure

TABLE 18.6. Symptom Status at Discharge for Bulimia Nervosa Patients (n = 224)

Status	%
Abstinent (0 BP/week)	49.1
Subthreshold (<2 BP/week)	32.1
Threshold (≥2 BP/week)	18.8

Note. The data pertain to symptoms assessed over the last 4 weeks of the program. BP, binge–purge episodes.

TABLE 18.8. Change in Bingeing and Vomiting Frequency over Treatment in Anorexia Bingers–Purgers (n = 61)

	No. of episodes per week	
	Admission	Discharge
Bingeing	10.0 (10.5)	0.8 (1.5)°
Vomiting	16.8 (15.2)	0.9 (1.8)°

°p = .0001.

of the program and the therapeutic model are unchanged, as is the length of stay for anorexia nervosa patients. These reductions in intensity and length of DHP treatment have been offset by a new transition program, which is available to patients immediately following the DHP. The transition program consists of three 90-minute group sessions weekly for up to 6 months. Patients may initially attend one to three times per week, but are expected to taper down to one session per week at some point during the 6 months. The goal of the program is to help patients maintain gains made in the DHP while they return to the demands of life. It is too soon to determine how well these revisions meet the primary objective of providing better long-term outcome for more patients.

REFERENCES

Kaplan, A. S., & Garfinkel, P. E. (1995). General principles of outpatient treatment. In G. Gabbard (Ed.), *Treatments of psychiatric disorders* (2nd ed., pp.). Washington, DC: American Psychiatric Press.

Kaplan, A. S., Kerr, A., & Maddocks, S. (1992). Day hospital group treatment for eating disorders. In R. MacKenzie & H. Harper (Eds.), *Group therapies for eating disorders* (pp. 161–181). Washington, DC: American Psychiatric Press.

Kaplan, A. S., & Spivak, H. (1996). Treatment of a patient with bulimia nervosa in a multigroup day hospital program. In J. Werne (Ed.), *Treating eating disorders* (pp. 259–288). San Francisco: Jossey-Bass.

Kaye, W. H., Kaplan, A. S., & Zucker, M. L. (1996). Treating eating disorder patients in a managed care environment. *Psychiatric clinics of North America* (pp. 793–810).

Kennedy, S., Kaplan, A. S., & Garfinkel, P. E. (1992). Intensive hospital treatment of anorexia nervosa and bulimia nervosa. In P. J. Cooper & A. Stein (Eds.), *Feeding problems and eating disorders* (pp. 161–181). London: Harwood.

Maddocks, S., & Kaplan, A. S. (1991). The prediction of positive treatment response in bulimia nervosa: A study of patient variables. *British Journal of Psychiatry, 159,* 846–849.

Maddocks, S., Kaplan, A. S., Woodside, D. B., Langdon, L., & Piran, N. (1992). Two year follow-up of bulimia nervosa: The importance of abstinence as the criterion of outcome. *International Journal of Eating Disorders, 12,* 133–141.

Olmsted, M. P., Kaplan, A. S., Jacobsen, M., & Rockert, W. (1996). Rapid responders to treatment of bulimia nervosa. *International Journal of Eating Disorders, 19,* 279–285.

Olmsted, M. P., Kaplan, A. S., & Rockert, W. (1994). Rate and prediction of relapse in bulimia nervosa. *American Journal of Psychiatry, 151,* 728–743.

Piran, N., & Kaplan, A. S. (Eds.). (1990). *A day hospital group treatment program for anorexia nervosa and bulimia nervosa.* New York: Brunner/Mazel.

CHAPTER 19

Behavioral Treatment to Promote Weight Gain in Anorexia Nervosa

STEPHEN W. TOUYZ
PIERRE J. V. BEUMONT

Many forms of treatment for anorexia nervosa have been advocated over the years, but few have stood the test of time. Nevertheless, Venables (1930) suggested practical guidelines for management that make interesting reading even today. He suggested that (1) every patient could be persuaded to eat normally; (2) the condition is hysterical, and no patient should remain uncured; (3) the doctor should sit down with the patient and fight for every mouthful of food, which could take an hour or two per meal; (4) the doctor should never lose his [*sic*] temper; and (5) the anorexia must be cured before the doctor starts on the psychology of symptoms. Venables was optimistic about the outcome in anorexia nervosa, and believed that all patients would eventually eat normally and everyone could be cured. Unfortunately, we now know that this is not the case. The admonition to therapists not to lose their tempers has been echoed in the writings of more recent authors. Garner (1985), warning of the iatrogenic dangers in treating patients with anorexia nervosa, quotes from Morgan's (1977) paper to illustrate his concern. Morgan examined the attitudes toward "fasting girls" and concluded that clinicians

> have great difficulty . . . in disengaging . . . from an attitude which implies that resistance to eating could be controlled with adequate exercise of will

on [the patients'] part. We are of course anxious to feed those who take insufficient food, but if frustrated, our anxiety quickly turns to hostility at what seems to be unnecessary self-imposed disease. (p. 1655)

Venables had also stated that meaningful psychotherapy can only be achieved once a patient has commenced regaining weight. The work of Keys, Brozek, Henschel, Mickelsen, and Taylor (1950) is relevant to this assertion: They found that many of the symptoms reported by patients with anorexia nervosa were also found in volunteers who were starved to about 75% of their original body weight. Most clinicians treating patients with anorexia nervosa would now agree that certain aspects of the psychopathology of anorexia nervosa are directly related to the effects of starvation per se, and that meaningful psychotherapy is best achieved once refeeding has commenced (Garner, Rockert, Olmsted, Johnson, & Coscina, 1985; Danziger, Carel, Tyano, & Mimounty, 1989; Beumont, Russell, & Touyz, 1993).

So how do clinicians overcome the difficulty of getting patients with anorexia nervosa to reverse their weight-losing behaviors and to eat in a more appropriate manner, without losing their own tempers? Many patients refuse to cooperate with treatment and even continue to lose weight while in the hospital, despite encouragement to the contrary. A dedicated nurse may spend an hour or more with a patient who slowly and painstakingly eats a meal, endeavoring to allay the patient's fears of losing control over eating and becoming fat. It is not difficult to understand the nurse's frustration and feelings of impotence upon discovering that the patient has induced vomiting 5 minutes after completing the meal! It is therefore not surprising that behavioral techniques have been introduced in order (1) to facilitate weight gain in hospitalized patients with anorexia nervosa, (2) to avoid lengthy periods of hospitalization, (3) to avert the prescription of medication, and (4) to minimize the necessity of resorting to more intrusive methods (e.g., nasogastric feeding).

BEHAVIOR MODIFICATION OF ANOREXIA NERVOSA

Behavioral therapies are now well accepted in clinical psychology and psychiatry. Phares (1992) has summarized the current situation well: "Behavior therapy has truly come of age and is now a force to be reckoned with. In fact, it has reached the stage of maturity where it can boast not only of its successes but also admit to its failures" (p. 356). There have been several comprehensive reviews of operant techniques to promote weight gain in patients with anorexia nervosa (Garfinkel & Garner, 1982; Agras & Kraemer, 1983; Halmi, 1985; Agras & Werne, 1978; Fairburn & Cooper, 1987; Bemis, 1987; Schmidt, 1989). One might well ask this question, however: How well have behavioral techniques been refined to address the specific problems of the anorexia nervosa patient, and is there still room for improvement? Unfortunately, much of the behavioral research on anorexia nervosa has been directed at specific aspects of the disorder in a rather fragmentary manner, without the development of a comprehensive treatment program in mind.

The aim of this chapter is to examine the efficacy of using behavioral strategies to promote weight gain in patients with anorexia nervosa, and to provide some insights into the management of this difficult disorder as we progress toward the year 2000. Historically, the basic operant paradigm for refeeding patients with anorexia nervosa has consisted of isolating patients from material and social reinforcers, and making the return of these reinforcers contingent upon specified amounts of weight gain or

caloric intake. In most instances, the decision to implement such programs has been pragmatic and atheoretical (Bemis, 1987).

The Introduction of Operant Conditioning Programs

Bachrach, Erwin, and Mohr (1965) were the first to introduce operant techniques in the management of a patient hospitalized with anorexia nervosa. The successful use of this new behavioral technology in promoting weight gain spawned a plethora of reports in the published literature. The data emanating from these studies tended to confirm that the majority of patients did in fact gain weight without any documented harmful side effects. Bruch (1974, 1978), however, disagreed with this contention and expressed grave concern regarding the use of behavior modification in treating patients with anorexia nervosa. It was her impression that most behaviorally oriented programs failed to take into account the major deficits in the personality development of these patients—namely, low self-esteem, self-doubt, lack of autonomy, and an inability to lead a self-directed life. She also indicated that behavioral programs had an adverse psychological effect on patients, who would gain weight under the "pressure of persuasion, force or threats" and would literally "eat their way out of [the] hospital" (1974, p. 1421). Bruch concluded: "It is generally known that true benefit is derived from such weight gain only if it is part of an integrated treatment program with correction of the underlying family problems and the inner psychological difficulties" (1978, p. 652). In a more positive vein, Stunkard (1972) portrayed behavior modification as a creative approach, but he emphasized the need to tailor each patient's program *individually* to the specific variables maintaining the patient's behavior.

Operant Conditioning: A Lenient, Flexible Approach

Most of the traditional operant programs developed for anorexia nervosa patients during refeeding have tended to be unnecessarily harsh. Garner (1985, p. 706) has alluded to reports in the literature that "capture the extraordinary degree of frustration, anger and maltreatment which have prevailed under the guise of behavior modification." There is no justification whatsoever for implementing harsh behavioral regimens to punish patients who have not complied with treatment. To this end, we compared the effects of "strict" and "lenient" operant conditioning programs in promoting weight gain in 65 anorexia nervosa patients (Touyz, Beumont, Glaun, Phillips, & Cowie, 1984). Thirty-one consecutive patients were treated using a traditional program of strict bed rest, with an individualized schedule of reinforcers for each 0.5 kg of weight gained. By contrast, the next 34 patients were treated with a lenient and flexible behavioral program. After an initial week of bed rest, a contract was made with each patient to gain a minimum of 1.5 kg per week. Provided that they complied with this requirement, patients were free to move around the unit. They understood that if they failed to achieve the weekly target of weight gain, they would be required to spend the following week on bed rest. No further restrictions were imposed, and patients had unlimited access to their personal possessions. In all other aspects, the treatment regimens for the two groups were similar. All the patients received nutritional counseling, supportive psychotherapy, group therapy, and occupational therapy, and the duration of hospital stay was approximately 9 weeks for both treatment groups. The mean daily weight gain did not differ significantly between the strict and lenient programs, and a similar proportion of patients in each group reached their target weight. The mean daily weight gain during refeeding (strict program = 0.21 kg per day; lenient program = 0.20 kg per day) on both programs compared favorably with the best figures reported by other authors using behavioral techniques (Agras, Barlow, Chapin, Abel, & Leitenberg, 1974; Halmi, Powers, & Cunningham, 1975; Bhanji & Thompson, 1974; Agras & Werne, 1978).

There were practical advantages in using the lenient program as opposed to the strict one. Most of our patients viewed the lenient program as more acceptable, and there was a general consensus among staff members that patients on the lenient program were better motivated for other aspects of treatment than those on the strict program. The lenient program also required less nursing time, and so was more economical; in addition, it provided less opportunity for patients to manipulate individual staff members in connection with their treatment. As a result, the staff members were able to use their time more constructively in both group therapy and supportive psychotherapy with pa-

tients. This was very much in keeping with our overall aim of providing a comprehensive, integrated approach to treatment.

We believe that our lenient treatment program, despite its behavioral basis, provides sufficient opportunity for psychotherapeutic contact and for patients to maintain their autonomy during treatment (Touyz et al., 1984; American Psychiatric Association, 1993; Beumont et al., 1993). However, the ultimate test of treatment programs in patients with anorexia nervosa is to demonstrate improvement at longer-term follow-up, and this aspect of the study has yet to be undertaken.

TARGET SYMPTOMS FOR BEHAVIOR MODIFICATION

Modification of Eating Behavior

One of the most importunate questions confronting behavior therapists has been the dilemma as to the choice of target behavior to be reinforced (Bemis, 1987). The applications of operant conditioning techniques have in fact focussed on some aspect of eating behavior (calories consumed, mouthfuls of food ingested, or meals completed) or weight gain. Bemis (1987) has documented both the advantages and disadvantages of using eating behavior as the basis for reinforcement. Behavior therapists who favor rewarding eating behavior per se to promote weight gain argue that (1) adaptive eating behaviors are acquired, and patients learn more about calorie–weight relationships; (2) reinforcements can be provided soon after the desired response has been performed; and (3) if the criterion includes having to consume all food, then more consistent weight gain may eventuate. The disadvantages are as follows: (1) patients may engage in surreptitious hoarding or disposal of food; (2) self-induced vomiting may permit patients to receive a reward for their eating, but then to fail to gain weight; (3) a pathological preoccupation with calories may develop, leading to an attempt to regulate food intake in a precise manner; (4) such aspects of eating behavior as size of portions, number of meals, and caloric content of foods are notoriously difficult to quantify in a meaningful and reliable manner; and, finally, (5) 24-hour supervision may be necessary to quantify caloric intake and prevent purging.

There are several other major concerns and

compelling reasons not to focus on eating as a target behavior to promote weight gain. Surely the ultimate aim is to teach anorexia nervosa patients normal eating behavior, and this is hardly achieved by insisting that patients keep track of each bite of food with a hand counter (Cincirpini, Kornblith, Turner, & Hersen, 1983; McGlynn, 1980). Furthermore, Agras et al. (1974) and Elkin, Hersen, Eisler, and Williams (1973) have investigated the relationship between meal size and calories consumed, and concluded that a greater amount of food served does in fact result in more being consumed. Agras et al. (1974) reported that their subjects consumed 2,306 calories per day when 3,000 calories were presented, and 2,882 when 6,000 calories were offered. This practice should be discouraged in the strongest possible manner even if it does facilitate weight gain. Bemis (1987) has thoughtfully argued this point: "Serving an anorexic portions that a lumberjack or a bulimic on a slow day would be hard pressed to consume teaches her little about normal eating behavior and may not be justified by a 500 calorie increase in intake" (p. 441). Casper (1982) has suggested that patients be offered only slightly more than they need to consume, as patients may find it reassuring to eat slightly less than they are prescribed. Once again, however, this practice is problematic: It inadvertently reinforces dieting behavior, the very behavior that treatment is aimed at extinguishing!

Should anorexia nervosa patients be discouraged from talking incessantly about food, and if this should be achieved, would it facilitate weight gain? In two published studies where staff members ignored comments and concerns pertaining to eating behavior, no direct effect on weight gain was achieved. Schlemmer and Barnett (1977) have come to the conclusion that it is virtually impossible to extinguish all talk about food. For this reason, it is imperative that a dietitian be an integral member of the multidisciplinary team and be involved in data collection, assessment, planning, supervision, and counseling, so that clinicians can focus more effectively on the underlying concerns rather than arguing about whether butter or margarine may be preferable in one's diet (Williams, Touyz, & Beumont, 1985; Beumont, O'Connor, Touyz, & Williams, 1987; Beumont, Touyz, Williams, & Russell, 1994; Touyz & Beumont, 1991).

Finally, the assumption that abnormal eating behavior will correct itself once a patient has received the necessary psychotherapy has not been borne out in clinical practice (Touyz, Williams, Marden, Kopec-Schrader, & Beumont, 1994) and has received scant attention in the literature. One possible reason for the lack of systematic research has been the absence of an appropriate instrument to quantify the extent of the phenomenon. Although several scales have been published (Slade, 1973; Van Strien, Frifters, Bergens, & Defares, 1986), most have not focused specifically on the eating behavior of anorexia nervosa patients. Because of these shortcomings, we developed an Eating Behavior Rating Scale (EBRS; Wilson, Touyz, Dunn, & Beumont, 1989). This scale was generated from a number of different sources, including observations of patients, clinicians' comments, and previously published literature. From the initial pool of behaviors, 12 were selected, and an observer's rating scale was constructed with a 6-point equal-interval scale to rate both the frequency and intensity of these behaviors (see Table 19.1). This instrument has been found to have a good interrater reliability coefficient of .86 and 24-hour and 4-month test–retest reliabilities of .90 and .85, respectively.

We recently used the EBRS in a study to assess whether direct informational feedback of eating behavior, via videotaped recording of meals, would improve abnormal eating behavior in patients with anorexia nervosa (Touyz et al., 1994). Thirty-two female inpatients were randomly assigned to two treatment groups, with only one group receiving regular videotape feedback of their eating behaviors. There was a greater improvement in the eating behaviors of patients who received regular videotape feedback of their meals than in those of patients who did not. Video recording of meals and feedback may therefore be a useful adjunct in treating patients with anorexia nervosa. However, a finding of much concern was that despite considerable attention to the eating behavior of all patients, their eating behavior remained worse than that of a nonanorexic population by the time of their discharge from the hospital. Furthermore, we recently investigated eating behaviors, nutritional intake, and anorexic psychopathology in 16 weight-recovered anorexia nervosa patients (Windauer, Lennerts, Talbot, Touyz, & Beumont, 1993). Body fat content and psychosocial adjustments were also assessed. The Eating Disorder Examination (Cooper & Fairburn, 1987) and a food diary were used to

TABLE 19.1. The Eating Behavior Rating Scale (EBRS): A Measure of Eating Pathology in Anorexia Nervosa

Behavior	Rating					
1. Global assessment of eating	0	1	2	3	4	5
2. Picking of food	5	4	3	2	1	0
3. Poor table manners involving eating utensils	0	1	2	3	4	5
4. Alternation between courses	0	1	2	3	4	5
5. Food disposal	5	4	3	2	1	0
6. Distaste for food	5	4	3	2	1	0
7. Abnormal verbalization during a meal	5	4	3	2	1	0
8. Preference for low-calorie foods	0	1	2	3	4	5
9. Abnormally slow eating	5	4	3	2	1	0
10. Abnormally rapid eating	0	1	2	3	4	5
11. Ritualistic eating	0	1	2	3	4	5
12. Excessive activity during the meal	5	4	3	2	1	0

Note. From Wilson, Touyz, Dunn, and Beumont (1989, p.). Copyright 1989 by the *International Journal of Eating Disorders.* Reprinted by permission.

assess outcome. Although body fat content and overall psychosocial adjustment had returned to normal in most patients, 12 continued to restrict their eating, with their nutritional intake below 90% of their energy requirements. These findings reflect the need to improve eating behavior while the patients are still hospitalized; they also provide further support for the invaluable role that dietitians play in the treatment of anorexia nervosa.

Modification of Excessive Exercise

Both Gull (1874/1964) and Lasègue (1873/1964) observed hyperactivity as one of the prominent symptoms in their series of patients with anorexia nervosa. Gull, in fact, commented that "this was in fact a striking expression of the nervous state, for it seemed hardly possible that a body so wasted could undergo the exercise which seemed agreeable." However, despite these comments over a century ago, the excessive exercising so commonly found in anorexia nervosa has received virtually no attention in the behavioral literature (Crisp, 1965; Blinder, Freeman, & Stunkard, 1970; Slade, 1973; Halmi, 1974; Touyz, Beumont, & Hook, 1987). Epling, Pierce, and Stefan (1983, p. 28) contend that the reason for this is that this behavior is viewed as "an interesting, but seemingly unimportant symptom [in] the anorexia syndrome." In practice, clinicians are often faced with a difficult dilemma pertaining to the question of exercise. Is there a need to treat the actual disturbed exercise behavior? If so, should anorexia nervosa patients be discouraged from exercising at all? Will policing patients' activity in the hos-

pital decrease or prevent them from overexercising after discharge? Is it realistic to expect patients to be completely inactive when moderate exercise is generally accepted as necessary for a healthy lifestyle? We have dealt specifically with these questions in our development of a supervised exercise program (Beumont, Arthur, Russell, & Touyz, 1994), which has not been found to compromise weight gain (Touyz, Lennerts, Arthur, & Beumont, 1993).

CURRENT CLINICAL PRACTICE

Despite the recurring controversy about the effectiveness of operant conditioning programs, they do form the basis for most inpatient treatment programs, as illustrated by the way our own efforts have evolved.

An Integrated Hospital-Based Behavioral Treatment Program

The hospital management of patients with anorexia nervosa can be divided into two stages: weight restoration and weight maintenance (Touyz & Beumont, 1985). The effects of starvation must be reversed if the patients are to benefit from other important aspects of treatment, such as individual, group, and family psychotherapy, as well as nutritional and exercise counseling.

A Lenient, Flexible Approach

At the time of admission, patients are encouraged to gain weight at an *average* rate of 1.5 kg per week. Patients are weighed three times per week (Monday, Wednesday, and Friday) at 7:00 A.M., prior to breakfast, in their nightclothes. Weighing patients three times per week instead of daily during refeeding does not compromise weight gain and may reduce the iatrogenic danger of intensifying these patients' already excessive concern with minor fluctuations in body weight (Touyz, Lennerts, Freeman, & Beumont, 1990). The weights for the 3 days are used to calculate an average weekly weight, and this weight is compared to the previous week's average weight. Reinforcers are made contingent upon the average weight gain; we have found this to result in a more consistent weight gain during refeeding, and it actively discourages idiosyncratic eating behaviors (e.g., overeating on Thursday in an attempt to obtain weekend leave by bolstering weight gained for the week). The reinforcers used are as follows. When weight is gained at an average rate of 1.5 kg per week or more, patients are permitted to dress in street clothes; to move freely around the unit and grounds of the hospital; and (when appropriate) to have time out of the unit, including both Saturday and Sunday from 8:30 A.M. to 10:30 P.M. When weight is gained at an average weekly rate of 1.0 to 1.4 kg, the reinforcers are the same, except that weekend leave is restricted to a morning or afternoon only on both Saturday and Sunday. When the average rate of weight gain is less than 1 kg per week, patients are placed on bed rest (in nightclothes), but retain all possessions and visiting privileges; leave of 3 hours only is permitted on weekends. Patients on bed rest attend only major psychotherapy groups and are denied attendance at more enjoyable activities (e.g., ward outings). All patients, regardless of their reinforcer status, attend all snacks and meals in the dining room, but can only attend our supervised anaerobic exercise program if they gain at least an average of 1 kg per week (Beumont, Arthur, et al., 1994). As stated previously, a program with relatively clear-cut objectives such as these reduces the opportunities for patients to manipulate staff members and thus to avoid focusing their attention on their underlying conflicts. Peer pressure within the therapeutic community also contributes significantly to patients' obtaining their weekly weight gain.

Patients eat all their snacks and meals in the dining room. Staff members are encouraged to eat meals with the patients, to provide role models for normal, healthy attitudes toward food and appropriate eating behavior. Patients with particular difficulties in their actual eating behavior are placed in a separate dining room and given more intensive supervision (a remedial eating program), in an attempt to better shape their eating behavior or lack of it. Patients are required to rest on their beds for 60 minutes following meals, as those with a previous history of self-induced vomiting are often tempted to do so after a meal, whereas those who have been exercising excessively may be inclined to "pay back the debt" (the meal consumed) by exercising strenuously. Bed rest in this context is utilized as a form of response prevention, in behavioral terms.

Minimum or Target Weight

There is no general consensus as to what constitutes an optimal weight for patients with anorexia nervosa, although most clinicians probably use a low average weight for height and sex as a general guideline. This often becomes the most contentious issue in therapy, and clinicians require both the wisdom of Solomon and the patience of Job in addressing it (Touyz & Beumont, 1991). Fortunately, there are some guidelines to use in coming to a decision about body weight in therapy (Garfinkel & Garner, 1982):

- It is preferable to specify the minimum target weight at the onset of treatment.
- The weight should be one the patient can maintain without continued dieting.
- There should be a range of approximately 2 kg rather than a specific set weight.

Quetelet's body mass index is a useful means of determining target weights (Beumont, Al-Alami, & Touyz, 1988). It is derived from a formula in which weight (in kilograms) is divided by squared height (in meters). For those patients aged 16 years or older, a body mass index of 20 should be used as a guide to minimum weight. For those aged between 14 and 15 years, a body mass index of 18.5–19.5 appears to be appropriate. However, for patients aged 13 years and under, it is best to consult standardized data. There will always be exceptions to any rule, and there is much to be said for using a pragmatic approach.

Once patients have reached their minimum weight, they should be "range"-weighed. That is, the scale should be set at the lowest acceptable weight and then at a weight 2 or 3 kg higher. This enables the clinician to document whether the patients are maintaining their weight within an acceptable range, without focusing upon a specific figure; this avoids reinforcement of the patients' preoccupation with weight as such.

Weight Maintenance

After patients have regained weight, it is advisable that they stay on for a further 2–3 weeks, so as to reduce their intake (under the supervision of the dietitian) from approximately 3,500 calories per day to a maintenance level of about 1,800 calories per day.

Patients should be encouraged to spend evenings and weekends at home, and to go out with friends and family members to eat in restaurants; these should include age-appropriate establishments (e.g., fast-food restaurants). Patients often feel safe eating out only when they know they can order foods such as salads, and they must be helped to cope in more demanding situations. They should also be permitted to go shopping and be encouraged, if finances permit, to buy a new wardrobe of clothes that will fit comfortably at their recently restored normal weight.

Once patients have successfully reduced their intake to a maintenance level, arrangements should be made for them to return to school or work; they may choose to attend work or classes for a week or so prior to discharge. Individual therapy as well as nutritional counseling should continue throughout this period, and a further therapy session should be scheduled at the time of discharge.

Once the maintenance period has been successfully negotiated, patients are discharged from the hospital. They should initially attend outpatient appointments on a weekly basis and, depending on their progress, move on to sessions every 2 weeks and then monthly. Because many patients relapse after treatment, consistent aftercare is most important. If relapse does occur, it is best to arrange prompt readmission, rather than to wait until the patient is again emaciated and in need of prolonged nutritional rehabilitation.

For a more detailed description of specific aspects of our integrated hospital-based behavioral program, the reader is referred to the following sources: Touyz and Beumont (1985);

Williams et al. (1985); Beumont et al. (1987, 1993); Beumont, Arthur, et al. (1994); Beumont, Touyz, et al. (1994); Touyz et al. (1984, 1990, 1993, 1994); Touyz, Beumont, and Hook (1987); Touyz, Garner, and Beumont (1995); and O'Connor, Touyz, and Beumont (1988).

Brief Reward Programs

Despite our cogent criticisms of the routine implementation of strict operant conditioning programs for refeeding patients with anorexia nervosa (Touyz et al., 1984; Touyz, Beumont, & Dunn, 1987), there is some justification for not abandoning this strategy altogether. When a recalcitrant patient in a hospital fails to gain weight on a more lenient program, we believe it to be both necessary and justifiable to implement a stricter operant conditioning program, but in a modified form. We recommend the introduction of "brief reward programs" (BRPs) as an adjunct to refeeding those patients who have not responded to a more lenient approach.

The major aim of the BRPs is to provide an incentive and/or a face-saving mechanism for the noncompliant patient to commence eating and gaining weight. Thus, instead of the traditional operant conditioning program (for an example, see Table 19.2)—which necessitated a patient's remaining in relative isolation on the ward, often for several months and at times for the entire admission—BRPs are developed to ensure that patients' confinement to their rooms is limited to a few weeks at most. The hierarchy of reinforcers is individualized, as in all operant programs but the entire hierarchy of reinforcers is restricted to a range of 4–5 kg (see Table 19.3). Thus, if the patient manages to gain 1 kg per week, then the entire duration of such a program is approximately 5 weeks. By this time, the patient is usually complying better with treatment and is able to continue to gain weight without the individualized program.

When we place patients on a BRP, we tell them at the outset that their progress will be reviewed on a regular basis. If they do well with regard to their weight gain, they may be given an opportunity to come off the program prior to completing it; however, if they fail to continue to gain an agreed-upon weekly weight, they will have to return to the BRP until it is successfully completed.

There are several advantages in using BRPs with patients who fail to respond to more lenient approaches to refeeding. First, patients,

TABLE 19.2. A Traditional Operant Conditioning Program for Refeeding Patients with Anorexia Nervosa (Commonly Used in the 1960s and 1970s)

Reward number	Weight (kg)	Reward provided
1.	33.5	Pen and writing paper
2.	34.0	Flowers
3.	34.5	Receive letters or postcards
4.	35.0	Radio for 1 hour/day
5.	35.5	Watch
6.	36.0	Jewelry
7.	36.5	Shower on Sundays, supervised (15 minutes)
8.	37.0	One magazine/week of own choice
9.	37.5	Moisturizer, scissors
10.	38.0	Own blanket and pillow
11.	38.5	Radio for 2 hours/day
12.	39.0	Comb and mirror
13.	39.5	Morning newspaper
14.	40.0	Shower on Thursdays, supervised (15 minutes)
15.	40.5	Crocheting material
16.	41.0	Visit from occupational therapist (15 minutes/week)
17.	41.5	Radio for 3 hours/day
18.	42.0	Shower on Mondays, supervised (15 minutes)
19.	42.5	Picture book
20.	43.0	Visit from staff member (15 minutes/day)
21.	43.5	Hair dryer
22.	44.0	Evening newspaper
23.	44.5	Visit from nonanorexic patient (15 minutes/day)
24.	45.0	Shower on Wednesdays, supervised (15 minutes)
25.	45.5	Phone call (15 minutes/week)
26.	46.0	Visit from parents (1 hour/week)
27.	46.5	Radio for 4 hours/day
28.	47.0	Visit from friend (1 hour/week)
29.	47.5	Radio to keep
30.	48.0	Shower each day, supervised (15 minutes)
31.	48.5	Two magazines/week of own choice
32.	49.0	Visit from parents (2 hours/week)
33.	49.5	Visit from occupational therapist (30 minutes/week)
34.	50.0	Visit from physiotherapist (on recommendation from department of physiotherapy)
35.	50.5	Eat lunch in dining room
36.	51.0	Eat dinner in dining room
37.	51.5	Attend socializing group
38.	52.0	Up and involved in ward program

Note. This program exemplifies the unnecessarily harsh and punitive aspects of such programs. The patient was aged 20 years, weighed 33 kg on admission, and was set a minimum or goal weight of 52 kg.

can see the "light at the end of the tunnel," in that such programs are designed to assist them in commencing the refeeding process and are therefore by nature short-lived. Traditional operant conditioning programs require patients to reach their goal weight before the programs are terminated, and the patients usually remain on the programs no matter how well they are doing. Second, since only a minority of patients will require BRPs, there is the added incentive of gaining weight so as to resume the normal ward program and not to be seen to be different

from the peer group. Third, there is less danger that patients will literally "eat their way out of [the] hospital" (Bruch, 1974). Finally, BRPs are seen as less punitive by the majority of our patients. It is our belief that such programs warrant further investigation.

CONCLUSION

With so much water under the bridge since Bachrach et al. (1965) introduced operant con-

TABLE 19.3. A Brief Reward Program (BRP)

Reward number	Weight (kg)	Reward provided
1.	46.0	Stereo to keep.
2.	46.5	TV for 4 hours/day. Modified stretching on Mondays and Tuesdays, subject to approval by physician.
3.	47.0	Extra visit from parents for 1 hour. May make one 2-minute phone call twice per week.
4.	47.5	Modified stretching: Mondays, Tuesdays, Wednesdays, and Thursdays. Unrestricted visits from other patients.
5.	48.0	Extra visit from parents for 1 hour. Modified stretching daily. May make one 10-minute phone call on alternate days.
6.	48.5	Extra visit from parents for 1 hour. Gym assessment. Friends from school may visit one afternoon a week.
7.	49.0	Modified gym program. Ward outings. May sit in the lounge room at dinner each night.
8.	49.5	Unrestricted visits from parents. May have day leave on Saturdays and Sundays.
9.	50.0	May go to a movie with parents one night during the week.
10.	50.5	Overnight leave (from Saturday after lunch to Sunday 5:30 P.M.) or a day at the races.
11.	51.0	Join in ward program.

While on this program the patient may have:

1. Shower every day for 10 minutes.
2. Books, cards, newspapers, puzzles, crafts, fluffy toys.
3. Attendance at therapy and groups as directed by nursing unit manager.
4. Two visits (1 hour each) from parents per week: one during the week, one on weekends.
5. Visits from other patients between 4:00 and 5:30 P.M. on weekdays and between 1:30 and 6:00 P.M. on weekends.
6. Daily weighings.
7. Phone calls as per the program (see above).

Note. This BRP was developed for an 18-year-old girl who was admitted to a hospital weighing 45.6 kg but failed to gain weight over several weeks. Her minimum or goal weight was 57 kg.

ditioning paradigms to the treatment of patients with anorexia nervosa over 30 years ago, one could be excused for expecting a general consensus as to the efficacy of this treatment strategy. Sadly, this is not the case.

Although the weight of evidence suggests that operant conditioning programs are effective in promoting weight gain in patients with anorexia nervosa, they may not have a distinct advantage over other hospital treatments. This lack of difference in outcome between operant conditioning programs and their less structured counterparts has been attributed to the fact that the latter include many behavioral elements without labeling them as such. Schmidt (1989) correctly asserts that this argument cannot be used to justify the superiority of operant conditioning programs per se. Notwithstanding this, Agras and Kraemer (1983) have argued rather cogently that operant conditioning programs do appear to result in facilitating faster weight gain in the shorter term, thereby significantly reducing the length of hospital stays and the subsequent costs involved. With the advent of managed care, this is particularly pertinent. However-

er, is it in the best interest of anorexia nervosa patients to gain weight rapidly? Bemis (1987) has concluded: "More is not necessarily better and . . . common sense suggests that at some point the short-term economic advantage of increasing speed is cancelled out by its clinical disadvantage." The risk of patients' developing bulimic symptoms under such circumstances should not be underestimated.

Despite Bruch's (1978) severe criticism, our patients responded favorably to the lenient, flexible approach to management (Touyz et al., 1984), although not all studies have reported such a universal acceptance (Kreipe & Kidder, 1986). Schmidt (1989) has argued for a second generation of studies to further investigate the behavioral treatment of anorexia nervosa. He refers to the study by Channon, deSilva, Hemsley, and Perkins (1989), which compared cognitive-behavioral and behavioral treatment of anorexia nervosa, as a good example of such research (it employed multiple outcome measures, had good follow-up data, and included standard outpatient treatment as a control procedure). Despite its general acceptance in clinical practice, cognitive-behavioral research in anorexia nervosa is still in its infancy, has yet to be systematically investigated, and is in urgent need of address. To conclude, the use of lenient operant programs within a humane framework does appear to add to the treatment of patients with anorexia nervosa, but in view of the relapse rates following treatment, the search for more effective treatment methods must continue in earnest.

REFERENCES

Agras, W. S., Barlow, D. H., Chapin, H. N., Abel, G. G., & Leitenberg, H. (1974). Behavior modification of anorexia nervosa. *Archives of General Psychiatry, 30,* 279–286.

Agras, W. S., & Kraemer, H. C. (1983). The treatment of anorexia nervosa: Do different treatments have different outcomes? *Psychiatric Annals, 13,* 928–935.

Agras, W. S., & Werne, J. (1978). Behavior therapy in anorexia nervosa: A data-based approach to the question. In J. P. Brady & H. K. H. Brodie (Eds.), *Controversy in psychiatry* (pp. 655–675). Philadelphia: W.B. Saunders.

American Psychiatric Association. (1993). Practice guidelines for eating disorders. *American Journal of Psychiatry, 150,* 212–228.

Bachrach, A. J., Erwin, W. J., & Mohr, J. P. (1965). The control of eating behavior in an anorexic by operant conditioning techniques. In L. P. Ullman & I. Krasner (Eds.), *Case studies in behavior modification* (pp. 153–163). New York: Holt, Rinehart & Winston.

Bemis, K. (1987). The present status of operant conditioning for the treatment of anorexia nervosa. *Behavior Modification, 11,* 432–463.

Beumont, P. J. V., Al-Alami, M., & Touyz, S. W. (1988). Relevance of a standard measurement of undernutrition to the diagnosis of anorexia nervosa: Use of Quetelet's body mass index. *International Journal of Eating Disorders, 7,* 399–406.

Beumont, P. J. V., Arthur, B., Russell, J. D., & Touyz, S. W. (1994). Excessive physical activity in dieting disorder patients: Proposals for a supervised exercise program. *International Journal of Eating Disorders, 15,* 21–36.

Beumont, P. J. V., O'Connor, M. O., Touyz, S. W., & Williams, H. (1987). Nutritional counseling in the treatment of anorexia and bulimia nervosa. In P. J. V. Beumont, G. D. Burrows, & R. C. Casper (Eds.), *Handbook of eating disorders: Part 1. Anorexia and bulimia nervosa* (pp. 349–359). Amsterdam: Elsevier.

Beumont, P. J. V., Russell, J., & Touyz, S. W. (1993). Treatment of anorexia nervosa. *Lancet, 341,* 1635–1640.

Beumont, P. J. V., Touyz, S. W., Williams, H., & Russell, J. (1994). The treatment of anorexia nervosa. In G. Andrews (Ed.), *Specialization in psychiatry* (pp. 47–118). Sidney: Ciba Geigy.

Bhanji, S., & Thompson, J. (1974). Operant conditioning in the treatment of anorexia nervosa: A review and retrospective study of 11 cases. *British Journal of Psychiatry, 124,* 166–172.

Blinder, B. J., Freeman, D. M., & Stunkard, A. J. (1970). Behavior therapy of anorexia nervosa: Effectiveness of activity as a reinforcer of weight gain. *American Journal of Psychiatry, 126,* 1093–1098.

Bruch, H. (1974). Perils of behavior modification in treatment of anorexia nervosa. *Journal of the American Medical Association, 230,* 1419–1422.

Bruch, H. (1978). Dangers of behavior modification in treatment in anorexia nervosa. In J. P. Brady & H. K. H. Brodie (Eds.), *Controversy in psychiatry* (pp. 245–254). Philadelphia: W.B. Saunders.

Casper, R. C. (1982). Treatment principles in anorexia nervosa. *Adolescent Psychiatry, 10,* 431–454.

Channon, S., de Silva, P., Hemsley, D., & Perkins, R. E. (1989). A controlled trial of cognitive-behavioural and behavioural treatment of anorexia nervosa. *Behaviour Research and Therapy, 27,* 529–535.

Cincirpini, P. M., Kornblith, S. J., Turner, S. M., & Hersen, M. (1983). A behavioral program for the management of anorexia and bulimia. *Journal of Nervous and Mental Disease, 171,* 186–186.

Cooper, Z., & Fairburn, C. G. (1987). The Eating Disorder Examination: A semi-structured interview for the assessment of the specific psychopathology of eating disorders. *International Journal of Eating Disorders, 6,* 1–8.

Crisp, A. H. (1965). Clinical and therapeutic aspects of anorexia nervosa: A study of thirty cases. *Journal of Psychosomatic Research, 9,* 67–78.

Danziger, Y., Carel, C. A., Tyano, S., & Mimounty, M. (1989). Is psychotherapy mandatory during the acute refeeding period in the treatment of anorexia nervosa? *Journal of Adolescent Health Care, 10,* 325–331.

Elkin, M., Hersen, M., Eisler, R. M., & Williams, J. G. (1973). Modification of caloric intake in anorexia nervosa: An experimental analysis. *Psychological Reports, 32,* 75–78.

Epling, W. F., Pierce, W. D., & Stefan, L. (1983). A theory of activity: Basic research. *International Journal of Eating Disorders, 3,* 7–46.

Fairburn, C. G., & Cooper, Z. (1987). Behavioral and cognitive approaches to the treatment of anorexia nervosa and bulimia nervosa. In P. J. V. Beumont, G. D. Burrows, & R. C. Casper (Eds.), *Handbook of eating disorders: Part 1. Anorexia and bulimia nervosa* (pp. 271–298). Amsterdam: Elsevier.

Garfinkel, P. E., & Garner, D. M. (1982). *Anorexia nervosa: A multidimensional perspective.* New York: Brunner/Mazel.

Garner, D. M. (1985). Iatrogenesis in anorexia and bulimia nervosa. *International Journal of Eating Disorders, 4,* 701–726.

Garner, D. M., Rockert, W., Olmsted, M. P., Johnson, G., & Coscina, D. V. (1985). Psychoeducational principles in the treatment of bulimia and anorexia nervosa. In D. M. Garner & P. E. Garfinkel (Eds.), *Handbook of psychotherapy for anorexia and bulimia* (pp. 513–572). New York: Guilford Press.

Gull, W. W. (1964). Anorexia nervosa (apepsia hysterica, anorexia hysterica). In R. M. Kaufman & M. Heiman (Eds.), *Evolution of a psychosomatic concept: Anorexia nervosa.* New York: International Universities Press. (Original work published 1874)

Halmi, K. A. (1974). Anorexia nervosa: Demographic and clinical features in 94 cases. *Psychosomatic Medicine, 36,* 18–26.

Halmi, K. A. (1985). Behavioral management for anorexia nervosa. In D. M. Garner & P. E. Garfinkel (Eds.), *Handbook of psychotherapy for anorexia nervosa and bulimia* (pp. 147–159). New York: Guilford Press.

Halmi, K. A., Powers, P., & Cunningham, S. (1975). Treatment of anorexia nervosa with behavior modification. *Archives of General Psychiatry, 32,* 93–96.

Keys, A., Brozek, J., Henschel, A., Mickelsen, O., & Taylor, H. L. (1950). *The biology of human starvation* (2 vols.). Minneapolis: University of Minnesota Press.

Kreipe, R. E., & Kidder, F. (1986). Comparison of two hospital treatment programs for anorexia nervosa. *International Journal of Eating Disorders, 5,* 649–657.

Lasègue, C. H. (1964). De l'anoréxie hystérique [On hysterical anorexia]. In R. M. Kaufman & M. Heiman (Eds.), *Evolution of a psychosomatic concept: Anorexia nervosa* (pp. 141–155). New York: International Universities Press. (Original work published in 1873)

McGlynn, F. D. (1980). Successful treatment of anorexia nervosa with self-monitoring and long distance praise. *Journal of Behavior Therapy and Experimental Psychiatry, 11,* 283–286.

Morgan, H. G. (1977). Fasting girls and our attitudes to them. *British Medical Journal, 24,* 1652–1655.

O'Connor, M. A., Touyz, S. W., & Beumont, P. J. V. (1988). Nutritional management and dietary counselling on bulimia nervosa: Some preliminary observations. *International Journal of Eating Disorders, 7,* 657–662.

Phares, J. E. (1992). *Clinical psychology: Concepts, methods and profession* (4th ed.). Pacific Grove, CA: Brooks/Cole.

Schlemmer, J. K., & Barnett, P. A. (1977). Management of manipulative behavior of anorexia nervosa patients. *Journal of Psychiatric Nursing, 15,* 35–41.

Schmidt, W. (1989). Behavioral psychotherapy of eating disorders. *International Review of Psychiatry, 1,* 215–256.

Slade, P. D. (1973). A short anorexic behavior scale. *British Journal of Psychiatry, 122,* 83–85.

Stunkard, A. (1972). New therapies for the eating disorders: Behavior modification of obesity and anorexia nervosa. *Archives of General Psychiatry, 26,* 391–398.

Touyz, S. W., & Beumont, P. J. V. (1985). A comprehensive, multidisciplinary approach for the management of patients with anorexia nervosa. In S. W. Touyz & P. J. V. Beumont (Eds.), *Eating disorders: Prevalence and treatment* (pp. 11–22). Sydney: Williams & Wilkins/Adis.

Touyz, S. W., & Beumont, P. J. V. (1991). The management of anorexia nervosa in adolescence. *Modern Medicine, 34,* 86–97.

Touyz, S. W., Beumont, P. J. V., & Dunn, S. M. (1987). Behavior therapy in the management of patients with anorexia nervosa: A lenient, flexible approach. *Psychotherapy and Psychosomatics, 48,* 151–156.

Touyz, S. W., Beumont, P. J. V., Glaun, D., Phillips, T., &

Cowie, I. (1984). A comparison of lenient and strict operant conditioning programs in refeeding patients with anorexia nervosa. *British Journal of Psychiatry, 144,* 517–520.

Touyz, S. W., Beumont, P. J. V., & Hook, S. (1987). Exercise anorexia: A new dimension in anorexia nervosa? In P. J. V. Beumont, G. D. Burrows, & R. C. Casper (Eds.), *Handbook of eating disorders: Part 1. Anorexia and bulimia nervosa* (pp. 145–159). Amsterdam: Elsevier.

Touyz, S. W., Garner, D. M., & Beumont, P. J. V. (1995). The inpatient management of the adolescent patient with anorexia nervosa. In H. C. Steinhausen (Ed.), *Eating disorders in adolescence: Anorexia and bulimia nervosa* (p. 247). New York: de Gruyter/Aldine.

Touyz, S. W., Lennerts, W., Arthur, B., & Beumont, P. J. V. (1993). Anaerobic exercise as an adjunct to refeeding patients with anorexia nervosa: Does it compromise weight gain? *European Eating Disorder Review, 1,* 177–182.

Touyz, S. W., Lennerts, W., Freeman, R., & Beumont, P. J. V. (1990). Frequency of weighing and rate of weight gain in patients with anorexia nervosa. *British Journal of Psychiatry, 157,* 752–754.

Touyz, S. W., Williams, H., Marden, K., Kopec-Schrader, E., & Beumont, P. J. V. (1994). Videotape feedback of eating behaviour in patients with anorexia nervosa: Does it normalise eating behaviour? *Australian Journal of Nutrition and Dietetics, 51,* 79–82.

Van Strien, T., Frifters, J. E. R., Bergens, G. P. A., & Defares, P. B. (1986). The Dutch Eating Behavior Questionnaire (DEBQ) for assessment of restrained, emotional, and external behavior. *International Journal of Eating Disorders, 5,* 295–315.

Venables, J. F. (1930). Anorexia nervosa: Study of the pathogenesis and treatment of nine cases. *Guy's Hospital Report, 80,* 213–226.

Williams, H., Touyz, S. W., & Beumont, P. J. V. (1985). Nutritional counselling in anorexia nervosa. In S. W. Touyz & P. J. V. Beumont (Eds.), *Eating disorders: Prevalence and treatment* (pp. 23–31). Sydney: Williams & Wilkins/Adis.

Wilson, A. J., Touyz, S. W., Dunn, S. M., & Beumont, P. J. V. (1989). The Eating Behavior Rating Scale (EBRS): A measure of eating pathology in anorexia nervosa. *International Journal of Eating Disorders, 8,* 583–592.

Windauer, U., Lennerts, W., Talbot, P., Touyz, S. W., & Beumont, P. J. V. (1993). How well are "cured" anorexia nervosa patients? An investigation of 16 weight recovered anorexia patients. *British Journal of Psychiatry, 163,* 195–200.

CHAPTER 20

Drug Therapies

PAUL E. GARFINKEL
B. TIMOTHY WALSH

Many treatments have been tried for anorexia nervosa and bulimia nervosa—in part because these conditions are difficult to treat; in part because of the wide variety of symptoms and impairments in people with eating disorders; and in part because of the differing theoretical perspectives health care professionals have brought to these problems. Medications have been widely tried since anorexia nervosa was related to primary endocrine illness early in this century (Garfinkel & Garner, 1982). Psychotropic drugs have been advocated for over 35 years (Dally & Sargant, 1960). Today, an empirically based literature is beginning to accumulate, and this should more properly inform and guide clinical decisions.

This area of investigation has been limited by several conceptual and methodological problems, including the definition of cases, the control of relevant variables, and methods of assessment and strategies for treatment outcome trials (Shaw & Garfinkel, 1990). In spite of these deficiencies, some tentative conclusions regarding the role of medications in the treatment of eating disorders can now be drawn:

1. Although medications have a role to play in helping some people with eating disorders, they should rarely become the exclusive mode of treatment. Their use should be coupled with nutritional restoration, education, and psychotherapy (Garfinkel & Garner, 1987).

2. The mechanisms of action of psychotropic medications in people with eating disorders are not well understood.

3. It is an error to assume that the pathophysiology of these disorders can be defined on the basis of patients' responsiveness to a particular group of medications and knowledge of how that medication works. All psychotropic medications affect multiple systems.

Although there has been significant progress in this area in the past decade, the ability to tailor treatments optimally to a person's individual needs is limited by a relative lack of good outcome studies that have identified specific predictors of outcome to particular treatments.

BULIMIA NERVOSA

Since the initial description of bulimia nervosa (Russell, 1979), there has been real progress in the development of effective therapies, including pharmacotherapies, for this condition—especially in contrast to anorexia nervosa. This is partly because bulimia nervosa is much more common, is usually less life-threatening, and is managed largely on an outpatient basis (Walsh, 1992).

Antidepressant Medications

The initial open trials of antidepressants in bulimia nervosa were reported in 1982 (Pope & Hudson, 1982; Walsh et al., 1982). These trials were based on the clinical observations that many bulimic patients displayed significant mood disorder. Later, bulimia nervosa and depression were linked by studies of family history (Kassett et al., 1989), longitudinal course (Toner et al., 1986), and biological changes (Goldbloom & Kennedy, 1993). At the same time, a body of knowledge about aminergic influences on hunger and satiety and on macronutrient selection was developing (Anderson & Kennedy, 1992); this provided an additional basis for the potential utility of psychotropic medication in eating disorders.

The earliest open trials were followed by a series of placebo-controlled studies, almost all of which showed a statistically significant short-term reduction in binge eating and purging, regardless of which specific medicine was examined (Walsh, 1992; Goldbloom & Kennedy, 1993). These studies as a whole revealed the following:

1. There were no clear difference in efficacy among the various drugs used. Various medications, including tricyclic antidepressants (Agras, Dorian, Kirkley, Arnow, & Bachman, 1987; Hughes, Wells, Cunningham, & Ilstrup, 1986; Walsh, Hadigan, Devlin, Gladis, & Roose, 1991), monoamine oxidase inhibitors (Walsh et al., 1988; Kennedy et al., 1988, 1993), and selective serotonin reuptake inhibitors (Fluoxetine Bulimia Nervosa Collaborative Study Group, 1992; Goldstein et al., 1995), have all been shown to produce benefits relative to placebo. The antidepressants examined in controlled trials appear to have roughly equal efficacy, but no studies have compared antidepressants directly.

2. Short-term abstinence rates (on average, 8 weeks) are about 30%, and overall reductions in bulimic behaviors are about 70% (Agras et al., 1992).

3. A significant relapse rate (30–45%) is observed if patients are followed for 4–6 months (Pyle et al., 1990; Walsh et al., 1991).

4. There are few predictors of who will respond to these medications. In particular, level of depression and family history of depression do not seem to help in such predictions.

5. Dropout rates tend to be high, in part because of side effects and in part because of some patients' attitudes toward medication use.

6. The doses used in these treatment studies have generally been similar to those employed in the treatment of depression, and, with a single exception, no dose–response study has been conducted. The exception was a multicenter fluoxetine study, which compared a high dose (60 mg) and a low dose (20 mg) of fluoxetine

with placebo. The high-dose regimen was clearly superior to both other treatments in this trial (Fluoxetine Bulimia Nervosa Collaborative Study Group, 1992).

More recent studies have examined the relative efficacy of antidepressant medication, psychotherapy, and their combination. In the first such study, Mitchell et al. (1990) found that an intensive form of group therapy was clearly superior to imipramine in reducing binge eating and purging. The combination of imipramine and intensive group therapy was no more effective in reducing these eating disorder symptoms than was the group therapy alone. However, there was some evidence of benefit from medication, in that patients receiving imipramine evidenced greater improvement in mood, whether or not they were receiving psychotherapy.

In a second study, Agras et al. (1992) compared desipramine to individual cognitive-behavioral psychotherapy given alone and to the combination of both treatments. Cognitive-behavioral therapy alone was clearly superior to medication alone, but there were suggestions that psychotherapy combined with medication for 24 weeks yielded the best results. Leitenberg et al. (1994) also compared cognitive-behavioral therapy with desipramine and with their combination. They found cognitive-behavioral psychotherapy to produce better results than desipramine alone, but the study was limited by a very small sample size and a high dropout rate on medication.

A fourth study was completed by Goldbloom, Olmsted, Davis, and Shaw (1994). Consistent with the work cited above, this study also found that psychotherapy was significantly better than medication alone, which in this case was fluoxetine. The combination of the two treatments produced added benefits over the two individual treatments on several parameters. Similar results have been reported in a preliminary fashion by Walsh and colleagues (1995). In a trial examining 120 patients, they found that cognitive-behavioral therapy alone was better than either supportive psychotherapy or antidepressant medication alone—in this case, desipramine (followed by fluoxetine for patients who had not adequately responded). Medication added modestly but significantly to the effect of psychotherapy.

All of the studies cited thus far were of outpatients. Fichter et al. (1991) compared fluoxetine to placebo among hospitalized patients who also received behavioral therapy. Gains from the addition of medication were not demonstrable, possibly because of the very high response induced by inpatient care.

In summary, the available studies are quite consistent in finding that cognitive-behavioral psychotherapy alone is superior to a single course of antidepressant medication, and in suggesting that the combination of medication and psychotherapy produces modest additional benefits. A question these findings leaves unresolved is the best sequence of treatments. Since cognitive-behavioral therapy has substantial short- and long-term benefits, it seems appropriate to recommend this as the initial treatment for patients when a qualified therapist is available. If patients do not respond adequately to such treatment, or if there is a serious associated mood disturbance, the use of antidepressant medication should be considered.

Which specific medication should be selected? At present, given no demonstrated differences among antidepressants in efficacy, selection is based on minimizing side effects and enhancing compliance. The newer selective serotonin reuptake inhibitors have advantages in this regard, since the troublesome anticholinergic and antihistaminic side effects are minimized.

The research of the past decade, though showing a clear benefit to these medications, raises a number of questions. Do the medications improve psychopathological attitudes as well as symptoms? Preliminary evidence from Goldbloom and Olmsted (1993) suggests that they do. How long should responders be maintained on medication? At present a period of 4–6 months would seem reasonable, but some people may require longer treatment, and others (as noted previously) relapse while on the drug. As is the case for major depressive disorder, it appears that some people with bulimia nervosa require maintenance therapy to prevent recurrence.

Finally, it should be noted that virtually all of the studies of the use of medication for binge eating have been conducted with individuals of normal weight who purge after binge eating. Little is known about the use of medications in people with the newly defined binge-eating disorder (American Psychiatric Association, 1994). Some, but not all, of the early work on this area suggests that obese individuals with binge-eating disorder may benefit from antidepressant medication (Alger, Schwalberg, Bigaouette, Michalek, & Howard, 1991; deZwaan, Nutzinger, & Schoenbeck, 1992; Marcus et al., 1990; McCann & Agras, 1990).

Mood Stabilizers

Lithium carbonate has been evaluated in a single placebo-controlled trial (Hsu, Clement, Santhouse, & Ju, 1991). The modest lithium levels (mean = 0.62 mEq/liter) achieved may have contributed to the negative findings in this study. Some earlier research led a neurophysiological abnormality to be hypothesized, which led in turn to the use of phenytoin (Green & Rau, 1974; Wermuth, Davis, Hollister, & Stunkard, 1977). Actual evidence of seizure activity on electroencephalography in bulimia nervosa is minimal, and a controlled trial failed to demonstrate clear superiority of phenytoin over placebo. Similarly, a controlled study of carbamazepine was negative, except for some benefit for a single patient with coexistent cyclothymia (Kaplan, Garfinkel, Darby, & Garner, 1983). Although these mood-stabilizing agents may play an adjunctive role when severe affective instability is an aggravating factor in the perpetuation of the bulimia nervosa, there is no evidence that most patients will benefit from their use.

Anxiolytics

Various affective states may trigger binge eating, including anxiety. There have been no careful investigations of the anxiolytic medications. And, because people with bulimia nervosa are at risk for developing substance abuse or dependence (Garfinkel et al., 1995), benzodiazepines and other drugs with a significant propensity for abuse should be used with caution.

Opiate Antagonists

Jonas and Gold (1987) conducted an open trial of naltrexone, based on the idea that alterations in central nervous system endogenous opiates might be linked to changes in appetite. Seven out of 10 subjects showed complete or partial benefit. However, placebo-controlled investigations of naltrexone found no evidence of benefit (Mitchell et al., 1989; Alger et al., 1991).

Fenfluramine

Trials of fenfluramine have been conducted in bulimia nervosa because of its effects in promoting satiety, presumably via enhancing serotonergic activity. An early study by Blouin et al. (1988) produced encouraging findings. But two subsequent trials in which fenfluramine was added to a cognitive-behavioral therapy did not support the utility of fenfluramine, possibly because the benefits of psychotherapy produced a ceiling effect (Russell, Checkley, Feldman, & Eisler, 1988; Fahy, Eisler, & Russell, 1993).

ANOREXIA NERVOSA

There have been major developments in pharmacological treatments in psychiatry in the past 40 years. However, the core psychopathology of anorexia nervosa remains relatively refractory to medication. Although this is so, it must be noted that physical therapies are critical to treating this condition. Many of the complications of the starvation state require medical intervention. Moreover, about 25% of patients go on to develop a chronic form of the illness, and they may display comorbidities that can be responsive to drug therapies. This section of the chapter deals primarily with psychotropic medications as they have been used since 1960 for anorexia nervosa, but we also comment on the possible use of prokinetic agents and on the role of estrogens for the prevention of osteoporosis.

Antipsychotic Medications

Shortly after chlorpromazine was introduced, Dally and Sargant (1960) reported on its use, together with insulin and bed rest, to promote weight gain in anorexia nervosa. Later, they suggested that the chlorpromazine was as effective without insulin (Dally & Sargant, 1966). In their original series they were impressed with the rate of weight gain, which they attributed to the medication. However, a significant minority of their patients developed seizures, bulimia, and other side effects, and on follow-up the outcome of patients treated with chlorpromazine was not superior to that of those treated without the medication. Later, it was learned that very rapid weight gain under such conditions was unnecessary and could be harmful (Russell, 1977).

Chlorpromazine also has other disadvantages. It has a propensity to lower blood pressure in a group of people who already have a tendency to hypotension; moreover, it produces a variety of gastrointestinal side effects and acute and chronic neurological sequelae, which far outweigh any established benefit from this medication. Other neuroleptic agents have also been examined. For example, pimozide and sulpiride have not been shown to offer any advantages over placebo in controlled trials (Vandereycken & Pierloot, 1982; Vandereycken, 1984).

Antidepressants

As in bulimia nervosa, there are a number of linkages between anorexia nervosa and depression (Strober & Katz, 1988), suggesting that antidepressant medication might be of use. However, many clinical features of depression can be the direct results of starvation, and many depressive symptoms and neurovegetative features resolve with improvement in nutrition. The clinical assessment of depressive symptoms in anorexia nervosa is therefore complex.

Twenty years ago, there were a few case reports and open studies of tricyclic antidepressants (Moore, 1977; White & Schnaultz, 1977; Needleman & Waber, 1977). These claimed success based on short-term weight gain and some reduction in levels of depression. There followed three placebo-controlled evaluations, which did not demonstrate any significant benefits of the medications (Lacey & Crisp, 1980; Biederman et al., 1985; Halmi, Eckert, LaDu, & Cohen, 1986). More recently, Kaye, Weltzin, Hsu, and Bulik (1991) have described an open trial of fluoxetine in a large group of anorexic subjects who displayed a high level of weight maintenance after nutritional restoration. Gwirtsman, Guze, Yager, and Gainsley (1990) reported on six patients with chronic anorexia nervosa who benefited from fluoxetine; their depressive symptoms were reduced, and their weights improved. Ferguson (1987) has also described fluoxetine as beneficial to a patient who was refractory to other medications. However, fluoxetine has also been reported to produce side effects, including the abuse of the drug to promote weight loss (Wilcox, 1987). These findings require careful follow-up examination in controlled trials.

There is at present no established benefit

from antidepressant medications in the acute treatment phase of anorexia nervosa. Furthermore, their use is likely to be associated with the development of unwanted side effects in this medically ill patient group. The notion that antidepressant medications may alleviate depression, reduce obsessionality, and thereby reduce relapse in patients with anorexia nervosa following refeeding is theoretically appealing, but at present unproven.

Anxiolytics

Anxiety is a common feature in anorexia nervosa, especially when patients are confronted with the need to gain weight. But these are also people with high rates of comorbidity for anxiety disorders (Garfinkel et al., 1996) and with high rates of these illnesses on long-term follow-up (Toner, Garner, & Garfinkel, 1976; Toner, et al., 1986). For people who are extremely anxious in spite of supportive measures, a small amount of a benzodiazepine (e.g., lorazepam, 0.25–0.50 mg) may be used 20–40 minutes before meals (Andersen, 1987). The use of minor tranquilizers in anorexia nervosa should be time-limited.

Appetite-Enhancing Agents

Cyproheptadine, a serotonin and histamine antagonist, was noted in the 1960s to promote weight gain. This observation led to three controlled trials in anorexia nervosa (Goldberg, Halmi, Eckert, Casper, & Davis, 1979; Vigersky & Loriaux, 1977; Halmi et al., 1986). Although the best designed of these studies (Halmi et al., 1986) suggested that cyproheptadine might be of benefit in a subgroup of patients, the overall evidence favoring the utility of medication was not impressive.

In another small study, Casper, Schlemmer, and Javaid (1987) found that clonidine was not effective in promoting weight gain in anorexics, in spite of some earlier work suggesting that it would induce eating behavior. Similarly, Gross et al. (1983) evaluated tetrahydrocannabinol (the active component of marijuana) relative to diazepam, and found no advantage of the former agent in inducing an enhanced appetite or weight gain. Furthermore, several patients experienced severe dysphoria.

Recently, research has focused on peptides such as growth-hormone-releasing factor (GRF). Studies in animals have found that central or intravenous administration of GRF enhanced food intake in both food-deprived and free-feeding animals (Vaccarino, Bloom, Rivier, Vale, & Koob, 1985). Findings such as these led Vaccarino, Kennedy, Ralevski, and Black (1994) to examine the effects of GRF in eight emaciated people with anorexia nervosa. The peptide enhanced weight restoration in this study, and this area requires further investigation.

However, the goal of pharmacological treatments of anorexia nervosa should not be simply to increase appetite. In fact, people with this disorder possess good appetites, but are terrified of giving in to this impulse. The goals of treatments such as these should be to encourage weight restoration without increasing appetite itself; the latter will merely increase the patients' fears of losing self-control.

Prokinetic Agents

Delayed gastric emptying, and the associated symptoms of early satiety and bloating, have been well documented in patients with anorexia nervosa through radionuclide studies (McCallum et al., 1985; Domstad et al., 1987). The delay is particularly pronounced for solids and hypertonic liquids (Domstad et al., 1987). Some studies have shown an improvement in gastric emptying with weight restoration (Szmukler, Lichtenstein, Young, & Andrews, 1990), although this has not always been the case (Dubois, Gross, Richler, & Ebert, 1981).

This delay in gastric emptying may contribute to the avoidance of food, and thus may be problematic in a treatment program. For this reason, a number of prokinetic agents have been examined, mostly in acute challenges. Intravenous or intramuscular administration of metaclopramide (McCallum et al., 1985; Domstad et al., 1987), intravenous domperidone (Stacher et al., 1986), and intravenous cisapride (Stacher et al., 1987) have all been shown to improve gastric emptying in the short term. Several of these drugs have significant central nervous system effects and have not been demonstrated to have a sustained clinical benefit. For example, one investigation of metaclopramide could not be completed because of the high frequency of depression produced by the central effects of the drug (Moldofsky, Jeuniewic, & Garfinkel, 1977).

Recently, Szmukler, Young, Miller, Lichtenstein, and Binns (1995) examined the effects of cisapride in an 8-week randomized double-blind placebo-controlled trial. Although gastric emptying improved over time in both the cisapride and the placebo groups, symptoms were more improved in the active drug group. Although patients also rated themselves as more improved on the drug, both groups gained similar amounts of weight. In a smaller study of outpatients, Stacher et al. (1993) found that cisapride appeared to accelerate gastric emptying, to improve symptoms associated with gastric retention, and perhaps to improve the rate of weight gain slightly.

The precise role for these prokinetic agents has not been well defined. At the present time, the conclusions of Szmukler et al. (1995) seem appropriate: Cisapride may be used for people with anorexia nervosa when they have significant distress associated with meals and when there is evidence of delayed gastric emptying. The subjective improvement afforded by the medication may improve compliance with overall treatment.

Estrogens for Bone Mineral Density

Several characteristic features of anorexia nervosa—low body weight and amenorrhea in female patients—serve as important risk factors for the development of osteoporosis. It should not be surprising that in recent years, with the increased frequency of the eating disorders and their not infrequent chronicity, more and more attention is being given to the problem of demineralization of bone. In the 1980s, alarming reports documented the presence of osteoporosis and pathological fractures in these patients (Rigotti, Nussbaum, Herzog, & Neer, 1984; Brotman, Rigotti, & Herzog, 1985).

As long ago as 1982, Garfinkel and Garner suggested that estrogen administration had no role in the management of chronic anorexia nervosa. Their rationale was based on the observation that the menses of most anorexic women return after a period of weight restoration and maintenance, and on the belief that an emphasis should be placed on the resumption of bodily functions in as natural a fashion as possible. Klibanski et al. (1995) recently reported that estrogen supplementation had no significant impact, compared to a placebo, on bone density in women with anorexia nervosa. Although there was a suggestion of some benefit from estrogen treatment among the lowest-weight patients, the greatest increase in bone density was evidenced by those patients who

had regained weight and whose normal menses had resumed.

CONCLUSIONS

The results of research over the past 15 years have contributed significantly to pharmacological treatment approaches for people with bulimia nervosa and, to a lesser extent, those with anorexia nervosa. Although the findings document that medications have a role to play in treating these disorders, the role is an adjunctive one—that of supplementing nutritional rehabilitation and psychotherapies. There is a pressing need to identify the best candidates for medication and the predictors of response.

REFERENCES

Agras, W. S., Dorian, B., Kirkley, B. G., Arnow, B., & Bachman, J. (1987). Imipramine in the treatment of bulimia: A double-blind controlled study. *International Journal of Eating Disorders, 6*, 29–38.

Agras, W. S., Rossiter, E. M., Arnow, B., Schneider, J. A., Telch, C. F., Raeburn, S. D., Bruce, B., Perl, M., & Koran, L. M., (1992). Pharmacologic and cognitive-behavioral treatment for bulimia nervosa: A controlled comparison. *American Journal of Psychiatry, 149*, 82–87.

Alger, S. A., Schwalberg, M. D., Bigaouette, J. M., Michalek, A. V., & Howard, L. J. (1991). Effect of a tricyclic antidepressant and opiate antagonist on binge-eating in normal weight bulimic and obese, binge-eating subjects. *American Journal of Clinical Nutrition, 53*, 865–871.

American Psychiatric Association. (1994). *Diagnostic and statistical manual of mental disorders* (4th ed.). Washington, DC: Author.

Andersen, A. E. (1987). Uses and potential misuses of antianxiety agents in the treatment of anorexia nervosa and bulimia nervosa. In P. E. Garfinkel & D. M. Garner (Eds.), *The role of drug treatments for eating disorders* (pp. 59–72). New York: Brunner/Mazel.

Anderson, G. H., Black, R. M., & Edmund, T. S. L. (1992). Physiological determinants of food selection: Association with protein and carbohydrate. In G. H. Anderson & S. H. Kennedy (Eds.), *The biology of feast and famine: Relevance to eating disorders* (pp. 73–88). Toronto: Academic Press Inc./Harcourt Brace Jovanovich.

Biederman, J., Herzog, D. B., Rivinus, T. N., Harper, G. P., Ferber, R. A., Rosenbaum, J. F., Harmatz, J. S., Tondorf, R., Orsulak, P., & Schildkraut, J. J. (1985). Amitriptyline in the treatment of anorexia nervosa. *Journal of Clinical Psychopharmacology, 5*, 10–16.

Blouin, A. G., Blouin, J. H., Aubin, P., Carter, J., Goldstein, C., Boyer, H., & Perez, E. (1992). Seasonal patterns of bulimia nervosa. *American Journal of Psychiatry, 149*, 73–81.

Blouin, A. G., Blouin, J. H., Perez, E. L., Bushnik, T., Zuro, C., & Mulder, E. (1988). Treatment of bulimia with fenfluramine and desipramine. *Journal of Clinical Psychopharmacology, 8*, 261–269.

Brotman, A. W., Rigotti, N. A., & Herzog, D. B. (1985). Medical complications of eating disorders. *Comprehensive Psychiatry, 26,* 258–272.

Casper, R. C., Schlemmer, R. F., & Javaid, J. I. (1987). A placebo-controlled crossover study of oral clonidine in anorexia nervosa. *Psychiatry Research, 20,* 249–260.

Dally, P., & Sargant, W. (1960). A new treatment of anorexia nervosa. *British Medical Journal, i,* 1770–1773.

Dally, P., & Sargant, W. (1966). Treatment and outcome of anorexia nervosa. *British Medical Journal, ii,* 793–795.

deZwaan, M., Nutzinger, D. O., & Schoenbeck, G. (1992). Binge eating in overweight women. *Comprehensive Psychiatry, 33,* 256–261.

Domstad, P. A., Shih, W. J., Humphries, L., DeLand, F. H., & Digenis, G. A. (1987). Radionuclide gastric emptying studies in patients with anorexia nervosa. *Journal of Nuclear Medicine, 28*(5), 816–819.

Dubois, A., Gross, H. A., Richler, J. E., & Ebert, M. H. (1981). Effect of bethanecol on gastric function in primary anorexia nervosa. *Digestive Diseases and Science, 26,* 598–600.

Fahy, T. A., Eisler, I., & Russell, G. F. M. (1993). A placebo-controlled trial of d-fenfluramine in bulimia nervosa. *British Journal of Psychiatry, 162,* 597–603.

Ferguson, J. M. (1987). Treatment of an anorexia nervosa patient with fluoxetine. *American Journal of Psychiatry, 144,* 1239.

Fichter, M. M., Leibl, K., Rief, W., Brunner, E., Schmidt-Auberger, S., & Engel, R. R. (1991). Fluoxetine versus placebo: A double-blind study with bulimic inpatients undergoing intensive psychotherapy. *Pharmacopsychiatry, 24,* 1–7.

Fluoxetine Bulimia Nervosa Collaborative Study Group. (1992). Fluoxetine in the treatment of bulimia nervosa. *Archives of General Psychiatry, 49,* 139–147.

Garfinkel, P. E., & Garner, D. M. (1982). *Anorexia nervosa: A multidimensional perspective.* New York: Brunner/Mazel.

Garfinkel, P. E., & Garner, D. M. (Eds.). (1987). *The role of drug therapies for the eating disorders.* New York: Brunner/Mazel.

Garfinkel, P. E., Lin, B., Goering, P., Spegg, C., Goldbloom, D., Kennedy, S., Kaplan, A., & Woodside, D. B. (1995). Bulimia nervosa in a Canadian community sample: Prevalence and co-morbidity. *American Journal of Psychiatry, 152,* 1052–1058.

Garfinkel, P. E., Lin, B., Goering, P., Spegg, C., Goldbloom, D., Kennedy, S., Kaplan, A., & Woodside, D. B. (1996). Is amenorrhea necessary for the diagnosis of anorexia nervosa? Evidence from a Canadian community sample. *British Journal of Psychiatry, 168,* 500–506.

Goldberg, S. C., Halmi, K. A., Eckert, E. D., Casper, R. C., & Davis, J. M. (1979). Cyproheptadine in anorexia nervosa. *British Journal of Psychiatry, 134,* 67–70.

Goldbloom, D. S., & Olmsted, M. P. (1993). Pharmacotherapy of bulimia nervosa with fluoxetine: Assessment of clinically significant attitudinal change. *American Journal of Psychiatry, 150,* 770–774.

Goldbloom, D. S., Olmsted, M. P., Davis, R., & Shaw, B. (1994). *A randomized control trial of fluoxetine and individual cognitive behavioural therapy for women with bulimia nervosa: Short-term outcome.* Paper presented at the Sixth International Conference on Eating Disorders, New York.

Goldstein, D. J., Wilson, M. G., Thompson, V. L., Potvin, J. H., Rampey, A. H., & The Fluoxetine Bulimia Nervosa Research Group. (1995). Long-term fluoxetine treatment of bulimia nervosa. *British Journal of Psychiatry, 166,* 660–666.

Green, R. S., & Rau, J. H. (1974). Treatment of compulsive eating disturbances with anticonvulsant medication. *American Journal of Psychiatry, 131,* 428–432.

Gross, H. A., Ebert, M. H., Faden, V. B., Goldberg, S. C., Nee, L. E., & Kaye, W. H. (1983). A double-blind trial of delta-9-tetrahydro-cannabinol in primary anorexia nervosa. *Journal of Clinical Psychopharmacology, 3,* 165–171.

Gwirtsman, H. E., Guze, B. H., Yager, J., & Gainsley, B. (1990). Fluoxetine treatment of anorexia nervosa: An open clinical trial. *Journal of Clinical Psychiatry, 51,* 378–382.

Halmi, K. A., Eckert, E., LaDu, T. J., & Cohen, J. (1986). Anorexia nervosa: Treatment efficacy of cyproheptadine and amitriptyline. *Archives of General Psychiatry, 43,* 177–181.

Hsu, L. K. G., Clement, L., Santhouse, R., & Ju, E. S. Y. (1991). Treatment of bulimia nervosa with lithium carbonate: A controlled study. *Journal of Nervous and Mental Disease, 179,* 351–355.

Hughes, P. L., Wells, L. A., Cunningham, C. J., & Ilstrup, D. M. (1986). Treating bulimia with desipramine: A double-blind placebo-controlled study. *Archives of General Psychiatry, 43,* 182–186.

Jonas, J. M., & Gold, M. S. (1987). Treatment of antidepressant-resistant bulimia with naltrexone. *International Journal of Psychiatry in Medicine, 16,* 305–309.

Kaplan, A. S., Garfinkel, P. E., Darby, P. L., & Garner, D. M. (1983). Carbamazepine in the treatment of bulimia. *American Journal of Psychiatry, 140,* 1225–1226.

Kassett, J. A., Elliot, M. P. H., Gershon, E. S., Maxwell, M. E., Guroff, J. J., Kazuba, D. M., Smith, A. L., Brandt, H. A., & Jimerson, D. C. (1989). Psychiatric disorders in the first degree relatives of probands with bulimia nervosa. *American Journal of Psychiatry, 146*(11), 1468–1471.

Kaye, W. H., Weltzin, T. E., Hsu, L. K. G., & Bulik, C. M. (1991). An open trial of fluoxetine in patients with anorexia nervosa. *Journal of Clinical Psychiatry, 52,* 464–471.

Kennedy, S. H., Goldbloom, D. S., Ralevski, E., Davis, C., D'Souza, J. D., & Lofchy, J. (1993). Is there a role for selective monoamine oxidase inhibitor therapy in bulimia nervosa? A placebo-controlled trial of brofaromine. *Journal of Clinical Psychopharmacology, 13,* 415–422.

Kennedy, S. H., Piran, N., Warsh, J. J., Prendergast, P. P., Mainprize, E., Whynot, C., & Garfinkel, P. E. (1988). A trial of isocarboxazid in the treatment of bulimia nervosa. *Journal of Clinical Psychopharmacology, 8,* 391–396.

Klibanski, A., Biller, B. M. K., Schoenfeld, D. A., Herzog, D. B., & Saxe, V. (1995). The effects of estrogen administration on trabecular bone loss in young women with anorexia nervosa. *Journal of Clinical Endocrinology and Metabolism, 80,* 898–904.

Lacey, J. H., & Crisp, A. H. (1980). Hunger, food intake and weight: The impact of clomipramine on a refeeding anorexia nervosa population. *Postgraduate Medical Journal, 56,* 79–85.

Lam, R. W., Goldner, E. M., Solyom, L., & Remick, R. A. (1994). A controlled study of light therapy for bulimia nervosa. *American Journal of Psychiatry, 151,* 744–750.

Leitenberg, H., Rosen, J. C., Wolf, J., Vara, L. S., Detzer, M. J., & Srebnik, D. (1994). Comparison of cognitive-behaviour therapy and desipramine in the treatment of bulimia nervosa. *Behaviour Research and Therapy, 32,* 37–45.

Marcus, M. D., Wing, R. R., Ewing, L., Kern, E., McDermott, M., & Gooding, W. (1990). A double-blind, placebo-controlled trial of fluoxetine plus behavior modification in the treatment of obese binge-eaters and non-binge-eaters. *American Journal of Psychiatry, 147,* 876–881.

McCallum, R. W., Grill, B. B., Lange, R., et al. (1985). Definition of a gastric emptying abnormality in patients with anorexia nervosa. *Digestive Diseases and Science, 30,* 713–722.

McCann, V. D., & Agras, W. S. (1990). Successful treatment of non-purging bulimia nervosa with desipramine: A double-blind, placebo-controlled study. *American Journal of Psychiatry, 147,* 1509–1513.

Mitchell, J. E., Christenson, G., Jennings, J., Huber, M., Thomas, B., Pomeroy, C., & Morley, J. (1989). A placebo-controlled, double-blind crossover study of naltrexone hydrochloride in outpatients with normal-weight bulimia. *Journal of Clinical Psychopharmacology, 9,* 94–97.

Mitchell, J. E., Pyle, R. L., Eckert, E. D., Hatsukami, D., Pomeroy, C., & Zimmerman, R. (1990). A comparison of antidepressants and structured intensive group psychotherapy in the treatment of bulimia nervosa. *Archives of General Psychiatry, 47,* 149–157.

Moldofsky, H., Jeuniewic, N., & Garfinkel, P. E. (1977). Preliminary report of metoclopramide in anorexia nervosa. In R. Vigersky (Ed.), *Anorexia nervosa* (pp. 373–375). New York: Raven Press.

Moore, D. C. (1977). Amitriptyline therapy in anorexia nervosa. *American Journal of Psychiatry, 134,* 1303–1304.

Needleman, H. L., & Waber, D. (1977). The use of amitriptyline in anorexia nervosa. In R. A. Vigersky (Ed.), *Anorexia nervosa* (pp. 357–362). New York: Raven Press.

Pope, H. G., Jr., & Hudson, J. I. (1982). Treatment of bulimia with antidepressants. *Psychopharmacology, 78,* 176–179.

Pope, H. G., Hudson, J. I., Jones, J. M., & Yurgelun-Todd, D. (1983). Treatment of bulimia with imipramine: A double-blind, placebo-controlled study. *American Journal of Psychiatry, 140,* 554–558.

Pyle, R. L., Mitchell, J. E., Eckert, E. D., Hatsukami, D., Pomeroy, C., & Zimmerman, R. (1990). Maintenance treatment and 6-month outcome for bulimic patients who respond to initial treatment. *American Journal of Psychiatry, 147,* 871–875.

Rigotti, N. A., Nussbaum, S. R., Herzog, D. B., & Neer, R. M. (1984). Osteoporosis in women with anorexia nervosa. *New England Journal of Medicine, 31,* 1601–1606.

Russell, G. F. M. (1977). General management of anorexia nervosa and difficulties in assessing the efficacy of treatment. In R. Vigersky (Ed.), *Anorexia nervosa.* New York: Raven Press.

Russell, G. F. M. (1979). Bulimia nervosa: An ominous variant of anorexia nervosa. *Psychological Medicine, 9,* 429–448.

Russell, G. F. M., Checkley, S. A., Feldman, J., & Eisler, I. (1988). A controlled trial of d-fenfluramine in bulimia nervosa. *Clinical Neuropharmacology, 22*(Suppl.), S146–S149.

Shaw, B., & Garfinkel, P. E. (1990). Problems of research on eating disorders. *International Journal of Eating Disorders, 5,* 545–555.

Stacher, G., Abatzi-Wenzel, T. A., Wiesnagrotzki, S., Bergman, H., Schneider, C., & Gaupmann, G. (1993). Gastric emptying, body weight and symptoms in primary anorexia nervosa: Long-term effects of cisapride. *British Journal of Psychiatry, 162,* 398–402.

Stacher, G., Bergmann, H., Wiesnagrotzki, S., Kiss, A., Schneider, C., Mittelback, G., Gaupmann, G., & Hobart, J. (1987). Intravenous cisapride accelerates delayed gastric emptying and increases antral contraction amplitude in patients with primary anorexia nervosa. *Gastroenterology, 92,* 1000–1006.

Stacher, G., Kiss, A., Wiesnagrotzki, S., Bergmann, H., Hobart, J., & Schneider, C. (1986). Oesophageal and gastric motility disorders in patients categorized as having primary anorexia nervosa. *Gut, 27,* 1120–1126.

Strober, M., & Katz, J. L. (1988). Depression in the eating disorders: A review and analysis of descriptive family and biological findings. In D. M. Garner & P. E. Garfinkel (Eds.), *Diagnostic issues in anorexia nervosa and bulimia nervosa* (pp. 80–111). New York: Brunner/Mazel.

Szmukler, G. I., Lichtenstein, M., Young, G. P., & Andrews, J. T. (1990). A serial study of gastric emptying in anorexia nervosa and bulimia. *Australian and New Zealand Journal of Medicine, 20,* 220–225.

Szmukler, G. I., Young, G. P., Miller, G., Lichtenstein, M., & Binns, D. S. (1995). A controlled trial of cisapride in anorexia nervosa. *International Journal of Eating Disorders, 17*(4), 345–357.

Toner, B. B., Garfinkel, P. E., & Garner, D. M. (1986). Long-term follow-up of anorexia nervosa. *Psychosomatic Medicine, 48,* 520–529.

Vaccarino, F. J., Bloom, F. E., Rivier, J., Vale, W., & Koob, G. F. (1985). Stimulation of food intake in rats by centrally administered hypothalamine growth-hormone-releasing factor. *Nature, 314,* 167–168.

Vaccarino, F. J., Kennedy, S. H., Ralevski, E., & Black, R. (1994). The effects of growth-hormone-releasing factor on food consumption in anorexia nervosa patients and normals. *Biological Psychiatry, 35,* 446–451.

Vandereycken, W. (1984). Neuroleptics in the short-term treatment of anorexia nervosa: A double-blind, placebo-controlled study with sulpiride. *British Journal of Psychiatry, 144,* 288–292.

Vandereycken, W., & Pierloot, R. (1982). Pimozide combined with behaviour therapy in the short-term treatment of anorexia nervosa: A double-blind placebo-controlled crossover study. *Acta Psychiatrica Scandinavica, 66,* 445–450.

Vigersky, R. A., & Loriaux, D. L. (1977). The effect of cyproheptadine in anorexia nervosa: A double-blind trial. In R. A. Vigersky (Ed.), *Anorexia nervosa* (pp. 349–356). New York: Raven Press.

Walsh, B. T. (1992). Pharmacological treatment. In K. A. Halmi (Ed.), *Psychobiology and treatment of anorexia nervosa and bulimia nervosa* (pp. 329–340). Washington, DC: American Psychiatric Press.

Walsh, B. T., Gladis, M., Roose, S. P., Stewart, J. W., Stetner, F., & Glassman, A. H. (1988). Phenelzine versus placebo in 50 patients with bulimia. *Archives of General Psychiatry, 45,* 471–475.

Walsh, B. T., Hadigan, C. M., Devlin, M. J., Gladis, M., & Roose, S. P. (1991). Long-term outcome of anti-depressant treatment for bulimia nervosa. *American Journal of Psychiatry, 148,* 1206–1212.

Walsh, B. T., Stewart, J. W., Wright, L., Harrison, W., Rosen, S. P., & Glassman, A. H. (1982). Treatment of bulimia with monoamine oxidase inhibitors. *American Journal of Psychiatry, 139,* 1629–1630.

Walsh, B. T., Wilson, G. T., Loeb, K., Devlin, M. J., Pike, K. M., Fleiss, J. L., & Watermaux, C. Psychological and pharmacological treatment of bulimia nervosa (submitted for publication, 1996).

Wermuth, B. M., Davis, K. L., Hollister, L. E., & Stunkard, A. J. (1977). Phenytoin treatment of the binge-eating syndrome. *American Journal of Psychiatry, 134,* 1234–1239.

White, J. H., & Schnaultz, N. L. (1977). Successful treatment of anorexia nervosa with imipramine. *Diseases of the Nervous System, 38,* 967–968.

Wilcox, J. A. (1987). Abuse of fluoxetine by a patient with anorexia nervosa. *American Journal of Psychiatry, 144,* 1100.

Wood, A. (1993). Pharmacotherapy of bulimia nervosa: Experience with fluoxetine. *International Journal of Clinical Psychopharmacology, 8,* 295–299.

V

SPECIAL TOPICS IN TREATMENT

CHAPTER 21

Managing Medical Complications

JAMES E. MITCHELL
CLAIRE POMEROY
DAVID E. ADSON

Patients with eating disorders represent unusual challenges to many mental health professionals, in that these patients commonly have physical signs and symptoms related to their eating disorders, and often develop significant medical complications that require evaluation and treatment (Comerci, 1990; Mitchell, Seim, Solon, & Pomeroy, 1987; Palla & Litt, 1988; Pomeroy & Mitchell, 1989; Sharp & Freeman, 1993). Such complications are fortunately infrequent in the management of bulimia nervosa, but they do occur, and on rare occasions can be life-threatening. In anorexia nervosa, serious medical complications are common. In general, patients with bulimia nervosa and anorexia nervosa require routine initial medical screening, and not uncommonly require ongoing medical monitoring (Harris, 1986). The purpose of this chapter is to briefly review the medical complications of eating disorders, and to offer practical suggestions for their assessment and management where appropriate.

SIGNS AND SYMPTOMS

In anorexia nervosa patients, many of the physical signs and symptoms are secondary to the starvation; however, in some anorexic patients and in bulimic patients, they may result from such behaviors as binge eating, vomiting, and/or laxative abuse. (The common signs and symptoms associated with both anorexia nervosa and bulimia nervosa are summarized in Table 21.1.) Generally the most striking thing when one interviews patients with anorexia nervosa is the relative paucity of physical complaints, despite their emaciated state. However, on physical examination the findings are often more revealing, and the state of semistarvation and its consequences are often obvious.

The clinical picture in anorexia nervosa patients is in many ways similar to that of patients who have been starved for other reasons, but there are important differences (Sharp & Freeman, 1993). For example, many patients with anorexia nervosa will indicate that their energy level is normal—an unusual finding in starvation for other reasons, and one that may correlate with the hyperactivity and excessive exercise that at times characterize the anorexic condition. Also, as one can surmise from the diagnostic criteria, patients with anorexia nervosa frequently minimize the physical consequence of their situation, whereas patients who are starved for other reasons usually have better insight into the risks associated with their physical state (Patton, 1988).

Interestingly, many patients with bulimia nervosa report more physical complaints than anorexia nervosa patients, despite the fact that their physical condition is usually not as seriously compromised. Many bulimic patients will be seen by other physicians and present with non-

TABLE 21.1. Physical Symptoms and Signs of Eating Disorders

Anorexia nervosa	Bulimia nervosa
Symptoms	
Agitation	Abdominal pain/bloating
Amenorrhea	Constipation
Constipation	Oligomenorrhea, irregular
Cold intolerance	menses
Fatigue	Swollen cheeks
Irritability	Dental complaints
Denial of illness	Weakness
Signs	
Bradycardia	Dental erosion
Dental erosion	Edema
Dry skin, yellow/orange	"Russell's sign" (lesions
skin	on dorsum of hand)
Edema	Salivary gland hypertrophy
Hair loss	
Hypotension	
Inanition	
Lanugo	
Low body temperature	
Low weight	

specific medical complaints, including such symptoms such as "heartburn" and feeling "bloated." The diagnosis of bulimia nervosa can be missed unless the clinician is particularly attuned to the possibility of this diagnosis (Pomeroy & Mitchell, 1989).

MEDICAL ASSESSMENT

When a diagnosis of an eating disorder is being entertained, it is particularly important for a physician to be involved in the patient's care. This may be a pediatrician, an internist, a family physician, or any other physician who is knowledgeable about eating disorders. Psychiatrists may also be qualified to fulfill this role and to understand the treatment of acute metabolic derangements, if they are properly trained to do so. Any eating disorders program that works with a substantial number of patients needs to include a physician on its team; the routine assessment should include a medical history and (in patients with anorexia nervosa and select patients with bulimia nervosa) a complete physical examination.

The initial medical history should include de-tailed questioning about eating behaviors that may be of particular importance to the medical state, including prolonged fasting and starvation, vomiting, the use of laxatives, the use of diuretics or diet pills, and any use of ipecac (Mitchell, Pomeroy, & Huber, 1988). Some patients abuse thyroid hormone for weight control, although this is uncommon. Questions should also be asked about menstrual function. Patients should be screened for the presence or absence of comorbid medical conditions that may complicate the clinical picture, including pancreatitis, diabetes mellitus, and prior problems with dehydration or electrolyte disturbances. In diabetic patients, it is important to assess whether or not they withhold insulin as a weight control technique.

The physical examination should include an accurate height and weight, as well as an assessment of the state of hydration by examining skin turgor, mucous membranes, and orthostatic blood pressure. An examination of the oral cavity can be useful, in that evidence of dental enamel erosion is often present in patients who engage in self-induced vomiting. Particular attention should be given to those major organ systems that may be adversely affected by an eating disorder, or in which other pathology might mimic signs of an eating disorder, especially the neurological and gastrointestinal systems. A neurological screening examination, including visual field testing (looking for the rare central nervous system tumor—e.g., a tumor of the hypothalamus) is also necessary.

The laboratory examination is dictated by the patients' history, their current complaints, and the results on physical examination, but most patients with eating disorders require at least some laboratory screening or evaluation. Typically, this should include tests of serum electrolytes for all patients (looking for evidence of alkalosis, hypochloremia, and particularly hypokalemia). Low-weight patients should also receive a complete blood count, as well as an evaluation of serum glucose, calcium, magnesium, and phosphorus; liver function tests; tests of albumin, transferrin, blood urea nitrogen (BUN), and creatinine; tests of thyroid functions; and urinalysis. A stool guaiac is useful to rule out blood loss in the stool, a possible complication of vomiting and/or laxative abuse. Low-weight patients should also receive an electrocardiogram (EKG), as should all patients who give a history of significant fluid and electrolyte abnormalities and/or ipecac usage.

Supplementary tests that may be considered, depending on a patient's individual history, include computed tomography (CT) or magnetic resonance imaging (MRI) of the head (when the symptoms are atypical or when physical examination suggests the possibility of a primary neurological lesion); tests of follicle-stimulating hormone (FSH), luteinizing hormone (LH), and prolactin (when history suggests an atypical pattern of gonadal dysfunction); tests of amylase (when pancreatitis is suspected or when evidence of salivary gland hypertrophy is present); bone densitometry (for low-weight patients); and muscle enzyme tests and echocardiogram (when ipecac use is documented or suspected). The use of other tests depends on the clinical presentation and results of the physical examination.

MEDICAL COMPLICATIONS

Both anorexia nervosa and bulimia nervosa are associated with serious, occasionally fatal medical complications. In particular, mortality in anorexia nervosa is unfortunately high, with 6–20% of patients eventually succumbing to the disorder; death in these cases is usually secondary to starvation or suicide (Crisp, Callender, Halek, & Hsu, 1992; Patton, 1988; Ratnasuriya, Eisler, Szmukler, & Russell, 1991; Rich, Caine, Findling, & Shaker, 1990). Mortality in patients with bulimia nervosa is rare, but has been reported, and morbidity in terms of medical complications and psychosocial disability remains a major problem. We approach this issue by discussing each of the various organ systems in turn (summarized in Table 21.2). (*Note:* Medical complications related to the misuse of laxatives, diuretics, diet pills, and ipecac are discussed in greater detail in Chapter 23 of this volume.)

Fluids, Electrolytes, and Kidneys

Electrolyte abnormalities are relatively common in patients with eating disorders, especially among bulimic patients who frequently purge by vomiting or by taking laxatives or diuretics (Mitchell, Pyle, Eckert, Hatsukami, & Lentz, 1983). Some of the deaths attributable to anorexia nervosa and bulimia nervosa can be linked to hypokalemia, which can result from both decreased oral fluid intake and increased potassium loss because of volume contraction,

vomiting, laxative abuse, or diuretic abuse. For these reasons, electrolytes need to be carefully assessed at baseline and monitored throughout the course of treatment. This is particularly true for low-weight anorexics and for bulimics who purge frequently. Hypokalemia can be associated with cardiac arrhythmias; kaliopenic nephropathy and myopathy have also been reported.

The dehydration that results from chronic vomiting, laxative abuse, or diuretic abuse results in stimulation of the renin–aldosterone system, which is activated in an attempt by the body to retain fluid and sodium to compensate for the hypovolemia (Mitchell, Pomeroy, Seppala, & Huber, 1988). This hyperaldolsteronism frequently results in reflex edema, which unfortunately often triggers further vomiting, laxative use, or diuretic use by the patient. This self-perpetuating cycle is common among patients who engage in these behaviors. Because of this, treatment should include withdrawal of laxatives and diuretics. Unfortunately, during this time it can be anticipated that patients will retain fluid. This can be minimized by salt restriction, but cannot be prevented altogether. Patients do best if they are seen frequently and reassured that the fluid retention is time-limited and will usually resolve within 7–10 days (Mitchell, Pomeroy, Seppala, & Huber, 1988).

Hypovolemia can also result in increased BUN and creatinine, and, rarely, in a decreased glomerular filtration rate (Boag, Weerakoon, Ginsburg, Havord, & Dandona, 1985). Other electrolyte abnormalities that can develop may include hypomagnesemia (which may be associated with hypocalcemia or hypokalemia, both of which will only resolve if magnesium deficiency is reversed) and hypophosphatemia. Refeeding early in the course of anorexia nervosa treatment often leads to further lowering of serum phosphorus levels, which can lead to severe myocardial dysfunction and neurological complications (e.g., seizures) (Wada, Nagase, Koike, Kugai, & Nagata, 1992).

Endocrine System

The endocrine system is frequently disrupted in eating disorders, but usually more profoundly in anorexia nervosa than in bulimia nervosa (Fichter & Pirke, 1990; Thomas & Rebar, 1990).

Amenorrhea is required for the diagnosis of anorexia nervosa (Devlin et al., 1989). This can result from weight loss, but the presence of

TABLE 21.2. Medical Complications Associated with Eating Disorders

	Anorexia nervosa			Bulimia nervosa		
	Rare	Occ.	Freq.	Rare	Occ.	Freq.
Fluids, electrolytes, kidneys						
Volume depletion			+			+
↓ Glomerular filtration rate	+				No data	
↓ Chloride, ↑ bicarbonate, ↓ potassium		+			+	
Edema	+			+		
Endocrine system						
Abnormal thyroid			+		+	
Abnormal hypothalamic–pituitary–gonadal axis			+		+	
Abnormal hypothalamic–pituitary–adrenal axis			+		+	
Abnormal menses			+		+	
Delayed puberty		+			No data	
Growth retardation		No data			No data	
Cardiovascular system						
Hypotension			+		+	
Bradycardia			+	+		
Congestive heart failure	+			+		
EKG abnormalities	+			+		
Myocardiopathy	+			+		
Pulmonary system						
Pneumomediastinum	+			+		
Aspiration pneumonitis	+			+		
Hematological system						
Anemia	+			+		
Leukopenia			+	+		
Thrombocytopenia	+			+		
Abnormal cytokines		+			No data	
Gastrointestinal system						
Salivary gland hypertrophy		+			+	
Hyperamylasemia		+			+	
Esophagitis	+				+	
↓ Gastric emptying			+		+	
Pancreatitis	+			+		
Constipation			+			+
Cathartic colon	+			+		
Bones and metabolism						
Osteoporosis		+		+		
↓ Calcium		+		+		
↓ Phosphorus		+		+		
↓ Magnesium		+		+		
↑ Cholesterol			+	+		
Skin						
Hair loss			+		+	
Lanugo		+			No data	
Dry skin			+		+	
"Russell's sign"	+				+	
Teeth						
Enamel erosion		+			+	
Neurological system						
↑ Ventricles			+		+	
Abnormal brain imaging studies		+		+		
Abnormal EEG	+			+		

amenorrhea is frequently difficult to predict in the presence of starvation. Moreover, amenorrhea has been reported prior to weight loss in some patients, suggesting that a change in diet prior to weight loss may be involved, or implicating a psychological etiology. Patients with anorexia nervosa generally evidence low levels of plasma estradiol, LH, and FSH, as well as an immature response of LH and FSH to growth-hormone-releasing factor. These endocrine disturbances generally normalize with weight gain, although regular menses may not return for several months. Patients with bulimia nervosa frequently also report irregular menses, but frank amenorrhea is rare (Pirke, Fichter, Chlond, & Doerr, 1987).

Abnormalities of the hypothalamic–pituitary–adrenal axis are well recognized in patients with anorexia nervosa (Gold et al., 1986; Gwirtsman et al., 1989; Hudson et al., 1983; Laue, Gold, Richmond, & Chrousos, 1991). These patients usually evidence hypercortisolism, which is attributable to both increased production and decreased clearance of cortisol (Boyar, Hellman, Roffwarg, Katz, Sumoff, O'-Connor, Bradlow, & Fukushima, 1977). Serum cortisol levels tend not to be suppressed on the dexamethasone suppression test (DST). Although plasma adrenocorticotropic hormone (ACTH) is commonly normal, ACTH in the cerebrospinal fluid has been reported to be low, suggesting that the hypercortisolism reflects a defect at or above the level of the hypothalamus, perhaps secondary to hypersecretion of corticotropin-releasing factor (CRF) (Mortola, Rasmussen, & Yen, 1989). In most studies, patients with bulimia nervosa have plasma cortisol levels that are similar to normal, although some bulimic women appear to have elevated levels of cortisol with a blunted response to CRF. Lack of suppression on the DST has also been reported in a subgroup of bulimic patients. However, this may be attributable in some bulimic patients to poor absorption of the dexamethasone, perhaps owing to abnormalities in gastrointestinal functioning.

Thyroid function tests are generally abnormal in patients with anorexia nervosa, who frequently demonstrate a decrease in T_3 with an elevation in reverse T_3, secondary to decreased peripheral conversion of T_4 to T_3 and preferential production of reverse T_3, which is less metabolically active than T_3 (Curran-Celentano, Erdman, Nelson, & Grader, 1985; Thomas & Rebar, 1990). This pattern has been termed "sick euthyroid syndrome," since patients are not deficient in thyroid hormones and should not receive hormone therapy. Secretion of thyroid-stimulating hormone (TSH) is normal, with a delayed but intact response of TSH to thyrotropin-releasing hormone (TRH) on provocative testing (Kiriike, Nishiwaki, Izumiya, & Kawakita, 1987; Levy, Dixon, & Malarkey, 1988). Other symptoms, however, suggest a resetting of the metabolism at a lower level, including bradycardia, dry skin, constipation, and cold intolerance. Bulimic patients in contrast generally have normal T_4 and T_3 levels, and only rarely evidence of blunting of the TSH response to TRH (Gwirtsman, Roy-Byrne, Yager, & Gerner, 1983; Kaplan, 1987). Another endocrine abnormality commonly described in patients with eating disorders is hypoglycemia (Rich, Caine, Findling, & Shaker, 1990). Abnormalities of prolactin in the fasting state are found inconsistently, as are baseline elevated growth hormone levels in some patients (perhaps reflecting decreased production of somatomedins). Results concerning insulin regulation have been inconsistent. Antidiuretic hormone (ADH) release is also at times erratic, which may predispose these patients to the development of partial diabetes insipidus.

Cardiovascular System

Various cardiac abnormalities have been described in eating disordered patients. Abnormalities of this organ system are usually of most concern in patients with anorexia nervosa (Isner, Roberts, Heymsfield, & Yager, 1985; Kriepe & Harris, 1992; Schocken, Holloway, & Powers, 1989). As discussed previously, some of the cardiac dysfunction may result from or be complicated by the electrolyte abnormalities (particularly hypokalemia) that characterize patients who vomit or use laxatives or diuretics. The starvation of anorexia nervosa is frequently accompanied by bradycardia and low blood pressure. At times the bradycardia can be profound and is often present despite restricted fluid volume.

Conduction abnormalities are occasionally described in eating-disordered patients; these may result from hypokalemia and less frequently from other fluid and electrolyte abnormalities, such as hypomagnesemia, hypocalcemia, and hypophosphatemia. Cardiomyopathy can result from excessively aggressive refeeding in patients with anorexia nervosa. In both bulimic and anorexic patients who use ipecac, the possibility of the development of cardiomyopathy must be considered and, if suspected, carefully evaluated, since this can be a fatal complication (Dresser, Massey, Johnson, & Bossen, 1992). The alkaloid emetine that is present in ipecac is also associated with toxicity to the skeletal muscles, which can lead to abnormalities on biopsy and electromyography, as well as to gait abnormalities secondary to proximal muscle weakness (Tolstoi, 1990). The weight loss seen in patients with anorexia nervosa can be associated with the development of mitral valve prolapse—a finding that appears to be reversible with weight gain (Meyers, Starke, Pearson, Wilken, & Ferrell, 1987).

EKG abnormalities may occur in patients with eating disorders, including prolongation of the QT interval, which may predispose very-low-weight anorexia nervosa patients to the development of life-threatening arrhythmias. More benign EKG changes, such as decreased QRS amplitude, nonspecific ST segment, and T-wave changes, are related to the decrease in left ventricular wall thickness and cardiac chamber size associated with loss of muscle mass (Isner et al., 1985).

Pulmonary System

Spontaneous pneumothorax and pneumomediastinum have been described in both anorexia nervosa and bulimia nervosa, although the exact pathophysiology of this is unclear; however, it perhaps results from rupture of a weakened bronchial area, which gives way under the pressure of vomiting (Ryan, Whittaker, & Road, 1992). Interestingly, however, it has been described in anorexics who do not vomit. Bulimic patients who engage in recurrent vomiting are also at risk for developing aspiration pneumonia, which fortunately appears to be quite rare.

Hematological System

Anorexia nervosa patients have often been characterized as having leukopenia with occasional thrombocytopenia and, in cases of extreme starvation, bone marrow atrophy (Howard, Leggat, & Chaudhry, 1992; Smith & Spivak, 1985). Relative lymphocytosis is generally seen, but the total lymphocyte count is usually decreased as well (Bowers & Eckert, 1978). Abnormalities of granulocyte function, including impaired chemotaxis and antimicrobial activity, have been described.

Other interesting immune abnormalities have been documented in anorexia nervosa patients, including reduced production of complement of the alternative pathway and reductions of immunoglobulin in some (but not all) patients. Absent delayed-type hypersensitivity is commonly seen in patients who weigh less than 60% of ideal body weight, and variably in those at higher weights. Lymphocyte types have been studied, with varying results. CD_4 cell counts usually have been found to be normal or low, while CD_8 counts have been found to be low. Recent research has suggested that the production of certain cytokines (such as gamma interferon) may be reduced, while levels of other cytokines (such as tumor necrosis factor, interleukin-6, and/or transforming growth factor-β) may be increased, in untreated anorexics (Pomeroy et al., in press). Despite obvious changes in immunity, these patients remain remarkably free from infection—an interesting observation that deserves more careful study.

Gastrointestinal System

Salivary gland hypertrophy, particularly swelling in the parotid glands, can be seen on physical examination in both bulimic and anorexic patients (Kinzl, Biebl, & Herold, 1993; Mandel & Kaynar, 1992; Ogren et al., 1987). The exact mechanism of this is unclear, although it has been linked by some to fluid and electrolyte abnormalities. However, it has also been described in malnourished anorexics who do not engage in binge eating or vomiting. It may take several months after the normalization of weight and eating behavior for parotid gland size to normalize.

Delayed gastric emptying is commonly encountered in patients with anorexia nervosa, and less commonly in bulimia nervosa patients; it may contribute to the postprandial "bloating" and feeling of fullness that are very aversive for many of these patients, and that tend to discourage them from further food intake (Ceuller & VanTheil, 1986; Ceuller et al., 1988; Geliebter et al., 1992). However, there is not a clear correlation between delayed gastric emptying and symptoms such as bloating, a feeling of "fullness," and early satiety (Ceuller & VanTheil, 1986). When delayed gastric emptying is present (and is associated with reduction in food intake), improvement in the emptying rate will take place quite early in the process of refeeding (Szmukler, Young, Lichtenstein, & Andrews, 1990).

The significant weight loss seen in anorexia nervosa also may be associated with what we and others term the "superior mesenteric artery (SMA) syndrome." There is some controversy regarding this syndrome's etiology, its nomenclature, its treatment, and in some circles even whether it exists (Marchant, Alvear, & Fagelman, 1989; Burrington, 1976; Shandling, 1976). Despite the contentious debate surrounding the issue, there appears to be sufficient evidence in support of a clinical picture wherein intestinal obstruction occurs at the level of the third portion of the duodenum in people who are invariably thin. A careful history (eliciting postprandial bloating and emesis) and barium imaging of the upper gastrointestinal tract will differentiate the syndrome from that of anorexia nervosa, though the literature makes many references to patients with SMA syndrome who have been misdiagnosed as having anorexia nervosa (Kornmehl, Weizman, Liss, Bar-Ziv, & Joseph, 1988; Burrington, 1976) and vice versa. In addition, patients with anorexia nervosa, because of their thin body habitus, are at risk of developing the SMA syndrome. Whatever the etiology of the condition, weight gain is curative in most cases (Gellis, 1976; Cohen, Field, & Sachar, 1985; Phillip, 1992), and only rarely should one resort to surgery.

Malnutrition and vomiting can result in gastrointestinal bleeding, which usually develops in the context of esophagitis and erosion (Ceuller & VanThiel, 1986). Also, esophageal rupture or Boerhoove syndrome has been described in patients with self-induced vomiting; this is an emergent, potentially fatal complication.

Acute dilatation of the stomach has been described in patients with bulimia nervosa and in patients with anorexia nervosa during refeeding (Abdu, Garritano, & Culver, 1987). A patient usually presents with the rather abrupt onset of abdominal pain, nausea, vomiting, and abdominal distention. Many times this can be treated by passing a nasogastric tube, but in rare cases surgical decompression may be necessary to prevent rupture.

Abuse of laxatives, particularly those of the stimulate type (containing phenolphthalein), may result in significant complications involving the colon; these include severe constipation and (rarely) so-called "cathartic colon," wherein the colon ceases to function because of degeneration of the ganglion cells of Auerbach's

plexi. This condition may require partial colonic resection (Mitchell, Pomeroy, Seppala, & Huber, 1988). Chronic recurrent use of laxatives has also been associated with gastrointestinal bleeding and with the development of steatorrhea, malabsorption, or protein-losing gastroenteropathy.

Acute pancreatitis has been described in association with bulimia nervosa, and, interestingly, bulimia nervosa has been discovered as an underlying disorder in some previously diagnosed patients with pancreatitis who do not respond to conservative medical intervention (Gavish et al., 1987). In such situations the presentation is fairly typical for pancreatitis. To distinguish whether hyperamylasemia is attributable to parotid gland hypertrophy or to pancreatitis, the measurement of amylase isoenzymes can be very helpful.

Bones and Metabolism

Delayed maturation of bone, decreased bone density, and pathological fractures have all been described in patients with anorexia nervosa (Rigotti, Nussbaum, Herzog, & Neer, 1984; Salisbury & Mitchell, 1991). The etiology of these complications is probably complex; however, the extent of demineralization generally correlates with both duration of illness and body mass index. Low estrogen levels appear to be important, as evidenced by the development of bone mineral density problems in older postmenopausal women. However, the exact mechanism by which hypogonadal function causes osteoporosis is unclear (Newman & Halmi, 1989). Abnormalities in osteoclast/osteoblast functioning and increased levels of interleukin-6 have been implicated, as has sustained hypercortisolism (Biller et al., 1989). Recent studies have shown a troublesome lack of restoration of bone density even in those anorexics who do regain weight (Rigotti et al., 1991; Bachrach, et al., 1991), despite restoration of menses and supplementation of calcium and estrogen.

Various other abnormalities—at times subtle, but at other times more serious—are occasionally described, including zinc deficiency and (rarely) vitamin or trace mineral deficiencies, including pellagra and scurvy. Interestingly, hypercholesterolemia has been reported frequently in patients with anorexia nervosa (Mira, Stewart, Vizzard, & Abraham, 1987), as opposed to other forms of starvation. It has been suggested that this is attributable to diminished bile acid secretion and diminished cholesterol turnover (Nestel, 1973).

Skin

Many patients with anorexia nervosa will develop lanugo, which is characterized by downy, soft body hair on the face, volar forearms, and other surfaces of the body (Gupta, Gupta, & Haberman, 1987). This is adaptational to the starvation; it may be accompanied by a loss of scalp hair. Many of these patients also report brittle nails and dry skin with yellowish discoloration, probably secondary to carotenemia. Elevated serum carotene levels are found in up to 72% of patients with anorexia nervosa (Gupta et al., 1987), although the reason for this is unclear.

The presence of lesions on the dorsum of the hand, caused by repeated trauma in using the hand to stimulate the gag reflex, can be one of the earliest clinical signs of bulimia nervosa; it is referred to as "Russell's sign" because it was first described by Gerald Russell (1979). Transient conjunctival hemorrhages have also been described, probably related to increasing intraocular pressure associated with vomiting.

Teeth

Self-induced vomiting exposes the surface of the tooth enamel to the highly acidic gastric contents (Simmons, Grayden, & Mitchell, 1986; Roberts & Li, 1987) . This usually results in decalcification of the lingual, palatal, and posterior occlusal surfaces of the teeth. The amalgams, which are relatively resistant to acid, end up projecting above the surface of the teeth. These signs are seen in the majority of patients who have been actively bulimic for at least 4 years, and they may constitute one of the best diagnostic clues to the presence of the illness (although the abnormalities are at times difficult to visualize). These changes can also be seen in patients with anorexia nervosa who engage in purging.

Neurological System

Brain imaging studies, including pneumoencephalograms, CTs, and MRIs, have generally shown enlarged ventricles and increased ventricle–brain ratios in patients with anorexia nervosa—and, interestingly, in a subgroup of patients with bulimia nervosa as well—compared to age- and sex-matched controls (Krieg, 1991; Krieg, Backmund, & Pirke, 1987; Krieg, 1989; Krieg, Pirke, Lauer, & Backmund, 1988; Lauer et al., 1989). These abnormalities are usually referred to as "pseudoatrophy" because they generally normalize with weight gain, but they can be quite dramatic when patients are very low in weight. The presence of these changes in normal-weight bulimia nervosa subjects suggests that their nutritional status may be compromised and may have adverse effects on major organ systems, despite their normal body weight.

MEDICAL MONITORING

The nature and extent of the monitoring of patients during ongoing therapy will depend on the underlying conditions and the baseline assessment. However, many of these patients will require the ongoing involvement of a physician skilled in the management of such problems. In particular, the physician must be alert to signs of organ system dysfunction in low-weight anorexics and in patients who abuse diuretics and laxatives.

The most common abnormalities that require repeated monitoring are those concerning electrolyte status and dehydration. Early in the course of refeeding, it is important first to examine at baseline and then periodically to reassess potassium, calcium, magnesium, and phosphate levels; phosphate levels in particular can decrease dramatically during the process of refeeding and weight gain.

Relative to electrolyte abnormalities there is no absolute guideline as to when potassium replacement should be initiated. Generally we start oral potassium if the serum level falls to 3.2 mg/liter or below. The physician needs to be aware of the serum bicarbonate level and mindful of its effect on extracellular potassium. In the case of metabolic acidosis (which occurs with loss of alkaline fluid from the bowel as a result of recent laxative abuse), hydrogen ions will move into the intracellular space, causing potassium levels in the serum to be raised. Rehydration, along with cessation of vomiting and laxative abuse, will restore the acid–base balance and move the serum potassium levels more into line with their intracellular values. Therefore, it is usually prudent to hold off on being overly aggressive in correcting potassium abnormalities associated with dehydration and acute acid–base disturbance. However, in the face of long-standing dehydration and hypovolemic metabolic alkalosis (the most common acid–base disturbance in eating-disordered patients), it is likely that total body potassium stores are diminished because of renal losses as the kidney preferentially reabsorbs sodium in order to retain water. Thus, adequate potassium replacement cannot be achieved until the contraction alkalosis has been corrected by attenuation or cessation of vomiting.

If the serum potassium levels remain low after correction of the acid–base disturbance, replacement is indicated. A drop of 1 mEq/liter in the serum potassium represents a total body deficit of approximately 350 mEq/liter. Assuming normal renal function, replacement is usually undertaken at 60–80 mEq/day (a liquid preparation containing 20 mEq/15 ml is available and well tolerated if mixed with orange juice), and the serum potassium and bicarbonate levels are checked frequently.

ADDITIONAL MANAGEMENT ISSUES

The treatment of hypoestrogenemia, and of the associated complications of amenorrhea and osteoporosis, has been insufficiently studied to allow us to make conclusive recommendations. The use of cyclic estrogen replacement (with or without progesterone) and/or oral calcium supplementation may need to be considered in very-low-weight anorexics with documented osteoporosis, although weight gain is obviously the preferred therapy.

Frequent dental evaluation is necessary for all eating-disordered patients who engage in recurrent vomiting. The use of bicarbonate rinses after vomiting may help alleviate the erosion of tooth enamel, although cessation of vomiting is the goal. Topical fluoride treatment should be considered.

The physician should also provide input into ongoing nutritional support, in collaboration with a trained dietitian and nursing personnel. A diet with adequate calories and with sufficient vitamin and mineral content is clearly desirable. In most cases, vitamin supplementation is not necessary.

Finally, the decision of when to hospitalize an eating-disordered patient can be quite challenging. Obviously, the development of medical emergencies (e.g., cardiac arrhythmias, symptomatic electrolyte disturbances, or significant gastrointestinal bleeding) requires admission and stabilization on a medical unit. Otherwise, the decision to hospitalize should be based on the severity of the eating disorder and on psychiatric or social factors. Most authorities will consider hospitalization if an anorexic has weight loss greater than about 25% of ideal body weight or rapidly decreasing weight, since serious medical problems are likely in these situations. In addition, patients with serious comorbid psychiatric conditions—especially suicidal ideation or intractable depression, poor social situations, or inadequate response to outpatient therapy—may require admission to an inpatient facility. Regardless of the setting, ongoing evaluation by the physician and other members of the eating disorders team is critical to the successful management of patients with anorexia nervosa (Stewart, 1992).

Infertility may result from untreated anorexia nervosa and bulimia nervosa. In addition, pregnancy may be problematic for women with eating disorders. Discomfort with body image may be exacerbated by the changes in body habitus associated with pregnancy; these can potentially worsen caloric restriction in anorectics and binge–purge episodes in bulimics. An increased risk of hyperemesis gravidarum has been described in eating-disordered patients. In some cases, it may be desirable to counsel the avoidance of pregnancy in women with active eating disorders; in any case, good communication among the patient, the obstetrician, and the eating disorder specialist is critical.

In summary, eating disorder patients can be challenging for mental health practitioners in that medical complications are common, particularly among patients with anorexia nervosa. Careful medical evaluation and ongoing medical management are important in the care of these patients; as a result, these patients require management strategies and resources not always available in offices and clinics that provide care for psychiatric patients. The involvement of medical staff members is therefore important in designing and implementing a comprehensive and thoughtful intervention plan for these patients.

REFERENCES

Abdu, R. A., Garritano, D., & Culver, O. (1987). Acute gastric necrosis in anorexia nervosa and bulimia. *Archives of Surgery, 122*, 830–832.

Bachrach, L. K., Katzman, D. K., Litt, I. F., Guido, D., & Marcus, E. (1991). Recovery from osteopene in adolescent girls with anorexia nervosa. *Journal of Clinical Endocrinology and Metabolism, 72*, 602–606.

Biller, B. M. K., Saxe, V., & Herzog, D. B. (1989). Mechanisms of osteoporosis in adult and adolescent women with anorexia nervosa. *Journal of Clinical Endocrinology and Metabolism, 68,* 548–554.

Boag, F., Weerakoon, J., Ginsburg, J., Havard, J., & Dandona, P. (1985). Diminished creatinine clearance in anorexia nervosa: Reversal with weight gain. *Journal of Clinical Pathology, 38,* 60–63.

Bowers, T. K., & Eckert, E. (1978). Leukopenia in anorexia nervosa: Lack of increased risk of infection. *Archives of Internal Medicine, 138,* 1520–1523.

Boyar, R. M., Hellman, K. L., Roffwart, H. P., Katz, J., Zumoff, B., O'Connor, J., Bradlow, H. L., & Fukushima, D. K. (1977). Cortisol secretion and metabolism in anorexia nervosa. *New England Journal of Medicine, 296,* 190–193.

Burrington, J. D. (1976). Superior mesenteric artery syndrome in children. *American Journal of Diseases of Children, 130,* 1367–1370.

Ceuller, R., et al. (1988). Upper gastrointestinal tract dysfunction in bulimia. *Diagnosis, Digestive Diseases and Science, 33,* 1549–1553.

Ceuller, R. E., & VanThiel, D. H. (1986). Gastrointestinal consequences of the eating disorders. Anorexia nervosa and bulimia. *American Journal of Gastroenterology, 81,* 1113–1124.

Cohen, L. B., Field, S. P., & Sachar, D. B. (1985). The superior mesenteric artery syndrome: The disease that isn't, or is it? *Journal of Clinical Gastroenterology, 7(2),* 113–116.

Comerci, G. (1990). Medical complications of anorexia nervosa and bulimia. *Medical Clinics of North America, 74,* 1293–1310.

Crisp, A. H., Callender, J. S., Halek, C., & Hsu, L. K. G. (1992). Long-term mortality in anorexia nervosa. *British Journal of Psychiatry, 161,* 104–107.

Curran-Celentano, A., Erdman, J. W., Nelson, R. A., & Grader, S. J. E. (1985). Alteration in vitamin A and thyroid hormone status in anorexia nervosa and associated disorders. *American Journal of Clinical Nutrition, 42,* 1183–1191.

Devlin, M. J., Walsh, B. T., Katz, J. L., Roose, S. P., Linkie, D. M., Wright, L., Van de Wiele, R., & Glassman, A. H. (1989). Hypothalamic–pituitary–gonadal function in anorexia nervosa and bulimia. *Psychiatry Research, 128,* 11–24.

Dresser, L. P., Massey, E. W., Johnson, E. E., & Bossen, E. (1992). Ipecac myopathy and cardiomyopathy. *Journal of Neurology, Neurosurgery and Psychiatry, 55,* 560–562.

Fichter, M. M., & Pirke, K. M. (1990). Endocrine dysfunction in bulimia nervosa. In M. M. Fichter (Ed.), *Bulimia nervosa: Basic research, diagnosis, and therapy* (pp. 235–257). Chichester, England: Wiley.

Gavish, D., Eisenberg, S., Berry, E. M., Kleinman, Y., Witztum, E., Norman, J., & Leitersdorf, E. (1987). Bulimia: An underlying behavioral disorder in hyperlipidemic pancreatitis. A prospective multidisciplinary approach. *Archives of Internal Medicine, 147,* 705–708.

Gellis, S. S. (1976). Editorial comment. *American Journal of Diseases of Children, 130,* 1373.

Geliebter, A., Melton, P. M., McCray, R. S., Gallagher, D. R., Gage, D., & Hashim, S. A. (1992). Gastric capacity, gastric emptying, and test-meal intake in normal and bulimic women. *American Journal of Clinical Nutrition, 56,* 656–661.

Gold, P. W., Gwirtsman, H., Avgerinos, P. C., Nieman, L. K., Galluci, W. T., Kaye, W., Jimerson, D., Ebert, M.,

Rittmaster, R., & Loviaux, D. L. (1986). Abnormal hypothalamic–adrenal function in anorexia nervosa. *New England Journal of Medicine, 314,* 1335–1342.

Gupta, M. A., Gupta, A. K., & Haberman, H. F. (1987). Dermatologic signs in anorexia nervosa and bulimia nervosa. *Archives of Dermatology, 123,* 1386–1390.

Gwirtsman, H. E., Kaye, W. H., George, D. T., Jimerson, D. C., Ebert, M. H., & Gold, P. W. (1989). Central and peripheral ACTH and cortisol levels in anorexia nervosa and bulimia. *Archives of General Psychiatry, 46,* 61–69.

Gwirtsman, H. E., Roy-Byrne, P., Yager, J., & Gerner, R. H. (1983). Neuroendocrine abnormalities in bulimia. *American Journal of Psychiatry, 140,* 559–563.

Harris, R. T. (1986). Eating disorders: Diagnosis and management by the internist. *Southern Medical Journal, 79,* 871–878.

Howard, M. R., Leggat, H. M., & Chaudhry, S. (1992). Haematological and immunological abnormalities in eating disorders. *British Journal of Hospital Medicine, 48,* 234–239.

Hudson, J., Pope, H. G., Jonas, J. M., Laffer, P. S., Hudson, M. S., & Melby, J. C. (1983). Hypothalamic–pituitary–adrenal axis hyperactivity in bulimia. *Psychiatry, 8,* 111–117.

Isner, J. M., Roberts, W. C., Heymsfield, S. B., & Yager, J. (1985). Anorexia nervosa and sudden death. *Annals of Internal Medicine, 102,* 49–52.

Kamal, N., Chami, T., Andersen, A., Rosell, F. A., Schuster, M. S., & Whitehead, W. E. (1991). Delayed gastrointestinal transit times in anorexia nervosa and bulimia nervosa. *Gastroenterology, 101,* 1320–1324.

Kaplan, A. S. (1987). Thyroid function in bulimia. In J. T. Hudson & H. G. Pope (Eds.), *The psychobiology of bulimia* (pp. 15–28). Washington, DC: American Psychiatric Press.

Kinzl, J., Biebl, W., & Herold, M. (1993). Significance of vomiting for hyperamylasemia and siadalenosis in patients with eating disorders. *International Journal of Eating Disorders, 13,* 117–124.

Kiriike, N., Nishiwaki, S., Izumiya, Y., & Kawakita, Y. (1987). Thyrotropin, prolactin, and growth hormone responses to thyrotropin-releasing hormone in anorexia nervosa and bulimia. *Biological Psychiatry, 22,* 167–186.

Kornmehl, P., Weizman, Z., Liss, Z., Bar-Ziv, J., & Joseph, A. (1988). Superior mesenteric artery syndrome presenting as an anorexia nervosa-like illness. *Journal of Adolescent Health Care, 9,* 340–343.

Kreipe, R. E., & Harris, J. P. (1992). Myocardial impairment resulting from eating disorders. *Pediatric Annals, 21,* 760–768.

Krieg, J. C. (1991). Eating disorders as assessed by cranial computerized tomography. In M. Vranic (Ed.), *Fuel homeostasis and the nervous system* (pp. 223–229). New York: Plenum Press.

Krieg, J. C., Backmund, H., & Pirke, K. M. (1987). Cranial computed tomography findings in bulimia. *Acta Psychiatrica Scandinavica, 75,* 144–149.

Krieg, J. C., Lauer, C., Leinsinger, G., Pahl, J., Schreiber, W., Pirke, K. M., & Moser, E. A. (1989). Brain morphology and regional cerebral blood flow in anorexia nervosa. *Biological Psychiatry, 25,* 1041–1048.

Krieg, J. C., Pirke, K. M., Lauer, C., & Backmund, H. (1988). Endocrine, metabolic, and cranial computed tomography findings in anorexia nervosa. *Biological Psychiatry, 23,* 377–387.

Laue, L., Gold, P. W., Richmond, A., & Chrousos, G. P. (1991). The hypothalamic–pituitary–adrenal axis in anorexia nervosa and bulimia nervosa: Patholphysiologic implications. *Advances in Pediatrics, 38,* 287–316.

Lauer, C., Schreiber, W., Berger, M., Pirke, K. M., Holsboer, F., & Krieg, J. C. (1989). The effect of neuroendocrine secretion on brain morphology and EEG sleep in patients with eating disorders. *European Archives of Psychiatry and Neurological Sciences, 238,* 208–212.

Levy, A. B., Dixon, K. N., & Malarkey, W. B. (1988). Pituitary response to TRH in bulimia. *Biological Psychiatry, 23,* 476–484.

Mandel, L., & Kaynar, A. (1992). Bulimia and paratoid swelling: A review and case report. *Journal of Oral and Maxillofacial Surgery, 50,* 1122–1125.

Marchant, E. A., Alvear, D. T., & Fagelman, K. M. (1989). True clinical entity of vascular compression of the duodenum in adolescence. *Surgery, Gynecology, and Obstetrics, 168*(5), 381–386.

Meyers, D. G., Starke, H., Pearson, P. H., Wilken, M. K., & Ferrell, J. R. (1987). Leaflet to left ventricular size disproportion and prolapse of a structurally normal mitral valve in anorexia nervosa. *American Journal of Cardiology, 60,* 911–914.

Mira, M., Stewart, P. M., Vizzard, J., & Abraham, S. (1987). Biochemical abnormalities in anorexia nervosa and bulimia. *Annals of Clinical Biochemistry, 24,* 29–35.

Mitchell, J. E., Pomeroy, C., & Huber, M. (1988). A clinician's guide to the eating disorders medicine cabinet. *International Journal of Eating Disorders, 7,* 211–223.

Mitchell, J. E., Pomeroy, C., Seppala, M., & Huber, M. (1988). Pseudo-Bartter's syndrome, diuretic abuse, idiopathic edema, and eating disorders. *International Journal of Eating Disorders, 7,* 225–237.

Mitchell, J. E., Pyle, R. L., Eckert, E. D., Hatsukami, D., & Lentz, R. (1983). Electrolyte and other physiological abnormalities in patients with bulimia. *Psychiatric Medicine, 13,* 273–278.

Mitchell, J. E., Seim, H. C., Colon, E., & Pomeroy, C. (1987). Medical complications and medical management of bulimia. *Annals of Internal Medicine, 107,* 71–77.

Mortola, J. F., Rasmussen, D. D., & Yen, S. S. C. (1989). Alterations of the adrenocorticotropin–cortisol axis in normal weight bulimic women: Evidence for a central mechanism. *Journal of Clinical Endocrinology and Metabolism, 68,* 517–522.

Nestel, P. J. (1973). Cholesterol metabolism in anorexia nervosa and hypercholesterolemia. *Journal of Clinical Endocrinology and Metabolism, 38,* 325–328.

Newman, M. M., & Halmi, K. A. (1989). Relationship of bone density to estradiol and cortisol in anorexia nervosa and bulimia. *Psychiatry Research, 29,* 105–108.

Ogren, F. P., Heurter, J. V., Pearson, P. H., Antonson, C. W., & Moore, G. F. (1987). Transient salivary gland hypertrophy in bulimics. *Laryngoscope, 97,* 951–953.

Palla, B., & Litt, L. F. (1988). Medical complications of eating disorders in adolescents. *Pediatrics, 81,* 613–623.

Patton, G. C. (1988). Mortality in eating disorders. *Psychiatric Medicine, 18,* 947–951.

Pirke, K. M., Fichter, M. M., Chlond, C., & Doerr, P. (1987). Disturbances of the menstrual cycle in bulimia nervosa. *Clinical Endocrinology, 27,* 245–251.

Phillip, P. A. (1992). Superior mesenteric artery syndrome: An unusual cause of intestinal obstruction in brain-injured children. *Brain Injury, 6*(4), 351–358.

Pomeroy, C., Eckert, E., Hu, S., Eiken, B., Mentink, M., Crosby, R., & Chao, C. C. (1996). Role of interleukin-6 and transforming growth factor-β in anorexia nervosa. *Biological Psychiatry, 36,* 836–839.

Pomeroy, C., & Mitchell, J. E. (1989). Medical complications and management of eating disorders. *Psychiatric Annals, 19,* 488–493.

Ratnasuriya, R. H., Eisler, I., Szmukler, G. I., & Russell, G. F. M. (1991). Anorexia nervosa: Outcome and prognostic factors after 20 years. *British Journal of Psychiatry, 158,* 495–502.

Rich, L. M., Caine, M. R., Findling, J. W., & Shaker, J. L. (1990). Hypoglycemic coma in anorexia nervosa. *Archives of Internal Medicine, 150,* 894–895.

Rigotti, N. A., Neer, R. M., Skates, S. J., Herzog, D. B., & Nussbaum, S. R. (1991). The clinical course of osteoporosis in anorexia nervosa. *Journal of the American Medical Association, 265,* 1133–1138.

Rigotti, N. A., Nussbaum, S. R., Herzog, D. B., & Neer, R. M. (1984). Osteoporosis in women with anorexia nervosa. *New England Journal of Medicine, 311,* 1601–1606.

Roberts, M. W., & Li, S. H. (1987). Oral findings in anorexia nervosa and bulimia nervosa: A study of 47 cases. *Journal of the American Dental Association, 142,* 482–485.

Russell, G. (1979). Bulimia nervosa: An ominous variant of anorexia nervosa. *Psychological Medicine, 9,* 429–448.

Ryan, C. F., Whittaker, J. S., & Road, J. D. (1992). Ventilatory dysfunction in severe anorexia nervosa. *Chest, 102,* 1286–1288.

Salisbury, J. J., & Mitchell, J. E. (1991). Bone mineral density and anorexia nervosa in women. *American Journal of Psychiatry, 148,* 768–774.

Schocken, D. D., Holloway, J. D., & Powers, P. S. (1989). Weight loss and the heart. *Archives of Internal Medicine, 149,* 877–881.

Shandling, B. (1976). The so-called superior mesenteric artery syndrome. *American Journal of Diseases of Children, 130,* 1371–1373.

Sharp, C. W., & Freeman, C. P. L. (1993). The medical complications of anorexia nervosa. *British Journal of Psychiatry, 162,* 452–462.

Simmons, M. S., Grayden, S. K., & Mitchell, J. E. (1986). The need for psychiatric–dental liaison in the treatment of bulimia. *American Journal of Psychiatry, 143,* 783–784.

Smith, R. R. L., & Spivak, J. L. (1985). Marrow cell necrosis in anorexia nervosa and involuntary starvation. *British Journal of Haematology, 60,* 525–530.

Stewart, D. E. (1992). Reproductive functions in eating disorders. *Annals of Internal Medicine, 24,* 287–291.

Szmukler, G. I., Young, G. P., Lichtenstein, M., & Andrews, J. T. (1990). A serial study of gastric emptying in anorexia nervosa and bulimia. *Australian and New Zealand Journal of Medicine, 20,* 220–225.

Thomas, M. A., & Rebar, R. W. (1990). The endocrinology of anorexia nervosa and bulimia nervosa. *Current Opinion in Obstetrics and Gynecology, 2,* 831–836.

Tolstoi, L. G. (1990). Ipecac-induced toxicity in eating disorders. *International Journal of Eating Disorders, 9,* 371–375.

Wada, S., Nagase, T., Koike, Y., Kugai, N., & Nagata, N. (1992). A case of anorexia nervosa with acute renal failure induced by rhabdomyolysis: Possible involvement of hypophosphatemia or phosphate depletion. *Internal Medicine, 31,* 478–482.

CHAPTER 22

Sexual Abuse and Other Forms of Trauma

PATRICIA FALLON
STEPHEN A. WONDERLICH

There have been many changes in the field of eating disorders in recent years, as evidenced by this second-generation book on the etiology and treatment of eating disorders. Nowhere have changes been more profound than in the area of sexual trauma and abuse. In 1985, there were virtually no references to sexual abuse in the eating disorder literature (Wooley, 1994a), and those that were found were ancillary or casual comments. Reports began to surface in the late 1980s (e.g., Goldfarb, 1987; Root & Fallon, 1988; Sloan & Leichner, 1986; Wooley & Kearney-Cooke, 1986), and the link between childhood sexual abuse and eating disorders became an important though controversial topic in the literature and at national conferences. Empirical studies have yielded differing results, and both clinicians and researchers have struggled to understand their meanings. Meanwhile, women with eating disorders and a history of sexual trauma have continued to come to treatment facilities, outpatient programs, and private therapy. (Note that because the majority both of eating-disordered individuals and of sexual abuse survivors are female, we use feminine nouns and pronouns throughout the chapter to refer to such individuals.) They have proven at times to be difficult to treat; consequently, modified treatment techniques that address the abuse as well as the eating-disordered behavior have begun to emerge.

The focus of this chapter is twofold. First, empirical studies of the relationship of childhood sexual abuse and eating disorders are reviewed, with an emphasis on common clinical and scientific questions raised in this literature. The second focus of this chapter is on the assessment and treatment of both sexual abuse and other forms of trauma, with an emphasis on ways to link the disordered eating behavior to the trauma, and a broad array of treatment techniques addressing the special needs of trauma survivors.

LITERATURE REVIEW

In recent years, sexual abuse has been recognized as a national problem with profound implications for the criminal justice, child protection, and health care delivery systems (Finkelhor, 1994; Larson, Terman, Gomby, Quinn, & Behrman, 1994). Numerous clinical and empirical studies have examined the relationship between reported sexual abuse and various types of psychopathology. Results have indicated that sexual abuse appears to be associated with symptoms of depression, anxiety, sleep disturbance, sexual difficulties, substance abuse, and other self-destructive behaviors (Briere & Elliott, 1994; Kendall-Tacket, Meyer-Williams, & Finkelhor, 1993).

However, studies examining whether or not sexual abuse is a risk factor for the eating disorders have been contradictory and controversial. Early clinical reports noted the potential relationship between sexual abuse and the eating disorders (e.g., Goldfarb, 1987; Sloan & Leichner, 1986), and the prevalence of sexual abuse in several clinical case series of eating-disordered individuals ranged from 5% to 75% (e.g., Folsom et al., 1993; Palmer & Oppenheimer, 1992; Root & Fallon, 1988; Waller, 1991). Clinical theorists hypothesized that the binge–purge behaviors of bulimic individuals may represent efforts to regulate extreme affective states related to a history of earlier abuse (Briere, 1992; Root & Fallon, 1989). Similarly, others suggested that sexually abused individuals may engage in starvation efforts in an attempt to attain a body shape that will help them regulate interpersonal factors related to the abuse, particularly when the abuse was incestuous (Calam & Slade, 1989).

Empirical examinations of the idea that sexual abuse is associated with eating disorders have been summarized in several separate reviews (Connors & Morse, 1993; DeGroot, 1991; Everill & Waller, 1995; Pope & Hudson, 1992). Each review notes the considerable methodological problems that complicate this empirical literature, including varying definitions of sexual abuse, absence of blind interviewing conditions, reliance on cross sectional designs that do not address possible third-variable confounding, and instrumentation problems for measures of sexual abuse and eating disorders. Three of these reviews examined the relationship between sexual abuse broadly defined (i.e., occurring in either childhood or adulthood) and the eating disorders (Connors & Morse, 1993; DeGroot, 1991; Everill & Waller, 1995). The authors of these reviews concluded that there was an absence of evidence indicating that sexual abuse occurred more often in eating disorder groups than would be expected in the general population. Although there was not evidence to suggest that sexual abuse is a necessary and sufficient causal variable for the eating disorders, these authors concluded that sexual abuse may have causal status in multifactorial causal models of the eating disorders, and may be particularly relevant in eating disorder cases where there is high psychiatric comorbidity. Everill and Waller (1995) strongly suggest that more complex detailed analyses are needed to properly study this relationship.

The review by Pope and Hudson (1992) summarized the literature examining the relationship between *childhood* sexual abuse and bulimia nervosa. This review focused on six controlled studies and numerous uncontrolled examinations of the relationship between childhood sexual abuse and bulimia nervosa. Like the authors of the other reviews, Pope and Hudson concluded that the rates of childhood sexual abuse in uncontrolled studies were not higher than would be expected in the general population. Furthermore, the authors identified several methodological problems (e.g., inadequate control groups) in the three controlled studies that had at least partially supported the hypothesis that childhood sexual abuse is associated with bulimia nervosa (Hall, Tice, Beresford, Wooley, & Hall, 1989; Steiger & Zanko, 1990; Stuart, Laraia, Ballenger, & Lydiard, 1990). The other three controlled studies (Finn, Hartmann, Leon, & Lawson, 1986; Folsom et al., 1993; Ross, Heber, Norton, & Anderson, 1989) failed to find a statistically significant relationship between childhood sexual abuse and bulimia nervosa. In their conclusions, these authors suggested that there was not evidence to support the hypothesis that childhood sexual abuse is a risk factor for bulimia nervosa.

However, there continues to be debate on this topic (Wooley, 1994a), and two specific arguments suggest that a definitive conclusion may be premature at this time. First, the three controlled studies in the review that *failed* to find a relationship between childhood sexual abuse and bulimia nervosa also appear quite methodologically limited.[1] Second, the *uncontrolled* comparison of rates of childhood sexual abuse in clinical samples of bulimic individuals to the rates of sexual abuse in large-scale community samples offers a limited test of the hypothesis.[2] We would conclude, in partial contrast to Pope and Hudson (1992), that none of the six controlled studies in their review adequately tested the hypothesis that childhood sexual abuse is a risk factor for bulimia nervosa, and consequently that no strong inference can be drawn from these studies. Below, we provide a review of this literature that includes several studies published since these earlier reviews appeared. This review is part of an ongoing project being conducted at the University of North Dakota in collaboration with researchers at the Medical University of South Carolina. Although this project will ultimately provide multiple ratings of the studies in this literature and an assessment of interrater reliability, this current version of the review only represents the conclusions of one rater (Stephen A. Wonderlich).

In the present literature review, several approaches were used to identify relevant papers. First, literature searches were conducted in Index Medicus and PsychLit with key words including "childhood abuse," "eating disorders," "anorexia nervosa," and "bulimia nervosa." Also, research centers that were known to be conducting research on this topic were contacted and asked to send any manuscripts or preprints addressing this topic. Finally, several articles were identified by reviewing the reference lists in other articles. This procedure resulted in the identification of 54 studies that were completed by April 1994 and had in some way examined the relationship between sexual abuse and eating disturbance. Inclusion and exclusion criteria were established for all studies that purported to examine the relationship of sexual abuse and eating disorders. Inclusion criteria were as follows:

1. Measurement of eating disorders had to be based on an interview utilizing *Diagnostic and Statistical Manual of Mental Disorders,* third edition or revised third edition (DSM-III or DSM-III-R) criteria for anorexia nervosa or bulimia/bulimia nervosa, or a self-report questionnaire with adequate reliability and validity (e.g., the Eating Attitudes Test, the Eating Disorder Inventory, the Bulimia Test—Revised).

2. Measurement of *childhood* sexual abuse had to be based on an interview or self-report questionnaire that explicitly asked whether the subject had sexual experiences with a family member at or before age 18, an unwanted or forced sexual experience with a nonfamily member at or before age 18, or sexual experiences at or before age 18 with an individual 5 or more years older than the subject. Typical measures included clinical or semistructured interviews, or self-report measures such as the Sexual Life Events Questionnaire (Finkelhor, 1979) or the Sexual Experiences Questionnaire (Calam & Slade, 1989).

3. All studies needed to include a control condition that provided a precise test of the hypothesis being addressed.

4. Subject sample size had to be at least 10 subjects per cell.

Studies were excluded for the following reasons: (1) subject selection bias (e.g., exclusion of normal controls whose first-degree relatives had a history of mental disorder); (2) the presence of a confound of the between-groups comparison (e.g., gender differences between comparison groups); and (3) absence of statistical analyses or inappropriate analysis for type and level of the data.

The current review is organized according to several clinical and scientific questions regarding the relationship between childhood sexual abuse and the eating disorders. These questions were derived before the formal literature review was conducted by examining the experimental questions and research designs in the available studies. Although this is not an exhaustive list of the experimental questions or issues that have been addressed in this literature, the questions posed below represent the most common issues that have been empirically examined.

Is Childhood Sexual Abuse Associated with Bulimia Nervosa?

The question of whether or not childhood sexual abuse is associated with bulimia nervosa has been addressed in 13 studies that have been published or presented at national meetings. Ten of these studies have supported the hypothesis that there is a relationship between sexual abuse in childhood and bulimic behavior or bulimia nervosa, and the other three have failed to support this relationship. Studies using three different research designs have addressed this question, which was the fundamental question addressed in the review by Pope and Hudson (1992). The first design compares the prevalence of reported childhood sexual abuse for a sample of clinical bulimic subjects with the rates for a normal control group. It is important that this be a normal control group if the question of whether there is *any* relationship between these two variables is to be adequately addressed. The use of a psychiatric control group would provide a test of specificity of the risk factor to eating disorders, which will be covered later. The two studies of this type that were included in the review provided somewhat contradictory results.[3] Steiger and Zanko (1990) did find that bulimic anorexics and normal-weight bulimics reported significantly more childhood sexual abuse than normal controls. On the other hand, Rorty, Yager, and Rossotto (1994) did not find that childhood sexual abuse alone was associated with bulimia nervosa. However, they did find that in conjunction with other childhood abuse (physical abuse or psychological abuse), childhood sexual abuse was significantly associated with bulimia nervosa.

A second design that has been used to examine this question is the comparison of sexually abused individuals to nonabused controls in terms of eating disorder behaviors and symptomatology.[4] Pribor and Dinwiddie (1992) compared 52 incest victims with 23 treatment control subjects in terms of lifetime bulimia diagnoses based on DSM-III criteria. Although the statistical test of differences between these groups was not significant, and consequently is viewed as not supporting the hypothesis, the authors noted that the 23% rate of bulimia in the incest victims (vs. 4% in controls) was "higher than expected rates" based on previous prevalence studies. In another study using this approach, Wonderlich et al. (1996) also compared 38 incest victims to 27 nonabused control subjects. The incest victims were more likely to self-report symptoms consistent with the DSM-III-R bulimia nervosa diagnostic criteria than were controls. Similarly, Mallinckrodt, McCreary, and Robertson (1993) found that eating disturbance was greater in women abused before age 14 than in a comparison group of women who did not experience abuse or were abused after age 14.

Finally, a third design that has been used to address this question relies on the comparison of nonclinical bulimic subjects with normal control subjects. Often this approach relies on general population samples or college student samples.[5] Of the eight studies included in the review, seven found a significant relationship between a history of childhood sexual abuse and eating disturbance (Bushnell, Wells, & Oakley-Browne, 1992; Calam & Slade, 1989; Dansky, Brewerton, Kilpatrick, & O'Neill, 1994; Hastings & Kern, 1994; Miller, McClusky-Fawcett, & Irving, 1993; Smolak, Levine, & Sullins, 1990; Wonderlich, Wilsnack, Wilsnack, & Harris, 1996). It is worth noting that two of these studies employed national representative samples of women in the United States (Dansky et al., in press; Wonderlich, Wilsnack et al., 1996). One study (Kinzl, Traweger, Guenther, & Biehl, 1994) failed to find a relationship between a history of childhood sexual abuse and self-reported eating disorder symptomatology.

Is Sexual Abuse More Common in Bulimia Nervosa Than in Anorexia Nervosa?

Twelve studies have addressed the question of whether sexual abuse is more common among bulimics than among anorexics by either comparing anorexics and bulimics in terms of reported histories of childhood sexual abuse, or comparing rates of both bulimic symptoms/bulimia nervosa and anorexia nervosa in samples of sexually abused individuals.[6] Overall, there is somewhat more evidence to suggest that childhood sexual abuse shows a stronger relationship to bulimic symptoms than to restricting anorexic symptomatology, although further study of this issue is clearly needed. Of the six studies included in the review, four supported the hypothesis that childhood sexual abuse shows a stronger association with bulimia/bulimia nervosa than with anorexia nervosa (Bushnell et al., 1992; Pribor & Dinwiddie, 1992; Steiger & Zanko, 1990; Waller, 1991). Two studies found no difference between bulimic and anorexic groups in histories of childhood sexual abuse (Palmer, Oppenheimer, Dignon, Chaloner, & Howells, 1990; Hall et al., 1989). In studies where a broader definition of abuse was used (including rape in adulthood and physical abuse), the relationship is not clarified. One study reported more trauma in bulimic than in anorexic individuals (Vanderlinden et al., 1993), but another found no differences between anorexic and bulimic individuals in rates of sexual abuse (DeGroot et al., 1992).

Is Childhood Sexual Abuse a Specific Risk Factor for Eating Disorders?

The question of whether childhood sexual abuse is a specific risk factor for eating disorders is examined by studies in which eating-disordered individuals are compared to other psychopathological control groups in rates of childhood sexual abuse. The degree of specificity can be judged by the degree to which eating-disordered individuals report childhood sexual abuse more often than other psychopathological controls. An alternative strategy for addressing this question is to measure numerous psychopathological conditions, including eating disorders, in victims of childhood sexual abuse. Here specificity is evident if childhood sexual abuse victims report eating disorder symptoms more frequently than other disorders. Overall, there is no evidence to suggest that childhood sexual abuse is a specific risk factor for eating disorders.

Eight studies were identified that compared eating disorder groups to psychopathology controls in rates of childhood sexual abuse or, alternatively, examined multiple disorders in victims of childhood sexual abuse.[7] In the six studies that employed one of these strategies and were included in the review (Bushnell et al., 1992; Folsom et al., 1993; Palmer & Oppenheimer, 1992; Pribor & Dinwiddie, 1992; Ross et al., 1989; Stuart et al., 1990), there was strong evidence that the relationship between childhood sexual abuse and the eating disorders is *nonspecific*. None of the four studies using eating disorder samples found rates of childhood sexual abuse to be higher in the eating-disordered individuals than in psychiatric controls. Furthermore, in the two studies that examined rates of various psychiatric disorders among sexual abuse victims, eating disorders were only one of a number of disorders associated with a history of abuse. Using a slightly broader definition of sexual abuse (i.e., not necessarily childhood abuse), Welch and Fairburn (1994) also failed to find evidence of specificity in their community-based case–control design.

Is a History of Childhood Sexual Abuse Related to More Severe Eating Disorder Symptomatology?

The critical relationship underlying the question of whether childhood sexual abuse is related to more severe eating disorder symptoms is the comparison of eating-disordered individuals with and without childhood sexual abuse on measures of eating disorder severity. Eleven studies were identified that used this design.[8] In the two studies that met inclusion criteria, there was no evidence to suggest that the presence of childhood sexual abuse was associated with severity of the eating disorder. Pope, Mangweth, Negrao, Hudson, and Cordas (1994) found that abused and nonabused subjects did not differ in body mass index, frequency of bingeing, or satisfaction with the body. Similarly, Folsom et al. (1993) found that abused and nonabused eating disordered individuals did not differ on any of the scales of the Eating Disorder Inventory.

This finding is strengthened further when the studies using a broader definition of sexual abuse (i.e., adult abuse) are included. Most of these studies found no evidence that a history of abuse was associated with severity of the eating disorder (e.g., Bulik et al., 1989; Waller, 1992a). Furthermore, in those where there was a difference, it was relatively modest in size (e.g. DeGroot et al., 1992; Waller, 1992b). One interesting finding was presented by Waller, Halek, and Crisp (1993), who found that among

restricting anorexics, the presence of sexual abuse at any age was associated with greater levels of purging behavior. Nonetheless, there is currently very little evidence to support the hypothesis that childhood sexual abuse is associated with severity of eating disorder symptoms.

Waller and his colleagues have examined a variation of the severity question in several studies. These researchers suggest that a more fine-grained approach to the sexual abuse variable needs to be utilized in attempting to predict eating disorder symptoms. Therefore, they have examined how specific *qualities* of the abuse experience are related to eating disorder severity. For example, Waller and Ruddock (1993) found that among both bulimic and anorexic individuals, a perceived negative interpersonal response to the disclosure of their childhood sexual abuse predicted higher levels of vomiting. Several other studies, which have not specifically examined childhood sexual abuse, have revealed other mediating factors between sexual abuse (at any age) and severity of eating disturbance, including earlier age of abuse, intrafamilial abuse, level of negative personal beliefs about the abuse, recency of the abuse, and the presence of physical force (Pitts & Waller, 1993; Waller, 1992a, 1992b, 1993, 1994; Waller & Ruddock, 1993; Waller, Hamilton, et al., 1993). Further examination of these and other potential mediators in samples of child sexual abuse victims is needed.

Is the Presence of Childhood Sexual Abuse Associated with Higher Levels of Comorbidity in Eating Disorder Patients?

To address the question of whether childhood sexual abuse is linked to higher levels of comorbidity in those with eating disorders, 12 studies were identified that compared sexually abused eating-disordered individuals with nonabused eating-disordered individuals in terms of the presence of other forms of concurrent psychopathology.[9] Of the six studies included in the review, five found higher levels of various forms of comorbidity in abused than in nonabused eating-disordered subjects (Bushnell et al., 1992; Folsom et al., 1993; McClelland et al., 1991; Rorty et al., 1994; Vanderlinden et al., 1993). Comorbid conditions associated with childhood sexual abuse in these studies included mood disorders, anxiety disorders, conduct disorder, various forms of personality disorder, dissociative disorders, and greater overall levels of psychopathology. One study failed to find differences between abused and nonabused bulimic subjects in the presence of comorbid depression (Pope et al., 1994). Overall, the bulk of the evidence suggests that eating-disordered individuals who report a history of childhood sexual abuse present with greater levels of psychiatric comorbidity than do nonabused eating disorder individuals.

Are Specific Features of Childhood Sexual Abuse Associated with the Level of Eating Disorder Disturbance?

In addressing the question of whether any particular features of childhood sexual abuse are linked to the level of eating disorder disturbance, studies were examined that correlated specific qualities of childhood sexual abuse (e.g., age at abuse) with level of eating disorder symptomatology in a sample that varied in degree of eating disturbance (typically a sample of sexually abused women or university students). Ten studies were identified that used such a design.[10] In the six studies included in the review, several variables were found to predict level of eating disorder disturbance, including social competence and perceptions of the quality of the maternal relationship (Mallinckrodt et al., 1993), severity of the abuse (Hastings & Kern, 1994), and self-reported features of posttraumatic stress disorder (PTSD) (Wonderlich & Donaldson, 1994). Family stability has produced mixed results as a mediator, with one study indicating that it did significantly mediate between a history of sexual abuse and level of eating disturbance (Smolak et al., 1990), and another study failing to find this relationship (Hastings & Kern, 1994). Interestingly, and in partial contrast to their findings with clinical subjects, Everill and Waller (1995) found only a limited relationship between reaction to disclosure of the abuse and level of eating disorder symptomatology.

Are Other Forms of Abuse or Maltreatment Associated with Eating Disorders?

Although most empirical studies of the relationship of trauma and eating disorders have focused on sexual abuse in childhood, recent preliminary data have suggested that other forms of trauma may be related to eating disorders.

For example, several studies suggest that childhood physical abuse (Rorty et al., 1994; van der Kolk et al., 1991), psychological abuse (Rorty et al., 1994), and various forms of victimization in adulthood (Dansky et al., in press) may be associated with eating disorders. Furthermore, studies that have simply attempted to examine the relationship of the overall level of collective traumatic experiences and eating disorders have suggested that eating disturbance may be part of a larger trauma response (Dansky et al., in press; Vanderlinden et al., 1993). Although this literature was not formally included as part of the present review, there is sufficient suggestive evidence to support further examination of the relationship of a broader spectrum of traumatic experiences and eating disturbance.

Summary

The results of this review provide preliminary support for the idea that childhood sexual abuse is a nonspecific risk factor for bulimia nervosa. Although such abuse may be associated with various forms of psychopathology, it may be more common in bulimic individuals than in restricting anorexic individuals. The presence of childhood sexual abuse does seem to be associated with greater levels of comorbidity in eating-disordered individuals; however, there is not strong evidence that it predicts a more severe eating disorder, although examination of specific qualities of the abuse may demonstrate an association with severity. Finally, a more complex approach to the definition of childhood sexual abuse has helped identify several possible features that are particularly predictive of later disturbances in eating. Methodological issues (appropriate definitional properties of childhood sexual abuse; potential biases in both underreporting and overreporting histories of abuse; and the limitations of a general reliance on small, clinical, cross sectional designs) continue to limit this literature. As is often the case, prospective longitudinal studies of children who have been abused will ultimately provide the best information regarding the relationship of childhood sexual abuse and the eating disorders.

Unfortunately, few empirical studies have examined the relationship of a history of childhood sexual abuse to treatment outcome in traditional eating disorder interventions. One report bearing on this topic has suggested that a history of childhood sexual abuse is associated with poor prognosis (Gleaves & Eberenz, 1994), but another has not (Fallon, Sadik, Saoud, & Garfinkel, 1994); this second study suggests that the presence of *physical* abuse predicts a poor outcome of treatment (Fallon et al., 1994). At this time, however, it remains generally unclear whether the presence of sexual abuse or other traumas is significantly predictive of the outcome of standardized, traditional eating disorder treatments. We would agree with authors such as Beutler and Alexander (1992), who suggest that the effectiveness of eating disorder treatments in victims of childhood sexual abuse needs to be more rigorously studied.

ASSESSMENT AND TREATMENT OF TRAUMATIC EXPERIENCES IN THE EATING-DISORDERED PATIENT

It is difficult to discuss the assessment of childhood sexual abuse and its sequelae without addressing the topic of possible false-memory induction, about which much has recently been written (e.g., Berliner & Williams, 1994; Lindsay & Read, 1994; Loftus, 1993). Paralleling these findings has been a similarly fascinating series of studies and commentaries addressing the possibility that childhood sexual abuse victims may in fact *fail* to recall abuse that occurred previously (e.g., Loftus, Garry, & Feldman, 1994; Meyer-Williams, 1994a, 1994b). This is a very important debate for both reported victims of childhood sexual abuse and their families. However, the present chapter does not address the topic of memory recovery techniques; it is most relevant to cases in which the patient is aware that she is a victim of childhood sexual abuse or some other trauma, without prompting or guiding from her therapist. Therefore, the treatment principles presented below are most appropriate when the patient and the therapist have freely agreed that some sort of abuse is a significant problem for the patient and that it is interfering with her efforts to recover from her eating disorder.

The literature review above has focused on childhood sexual abuse and eating disorders. However, in this section on assessment and treatment, we offer theory and techniques that are applicable to eating-disordered patients with a broader range of traumas, including physical abuse as a child or adult, stranger and date rape, and extreme emotional abuse and neglect. In the absence of data indicating whether or not traditional eating disorder treatments are effective for victims of abuse or trauma, it seems reasonable for practicing clinicians to consider such abuse carefully in their assessment and treatment planning. Clinicians should be alert to the possibility that a history of such abuse may be particularly relevant for individuals with a high degree of comorbidity, and also for those with whom more traditional approaches have previously proven ineffective. Furthermore, a patient's history of abuse may assert itself in ways that interfere with traditional eating disorder treatment (e.g., flashbacks, dangerous and abusive ongoing relationships). Therefore, it is important for clinicians to be familiar with approaches to the assessment and treatment of complications of abuse. Below, we review several intervention strategies used to treat individuals with a history of childhood sexual abuse or other forms of trauma. This is clearly not an exhaustive discussion, but we hope that it will provide the reader with general strategies for such intervention.

The Role of Assessment

Assessing the abuse begins in the initial interview and usually continues throughout the process of therapy. The assessment process may be an ongoing one for a number of reasons. Many survivors do not feel comfortable and safe enough to acknowledge that the abuse has happened to them, especially in an initial clinical interview. Others have not yet named their experiences as abuse because of the silence, isolation, and shame that surround these experiences. Still others feel so emotionally disconnected from the abuse that they are unable to link these events with current distress or symptoms in their lives. For some, the abuse continues and they fear that disclosure may bring harm to themselves and retaliation to their loved ones. Often, coming to therapy to work on their eating disorder is the beginning of the process of understanding the impact of the abuse on the survivors' sense of self, their world view, and their past and current relationships. One survivor put it this way:

> I thought for a long time that what my dad did to me wasn't related to my bulimia. I managed to keep it a secret from two therapists, and I only told because I felt like I was dying from my bulimia and I was desperate.

It was a terrible time for me—I felt like I was losing my father all over again—but now, looking back, it was the beginning of my climb out of hell.

The Initial Interview

In the initial interview, the clinician may explore the issue of past abuse or trauma in a variety of ways, while still being sensitive to the issues surrounding disclosure.[11] It is helpful to ask questions about childhood sexual abuse and other forms of trauma both in a direct interview and as part of a written intake form. More information may be obtained when patients are asked to respond either "Yes," "No," or "Unsure" to questions on a written form (Root, Fallon, & Fredrich, 1986). Interview questions can begin with general questions, such as "Paint a picture of your family in words—the ways people communicate with each other; the ways they express feelings, especially anger; and the closeness and/or distance between members." Asking patients to describe important experiences or people that have shaped or defined them is another technique to elicit information.

After the interviewer has gained a general understanding of the patient's family history, specific questions can help the patient disclose information about abuse. Root and Fallon (1988, p. 165) suggest that the following questions may be useful:

- When you were a child, did anyone ever touch your breasts or genitals, or ask you to touch them in ways that made you feel uncomfortable, "dirty," or scared?
- Have you ever been threatened or physically forced into sex as a child or an adult?
- When you were a child or teenager, did your teachers or other adults ever question you about bruises you received from an adult?
- Have you ever dressed in such a way to hide bruises?

Battered women are often neglected in clinical discussions concerning abuse and an eating disorder. A recent study underscores the clinician's need to be sensitive to the possibility that battery by a partner may currently be present, particularly in women with childhood sexual or physical abuse (Kaner, Bulik, & Sullivan, 1993). These researchers found that the majority of battered eating-disordered women in their study blamed themselves for their partners' abuse of them—a finding with significant clinical and treatment implications. They further recommend a list of written questions to assess the battery frequency, including severity, types of abuse, and attributions of self-blame.

Assessment as an Ongoing Process

Ongoing assessment is an integral part of any effective treatment, and this is particularly true in the area of abusive or traumatic experiences. As noted earlier, the therapeutic relationship needs to be perceived as strong and safe for disclosure of abuse to take place, and this may take a considerable amount of time to accomplish. Studies have found that fewer than 50% of abused women disclose their abuse in the initial clinical interview, even if the interview is conducted by an experienced clinician (Briere & Runtz, 1987; Kelly, 1988).

One of the clinician's roles during the assessment of past abuse is to serve as a "witness" (Herman, 1992), and to ask about and listen to the details of the abuse. It is a statement to the patient that the clinician can, at the very least, tolerate hearing about what she had to endure. Such details may be disclosed only after months in therapy, but may also be part of the initial assessment phase. In these cases, it is as though once patients decide to tell someone about the abuse, the details come tumbling out. Asking how others responded when told about the abuse, and getting the patients' thoughts about who knew what was happening to them, also provides essential therapeutic information (Waller & Ruddock, 1993).

Many survivors talk about the phenomenon of others' "knowing but not knowing." It may be particularly important to ask about specific details with these survivors, in order for the therapist to avoid recreating their "knowing but not knowing" experiences. There are two ways in which such experiences can be replicated in therapy. First, the therapist may fail to inquire about past or present abuse. Second, the therapist may inquire briefly and get a few details, or may have one intense disclosure session and then never mentions the abuse again. This second scenario is much like the childhood experience many trauma survivors relate: They told an adult about the abuse and were briefly reassured, but it was never mentioned again—seemingly thrust into the pit of undiscussed family secrets.

If a patient discloses that she has been abused, the therapist should ask her for more specific information. The timing of this, of course, is mediated by the survivor's ability to tolerate disclosure and related feelings. Possible questions include the following:

- What specifically happened?
- Who did it? What was this person's relationship to you?
- How did it begin?
- What degree of force was used?
- Were you or someone else threatened if you disclosed?
- How long did it go on?
- Did you tell anyone? If so, what happened?
- How old were you?
- Who else have you told?
- How did it end?
- Did it happen to anyone else? (This question moves the blame from the victim to the perpetrator.)
- Why do you think it happened?
- What did you feel?
- Do you feel that there is any connection to either the onset of your eating disorder or its current maintenance?

These questions are a part of both the assessment process and treatment interventions. Shifting self-blame, connecting the abuse to the eating-disordered behavior, bearing witness to the patient's experience, and understanding the development of her sense of self and her view of the world are all facilitated by this questioning process.

Therapy with Eating-Disordered Trauma Survivors

A number of different therapies have been used successfully both to treat the effects of trauma and to treat eating disorders. Regardless of the orientation of the treatment, attention must be given to the feelings of powerlessness, shame, isolation, and loss experienced by the eating-disordered trauma survivor. The type of therapy utilized may be a function of its match with both the patient and the clinician.

Linking the Disordered Eating Behavior to the Trauma

An essential part of therapy with eating-disordered trauma survivors is helping them to understand possible connections between their eating behavior and the trauma. This is important for several reasons. First, the patients may have sought treatment specifically for their eating behavior. Unless they understand how the trauma may be related to their disordered eating behavior, they may drop out of treatment if their trauma history is focused on and connections with their eating disorder are left unexplored. Second, clinical reports suggest that without resolution of the impact of the trauma, the disordered eating behavior will continue, or it will improve briefly and then the patient will relapse (Root & Fallon, 1989). Third, if the eating disorder improves with treatment, but the abuse has not been addressed, other impulsive or self-destructive behaviors may arise (Everill & Waller, 1995). Fourth, observing the connections between thoughts or feelings about the abuse and the eating disorder symptoms may allow for more stability in the eating behavior. It has been our experience that when the trauma is being addressed in therapy, the eating behavior may temporarily fluctuate and worsen in order to allow the patient to avoid the feelings connected with the trauma. However, the therapist should remind the patient that as she works through these issues, she will ultimately gain more control over her eating behavior.

Disordered eating behaviors and other "acting-out" strategies can be conceptualized as problem-solving responses, albeit potentially harmful ones, to a traumatic situation. Briere and Runtz (1993) see these types of behaviors as ways for trauma survivors to distract themselves and to decrease their guilt, dysphoria, and self-hatred. Disordered eating behaviors are generally effective in interrupting these feelings, and the survivors experience a temporary but extremely reinforcing sense of emotional relief. Briere and Runtz's description of the function of acting-out behavior in trauma victims are strikingly similar to Root and Fallon's (1989) description of the functions of bulimia in traumatized patients. Kaner et al. (1993) also outlines the different reactive and coping strategies utilized by battered bulimics. An understanding of these functions is essential for both the therapist and the patient.

Making the link between the functions of the eating disorder and the unresolved trauma needs to take many forms over a period of time. The use of both cognitive and affective strategies can help patients make the connections at several different levels. Journal entries about feelings experienced during and after the abuse can be compared to feelings before and after a binge–purge cycle. Helping patients describe what happens to them when they reach a certain weight (such as feeling more sexual and being responded to sexually by others) can provide an insight into their need to keep their weight at a prepubescent level. The use of an art therapy activity, such as sculpting or drawing the eating disorder, can help patients to unmask the abuse or make important connections (Coffman & Fallon, 1990). As a patient begins to connect the two, she will have less of a need to turn automatically to eating behaviors when abuse-related memories or feelings arise.

Cognitive-Behavioral Therapy

A number of authors suggest using cognitive-behavioral therapy (CBT) with abuse survivors (e.g., Briere, 1992; Frank et al., 1988; Kilpatrick, Veronen, & Resick, 1982), as well as with eating-disordered patients (Wilson, Fairburn, & Agras, Chapter 6, and Garner, Vitousek, & Pike, Chapter 7, this volume). The educational nature of CBT, along with its collegial approach, can serve as a way to empower survivors, decrease their passivity, and provide them with the experience of being in an equal partnership with another adult. CBT can result in both symptom relief and long-term changes in beliefs about themselves and the world for survivors (Fallon & Coffman, 1991).

For some survivors, core positive beliefs about themselves and the world were never allowed to develop; for others, such beliefs have been shaken to their foundation. Addressing underlying cognitive schemas plays a primary role in the resolution of trauma, and the development of healthier assumptions is the primary task of recovery. Roth and Newman (1993) suggest that when core beliefs are invalidated by trauma, there is a compensatory search for a new belief system. The individual can construct either an adaptive or a maladaptive set of beliefs, and, as Pitts and Waller (1993) indicate, negative beliefs about abuse may mediate the relationship between abuse and eating disturbances. The person who has experienced abuse or abandonment at an early age is likely to struggle significantly with the construction of an adaptive belief system, because she has had little experience to counter her negative schemas.

CBT is frequently utilized as a short-term intervention, in which the presenting complaint is treated, but the origin of the patient's belief system is often neglected. However, trauma survivors have intense, unremitting, and pervasive negative beliefs. If the origins of these beliefs are not addressed explicitly in therapy and the roots are not extracted, superficial changes will result and relapse often occurs. Elucidating a patient's core beliefs about the abuse, and issuing cognitive challenges to such thoughts, can result in new beliefs about herself and the abuse (Marmar, Foy, Kagan, & Pynoos, 1993). Core themes in the schemas of survivors include unworthiness, guilt, powerlessness, hopelessness, and unlovability (Fallon & Coffman, 1991). Briere (1989) states that negative self-evaluation, guilt, perceived helplessness and hopelessness, and distrust of others are cognitions frequently observed in survivors. Asking a survivor to list five endings to each of the following sentences can help identify her core beliefs:

- I deserved the abuse because . . .
- He couldn't help it because . . .
- I should have stopped it because . . .
- He did it because . . .

Also, self-report instruments such as Jehu's (1988) Belief Inventory may help further clarify survivors' beliefs about their abuse experience.

Working with a patient's belief system in an effort to make long-term changes in thinking can be a challenge. Abuse survivors tend either to be overly compliant as they seek safety and approval, or to engage in numerous power struggles as they attempt to assert themselves in a treatment relationship that replicates (in part) the power dynamics of their abusive relationships. Common interventions with eating-disordered patients, such as logging thoughts, feelings, and situations related to bulimic episodes or keeping a food diary, may feel intrusive or frightening for survivors. Exhibiting a willingness to process these issues at a patient's own pace may ultimately change the patient's beliefs about relationships and facilitate her recovery from the eating disorder.

Systematic desensitization has been used in the treatment of rape victims to decrease their fearfulness (Foa, Rothbaum, Riggs, & Murdock, 1991; Foa & Danca, 1994). Identifying feared thoughts and images about the rape, a patient works through the experience in a structured, safe, and controlled environment. Foa and Danca (1994) suggest that PTSD is likely to occur if existing rigid schemas are violated by the trauma (e.g., "I'll never be raped") or if new trauma restimulates preexisting memory records of similar trauma. In the systematic desensitization model, the exposure allows cognitive reprocessing to occur. It allows the memory of the trauma to become more organized and less confused as irrelevant details disappear. There is a move from the vague to the concrete, as verbal expressions of shock, confusion, and incomprehension are replaced by realizations of places and events.

A caveat about CBT is in order. If the impact of irrational thinking on mood is overemphasized, some patients become demoralized if they conclude that they must be "irrational" to feel the way they do. Validating certain situationally induced thoughts and feelings can help such a patient understand how the shattering of her basic assumptions has left her vulnerable, frightened, and guilty.

Experiential Therapy: Affect-Generating Techniques

The use of experiential techniques to treat eating disorders has increased in the past decade, as evidenced by a growing body of literature in this area (e.g., Hornyak & Baker, 1989; Kearney-Cooke & Striegel-Moore, 1994; Wooley, 1994b). Experiential therapy has been difficult to define, although many of the techniques have been widely used for many years by clinicians who treat both trauma and eating disorders. Hornyak and Baker (1989) have defined experiential therapy as "treatment techniques based on psychological principles, that are developed and used with the specific intention of increasing the client's present awareness of feelings, perceptions, cognitions, and sensations" (p. 3). Because experiential therapy has also been referred to by various authors as "the expressive therapies," "experiential techniques," and "experiential treatment methods," there is some confusion as to whether this is a theory, a type of therapy, or a specific treatment technique that can be utilized by clinicians with varying theoretical stances. Typically included in the expressive therapies are interventions that rely on art, music, dance, guided imagery, and psychodrama (including Gestalt therapy). Little empirical research exists in this area, although many clinicians firmly believe in the utility of experiential therapy, especially with trauma survivors. The experiential therapies are

particularly well suited to the traumatized eating-disordered patient. Many of such a patient's early experiences have been encoded on a preverbal level, or her memories are so intense that she does not have an adult cognitive framework for discussing them. Experiential therapy, which uses nonverbal techniques, attempts to relax the patient's defenses so that long-unexpressed feelings may be understood.

The therapist must facilitate a complex alternation between generating affect and providing containment strategies (which are discussed later). This sequencing needs to be tailored to each patient. The intensity and duration of affect-generating interventions depend on the patient's current level of functioning, her current life demands, and the type of treatment structure being provided. A woman who is working, parenting young children, and meeting with a therapist once a week will require different intervention strategies than will someone at an intensive outpatient program or an inpatient treatment program. Nonetheless, experiential techniques can be utilized with all kinds of patients in assorted situations. The use of these affect-generating techniques require care and thoughtfulness on the part of the therapist.

1. *Guided imagery.* Guided imagery has been used in the treatment of negative body image and eating disorders (e.g., Hutchinson, 1994; Kearney-Cooke, 1989). Relaxation techniques are often taught as a prelude to guided imagery and can be used to cope with overwhelming affect. Images about early sexual experiences, the family house, the transition to puberty, and recent sexual experiences may be employed to evoke connections between the abuse and a survivor's present feelings and eating patterns. Guided imagery can also be tied into the survivor's cognitive schemas as she learns how her typical images have influenced her current belief system.

2. *Family photographs.* Briere (1989) describes the technique of having survivors bring in old family photographs. He suggests looking at the following themes: (a) How do people relate? (b) Who are the central people in the family? (c) Who was absent and why? (d) When and how did people touch each other? Patients can also bring in any old photographs related to food and can look at the ways in which food was used and misused in the family.

Carol brought in pictures of herself as a child. As she studied the old photographs, they revealed that she was either alone or with her dad.

CAROL. Where were my parents? Where was my mom? My dad? They couldn't both be taking the picture.

THERAPIST. Where was your mom? Where was your dad?

CAROL. My mom was gone! (*Begins to cry angrily*) She was always taking care of my brother or moaning and groaning about her aches and pains. I only remember taking care of her. I don't remember her taking care of me. Look at that kid . . . she looks so sad and alone . . .

THERAPIST. Where was your dad?

CAROL. He was out of the house with his buddies. When he was home, he was either angry or stomping and yelling at my mom and us . . . or trying to touch me or coming into my room at night (*voice gets tight, scared*). He was never there *for me.*

THERAPIST. The little kid looks so sad. What did she need?

The session continued with Carol and the therapist talking about what she needed as a child and what she needs now as an adult. She began to make connections with how bingeing and purging kept her from feeling needy and subsequently vulnerable to others.

3. *Drawings.* Asking the patient to draw a family picture, a floor plan of her childhood home, or a symbol of her eating disorder can open an emotional door that has long been locked. It can also be enlightening to ask her what picture she decided *not* to draw or what was left out of the picture. Drawing, as well as sculpting (see below), can follow guided imagery to capture the most intense or important images (Wooley & Kearney-Cooke, 1986; Kearney-Cooke & Striegel-Moore, 1994).

Jackie brought in her family drawing to share in therapy. It showed her father looking large, the central figure in the family. Jackie, her sister, and her mother were drawn faceless and futilely attempting to run away from him. Jackie spoke of her terror when he turned his anger on her, and her guilt when she escaped and he turned on her sister or mom.

JACKIE. You know, it's still going on; we're all still scared to death of him.

THERAPIST. So the picture captures what it was like growing up and what it still feels like to be with your family.

JACKIE. Yeah, and then I go home [to her own apartment] and throw up over and over and get every bit of their food out of me. It's the only way I can get to sleep.

THERAPIST. The bulimia helps you to survive.

JACKIE. Yeah, but it's not much of a life . . .

THERAPIST. How do you think the picture will change when you recover from your eating disorder?

JACKIE. (*Pauses, tears up*) I think—I hope that my dad may still look the same, but my sister and I and maybe my mom too will be over here (*points to a corner of the paper*), holding hands and laughing and ignoring him. He won't have so much power over all of us, and we'll be strong together.

THERAPIST. How does your bulimia keep this picture the same as always.

JACKIE. Every time I throw up, I give up some power. I feel a bit crazier, sicker, more screwed up, and like I'll never have a relationship . . . just like my dad always says.

Jackie came into the session the next week with what she called her "recovery drawing." She made her father smaller, and drew strength and connection between the women in the family. She taped this picture on her refrigerator, taking down the picture of the thin model that was supposed to help her develop the "willpower" to diet. She also began to take the drawing with her when she visited her family; she reported feeling stronger and less intimidated around her father, and she was able to stop vomiting after family visits.

4. *Telling the story.* A survivor may need to tell and retell her story a number of times. Telling the story to different people and in different ways helps her to process a myriad of feelings and beliefs, and also helps her to make connections between her eating disorder and the trauma. Writing the story, reading the story, telling the story to a group, drawing a picture of the story, reenacting key parts, and describing what was lost in her life are different ways of telling the story. Each allows her to connect in a different way with what happened.

Focusing on the connections between her anorexia or bulimia and the abuse allows her to make the connections essential to long-term change.

5. *Sculpting.* Many clients, at first reluctant to sculpt in clay (perhaps because of perfectionistic expectations), are able to create intense and powerful images that speak volumes where words fail. Sculpting the eating disorder, the abuse, or an intense image of a memory and then sharing it with the therapist and/or the group can reduce the influence of the image and supply healing connections. Sculpting and the other expressive therapies often evoke an intense outpouring of feelings, and the patient and therapist may need to have healthy containment strategies available, such as the ones outlined below.

Adaptive Containment Strategies

As noted previously, effective therapy with trauma survivors involves an intricate interplay between the generation of suppressed affect and healthy strategies to contain feelings so that the patient can continue to function. As the survivor's denial, avoidance, and other defenses decrease, her feelings may become overwhelming, and cognitively oriented thought-stopping techniques or any of the approaches described below may become essential for the patient to have in her repertoire. All of these strategies can be useful in dealing with urges to binge and purge as well.

1. *Relaxation techniques.* Simple relaxation or breathing techniques can be taught, with adjustments made for abused eating disorder patients. For example, it can be difficult for some women to feel safe enough to close their eyes in a room with someone else; they can be encouraged to look at the floor or at a certain spot in the room. As noted above, learning such relaxation skills may be helpful for containing overwhelming feelings associated with the abuse, as well as urges to binge and purge.

2. *Memory box.* This technique, described elsewhere (Kearney-Cooke & Striegel-Moore, 1994), involves the use of in-session imaging skills to help a patient construct a "box" in which she can place her memories and/or feelings. She may decide to lock the box and then to hide it. She may decide to keep the only key or offer a key to someone she trusts, such as her

therapist. The emphasis here is on the patient as the one who is in charge of taking her memories in and out of the box, rather than having them intrude upon her. The therapist may also serve as a container for her memories. Construction of an actual memory box in the session, which she leaves with the therapist or takes with her, can be used. Also, the patient may decide to leave letters, sculptures, drawings, or descriptions of the abuse with the therapist, knowing that she can retrieve them when she feels ready. Patients may express many fears during expressive phases of the treatment, including the possibility that the memories will harm or contaminate the therapist. At this point, patients may need reassurance that the therapist is strong enough to handle the memories.

3. *Multimedia strategies.* Many survivors like the idea of carrying either an imaginary or a real VCR remote control with them. As disturbing images flash onto the "screen" in their heads, they can use the remote control to fast-forward, go in slow motion, progress frame by frame, change the "channel," or turn it off altogether. They can also imagine their memories as stored in a computer, safeguarded by a password known only to them. The therapist can help a patient to think about ways (either real or imagined) to hide files with a command known only to her; this allows her an increased feeling of safety and may allow more feelings to surface. This can be extremely important for a woman who is currently in an abusive or volatile relationship, or in a family situation where the discovery of journals could potentially place her in increased danger.

4. *Prediction.* A powerful containment strategy that can be used with both flashbacks and urges to binge and purge is for the patient to predict the type of feelings she will experience. This allows her to make connections between her eating disorder and the intense memories and feelings connected to the trauma. A variation on this is to have her decide in advance what days or times she will take the time to feel her most intense feelings. She may also be able to predict when she may binge or purge in response to the feelings. For example, incest survivors are often bulimic right after family interactions. Asking such a survivor to predict this and then delay her bulimic episode for 2 hours allows her to feel some otherwise repressed feelings, but then can allow her to escape them. Working toward the eventual use of other,

healthier containment strategies would of course be a goal of treatment.

5. *Distraction.* The use of distraction techniques, such as walking, watching television, playing with a pet, working on a project, or talking on the telephone can provide important distractions for patients when they feel overwhelmed (Kearney-Cooke & Striegel-Moore, 1994). It is important to stress, however, that it is essential for patients to be in charge of deciding to be distracted, rather than to float into distractions and feel lost and dissociated.

6. *Increased supportive connections.* A goal of therapy is to increase connections with friends, partners, children, and coworkers—relationships that are healthy and remind the survivor that she is an adult and is safe. Some of these connections may involve talking about the trauma, but others may simply reaffirm her here-and-now experience as an adult. It may also be helpful to increase the frequency of therapy as a way to help a patient cope with the increasing intensity of feelings and urges to binge and purge, and to allow her to experience a safe, healthy connection with her therapist.

7. *Safety plan.* All survivors and patients with a history of acting-out behaviors should construct a safety plan. Often feelings of wanting to restrict food intake severely or binge and purge follow contact with those connected to the trauma, or are ways to cope with PTSD symptoms. It can be helpful for a patient to write out her safety plan so that she can refer back to it as needed. In addition, having something written by the therapist can function as a transitional object for the survivor in times of severe stress.

It is likely that containment strategies may be needed more frequently in an outpatient setting where a patient is meeting with a therapist once or twice a week. However, all survivors benefit from having a repertoire of these skills, as they are likely to need them throughout the process of recovery.

Group and Family Therapy

The therapy setting may be the first place where a survivor has felt some sense of interpersonal trust, safety, and protection. Although the disclosure of the trauma and its details is often necessary for recovery, it does not necessarily address the interpersonal aspects associated with the trauma. Group therapy and family sessions are two ways in which this relational aspect can be addressed.

Group Therapy. Resolution of abuse and trauma can be facilitated in a group setting where survivors can share their experiences. Group therapy decreases shame, as members are able to empathize with others who have similar histories. Group therapy can also increase hope, as patients see others managing significant distress and difficult situations in their lives. Group therapy serves as a healing relational context—sometimes the first place beyond the individual therapy setting in which mutual, nonexploitative relationships are experienced. Hearing stories of other people often helps patients to experience suppressed affect. Furthermore, hearing others' stories may also provide some important emotional distance for the survivors as they vicariously experience their own histories.

Development of empathy for others can facilitate the development of empathy for the self. Group therapy can help a survivor to see that even though she may feel responsible, she was not actually responsible for what happened to her. One such survivor stated:

> For me, group was an eye-opening experience. I listened to other women, cried as they talked, felt anger and rage for them. Then later, as I told my story, I saw that others felt the same for me. It was the beginning of my realizing that I deserved some tears and anger. I don't know how I would have really gotten that otherwise.

In addition, the specific interchanges that can take place between members can have a profound impact on their recovery.

> In one such interaction, group members were asked to sculpt with clay after guided imagery about sexuality and early sexual messages. Karen sculpted her father raping her in vivid detail, her first disclosure of this experience to anyone besides her therapist. Shannon sculpted a circle with a slash through it to signify that there was no talking in her family about sex. After each had talked, Shannon tenderly reached toward Karen and offered her the "No" symbol, saying, "I don't want this any more. I don't want the shame of my parents about sex. I want

you to have this big 'No' so you'll know that this should never have happened to you." Sobbing together, they placed the symbol tenderly over the rape scene. Both women later described this interaction as one of the most powerful connections in their recovery.

Through group therapy, members can forge connections and experience reenactments of past events and family interactions. These links can provide a basis for future family work; in some cases, the group setting may be the place to work through family issues. Wooley and Kearney-Cooke (1986) see group therapy as the essence of the psychotherapy experience. They suggest that in an effective group, the patient's problematic relationships with others will surface and her role within her family will become apparent. Group therapists and members become symbolic parents and siblings, helping the patient address her grief, anger abandonment, and guilt.

Family Sessions. Helping the patient confront or work through issues of abuse with her family is complex and difficult work. The involvement of family members can be a powerful intervention that speeds up the recovery process if handled appropriately. Many therapists never see the family members who are so frequently discussed in the therapy sessions. Other therapists bring in family members before the patient is prepared for this, and in their zeal create new wounds without healing old ones.

Family members can provide important information about the abuse and the family dynamics in childhood. Relationships with one or more family members may be improved through the process of communicating about the abuse. Family work can help the patient understand more about the story of the trauma and help her "put the pieces together." This can reduce her guilt and help her to reconstruct a belief system that includes a more complete understanding of the trauma (Herman, 1992). Asking family members to attend sessions also sends a powerful message to the survivor. The therapist affirms a belief in the survivor as a person who is strong and healthy enough to confront the family members, and who will be able to handle whatever response is given. It is ultimately a statement of a new era in the family relationships. This era is one

in which the survivor experiences a sense of power rather than shame, clarity of responsibility rather than guilt, safety rather than vulnerability, and connection rather than isolation.

Family sessions can also serve as a symbolic ritual in the patient's efforts to overcome the effects of the abuse. Speaking about the loss and pain directly in front of others is a symbolic reenactment of what was needed when the abuse occurred. In the sessions, the nonoffending family members can listen to, support, and protect each other in ways they may not have been able to do in the past. The therapist can help the family members by modeling this behavior and teaching them how to listen to each other.

The preparatory work done prior to the actual family sessions often constitutes the majority of therapeutic work for the survivor. As in individual therapy, the pacing, control, and timing need to be matched to the needs of the survivor, so that the family sessions represent progress toward recovery rather than a reexperiencing of the trauma (Herman, 1992). Before family members are invited in, the patient needs to be able to define the abuse as abuse and to have told her story to others. She will also benefit from having worked on methods for releasing and containing affect as a means of control in the session. She needs to decide which family members to invite and what she wants to disclose (sorting out privacy vs. secrecy issues). She should also have some specific goals for the session and should have a safety plan in place for the time immediately following the session (Fallon, 1994).

The patient also needs to prepare for not getting what she needs or hopes for from her family. The therapist should prepare the patient for the types of denial commonly expressed by an abusive family. Denial of the abuse, denial of its impact, and denial of lack of consent can often be the responses of either the offender or the nonoffending family members. Preparing a response to each of these scenarios can be facilitated most effectively in a group therapy setting, but it can also be worked on in individual therapy, especially with the use of an empty-chair technique.

Katie, a 23-year-old survivor of years of sexual abuse by her stepfather, was lost in a fog of drugs, alcohol, bulimia, and prostitution during her adolescence. Her mother, Fran, a recovering alcoholic and heroin addict, agreed to come in for a few sessions. She had divorced Katie's stepfather when he was convicted and imprisoned for molesting a neighbor girl after Katie left home at age 14. Katie set these goals for the mother–daughter sessions:

1. To acknowledge the problems in the relationship.
2. To feel some boundaries with my mother.
3. To express my anger and feelings about Fred's molesting me.
4. To become more clear about my mom's knowledge of what was happening with me and Fred.
5. For my mom to listen and acknowledge my pain—as my mother—and to not automatically go on to talking about her pain and bad childhood.

Katie's mother was invited to come in for three sessions rather than on a continuing basis; this allowed the therapist to evaluate both her capacity for connection with Katie and her ability to tolerate confrontation about the abuse. The most difficult goal proved to be helping Fran to listen to Katie without immediately talking about how she too was molested as a child—a story that Katie had heard numerous times and experienced as abandoning and self-absorbed. A decision was made to devote 15 minutes of each session to Fran's childhood experiences, with the agreement that for the rest of the session, she would listen and respond to Katie. Fran also began to see an individual therapist to work on her own abuse issues.

In the family sessions, it can also be helpful to gather information about members' thoughts as to the connection between the trauma and the eating disorder. Asking what the eating disorder indicates about what the family has experienced can be a way to foster communication. Hearing other members talk about possible links between the two affords the patient other views of the connections between her emotional pain and her disordered eating (Root et al., 1986).

Family sessions are among the most powerful of psychotherapeutic interventions. Thought, care, and skill on the part of the therapist must go into every move. Helping the patient to forge new connections with one or more family members can soften the effect of early betrayal and loss, ease her self-hatred and body hatred, and ultimately move her toward a more solid identity.

Medication

Special consideration should be given to issues of medication with eating-disordered trauma survivors. Awareness of the power differential between the physician and the patient, and of how this may replicate the dynamics of childhood or adult trauma, is essential to the establishment of a therapeutic alliance with any patient. However, the traumatized eating-disordered female patient may be even more likely than other patients to project and/or experience the power differential and may actively feel the replication of painful experiences. The "silent expert" approach (Kearney-Cooke & Striegel-Moore, 1994), in which the physician knows the answer but doesn't tell the patient, is more likely to be experienced negatively than a collaborative relationship. Experiencing the physician as a positive ally who will work with the patient to manage her symptoms can itself provide an important therapeutic experience.

Medications can also change the patient's affective experience in the world, and she may experience dissociation, disorientation, or numbing, as she did during the trauma (Raymond, Mitchell, Fallon, & Katzman, 1994). Prediction of possible side effects and how to cope with them allows her to feel a sense of control. Listening to her fears, increasing the dosage slowly, and explicitly giving her as much control as possible in the process can help her to have a positive experience. As in psychotherapy, the pacing, timing, and control should rest in the hands of the survivor, with the physician functioning as an expert ally and collaborator.

Summary

Working with an eating-disordered trauma survivor requires flexibility, a willingness to give the patient significant amounts of control over certain aspects of the assessment and treatment, and a respect for the experiences she has shared. The therapist must be willing to work with issues of power and powerlessness, and must be willing to offer reassurances of safety and protection. The role of the therapist as a witness, an ally, an educator, a collaborator, and a consistent, feeling human being can be exhausting and exhilarating. Recovery from trauma involves managing PTSD symptoms, tolerating numerous intense feelings, reestablishing important relationships, and constructing a coherent story about the meaning of the trauma (Herman, 1992). Recovery from an eating disorder entails taking responsibility for oneself and the eating disorder, establishing meaningful connections, and feeling a sense of personal power (Peters & Fallon, 1994). The assessment and treatment of eating-disordered trauma survivors often strain the limits of our clinical training and experience. It can be disheartening and discouraging at times, although this is often balanced by the transformation that can take place as such a patient moves from being a victim to a genuine survivor, who can see herself as an adult to whom something horrible happened in the past (Roth & Newman, 1993). As she reclaims the identity that was taken away or never given to her, meaningful connections multiply, and the need to express herself through starving, bingeing, and purging is often reduced.

NOTES

1. For example, one study (Ross et al., 1989) compared the prevalence of childhood sexual abuse in a *mixed* sample of anorexic and bulimic individuals to other psychiatric control groups and found no differences. However, mixing anorexic and bulimic individuals in one group is not a precise test of the premise of the review—namely, that childhood sexual abuse is a risk factor for *bulimia nervosa*. Given that childhood sexual abuse may be less common in anorexia nervosa than in bulimia nervosa (Pribor & Dinwiddie, 1992; Waller, 1991), such a mixed eating disorder sample may dilute any potential effect. Similarly, another study did not provide a precise test of the hypothesis because it included individuals in the design who were abused in adulthood (Finn et al., 1986). Sexual abuse of adults, though significant in its own right, may very well be a different phenomenon from sexual abuse that occurs during childhood. Also, two of these studies (Folsom et al., 1993; Ross et al., 1989) did not include a normal control group, and comparisons were made to psychiatric control groups; thus, notions of specificity were tested, but the potential causal significance of childhood sexual abuse as a general risk factor was not examined.

2. Different definitions of childhood sexual abuse, and variability in measurement and instrumentation between clinical studies and community-based surveys, limit the strength of the interpretation that can be drawn from this procedure. Furthermore, the large-scale community-based studies of childhood sexual abuse prevalence that Pope and Hudson (1992) cite in their review also have methodological limits. For example, Finkelhor (1994) notes that the vague probes assessing childhood sexual abuse in his national study (Finkelhor, Hotaling, Lewis, & Smith, 1990) may have significantly influenced the estimate of the rate of childhood sexual abuse in that study. Similarly, Finkelhor (1994) suggests that the community surveys by Wyatt (1985) and Russell (1986) may also be limited by the fact that they were conducted on the West coast of the United States, where report rates of childhood sexual abuse appear to be higher than in other parts of the United States (Finkelhor et al., 1990). As Finkelhor (1994) points out, a recent study using a national representative sample of women and Russell's definition of sexual abuse found a considerably lower rate of abuse than Russell did in her San Francisco sample (Wilsnack, Klassen, Vogeltanz, & Harris, 1994). Finkelhor (1994) concludes that approximately 20% of women in North America have experienced contact *or* noncontact childhood sexual abuse, thus representing a rough estimate for Pope and Hudson's (1992) "intermediate" definition of childhood sexual abuse. Clearly, controlled national representative studies with appropriate methodologies will clarify many of these problems. Two such studies are reviewed later in this chapter.

3. Of the four identified studies that have employed this design, two were excluded because of either potential bias in the recruitment of the control groups (Stuart et al., 1990), or uncertainty about whether or not the sexual abuse took place in childhood (Vanderlinden, Vandereycken, van Dyck, & Vertommen, 1993).

4. Of the four studies that have utilized this design, one was excluded for including subjects with adult-onset abuse in the abused group (Finn et al., 1986).

5. Of the 12 studies that have utilized this design, three were excluded because of a lack of clarity regarding the definition of childhood sexual abuse (Bailley & Gibbons, 1989; Beckman & Burns, 1990; van der Kolk, Perry, & Herman, 1991). One study (Welch & Fairburn, 1994), although using a strong methodology, was also excluded because the abuse did not necessarily occur during childhood.

6. For the present review, six of these studies were excluded because they either did not report a clear statistical comparison of anorexic and bulimic individuals (Folsom et al., 1993; McClelland, Mynor-Wallis, Fahy, & Treasure, 1991; Vanderlinden et al., 1993), used definitions of sexual abuse that were not specific to childhood (DeGroot, Kennedy, Rodin, & McVey, 1992; van der Kolk et al., 1991), lacked adequate sample size (Herzog, Staley, Carmody, Robbins, & van der Kolk, 1993), or did not clearly sepa-

rate childhood sexual abuse from other forms of psychological trauma (Vanderlinden et al., 1993).

7. Two studies were excluded because either they did not focus specifically on childhood sexual abuse (Welch & Fairburn, 1994), or there was a significant confound between the two comparison groups (Hall et al., 1989).

8. Nine of these studies were excluded for reasons including abuse definitions that were not specific to childhood (Bulik, Sullivan, & Rorty, 1989; Dansky et al., 1993; DeGroot et al., 1992; Pitts & Waller, 1993; Waller, 1992a, 1992b; Waller, Halek, & Crisp, 1993; Waller, Hamilton, Rose, Sumra, & Baldwin, 1993), the combination of physical abuse and sexual abuse into one abuse category (Fullerton, Wonderlich, & Gosnell, 1995), and an absence of a statistical test of the critical comparison (Pitts & Waller, 1993).

9. Twelve studies were examined in the review, but six were not included because of either definitions of abuse that did not fit the criteria for the study (Bulik et al., 1989; Dansky et al., in press; Fullerton, et al., 1995; Waller, 1993; Wonderlich & Swift, 1990) or inadequate sample size (Herzog et al., 1993).

10. Four of these studies were not included in the review because they either had inadequate sample size (Williams, Wagner, & Calam, 1992) or did not clearly represent childhood sexual abuse (Abramson & Lucido, 1991; Byram, Wagner, & Waller, 1994).

11. Therapists engaging in clinical practice of any kind should be familiar with state and national guidelines and laws relating to informed consent and mandatory reporting of abuse. A written statement detailing the limits of confidentiality should be provided to each patient and discussed at the beginning of treatment. This is particularly important for an individual with a current or past history of abuse, as disclosures in therapy may necessitate the breaking of therapist–patient confidentiality in order to ensure the safety of the individual or others who may be victims of the offender.

REFERENCES

Abramson, E. A., & Lucido, G. M. (1991). Childhood sexual experience and bulimia. *Addictive Behaviors, 16,* 529–532.

Bailley, C. A., & Gibbons, S. G. (1989). Physical victimization and bulimic-like symptoms: Is there a relationship? *Deviant Behavior, 10,* 335–352.

Beckman, K. A., & Burns, G. L. (1990). Relation of sexual abuse and bulimia in college women. *International Journal of Eating Disorders, 9,* 487–492.

Berliner, L., & Meyer-Williams, L. (1994). Memories of childhood sexual abuse: A response to Lindsey and Read. *Applied Cognitive Psychology, 8,* 379–387.

Beutler, L. E., & Hill, C. E. (1992). Process and outcome research in the treatment of adult victims of childhood sexual abuse: Methodological issues. *Journal of Consulting and Clinical Psychology, 60,* 204–212.

Briere, J. N. (1989). *Therapy for adults molested as children: Beyond survival.* New York: Springer.

Briere, J. N. (1992). *Child abuse trauma.* Newbury Park, CA: Sage.

Briere, J. N., & Elliot, D. M. (1994). Immediate and long term impacts of child sexual abuse. *Sexual Abuse of Children, 4,* 54–70.

Briere, J. N., & Runtz, M. (1987). Post sexual abuse trauma: Data and implications for clinical practice. *Journal of Interpersonal Violence, 2,* 367–379.

Briere, J. N., & Runtz, M. (1993). Childhood sexual abuse: Long term sequeloe and implications for psychological assessment. *Journal of Interpersonal Violence, 8(3),* 312–330.

Bulik, C. M., Sullivan, P. F., & Rorty, M. (1989). Childhood sexual abuse in women with bulimia. *Journal of Clinical Psychiatry, 50,* 460–464.

Bushnell, J. A., Wells, J. E., & Oakley-Browne, M. A. (1992). Long term effects of introfamilial sexual abuse in childhood. *Acta Psychiatrica Scandinavica, 85,* 136–142.

Byram, V., Wagner, H. L., & Waller, G. (1994). Sexual abuse and body image distortion. *Child Abuse and Neglect, 19,* 507–510.

Calam, R. M., & Slade, P. D. (1989). Sexual experiences and eating problems in female undergraduates. *International Journal of Eating Disorders, 8,* 391–397.

Coffman, S., & Fallon, P. (1990). Unmasking and treating victimization in women: Cognitive and nonverbal approaches. In P. Keller & S. Heyman (Eds.), *Innovations in clinical practice: A sourcebook* (Vol. 9, pp. 45–60). Sarasota, FL: Professional Resource Exchange.

Connors, M. E., & Morse, W. (1993). Sexual abuse and eating disorders: A review. *International Journal of Eating Disorders, 13,* 1–11.

Dansky, B. S., Brewerton, T. D., O'Neil, P. M., & Kilpatrick, D. G. (in press). The national women's study: Relationship of victimization and PTSD to bulimia nervosa. *International Journal of Eating Disorders.*

DeGroot, J. M. (1991). *Correlation between eating disorders and prior sexual abuse: Theory, evidence and future directions.* Paper presented at the North American Scientific Symposium on Eating Disorders in Adolescence, Seattle.

DeGroot, J. M., Kennedy, S., Rodin, G., & McVey, G. (1992). Correlates of sexual abuse in women with anorexia nervosa and bulimia nervosa. *Canadian Journal of Psychiatry, 37,* 516–518.

Everill, J., & Waller, G. (1994). Reported sexual abuse and eating psychopathology: A review of the evidence for a causal link. *International Journal of Eating Disorders, 18,* 1–12.

Everill, J., & Waller, G. (1995). Disclosure of sexual abuse and psychological adjustment in female undergraduates. *Child Abuse and Neglect, 19,* 93–100.

Fallon, B. A., Sadik, C., Saoud, J. B., & Garfinkel, R. S. (1994). Childhood abuse, family environment and outcome in bulimia nervosa. *Journal of Clinical Psychiatry, 55,* 424–428.

Fallon, P. (1994). Family therapy and the traumatized eating-disordered patient. In P. Fallon (Chair), *The Traumatized Eating Disordered Patient,* Plenary symposium presented at the Sixth Annual International Conference on Eating Disorders, New York.

Fallon, P., & Coffman, S. (1991). Cognitive-behavioral treatment of survivors of victimization. *Psychotherapy in Private Practice, 9(3),* 53–65.

Finkelhor, D. (1979). *Sexually victimized children.* New York: Free Press.

Finkelhor, D. (1994). Current information on the scope and nature of child sexual abuse. *Sexual Abuse of Children, 4,* 31–54.

Finkelhor, D., Hotaling, G., Lewis, I. A., & Smith, C. (1990). Sexual abuse in a national survey of adult men and women: Prevalence, characteristics and risk factors. *Child Abuse and Neglect, 14,* 19–28.

Finn, S. E., Hartman, M., Leon, G. R., & Lawson, L. (1986). Eating disorders and sexual abuse: Lack of confirmation for a clinical hypothesis. *International Journal of Eating Disorders, 5,* 1051–1060.

Foa, E., & Danca, C. (1994). *Cognitive-behavioral treatments for women with PTSD following sexual assault.* Workshop presented at the 28th Annual Convention of the Association for Advancement of Behavior Therapy, San Diego.

Foa, E., Rothbaum, B., Riggs, D., & Murdock, T. (1991). Treatment of posttraumatic stress disorder in rape victims: A comparison between cognitive-behavioral procedures and counseling. *Journal of Consulting and Clinical Psychology, 5,* 715–723.

Folsom, V., Krahn, D., Nairn, K., Gold, L., Demitrack, M. A., & Silk, K. R. (1993). The impact of sexual and physical abuse on eating disordered and psychiatric symptoms: A comparison of eating disordered and psychiatric inpatients. *International Journal of Eating Disorders, 13,* 249–257.

Frank, E., Anderson, B., Stewart, B. D., Dancu, C., Hughes, C., & West, D. (1988). Efficacy of cognitive behavior therapy and systematic desensitization in the treatment of rape trauma. *Behavior Therapy, 19,* 403–420.

Fullerton, D. T., Wonderlich, S. A., & Gosnell, B. A. (1995). Clinical characteristics of eating disorder patients who report sexual or physical abuse. *International Journal of Eating Disorders, 17,* 243–249.

Gleaves, D. H., & Eberenz, D. H. (1994). Sexual abuse histories among treatment resistant bulimia nervosa patients. *International Journal of Eating Disorders, 15,* 227–232.

Goldfarb, L. A. (1987). Sexual abuse antecedent to anorexia nervosa, bulimia and compulsive overeating: Three case reports. *International Journal of Eating Disorders, 6,* 675–680.

Hall, R. C. W., Tice, L., Beresford, T. P., Wooley, B., & Hall, A. K. (1989). Sexual Abuse in patients with anorexia nervosa and bulimia. *Psychosomatics, 30,* 73–79.

Hastings, T., & Kern, J. M. (1994). Relationships between bulimia, childhood sexual abuse and family environment. *International Journal of Eating Disorders, 15,* 103–111.

Herman, J. L. (1992). *Trauma and recovery.* New York: Basic Books.

Herzog, D. B., Staley, J. E., Carmody, S., Robbins, W. M., & van der Kolk, B. A. (1993). Childhood sexual abuse in anorexia nervosa and bulimia nervosa: A pilot study. *Journal of the American Academy of Child and Adolescent Psychiatry, 32,* 962–966.

Hornyak, L., & Baker, E. (Eds.). (1989). *Experiential therapies for eating disorders.* New York: Guilford Press.

Hutchinson, M. (1994). Imagining ourselves whole: A feminist approach to treating body image disorders. In P. Fallon, M. Katzman, & S. Wooley (Eds.), *Feminist perspectives on eating disorders* (pp. 152–168). New York: Guilford Press.

Jehu, D. (1988). *Beyond sexual abuse: Therapy with women who were childhood victims.* Chichester, England: Wiley.

Kaner, A., Bulik, C., & Sullivan, P. (1993). Abuse in adult relationships of bulimic women. *Journal of Interpersonal Violence, 8*(1), 52–63.

Kearney-Cooke, A. (1989). Reclaiming the body: Using guided imagery in the treatment of body image disturbances among bulimic women. In L. Hornyak & E. Baker (Eds.), *Experiential therapies for eating disorders* (pp. 11–33). New York: Guilford Press.

Kearney-Cooke, A., & Striegel-Moore, R. (1994). Treatment of childhood sexual abuse in anorexia nervosa and bulimia nervosa: A feminist psychodynamic approach. *International Journal of Eating Disorders, 15*(4), 305–319.

Kelly, L. (1988). How women define their experiences of violence. In L. Yllo & M. Bogard (Eds.), *Feminist perspectives on wife abuse* (pp. 114–132). Newbury Park, CA: Sage.

Kendall-Tackett, K. A., Meyer-Williams, L., & Finkelhor, D (1993). Impact of sexual abuse on children: a review and synthesis of recent empirical studies. *Psychological Bulletin, 113,* 164–180.

Kilpatrick, D. G., Veronen, L. J., & Resick, P. A. (1982). Psychological sequelae to rape: Assessment and treatment strategies. In D.M. Doleys, R.L. Meredith, & A.R. Ciminero (Eds.), *Behavioral medicine: Assessment and treatment strategies* (pp. 473–497). New York: Plenum Press.

Kinzl, J. F., Traweger, C., Guenther, V., & Biehl, W. (1994). Family background and sexual abuse with eating disorders. *American Journal of Psychiatry, 151,* 1127–1131.

Larson, C. S., Terman, D. L., Gomby, D. S., Quinn, L. S., & Behrman, R. E. (1994). Sexual abuse of children: Recommendations and analyses. *Sexual Abuse of Children, 4,* 4–30.

Lindsay, D. S., & Read, J. D. (1994). Psychotherapy and memories of childhood sexual abuse: A cognitive perspective. *Applied Cognitive Psychology, 8,* 281–338.

Loftus, E. F. (1993). The reality of repressed memories. *American Psychologist, 48,* 518–537.

Loftus, E. F., Garry, M., & Feldman, J. (1994). Forgetting sexual trauma: What does it mean when 38% forget? *Journal of Consulting and Clinical Psychology, 62,* 1177–1181.

Mallinckrodt, B., McCreary, B. A., & Robertson, A. K. (1993). Co-occurrence of eating disorders and incest: The role of attachment, family environment and social competencies. In B. Mallinckrodt (Chair), *Incest and eating disorders co-occurrence: Family environment and social sompetencies.* Symposium conducted at the meeting of the American Psychological Association, Toronto.

Marmar, C., Foy, D., Kagan, B., & Pynoos, R. (1993). An integrated approach for treating post-traumatic stress. *American Psychiatric Press review of psychiatry* (Vol. 12, pp. 239–272). Washington, DC: American Psychiatric Press.

McClelland, L., Mynor-Wallis, L., Fahy, T., & Treasure, J. (1991). Sexual abuse, disordered personality, and eating disorders. *British Journal of Psychiatry, 158,* 63–68.

Meyer-Williams, L. (1994a). Recall of childhood memories: A prospective study of women's memories of child sexual abuse. *Journal of Consulting and Clinical Psychology, 62,* 1167–1176.

Meyer-Williams, L. (1994b). What does it mean to forget child sexual abuse? A reply to Loftus, Garry, & Feldman

(1994). *Journal of Consulting and Clinical Psychology*, 62, 1182–1186.

Miller, D. A. F., McClusky-Fawcett, K., & Irving, L. M. (1993). The relationship between childhood sexual abuse and subsequent onset of bulimia nervosa. *Child Abuse and Neglect*, 17, 305–314.

Palmer, R. L., & Oppenhiemer, R. (1992). Childhood sexual experiences with adults: A comparison of women with eating disorders and those with other diagnoses. *International Journal of Eating Disorders*, 12, 359–364.

Palmer, R. L., Oppenheimer, R., Dignon, A., Chalmer, D. A., & Howells, K. (1990). Childhood sexual experiences with adults reported by women with eating disorders: An extended series. *British Journal of Psychiatry*, 156, 699–703.

Peters, L., & Fallon, P. (1994). The journey of recovery: Dimensions of change. In P. Fallon, M. Katzman, & S. Wooley (Eds.), *Feminist perspectives on eating disorders* (pp. 339–354). New York: Guilford Press.

Pitts, C., & Waller, G. (1993). Self denigratory beliefs following sexual abuse: Association with the symptomatology of bulimic disorders. *International Journal of Eating Disorders*, 13, 407–410.

Pope, H. G., & Hudson, J. I. (1992). Is childhood sexual abuse a risk factor for bulimia nervosa? *American Journal of Psychiatry*, 149, 455–463.

Pope, H. G., Mangweth, B., Negrao, A. B., Hudson, J. I., & Cordas, T. A. (1994). Childhood sexual abuse and bulimia nervosa: A comparison of American, Austrian and Brazilian women. *American Journal of Psychiatry*, 151, 732–737.

Pribor, E. F., & Dinwiddie, S. H. (1992). Psychiatric correlates of incest in childhood. *American Journal of Psychiatry*, 149, 52–56.

Raymond, N., Mitchell, J., Fallon, P., & Katzman, M. (1994). A collaborative approach to the use of medication. In P. Fallon, M. Katzman, & S. Wooley (Eds.), *Feminist perspectives on eating disorders* (pp. 231–250). New York: Guilford Press.

Root, M., & Fallon, P. (1988). The incidence of victimization experiences in a bulimic sample. *Journal of Interpersonal Violence*, 3(2), 161–173.

Root, M., & Fallon, P. (1989). Treating the victimized bulimic: The functions of binge-purge behavior. *Journal of Interpersonal Violence*, 4, 90–100.

Root, M., Fallon, P., & Friedrich, W. (1986). *Bulimia: A systems approach to treatment*. New York: Norton.

Rorty, M., Yager, J., & Rossotto, E. (1994). Childhood sexual, physical and psychological abuse in bulimia nervosa. *American Journal of Psychiatry*, 151, 1122–1126.

Ross, C. A., Heber, S., Norton, G. R., & Anderson, G. (1989). Differences between multiple personality disorder and other diagnostic groups on structured interview. *Journal of Nervous and Mental Disease*, 177, 487–491.

Roth, S., & Newman, E. (1993). The process of coping with incest for adult survivors. *Journal of Interpersonal Violence*, 8, 363–377.

Russell, D. (1986). *The secret trauma: Incest in the lives of girls and women*. New York: Basic Books.

Sloan, G., & Leichner, P. (1986). Is there a relationship between sexual abuse or incest and eating disorders? *Canadian Journal of Psychiatry*, 31, 656–660.

Smolak, L., Levine, M., & Sullins, E. (1990). Are child sexual experiences related to eating disorder attitudes and behaviors in a college sample? *International Journal of Eating Disorders*, 9, 167–178.

Steiger, H., & Zanko, M. (1990). Sexual traumata among eating disorderd, psychiatric, and normal female groups. *Journal of Interpersonal Violence*, 5, 74–86.

Stuart, G. W., Laraia, M. T., Ballenger, J. C., & Lydiard, R. B. (1990). Early family experiences of women with bulimia and depression. *Archives of Psychiatric Nursing*, 4, 43–52.

van der Kolk, B. A., Perry, C., & Herman, J. L. (1991). Childhood origins of self destructive behavior. *American Journal of Psychiatry*, 148, 1665–1671.

Vanderlinden, J., Vandereycken, W., van Dyck, R., & Vertommen, H. (1993). Dissociative experiences in eating disorders. *International Journal of Eating Disorders*, 13, 189–193.

Waller, G. (1991). Sexual abuse as a factor in eating disorders. *British Journal of Psychiatry*, 159, 664–671.

Waller, G. (1992a). Sexual abuse and bulimic symptoms in eating disorders: Do family interaction and self esteem explain the links? *International Journal of Eating Disorders*, 12, 235–240.

Waller, G. (1992b). Sexual abuse and the severity of bulimic symptoms. *British Journal of Psychiatry*, 161, 90–99.

Waller, G. (1993). Sexual abuse and eating disorders: Borderline personality disorder as a mediating factor. *British Journal of Psychiatry*, 162, 771–775.

Waller, G. (1994). Childhood sexual abuse and borderline personality disorder in the eating disorders. *Child Abuse and Neglect*, 18, 97–101.

Waller, G., Halek, G., & Crisp. A. H. (1993). Sexual abuse as a factor in anorexia nervosa. Evidence from two separate case series. *Journal of Psychosomatic Research*, 17, 873–879.

Waller, G., Hamilton, K., Rose, N., Sumra, J., & Baldwin, G. (1993). Sexual abuse and body image distortion in the eating disorders. *British Journal of Clinical Psychology*, 32, 350–352.

Waller, G., & Ruddock, A. (1993). Experience of disclosure of childhood sexual abuse and psychopathology. *Child Abuse Review*, 2, 185–195.

Welch, S. L., & Fairburn, C. G. (1994). Sexual abuse and bulimia nervosa: Three integrated case control comparisons. *American Journal of Psychiatry*, 151, 402–407.

Williams, H. J., Wagner, H. L., & Calam, R. M. (1992). Eating attitudes in survivors of unwanted sexual experiences. *British Journal of Clinical Psychology*, 31, 203–206.

Wilsnack, S. C., Klassen, A. D., Vogeltanz, N. D., & Harris, T. R. (1994). *Childhood sexual abuse and women's substance abuse: National survey findings*. Paper presented at the American Psychological Association Conference on Psychological and Behavioral Factors in Women's Health, Washington, DC.

Wonderlich, S. A., Donaldson, M. A., Carson, D. K., Staton, D., Gertz, L., Leach, L., & Johnson, M. (1996). Eating disturbance and incest. *Journal of Interpersonal Violence*, 11, 195–207.

Wonderlich, S. A., & Swift, W. J. (1990). Borderline versus other personality disorders in the eating disorders. *International Journal of Eating Disorders*, 9, 629–638.

Wonderlich, S. A., Wilsnack, S., Wilsnack, R., & Harris, T. R. (1996). *The relationship of sexual abuse and bulimic behavior: Results of a U.S. national survey*. Manuscript under review.

Wooley, S. C. (1994a). Sexual abuse and eating disorders: The concealed debate. In P. Fallon, M. Katzman, & S. Wooley (Eds.), *Feminist perspectives on eating disorders* (pp. 171–212). New York: Guilford Press.

Wooley, S. C. (1994b). The female therapist as outlaw. In P. Fallon, M. Katzman, & S. Wooley (Eds.), *Feminist perspectives on eating disorders* (pp. 171–211). New York: Guilford Press.

Wooley, S. C., & Kearney-Cooke, A. (1986). Intensive treatment of bulimia and body image disturbance. In K. Brownell & J. Foreyt (Eds.), *Physiology, psychology and the treatment of eating disorders* (pp. 476–506). New York: Basic Books.

Wyatt, G. (1985). The sexual abuse of Afro American and white American women in childhood. *Child Abuse and Neglect, 9,* 507–519.

CHAPTER 23

Management of Substance Abuse and Dependence

JAMES E. MITCHELL
SHEILA SPECKER
KAREN EDMONSON

The high rate of comorbid substance abuse and dependence was recognized early in the clinical descriptions of individuals with bulimia nervosa, and in early work characterizing the binge-eating/purging subpopulation of patients with anorexia nervosa (Casper, Eckert, Halmi, Goldberg, & Davis, 1980; Garfinkel, Moldofsky, & Garner, 1980; Russell, 1979). These descriptions focused on the misuse of traditional drugs of abuse, particularly alcohol. However, as information about eating disorders has accumulated, it has become clear that many affected individuals also have problems with the abuse of substances that would be considered atypical among other psychiatric patients. These substances include laxatives, diuretics, diet pills, and the over-the-counter emetic ipecac (Mitchell, Pomeroy, & Huber, 1988). In this chapter, we first briefly review the literature on traditionally defined substance abuse and dependence in individuals with eating disorders, and then discuss the assessment and management of these dual-diagnosis patients. After that, we discuss the atypical substances of abuse and describe how each type affects the management of eating-disordered patients.

SUBSTANCE ABUSE AND DEPENDENCE AS TRADITIONALLY DEFINED

Review of the Literature

In his initial description of bulimia nervosa, Russell (1979) noted that many patients tended to abuse drugs and alcohol. Also, in two seminal papers that focused attention on the binge-eating/purging versus the restricting subtypes of anorexia nervosa, substance use problems were noted to be associated with the former subgroup (Casper et al., 1980; Garfinkel et al., 1980). Since these early reports, various researchers have confirmed these associations (Beary, Lacey, & Merry, 1986; Brisman & Seigel, 1986; Bulik, 1987a; Hatsukami, Eckert, Mitchell, & Pyle, 1984; Hudson, Pope, Jonas, & Yurgelun-Todd, 1983b; Jones, Cheshire, & Moorhouse, 1985; Pyle, Mitchell, & Eckert, 1981; Stern et al., 1984; Walsh, Roose, Glassman, Gladis, & Sadik, 1985). For example, in a report by our group on 275 bulimic outpatients, 34% had a history of problems with alcohol or drugs, and 20.7% reported prior treatment for substance dependence—a very high rate, even allowing for the fact that treatment for substance abuse or dependence tends to be more common at a given level of severity in certain geographic areas (e.g., Minnesota) than in other areas (Mitchell, Hatsukami, Eckert, & Pyle, 1985). High comorbid rates of substance use disorders have been described in various bulimic samples, with prevalences ranging from 9% to 55%; however, a few studies have found no suggestions of comorbidity (Kagan & Albertson, 1986). The increased risk of comorbid substance use disorders appears in both normal-weight bulimic patients and the binge-eating/purging subtype of anorexia nervosa patients. The data regarding risk in the restricting subtype are mixed, with some studies finding increased risk and others not (Hall, Beresford, Wooley, Tice, & Hall, 1989; Laessle, Wittchen, Fichter, & Perke, 1989; Toner, Garfinkel, & Garner, 1986). An excellent recent review concluded that binge-eating/purging anorexics in general report more substance use disorders than restricting anorexics do. Also of note, higher rates of substance use disorders have been described among patients with bulimia nervosa than among those with major depressive disorder, again suggesting some specificity of this association (Hudson, Pope, Jonas, Yurgelun-Todd, & Frankenburg, 1987).

This issue of comorbidity has also been addressed via other methodologies, such as surveys of nonpatient samples. For example, a history of repeated episodes of drunkenness was associated with a comorbid history of purging behavior in a large survey of 10th-graders reported by Killen, Taylor, Telch, Robinson, et al. (1987). Frank, Serdula, and Adame (1991) found that female first-year college students who purged were also more likely to report drug use. Also, several studies examining the risk for eating pathology in groups of substance-dependent individuals have suggested this association. For example, Jonas, Gold, Sweeney, and Pottash (1987) reported that of 259 callers to a cocaine hotline, 32% met *Diagnostic and Statistical Manual of Mental Disorders*, third edition (DSM-III) criteria for an eating disorder. Beary et al. (1986) found high rates of eating disorders in alcoholic women. In a comparison study involving 1,355 college students and 440 substance-dependent patients, the prevalence of DSM-III bulimia coupled with the criterion of weekly binge eating and purging was 1% in the college sample but 6.7% among the substance-dependent patients (Pyle et al.,

1983). Other studies have found variable but generally high rates of eating disorders among alcoholic and drug-misusing women, with rates ranging from 8% (Corrigan, Johnson, Alford, Bergeron, & Lemmon, 1990) to 41% (Lacey & Moureli, 1986). Rates of anorexia nervosa in subjects misusing drugs and alcohol have been lower, as would be expected, but still substantial (Beary et al., 1986; Butterfield & LeClair, 1988; Jonas et al., 1987).

Some studies have also suggested a familial relationship between substance use disorders and eating disorders. Hudson, Pope, Jonas, and Yurgelun-Todd (1983a) reported an elevated risk for alcohol abuse and dependence among the first-degree relatives of bulimic patients, compared to a group of age-matched controls. Bulik (1987b) found an elevated risk for alcoholism in the families of bulimic subjects compared to the rate in control families, and later reported that bulimics who had themselves abused alcohol were more likely than other bulimics to have a possible family history of alcoholism (Bulik, 1991). In various other studies, the risk of substance use problems in the first-degree (and at times second-degree) relatives of patients with eating disorders has usually been high, although the significance (or lack of it) of the differences between eating disorder samples and controls has varied considerably (Hudson, Pope, Jonas, et al., 1987; Kassett et al., 1989; Keck et al., 1990; Logue, Crowe, & Bean, 1989).

In considering this association, it is also important to keep in mind the age of risk. For example, Beary et al. (1986) reported that the rate of alcoholism by age 35 was 50% in a population of bulimic patients, suggesting an increasing risk for the development of such comorbid problems as individuals grow older.

Assessment of Dual-Diagnosis Patients

A careful assessment of possible comorbid substance abuse or dependence needs to be included in the evaluation of every patient with an eating disorder. Also, as evidenced by modest research but substantial clinical experience, many patients with eating disorders—already reluctant to divulge their eating problems—may not be forthcoming regarding possible drug and alcohol misuse. In these cases, data from significant others/family members can be very helpful.

A direct, nonjudgmental, yet thorough approach is needed in eliciting such information from patients or relatives. Beginning the assessment for possible substance use in a 14-year-old anorexia nervosa patient with the question "You don't use drugs, do you?" will make for a brief interview but an inadequate and misleading assessment. An accepting, direct approach that emphasizes the possibility of positive answers is preferable.

When a diagnosis of comorbid alcohol or drug misuse is suspected or entertained, other diagnostic considerations come into play. Would a urine toxicology screen be useful? What about liver function tests? These are questions that need to be considered, often in consultation with a medical consultant if the interviewer is not a physician.

Management

Although comorbid substance use problems are frequently encountered in patients with eating disorders, very little is known about the treatment of these dual-diagnosis patients. Many of the available controlled treatment trials of individuals with bulimia nervosa and anorexia nervosa have excluded those with comorbid substance use problems.

A common clinical recommendation is that individuals with both types of disorders should receive treatment for their substance use disorder first, since it is difficult to involve patients meaningfully in eating disorder treatment if they are actively misusing alcohol or other substances. However, this model has never been empirically tested. The ideal treatment might be one that would combine interventions for both disorders. Nevertheless, to our knowledge, such a comorbid approach has never been systematically investigated.

Because of the similarities between substance use disorders and eating disorders (at least bulimia nervosa and the binge-eating/purging type of anorexia nervosa), some have argued that the programs that have evolved for the treatment of substance use disorders—many of which rely on the so-called "Twelve-Step" approach and reliance on a "higher power"—can be used for the treatment of eating disorders. There has been little or no research on such an approach, perhaps because of a bias against such research by some practitioners in the area. However, despite the lack of supportive data, such approaches are widely used and may actually constitute the most wide-

ly practiced treatment approach for these patients. The reasons for the popularity of such approaches are manifold; they include the number of practitioners and programs with experience of such programs, the relative ease with which such approaches can be adapted to new disorders, and the frustration of many mental health practitioners in dealing with eating disorder patients (and their attendant willingness to refer such patients to "specialized" programs). Some practitioners who have been interested in cognitive and/or dynamic approaches to the treatment of eating disorders have found such Twelve-Step programs somehow antithetical to their ways of thinking, and an interesting, at times volatile, and even occasionally destructive dialogue has ensued. Such skirmishes may be entertaining for onlookers and cathartic for participants, but opportunities for both sides to discuss and compare such approaches may have been lost.

Our intention here is not to recapitulate the arguments involved, or (because of the paucity of data in this area) to review the research. Rather, we offer as a model a program currently in place at the University of Minnesota, which is designed to treat patients who have both a substance use disorder and an eating disorder. Although controlled studies that compare sequential treatment to concomitant treatment are lacking, clinical experience and conventional wisdom indicate that there may be problems inherent in the sequential approach. Treatment of the identified "primary" disorder (whether this is the substance use disorder or the eating disorder), without addressing the other disorder, has led to patients' dropping out of treatment or simply switching from one problematic behavior to the other. Another clinical observation is that patients with both problems who are beginning treatment for just one of the disorders at times will deflect treatment efforts and state that their real problem is the other disorder. The advantages of concomitant treatment are a unified comprehensive approach, the elimination of concerns related to the question of "primary" versus "secondary" disorder, continuity of care, and cost-effectiveness.

Several aspects of this combined program make it different from many standard treatment protocols. The program meets daily during the week, in the evening from 5:00 to 8:00 P.M. This encourages individuals who are employed or in school to continue those pursuits, but the schedule also communicates that intensive involvement is important, providing a total of 15 hours of therapy a week. Also, evening programming, in addition to permitting other activities during the day, keeps patients occupied during the hours when they are most likely to engage in bulimic behaviors and/or substance misuse.

The therapists who conduct this program have backgrounds in substance use disorders or eating disorders. The combination of a "recovering" therapist and a therapist without a history of substance misuse or an eating disorder allows both to act as role models with different emphases. Judicious self-disclosure is not uncommon in treatment programs for substance abuse and dependence, whereas it is unusual in traditional psychiatric treatment programs. The combination of therapists with different backgrounds has worked well; for certain patients, it has also been helpful to have a therapist who has personally been through treatment and can empathize with the patients' struggles. Other patients identify with the therapist who has not been addicted or suffered from an eating disorder. This allows each therapist to have a more distinct clinical role without the risk of crossing boundaries. The therapists who currently direct the groups also have very different styles. The "recovering" therapist is a dynamic, directive therapist of the substance abuse/dependence tradition, whereas the other therapist is more facilitative and process-oriented. Although individual patients may prefer one style over another, many seem to find it beneficial to be exposed to both. Patients' reactions to these different styles are dealt with as therapeutic issues.

Standard cognitive-behavioral therapy (as is often used in eating disorder treatment) is integrated with a Twelve-Step program that focuses on substance misuse issues. These approaches are not always as disparate as they might initially appear. The Twelve-Step model incorporates many principles of cognitive-behavioral therapy by encouraging rational thinking and problem solving. Eating disorder patients often benefit from the addition of spirituality—an area often overlooked in eating disorder treatment (Mitchell, Erlander, Pyle, & Fletcher, 1990). Another element shared by Twelve-Step and cognitive-behavioral approaches that is integrated into our program is skill building, covering such topics as assertiveness training, relaxation therapy, and relapse prevention.

The psychiatrist responsible for the program attends the group on a weekly basis to monitor medications, provide direction to the therapists, and clarify diagnostic issues. This population has high rates of comorbidity other than substance use disorders and eating disorders—most frequently major depression, posttraumatic stress disorder, and avoidant, dependent, or borderline personality disorders. These other disorders require a comprehensive and individualized treatment approach with input from a psychiatrist.

The first hour of group sessions consists of a check-in time to see how clients have been doing with their substance use problems and eating problems, and to review self-monitoring and homework. The second hour involves a group dinner in the hospital cafeteria during which clients follow their prescribed meal plan, but make their own food choices. Following the meal, they return immediately to the group. During the third hour, therapists teach skill building. The skill-building section includes a cognitive-behavioral/behavioral psychotherapy component, in which cognitive restructuring, behavioral alternatives, and self-rewards are discussed. Patients do their individual First, Second, and Third Steps of a Twelve-Step program in the group, and are also required to atten outside Twelve-Step meetings weekly. In addition, patients are exposed to the concepts of spirituality, a "higher power," honesty, and meditation.

In many cases, relapses and lapses occur. These are not grounds for discharge under most circumstances; rather, they are regarded as opportunities to learn. However, as patients progress through the weeks of treatment, a strong expectation of abstinence from substance use and self-injurious behaviors develops, as does an expectation for a gradual reduction of eating disorder symptoms.

ATYPICAL SUBSTANCES OF ABUSE

Laxatives

The most common substances of abuse in patients with eating disorders are the over-the-counter laxatives. An early report by our group noted that a majority of bulimic patients reported prior laxative use (Pyle et al., 1981). Subsequent reports from our group and others have documented high prevalences of laxative abuse, ranging from 18% to 75% (Abraham & Beumont, 1982; Fairburn & Cooper, 1984). As an example, in our report on 275 bulimic outpatients, 19.7% admitted to having taken laxatives on at least a daily basis for weight control purposes, and 60.6% had at a minimum "tried" laxatives during the course of their illness (Mitchell et al., 1985).

Though many different types of laxatives are marketed in the United States, the ones used by patients with eating disorders are primarily the stimulant-type laxatives, which when used in sufficient quantity will produce a watery diarrhea and engender a sense of weight loss. In a more detailed examination of a series of 40 bulimic women who had abused laxatives, we found that the two most commonly misused agents were the stimulant-type laxatives Ex-Lax® and Correctol® (Mitchell, Boutacoff, Hatsukami, Pyle, & Eckert, 1986). In this series, 22 (55%) reported that their maximum frequency of usage had been several times a week; 12 (30%) reported a daily maximum frequency of usage; and 6 (15%) reported a maximum frequency of usage of several times a day. In terms of amounts used, 11 patients (27.5%) reported using an average of 11 to 20 pills per session, while 6 (15%) reported using an excess of 20 times the recommended amount, indicating high usage among a significant proportion.

Lacey and Gibson (1985) reported that patients who engaged in self-induced vomiting rather than using laxatives tended to eat more but weigh less, suggesting that laxatives are relatively ineffective as a purging technique. A report by Bo-Linn, Santa Ana, Morawaki, and Fordtran (1983) supports this observation, showing that the weight loss seen in patients who abuse laxatives results primarily from the loss of fluid from the bowel, rather than the loss of ingested food.

Our group has previously reviewed some of the complications associated with laxative abuse (Mitchell & Boutacoff, 1986), and we briefly summarize them here. Fluid and electrolyte abnormalities are common. Laxative-induced diarrhea markedly increases the electrolyte content of the feces. Hypokalemia and acidosis (because of bicarbonate loss in the stool) are acute results, whereas alkalosis may result secondary to the chronic fluid depletion (Cooke, 1977; Mitchell, Pyle, Eckert, Hatsukami, & Lentz, 1983). The fluid loss experienced by these patients results in volume depletion and secondary hyperaldosteronism, which then result

in reflex peripheral edema—a problem that is heightened during laxative withdrawal (Ullrich & Lizarralde, 1978; Gross, Chetrit, Stein, Rosler, & Eliakim, 1980). Constipation is common, and again this becomes particularly problematic during laxative withdrawal (Cooke, 1977). Other rare complications include the development of cathartic colon, wherein chronic abuse of stimulant-type laxatives results in permanent impairment of colonic function; the development of steatorrhea or of protein-losing gastroenteropathy (Larusso & McGill, 1975); pancreatic dysfunction (Lesna, Hamlyn, Venables, & Record, 1977); osteomalacia (Cummings, 1974); and hypomagnesemia (Swift, 1979).

The discontinuation of laxatives can be quite problematic for patients. In particular, it is not uncommon for patients to gain 2–5 kg in reflex edema. Although this will usually resolve in a week to 10 days, it is very worrisome to patients, who are convinced that they are gaining a large amount of body fat. Issues related to laxative withdrawal have previously been reviewed (Mitchell & Boutacoff, 1986) and are briefly summarized here:

1. Patients should be instructed to discontinue the laxative abruptly. Although some clinicians advocate a tapering withdrawal, this has never been shown to improve the likelihood of compliance and may simply prolong the process. If something is needed to promote bowel function, lactulose can be prescribed to prevent fecal impaction.

2. High fiber intake should be encouraged, as should regular physical exercise to regulate bowel function.

3. Patients should be carefully educated about fluid retention. They should be instructed not to limit fluid intake, since this will only promote constipation. If necessary, temporary sodium restriction can be recommended.

4. Patients need to be seen quite frequently during the period of laxative withdrawal, since the temptation to return to the use of laxatives is strong, particularly during the phase of water weight gain.

Studies have shown that eating-disordered patients who abuse laxatives are likely to be among the most difficult to treat, since they evidence high rates of comorbid psychopathology and marked comorbidity with other problems, such as suicide attempts (Mitchell et al., 1986).

Diet Pills

The second type of over-the-counter medication commonly used by patients with eating disorders is diet pills. Fortunately, the abuse of prescription diet pills is rare. We found that 52.2% of our series of 275 bulimic patients reported using over-the-counter diet pills, and that 25.1% reported using at least one pill a day for a period of time during the course of their eating disorder (Mitchell et al., 1985). In a series of 100 consecutive women evaluated for bulimia nervosa, 26 reported having used diet pills in the month prior to evaluation (Mitchell, Pyle, & Eckert, 1991). Of particular interest, eight patients revealed that they took diet pills at least several times a day, and seven patients admitting using more than two diet pills at a given time. The most commonly used agents in our area include Dexatrim® (92.3%), Dietac® (11.5%), and Acutrim® (7.7%).

Over-the-counter diet pills contain phenolpropanolamine, and when they are taken as instructed on the package, the user will consume a total of 75 mg per day (Mitchell, Pomeroy, & Huber, 1988). These drugs have been the source of considerable debate. There is a large clinical literature suggesting possible side effects and toxicity, but because of their widespread usage, many experts believe that they are relatively safe. However, their use in higher-than-recommended amounts has not been systematically investigated, and this usage is of greatest concern in the treatment of eating disorder patients. Anecdotal reports and studies suggest various problems, including transient neurological problems (Johnson, Eitter, & Reeves, 1985), cerebrovascular hemorrhage (Kitka, Devareau, & Chandar, 1985), seizures (Howrie & Wolfson, 1983), and renal failure (Swenson, Golper, & Bennett, 1982). The most consistently reported potential problem has been elevation in blood pressure (Cuthbert, 1980; Horowitz et al., 1980).

Management of diet pill usage consists of educating patients about the pills' possible adverse effects and having the patients discontinue them. Fortunately, most patients who use these compounds do not do so consistently in high quantities.

Diuretics

Various clinical reports have substantiated that some patients with eating disorders abuse diuretics. This generally involves over-the-counter diuretics, which are relatively impotent and usually not sufficiently reinforcing to result in protracted use. In Russell's initial 1979 paper, he described a patient who "misappropriated" diuretics, and in our subsequent report of 34 cases, 10 patients reported having used diuretics as a means of weight control (Mitchell & Eckert, 1981, p. 6). In our series of 275 bulimic patients, 90 (33.9%) indicated that they had used diuretics for weight control, and 27 (10.2%) reported doing so on a daily basis (Mitchell et al., 1985). In a series of 355 college students, Halmi, Falk, and Schwartz (1981) found that 4.2% reported that they had used diuretics, and a survey of 1,268 high school students indicated that 4% used diuretics (Johnson, Lewis, Love, Stuckey, & Lewis, 1984). These findings suggest that diuretic use is not uncommon in the general population of late adolescent and young adult women, but it occurs more frequently in patients with eating disorders.

Many types of diuretics are available, either over the counter or by prescription. Over-the-counter diuretics usually use pamabrom or caffeine as the active diuretic agent; however, these are not very potent (Mitchell, Pomeroy, & Huber, 1988). By contrast, prescription diuretics such as thiazides, loop diuretics, and potassium-sparing diuretics are potent and have serious adverse consequences, including weakness, nausea, palpitations, polyuria, constipation, hypokalemia, cardiac conduction defects, nephropathy, and abdominal pain (Mitchell, Pomeroy, Seppala, & Huber, 1988).

The management of diuretic abuse is very similar to the management of laxative abuse. Both result in reflex fluid retention, with the same implications for management. Patients should be seen frequently and told to restrict sodium intake if necessary, but they should not restrict fluid intake.

Ipecac

Ipecac syrup is dispensed in bottles containing 30 cc of the drug, equivalent to 21 mg of emetine base. The ipecac alkaloid emetine can be responsible for serious myopathies, including cardiomyopathies (Manno & Manno, 1977). Serious and at times fatal myopathies have been reported in patients with eating disorders (Brotman, Forbath, Garfinkel, & Humphrey, 1981; Bennett, Spiro, Pollack, & Zucker, 1982; Palmer & Guay, 1985).

Pope, Hudson, Nixon, and Herridge (1986) reported that of 100 consecutive eating disorder patients, 28 had used ipecac to induce vomiting. Of these, 17 had used the drug 1 to 9 times; 7 had used it 10 to 90 times; and 4 had used it more than 100 times. In another series of 851 outpatients who were evaluated for eating disorders, 7.6% had experimented with the drug, while 1.1% were regular users (Greenfeld, Mickley, Quinlan, & Roloff, 1993). Therefore, though high-frequency usage is uncommon, experimentation with this drug is not unusual.

When the use of ipecac is suspected or discovered, it is important that the patient be very carefully assessed for evidence of myopathy. This should include a careful examination of cardiovascular status, including electrocardiogram and echocardiogram, as well as a careful neuromuscular examination. The drug should be abruptly discontinued, and if acute toxicity has not developed, it can be anticipated that the patient should make a good recovery as the drug is gradually eliminated from the body.

SUMMARY AND CONCLUSIONS

It is not uncommon for patients with eating disorders to misuse both typical (e.g., alcohol, street drugs) and atypical (e.g., laxatives, diuretics, diet pills, and ipecac) substances. Comorbid use of either type of substance has significant implications for the history, medical assessment, and treatment of these patients. Careful assessment for the use of such substances should be included as a part of every diagnostic evaluation. Additional testing may be indicated, depending on the history that is obtained. Since asking about the use of various substances may suggest their use to certain patients, there should be a strong emphasis on educating patients about the risks associated with their use.

REFERENCES

Abraham, S. F., & Beumount, P. J. V. (1982). How patients describe bulimia or binge-eating. *Psychological Medicine, 12,* 625–635.

Beary, M. D., Lacey, J. H., & Merry, J. (1986). Alcoholism and eating disorders in women of fertile age. *British Journal of Addiction, 81,* 685–689.

Bennett, H. S., Spiro, A. J., Pollack, M. A., & Zucker, P. (1982). Ipecac-induced myopathy simulating dermatomyositis. *Neurology, 32,* 91–94.

Bo-Linn, G., Santa Ana, C., Morawaki, S., & Fordtran, J. (1983). Purging and caloire absorption in bulimic patients and normal women. *Annals of Internal Medicine, 99,* 14–17.

Brisman, J., & Siegel, M. (1986). Bulimia and alcoholism— Two sides of the same coin? *Journal of Substance Abuse and Treatment, 1,* 113–118.

Brotman, M. C., Forbath, N., Garfinkel, P. E., & Humphrey, S. G. (1981). Myopathy due to ipecac syrup poisoning in a patient with anorexia nervosa. *Canadian Medical Assocation Journal, 125,* 453–473.

Bulik, C. M. (1987a). Alcohol use and depression in women with bulimia. *American Journal of Drug and Alcohol Abuse, 13,* 343–355.

Bulik, C. M. (1987b). Drug and alcohol abuse by bulimic women and their families. *American Journal of Psychiatry, 144,* 1604–1606.

Bulik, C. M. (1991). Family histories of bulimic women with and without comorbid alcohol abuse or dependence. *American Journal of Psychiatry, 148,* 1267–1268.

Butterfield, P. S., & LeClair, S. (1988). Cognitive characteristics of bulimia and drug-abusing women. *Addictive Behaviors, 13,* 131–138.

Casper, R. C., Eckert, E. D., Halmi, K. A., Goldberg, S. C., & Davis, J. M. (1980). Bulimia: Its incidence and clinical importance in anorexia nervosa. *Archives of General Psychiatry, 37,* 1030–1035.

Cooke, W. T. (1977). Laxative abuse. *Clinical Gastroenterology, 6,* 659–673.

Corrigan, S. A., Johnson, W. G., Alford, G. S., Bergeron, K. C., & Lemmon, C. R. (1990). Prevalence of bulimia among patients in a chemical dependency treatment program. *Addictive Behaviors, 15,* 581–585.

Cummings, J. H. (1974). Progress report: Laxative abuse. *Gut, 15,* 758–766.

Cuthbert, M. F. (1980). Anorectic and decongestant preparations containing phenylpropanolamine. *Lancet, i,* 60.

Fairburn, C. G., & Cooper, P. J. (1984). Binge-eating, self-induced vomiting and laxative abuse: A community study. *Psychological Medicine, 14,* 401–410.

Frank, L. R. E., Serdula, M. K., & Adame, D. (1991). Weight loss and bulimic eating behavior: Changing patterns within a population of young adult women. *Southern Medical Journal, 84,* 457–460.

Garfinkel, P. E., Moldofsky, H., & Garner, D. M. (1980). Prognosis in anorexia nervosa: Bulimia as a distinct subgroup. *Archives of General Psychiatry, 37,* 1036–1040.

Greenfeld, D., Mickley, D., Quinlan, D. M., & Roloff, P. (1993). Ipecac abuse in a sample of eating disordered outpatients. *International Journal of Eating Disorders, 13,* 411–414.

Gross, D. J., Chetrit, E. B., Stein, P., Rosler, A., & Eliakim, M. (1980). Edema associated with laxative abuse and excessvie diuretic therapy. *Israel Journal of Medical Science, 16,* 787–789.

Hall, R. C. W., Beresford, T. P, Wooley, B., Tice, L., & Hall, A. K. (1989). Covert drug abuse in patients with eating disorders. *Psychiatric Medicine, 7,* 247–256.

Halmi, K. A., Falk, J. R., & Schwartz, E. (1981). Binge-eating and vomiting: A survey of a college population. *Psychological Medicine, 11,* 697–706.

Hatsukami, D., Eckert, E., Mitchell, J. E., & Pyle, R. (1984). Affective disorder and substance abuse in women with bulimia. *Psychological Medicine, 14,* 701–704.

Horowitz, J. D., Howes, L. G., Christophidis, N., Lang., W. J., Fennessy, M. R., Rand, M. S., & Lewis, W. J. (1980).

Hypertensive responses induced by phenyl-propanolamine in anorectic and decongestant preparations. *Lancet, i,* 60–61.

Howrie, D. L., & Wolfson, J. H. (1983). Phenylpropanoliamine-induced hypertensive seizures. *Journal of Pediatrics, 102,* 143–145.

Hudson, J., Pope, H., Jonas, J. M., Yurgelun-Todd, D., & Frankenburg, F. R. (1987). A controlled family history study of bulimia. *Psychological Medicine, 17,* 883–890.

Hudson, J., Pope, H., Jonas, J. M., & Yurgelun-Todd, D. (1983a). Family history study of anorexia nervosa and bulimia. *British Journal of Psychiatry, 142,* 133–138.

Hudson, J., Pope, H., Jonas, J. M., & Yurgelun-Todd, D. (1983b). Phenomenologic relationship of eating disorders to major affective disorder. *Psychiatry Research, 9,* 345–354.

Hudson, J., Pope, H., Wurtman, J., Yurgelun-Todd, D., Mark, S., & Rosenthal, N. E. (1988). Bulimia in obese individuals: Relationship to normal-weight bulimia. *Journal of Nervous and Mental Disease, 176,* 144–152.

Hudson, J., Pope, H., Yurgelun-Todd, D., & Jonas, J. M. (1987). A controlled study of lifetime prevalence of affective and other psychiatric disorders in bulimia outpatients. *American Journal of Psychiatry, 144,* 1283–1287.

Johnson, C. L., Lewis, C., Love, S., Stuckey, M., & Lewis, L. (1984). A descriptive survey of dieting and bulimic behavior in a female high school population. In *Report of the Fourth Ross Conference in Medical Research, September, 1983* (pp. 14–18).

Johnson, D. A., Eitter, H. S., & Reeves, D. J. (1985). Stroke and phenylpropanolamine use. *Lancet, ii,* 970.

Jonas, J. M., Gold, M. S., Sweeney, D., & Pottash, A. L. C. (1987). Eating disorders and cocaine abuse: A survey of 259 cocaine abusers. *Journal of Clinical Psychiatry, 48,* 47–50.

Jones, D. A., Cheshire, N., & Moorhouse, H. (1985). Anorexia nervosa, bulimia and alcoholism: Association of eating disorder and alcohol. *Journal of Psychiatric Research, 19,* 377–380.

Kagan, D. M., & Albertson, L. M. (1986). Scores on the MacAndrew factor: Bulimics and other addictive populations. *International Journal of Eating Disorders, 5,* 1095–1101.

Kassett, J. A., Gershon, E. S., Maxwell, M. E., Guroff, J. J., Kazuba, D. M., Smith, A. L., Brandt, H. A., & Jimerson, D. C. (1989). Psychiatric disorders in the first-degree relatives of probands with bulimia nervosa. *American Journal of Psychiatry, 146,* 1468–1471.

Keck, P. E., Pope, H. G., Hudson, J. L., McElroy, S. L., Yurgelun-Todd, D., & Hundert, E. M. (1990). A controlled study of phenomenology and family history in outpatients with bulimia nervosa. *Comprehensive Psychiatry, 31,* 275–283.

Killen, J., Taylor, C., Telch, M. J., Robinson, T. N., Maron, D. J., & Saylor, K. E. (1987). Depressive symptoms and substance use among adolescent binge eaters and purgers: A defined population study. *American Journal of Public Health, 77,* 1539–1541.

Kitka, D .G., Devereaux, M. W., & Chandar, K. (1985). Intracranial hemorrhages due to phenylpropanolamine. *Stroke, 16,* 510–512.

Lacey, J. H., & Gibson, E. (1985). Controlling weight by purgation and vomiting: A comparative study of bulimis. *Journal of Psychiatric Research, 19,* 337–341.

Lacey, J. H., & Moureli, E. (1986). Bulimic alocholics:

Some findings of a clinical subgroup. *British Journal of Addiction, 81,* 389–393.

Laessle, R., Wittchen, H., Fichter, M., & Pirke, K. M. (1989). The significance of subgroups of bulimia and anorexia nervosa: Lifetime frequency of psychiatric disorders. *International Journal of Eating Disorders, 8,* 569–574.

Larusso, N. F., & McGill, D. B. (1975). Surreptitious laxative ingestion: Delayed recognition of a serious condition. A case report. *Mayo Clinic Proceedings, 50,* 706–708.

Lesna, M., Hamlyn, A. N., Venables, C. W., & Record, C. O. (1977). Chronic laxative abuse associated with pancreatic islet cell hyperplasia. *Gut, 18,* 1032–1035.

Logue, C. M., Crowe, R. R., & Bean, J. A. (1989). A family study of anorexia nervosa and bulimia. *Comprehensive Psychiatry, 30,* 179–188.

Manno, R. R., & Manno, J. E. (1977). Toxicology of ipecac: A review. *Clinical Taxicology, 10,* 221–242.

Mitchell, J. E., & Boutacoff, L. I. (1986). Laxative abuse complicating bulimia: Medical and treatment implications. *International Journal of Eating Disorders, 5,* 325–334.

Mitchell, J. E., Boutacoff, L. I., Hatsukami, D., Pyle, R. L., & Eckert, E. D. (1986). Laxative abuse as a variant of bulimia. *Journal of Nervous and Mental Disease, 174,* 174–176.

Mitchell, J. E., Erlander, R. M., Pyle, R. L., & Fletcher, L. A. (1990). Eating disorders, religious practices and pastoral counseling. *International Journal of Eating Disorders, 9,* 589–593.

Mitchell, J. E., Hatsukami, D., Eckert, E. D., & Pyle, R. L. (1985). Characteristics of 275 patients with bulimia. *American Journal of Psychiatry, 142,* 482–485.

Mitchell, J. E., Pomeroy, C., & Huber, M. (1988). A clinician's guide to the eating disorders medicine cabinet. *International Journal of Eating Disorders, 7,* 211–223.

Mitchell, J. E., Pomeroy, C., Seppala, M., & Huber, M. (1988). Pseudo-Bartter's syndrome, diuretic abuse, idiopathic edema, and eating disorders. *International Journal of Eating Disorders, 7,* 225–237.

Mitchell, J. E., Pyle, R. L., & Eckert, E. D. (1991). Diet pill usage in patients with bulimia nervosa. *International Journal of Eating Disorders, 2,* 233–237.

Mitchell, J. E., Pyle, R. L., Eckert, E. D., Hatsukami, D., & Lentz, R. (1983). Electrolyte and other physiological abnormalities in patients with bulimia. *Psychological Medicine, 13,* 273–278.

Palmer, E. P., & Guay, A. T. (1985). Reversible myopathy secondary to abuse of ipacac in patients with major eating disorders. *New England Journal of Medicine, 313,* 1457–1459.

Pope, H. G., Hudson, J. I., Nixon, R. A., & Herridge, P. L. (1986). The epidemiology of ipecac abuse. *New England Journal of Medicine, 314,* 245.

Pyle, R. L., Mitchell, J. E., & Eckert, E. D. (1981). Bulimia: A report of 34 cases. *Journal of Clinical Psychiatry, 42,* 60–64.

Pyle, R. L., Mitchell, J. E., Eckert, E. D., Halvorson, P. A., Neuman, P. A., & Goff, G. M. (1983). The incidence of bulimia in freshman college students. *International Journal of Eating Disorders, 2,* 75–85.

Russell, G. (1979). Bulimia nervosa: An ominous variant of anorexia nervosa. *Psychological Medicine, 9,* 429–448.

Stern, S. L., Dixon, K. N., Nemzer, E., Lake, M. D., Sansome, R. A., Smeltzer, D. J., Lantz, S., & Schrier, S. S. (1984). Affective disorder in the families of women with normal weight bulimia. *American Journal of Psychiatry, 141*, 1224–1227.

Strober, M. (1981). The signficiance of bulimia in juvenile anorexia nervosa: An exploration of possible etiologic factors. *International Journal of Eating Disorders, 1*, 28–43.

Swenson, R. D., Golper, R. A., & Bennett, W. M. (1982). Acute renal failure and rhabdomyolysis after ingestion of phenylpropanolamine-containing diet pills. *Journal of the American Medical Association, 248*, 1216.

Swift, T. R. (1979). Weakness from magnesium-containing cathartics: Electrophysiological studies. *Muscle and Nerve, 2*, 295–298.

Toner, B. B., Garfinkel, P. E., & Garner, D. M. (1986). Long-term follow-up of anorexia nervosa. *Psychosomatic Medicine, 48*, 520–529.

Ullrich, I., & Lizarralde, G. (1978). Amenorrhea and edema. *American Journal of Medicine, 64*, 1080–1083.

Walsh, B. T., Roose, S., Glassman, A., Gladis, M., & Sadik, C. (1985). Bulimia and depression. *Psychosomatic Medicine, 47*, 123–131.

CHAPTER 24

Management of Patients with Comorbid Medical Conditions

PAULINE S. POWERS

Eating disorder patients frequently present with comorbid medical conditions that may complicate treatment. Certain conditions, such as diabetes mellitus or hyperthyroidism, may precipitate eating disorders in vulnerable individuals (particularly during adolescence). Many illnesses that have been reported in association with eating disorders are connected in important ways with the classic symptoms of anorexia nervosa or bulimia nervosa. The following are examples. In order to comply with treatment, patients with diabetes mellitus must follow a low-carbohydrate, low-fat diet; this type of diet is a known precursor of both anorexia nervosa and bulimia nervosa. Weight loss and emphasis on eating are typical symptoms in cystic fibrosis patients. The nausea and vomiting that may occur in pregnancy may merge with symptoms of bulimia nervosa. The diarrhea that occurs in the various inflammatory bowel diseases may precipitate weight loss, and in vulnerable patients may lead to eating disorders. Since some of the key symptoms of eating disorders may overlap with symptoms of the medical conditions to be discussed, diagnosis may be difficult.

In this chapter, the common themes seen in patients with comorbid medical conditions are described first, along with psychotherapeutic recommendations. Common iatrogenic complications that result from insistence upon "compliance" rather than "cooperation" are addressed. Then the comorbid conditions that may occur with eating disorders are discussed. For each of these, the relevant medical findings

are described; the specific psychotherapeutic and medical issues that must be addressed are also outlined.

COMMON THEMES

There are a number of common themes in the conditions to be reviewed. Although diabetes mellitus, cystic fibrosis, pregnancy, and thyroid disease may precipitate or complicate an eating disorder, there is currently little evidence that eating disorders are more likely in these groups. Most patients with other medical conditions who develop eating disorders appear to have been vulnerable prior to the onset of their other conditions and to have had multiple risk factors for eating disorders.

However, these patients do have unique and dangerous opportunities to misuse features of their conditions or medical treatments to facilitate weight loss or purging. Diabetic patients may withhold insulin, and cystic fibrosis patients may withhold their pancreatic enzymes to facilitate weight loss. Patients who must take thyroid replacement may take more than prescribed to increase metabolic rate and lose weight. The nausea and vomiting that occur during pregnancy may be used to facilitate weight loss or prevent weight gain. Hyperthyroid patients may fail to take antithyroid medication in order to facilitate weight loss. The possible methods for inappropriately facilitating weight loss or inducing purging are listed in Table 24.1.

TABLE 24.1. Methods Misused to Cause Weight Loss

Condition	Method	Effect
Insulin-dependent diabetes mellitus	Omission of insulin	Glycosuria
Cystic fibrosis	Omission of pancreatic enzymes	Steatorrhea
Inflammatory bowel disease	Omission of steroids Consumption of lactose-containing foods	Diarrhea Malabsorption
Crohn's disease	Omission of sulfasalazine	Diarrhea
Pregnancy	Use of pregnancy-related nausea to facilitate vomiting	Vomiting
Hypothyroidism	Use of more thyroid than described	Increased metabolism
Hyperthyroidism	Omission of antithyroid medications	Increased metabolism

In patients with most of the conditions to be discussed, several of the psychological themes are the same as those in other patients with eating disorders. Denial of illness is a common problem in eating disorder patients, especially in those with anorexia nervosa. Patients may also deny certain aspects of their comorbid medical conditions as well. Denial and avoidance of conflict are also common in families with an eating disorder patient, and these traits may interfere with the management of both the medical condition and the eating disorder.

Grief is a second important issue that is commonly seen in patients with eating disorders who have comorbid physiological disorders. For example, patients with diabetes mellitus and cystic fibrosis have shortened life expectancies and must alter their lifestyles significantly to manage their illnesses. For adolescents, these adjustments may be difficult. Patients may need to grieve for the loss of a normal lifestyle and of normal life expectancy; their recognizing and experiencing their feelings of sadness and anger about these losses may add to the difficulties inherent in the treatment of their eating disorders.

Another theme common to medical conditions and to eating disorders relates to compliance with medical regimens. In the conditions to be discussed, patients are expected to be "compliant"—a term implying that the patients will dutifully follow the treatments prescribed. Since eating disorders typically occur in adolescents, when teenagers are attempting to emancipate themselves from parental control, compliance with authority is at best problematic. A more helpful concept is "cooperation," in which there is a less hierarchical use of power and authority by the care provider, and more emphasis on a shared responsibility for the management of the condition. Eating disorder patients may expect that they will be ordered to comply rigidly with the expectations of authority figures; in the long run, however, cooperation rather than compliance will facilitate optimal management of both eating disorders and comorbid physiological conditions.

CYSTIC FIBROSIS

Cystic fibrosis (CF) is an autosomal recessive disorder and is the most common genetic disease among Caucasians; 1 in 25 Caucasians is a carrier of the CF gene. The disorder affects 1 in 2,000 children born each year in the United States. The gene encodes for a membrane protein that interferes with ion transport in epithelial cells; this results in airway obstruction in the lungs and duct obstruction in the pancreas (Aitken & Fiel, 1993), together with abnormalities in many other organ systems. The average life expectancy of an individual with CF is 29 years. Malabsorption secondary to exocrine pancreatic malfunction results in steatorrhea, which contributes to malnutrition and growth failure. There is a documented connection between malnutrition and poor lung function (Durie & Pencharz, 1989; Heijerman, 1993), which is significant, since undernourished patients have shorter long-term survival. Several studies have documented the multiple losses and adjustments that patients with CF and their families experience, resulting in an increased likelihood of psychiatric symptomatology (e.g., Pearson, Pumariega, & Seilheimer, 1991).

Association between Eating Disorders and CF

The relationship between CF and eating disorders has been the focus of several reports. Undernutrition, which is common in adolescent CF patients, may both facilitate the emergence of an eating disorder and complicate the diagnosis. Pumariega, Pursell, Spock, and Jones (1986) described 13 CF patients with atypical eating disorders, similar (but not identical) to anorexia nervosa. These 13 patients represented 12% of the adolescent CF patients seen during a 3-year period. The patients were all more than 25% below ideal body weight (IBW) and had lost weight despite normal pancreatic function or adequate enzyme replacement. The precipitant for the weight loss was usually a pulmonary infection during which there was true loss of appetite (i.e., anorexia). The patients then resisted weight gain and avoided discussion of their feelings about their chronic illness. These patients did not have the typical body image disturbance seen in eating disorders, and none of the patients exhibited binge-eating or purging behavior. In a second study by the same group (Pearson et al., 1991), 61 patients were given the Eating Attitudes Test (EAT; Garner & Garfinkel, 1979); 16.4% reported symptoms consistent with anorexia nervosa in the younger group (ages 8 to 15), as did 28% in the older group (ages 16 to 40 years). There were several problems with this study, including sole reliance on self-report measures rather than interviews. Steiner, Rahimzadeh, and Lewiston (1990) compared 10 patients with anorexia nervosa to 10 patients with CF. The anorexia nervosa patients and their families had significantly more evidence of psychopathology than patients with CF and their families.

Implications for Psychotherapy

Patients with CF face premature death preceded by complex, frightening, and painful symptoms. During adolescence—the time when abstract reasoning and planning for adult life assume central importance—CF patients must grapple with the fact that they will probably die prematurely. A family environment in which the open discussion of sadness and anger is permitted is most likely to help a young CF patient accept the loss of a normal life potential, and at the same time to allow the adolescent to accomplish some of life's goals and enjoy the process. The psychotherapist working with a patient with an eating disorder and CF needs to be knowledgeable about both illnesses and to encourage frank discussion of feelings and thoughts about the losses that are being faced. By adolescence, most CF patients have had to alter their lifestyles significantly in order to comply with treatment regimens. These alterations may make peer interactions more difficult. Encouraging patients to participate in normal activities as much as possible is very important.

The family attitude toward CF management is crucial for treatment. Pearson et al. (1991) have posited that patients with the best adaptation have families with moderate compliance; that is, they neither neglect the illness nor become preoccupied with it. Likewise, Johnson, Gershowitz, and Stabler (1981) found highest levels of self-concept in children with CF whose mothers were moderately compliant with treatment.

Medical Issues

Adolescent patients usually possess the intellectual skills to benefit from psychoeducation regarding the relationship among weight loss, pulmonary complications, and death. The CF literature is replete with practical guidelines for nutritional intervention. Most undernutrition in CF is protein calorie malnutrition and is a consequence of one or more of the following factors: loss of appetite, malabsorption, and an increase in resting expenditure. Rapid correction of respiratory infections and adequate enzyme replacements to correct steatorrhea must be achieved first. Then oral supplementation should be undertaken. Behavioral treatments to restore weight have been shown to be effective and have included nutritional education, contingency management, and relaxation therapy (Stark et al., 1993). A consensus conference (Ramsey, Farrell, Pencharz, and the Consensus Committee, 1992) has recommended supplementation in patients with decreased weight velocity and/or weight–height index of 85–90% of IBW. Patients who are at less than 85% of IBW will also require enteral supplements, and those at less than 75% of IBW will require parenteral nutrition.

INFLAMMATORY BOWEL DISEASE

Crohn's disease and ulcerative colitis are two distinct inflammatory conditions affecting the gastrointestinal tract. Crohn's disease may involve any segment of the gastrointestinal tract with a chronic granulomatous inflammation of all layers of the bowel wall, whereas ulcerative colitis affects only the mucosa of the large bowel. Crohn's disease frequently results in fistulas, which require resection of the bowel. Both conditions are chronic and are treated symptomatically with corticosteroids and sulfasalazine. The presenting symptoms include weight loss, growth failure, loss of appetite, diarrhea, nausea, and vomiting. These symptoms may overlap with symptoms of eating disorders; several reports have described patients with inflammatory bowel disease who have been initially misdiagnosed as having anorexia nervosa (Gryboski, Katz, Sangree, & Herskoovic, 1968; Rickards, Prendergast, & Booth, 1994), and recently there have been reports of patients with both inflammatory bowel disease and eating disorders (Gryboski, 1993; Meadows & Treasure, 1989).

Malnutrition is a common finding in inflammatory bowel disease and is a consequence of several factors (Rosenberg, Bengoa, & Sitrin, 1985). These include decreased oral intake (because of abdominal pain, nausea, and loss of appetite), malabsorption (because of decreased absorption caused by the disease or by bowel resection, or because of lactose intolerance secondary to lactase deficiency), and increased caloric requirements (because of fever and inflammation).

Gryboski et al. (1968) described 11 adolescent girls who presented with symptoms of anorexia nervosa (fear of obesity, weight loss, and body image disturbances) who were later found to have Crohn's disease. More recently, Gryboski (1993) described three patients with inflammatory bowel disease (two with ulcerative colitis and one with Crohn's disease) who also had eating disorders (two had bulimia nervosa and one had the binge-eating/purging subtype of anorexia nervosa). Two of these patients, who were lactose-intolerant, used milk ingestion as a purgative to facilitate weight loss. Two patients failed to take either their steroids or sulfasalazine and developed diarrhea and weight loss. Rickards et al. (1994) described four cases of children who presented with growth failure and a variety of psychiatric symptoms; all were eventually diagnosed with Crohn's disease.

Case Report

The following case description is of a patient treated for anorexia nervosa for over a year before transfer to our unit; the diagnosis of Crohn's disease was made a week later.

Amy was a 13-year-old girl referred by her family physician for psychiatric treatment. For 14 months she had complained of abdominal pain, nausea, and intermittent nonbloody diarrhea, and her weight had dropped from 90 pounds to 71 pounds (at 5'0" in height). Six months earlier, she had been hospitalized on a psychiatric unit for 1 month and had failed to gain weight, but she had run a low-grade fever throughout her hospitalization. Outpatient treatment was ineffective in achieving weight gain. There was no evidence of a body image disturbance. She had regular menses. She had been started on amitryptyline several months earlier. Physical examination revealed marked tachycardia (140 beats per minute), normal temperature, slightly inflamed tonsils, and fat content by anthropometric evaluation (the four-site caliper method described by Westrate & Deurenberg, 1989) of 29%. The remainder of the physical examination was normal, but rectal and pelvic examinations were deferred. She was cooperative but appeared tired and ill. Her mother specifically requested family therapy. Laboratory testing revealed elevated platelets, elevated sedimentation rate, mild anemia, low iron, low albumin, and low cholesterol. Pediatric consultation was requested, and a rectal examination revealed a rectal fistula. The diagnosis of Crohn's disease was then made, and Amy received the appropriate treatment.

This case illustrates many of the findings that should alert a physician to the possibility of Crohn's disease. First, except for her weight loss, Amy did not have the classic symptoms of anorexia nervosa: She did not have a fear of weight gain or other body image disturbance, she had regular menses, and her fat content was normal. Second, the laboratory test results were not consistent with the findings typically seen in anorexia nervosa. Hypoalbuminemia and elevated sedimentation rates are rarely seen in anorexia nervosa (Palla & Litt, 1987), iron stores are usually not depleted, and cholesterol level is usually high rather than low. Third, gastrointestinal symptoms should have elicited a complete gastrointestinal workup, beginning with a rectal examination.

DIABETES MELLITUS

Diabetes mellitus is a clinically and genetically heterogeneous group of metabolic disorders characterized by glucose intolerance. Although various subtypes have been described, the most common are insulin-dependent diabetes mellitus (IDDM) and non-insulin-dependent diabetes mellitus (NIDDM). IDDM can begin at any age, but it usually starts in early childhood or adolescence. IDDM is one of the most common chronic disorders of childhood and adolescence; approximately 1 in 300 to 600 children is affected by age 20 (Drash, 1987).

There have been several studies of the relationship between IDDM and eating disorders. The recent literature is summarized, including the finding that although the eating disorders may be no more common among IDDM patients than among the general population, complications are more common among eating-disordered diabetics.

Prevalence of Eating Disorders

Initial studies suggested that there was a greater prevalence of eating disorders among IDDM adolescent patients (Hudson, Wentworth, Hudson, & Pope, 1985; Rodin, Daneman, Johnson, Kenshole, & Garfinkel, 1985). However, there were several problems with these early studies, including use of criteria that were probably too broad, and exclusive reliance on the 26-item form of the EAT (EAT-26; Garner, Olmsted, Bohr, & Garfinkel, 1982). Wing, Norwalk, Marcus, Koeske, and Finefold (1986) have shown that diabetic adolescents score higher on the Dieting subscale of the EAT-26, but this may be appropriate, since carbohydrate restriction is a necessary part of diabetic treatment; the diabetic adolescents had scores similar to or lower than those of normal controls on other subscales of the EAT-26. Later studies have found that the prevalence of formally diagnosed eating disorders is apparently no higher among IDDM pa-

tients (Birk & Spencer, 1989; Powers, Malone, Coovert, & Schulman, 1990). However, induction of glycosuria to lose weight occurs in 12–39% of female diabetic patients (Rodin, Craven, & Littlefield, 1991; Stancin et al., 1989).

Increased Likelihood of Complications

Patients with IDDM who also have eating disorders are more likely to have both short-term and long-term complications of their diabetes than non-eating-disordered diabetics. Insulin misuse and binge eating both contribute to poor diabetic control. The most common and best-known misuse of insulin is omission or reduction of the dose, causing glycosuria and weight loss. However, some patients who binge-eat may take large doses of insulin to compensate and may gain weight as a consequence. Anorexia nervosa patients who have severely restricted their diets or who overexercise may not reduce their insulin doses appropriately and may become hypoglycemic.

One means of assessing diabetic control is measurement of glycosylated hemoglobin (HbA1c), which gives an estimate of blood sugar over the previous 3 months. The principle behind this is that the amount of hemoglobin that has become conjugated with glucose is proportional to the average level of blood glucose during the life of the red blood cell (an average of 3 months). HbA1c levels are higher in diabetic patients with eating disorders than in diabetics without eating disorders (Wing et al., 1986; Birk & Spencer, 1989; Steel, Young, Lloyd, & Clarke, 1987). Since the risk of developing long-term complications can be significantly reduced by good diabetic control (Diabetes Control and Complications Trial Research Group, 1993), it is not surprising that eating-disordered IDDM patients develop long-term complications earlier than non-eating-disordered diabetics. Rydall, Rodin, Olmsted, Devenyi, and Daneman (1994) found that 90% of young women who had a previously suspected eating disorder had early signs of either diabetic retinopathy or nephropathy, compared to 40% without a suspected eating disorder. Cantwell and Steel (1996) confirmed that diabetic complications are more common in patients with eating disorders. Other long-term complications are growth failure and pubertal delay (Rodin et al., 1985).

The short-term complications include unexpected episodes of diabetic ketoacidosis or severe hypoglycemia (Powers, Malone, & Duncan, 1983; Hilliard & Hilliard, 1984). Both of these conditions are life-threatening. Patients with anorexia nervosa may develop acute painful neuropathy at the peak of weight reduction (Steel et al., 1987).

Diagnosis of an Eating Disorder in a Diabetic Patient

Unexpected, unexplained episodes of ketoacidosis or hypoglycemia, particularly in an adolescent female, should alert the clinician to the possibility of an eating disorder. If blood sugar is easily normalized in the hospital, under nursing supervision, this is another warning sign. Weight loss or weight gain should be carefully monitored, and the patient should be evaluated for other signs and symptoms of an eating disorder. More subtle indications include poor adherence to general management of the diabetes, high HbA1c levels, or growth failure. Diabetic patients with eating disorders may purge by vomiting, laxative abuse, or diuretic abuse, although purging appears to be less common than among eating disorder patients in general (Fairburn, Peveler, Davies, Mann, & Mayou, 1991). Binge eating may be less severe yet still very dangerous, since diabetic control can be impaired with small quantities of high-carbohydrate foods.

Pathogenesis

It was recognized in the early studies that IDDM usually preceded the onset of an eating disorder (Powers et al., 1983; Hilliard & Hilliard, 1984). This has recently been confirmed by Ward, Troop, Cachio, Watkins, and Treasure (1995). The actual precipitant for eating disorders in patients with IDDM may be the typical weight gain that occurs following the institution of insulin therapy. In predisposed adolescent females, this weight gain may trigger the onset of eating disorders, often with omission of insulin. The chronic dietary restraint and preoccupation with carbohydrate restriction may further foster the development of eating disorders. Lawson, Rodin, Rydall, Olmsted, and Daneman (1994) have diagrammed the relationship among various factors that can potentiate eating disorders in vulnerable adolescent females with IDDM (Figure 24.1).

Treatment

Patients with anorexia nervosa and IDDM almost always require hospitalization. Treatment should include weight restoration and normalization of eating, both individual and family therapy, and nutritional counseling. Initially, the nursing staff may need to inject each insulin

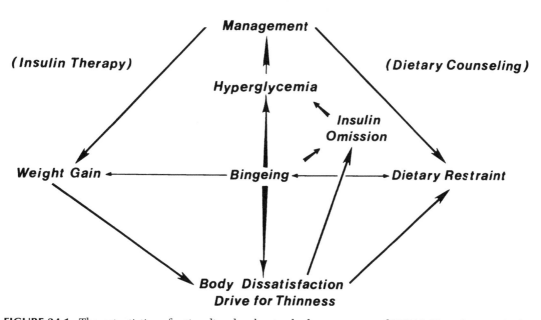

FIGURE 24.1. The potentiation of eating disorders by standard management of IDDM. From Lawson, Rodin, Rydall, Olmsted, and Daneman (1994). Copyright 1994 by J. B. Lippincott Company. Reprinted by permission.

dose; some patients may be so determined to lose weight that they surreptitiously dispose of insulin even if a nurse is supervising an injection. If there are unexplained variations in blood sugar, or if an anorexic patient fails to gain weight despite appropriate caloric intake, it may be helpful to have members of the nursing staff not only administer the insulin but sign for its administration as they would for a narcotic. The patient may report false blood sugar levels unless monitored closely. As the patient improves and is able to cooperate with the treatment, very close monitoring of blood sugars is necessary, as insulin requirements may change dramatically when weight is gained or when binge eating is discontinued.

Nutritional consultation can be very difficult. Many patients with eating disorders are unnecessarily rigid in their food choices, whereas others discount the effect of binge eating if they believe that omitting insulin (or taking a higher dose) has compensated for possible weight gain (or effect on blood glucose). It may be more difficult for an overweight bulimic to lose weight and still follow a diabetic diet. Body fat content is probably higher in diabetic patients than in age- and weight-matched peers. This higher fat content may mean that with normal caloric intake, especially in a patient with a long-standing history of bulimia, weight gain will occur. The patient may have to choose between a slightly lower caloric intake (which may increase hunger and thus vulnerability to binge eating) and a slightly higher weight (which may intensify body image dissatisfaction).

Individual psychotherapy is often characterized by denial of both the eating disorder and the diabetes or of their meanings, in terms of both decreased longevity and alteration in lifestyle. Some patients may believe that if they become thin enough, they will not have diabetes; this erroneous belief is given some credibility by the fact that insulin requirements do decrease with weight loss. The conflict between autonomy and dependence may be particularly difficult for diabetic adolescents. These young patients must assume responsibility for management of their illness early, yet they are dependent on treatment and care providers for their survival. Issues related to grief over loss of normal daily functioning are also important, particularly in patients who have difficulty expressing their emotions.

Family issues may be very important. Parents may feel guilty about their child's illness (espe-

cially if one or both parents have a family history of diabetes) and may overindulge a clinically ill child or teenager. On the other hand, parents may distance themselves inappropriately from a diabetic adolescent, who may appear pseudomature because of having to manage the diabetes. It may be difficult for a family to facilitate appropriate independence in a youngster with an eating disorder who is also diabetic. Family conflicts may be rerouted into conflicts over compliance with diabetic treatment.

Cognitive-behavioral techniques, typically in group settings, have been used for diabetic patients with bulimia nervosa (Peveler & Fairburn, 1992) or anorexia nervosa (Peveler & Fairburn, 1989). These techniques may be less effective in the IDDM population than in the general eating disorder population.

Prevention

Lawson et al. (1994) have recently proposed group psychoeducation to prevent eating disorders among newly diagnosed IDDM patients. These investigators propose a group lecture format. In this setting, the need for a flexible approach to treatment and for cooperative rather than compliant interaction with care providers can be stressed.

PREGNANCY

Several early psychodynamic theories posited the repudiation of a fantasized oral impregnation as the cause of anorexia nervosa (Jones 1938; Alexander, Bacon, Wilson, Levey, & Levine, 1934). Lindner (1955) conceptualized bulimic behavior as representing the wish to be impregnated and purging as the rejection of that wish. Although at present psychoanalytic drive theory is invoked less often as an explanation for anorexic and bulimic behavior, fears of adult heterosexuality, pregnancy, and motherhood are important themes in the individual psychotherapy of patients.

Onset of Eating Disorders during Pregnancy

Eating disorders can begin at any age, because onset can be precipitated by inability to master a developmental step. Pregnancy is a dramatic reminder that changes in status and responsibilities have occurred.

Weinfeld (1977) described a patient who was at a normal weight before pregnancy but who developed anorexia nervosa during her pregnancy. Price, Giannini, and Loiselle (1986) described a patient who began vomiting during pregnancy because she was afraid of becoming obese; following her pregnancy, she continued purging by vomiting and also began using laxatives. The authors posited that "morning sickness" and vomiting might lay the groundwork for future bulimic behavior.

Fairburn, Stein, and Jones (1992) studied an unselected community sample of 100 women who were pregnant for the first time. They found that five subjects developed eating disorders during pregnancy, although two had a past history of bulimia nervosa that had resolved prior to the pregnancy. Another three patients, who met criteria for eating disorders just prior to conception, had resolution of symptoms during the study. The authors note a decline in dietary restraint and increase in concern about body shape and weight by late pregnancy.

The following case description is of a patient who developed anorexia nervosa during pregnancy.

Catrina was a 31-year-old woman who weighed 85 pounds (at 5'4" in height). She had a 5-year-old son. Prior to her pregnancy, she weighed 125 pounds and was in an unhappy, conflicted marriage. Shortly after she conceived, the couple separated, and Catrina returned home to live with her parents. She became very concerned about weight gain and failed to consume adequate calories; she continued to work during her pregnancy and gained a mere 8 pounds during the pregnancy. Birth and delivery were normal. After delivery she lived with her parents and did not return to work. She felt completely overwhelmed by the needs of her son, and her parents provided most of his care. During the first postpartum month, she reduced her weight to 105 pounds. She then started to purge by vomiting and laxative abuse, and her weight dropped to 85 pounds. She was preoccupied with her son's eating behavior and attempted to restrict his food intake; in kindergarten, he was unruly with a short attention span. Despite repeated hospitalizations and multiple attempts to engage Catrina in treatment, she failed to maintain gains made in the hospital and was eventually lost to treatment.

Effects of Pregnancy on Patients with Eating Disorders

Although much remains to be known about the effects of pregnancy in patients with chronic eating disorders, what is known suggests that there may be dire consequences for both the mothers and their babies.

Although many underweight anorexia nervosa patients are infertile, some are not, and these patients may become pregnant. Usually anorexia nervosa patients fail to gain weight, and among several case reports (Stewart, Raskin, Garfinkel, MacDonald, & Robinson, 1987; Weinfeld, 1977; Brinch, Isager, & Tolstrup, 1988; Treasure & Russell, 1988), there were complications of pregnancy and birth in every case. Maternal complications included inadequate weight gain, hyperemesis, and vaginal bleeding; fetal and birth complications included low birth weight and prenatal death. Two other studies found that anorexia nervosa patients who gained weight during their pregnancies had normal deliveries, and that birth weights of the infants were normal (Namiri, Melman, & Yager, 1986; Rand, Willis, & Kuldau, 1987).

There are more studies of the effects of bulimia nervosa on pregnancy, since bulimic patients are more likely to be fertile. In a retrospective study, Mitchell, Seim, Glotter, Soll, and Pyle (1991), found that the risk of fetal loss was approximately twice as high in bulimics as in normal controls (although this difference did not reach statistical significance). Lacey and Smith (1987) found that the prevalence of binge eating and vomiting decreased sequentially during each trimester, but that symptoms returned after delivery in two-thirds of patients. They concluded that the increase in uterine size made binge eating physically more difficult. Other studies have confirmed that bulimic behaviors resume after delivery (Lemberg & Phillips, 1989; Willis & Rand, 1988).

Effects on the Children

Several studies have found long-term physiological and psychological consequences in children of patients with eating disorders. Hunt, Cooper, and Tooley (1988) found cognitive, sensory, and physical problems in children up to age 11. Mothers with eating disorders may be excessively concerned about the eating behavior and weights of their children (Stein & Fairburn, 1989; Woodside & Shekter-Wolfson,

TABLE 24.2. Possible Teratogenic Risks of Prescription Medications Used or Abused by Eating Disorder Patients

Generic name	Brand name	Use or abuse	Category[a]
Metoclopramide	Reglan	Facilitator of gastric emptying	B
Cisapride	Propulsid	Facilitator of gastric emptying	C
Fluoxetine	Prozac	Antidepressant	B
Paroxetine	Paxil	Antidepressant	B
Sertraline	Zoloft	Antidepressant	B
Lithium	Eskalith, others	Antimanic	D
Amphetamine	Dexedrine, others	Appetite suppressant	C
Furosemide	Lasix	Purge method	C
Chlorothiazide	Diuril	Purge method	C

[a]Federal Drug Administration (FDA) categories: A, controlled studies show no risk; B, no evidence of risk in humans; C, risk cannot be ruled out; D, positive evidence of risk.

1990). There is a report of one anorexic mother who starved her child to death (Seller, 1987).

Many patients with eating disorders need medications that may be teratogenic. Such patients may suffer from comorbid psychiatric conditions, which may require medications suspected to be teratogenic (e.g., lithium). Certain medications used as adjunctive treatments for physiological complications (e.g., metoclopramide for delayed gastric emptying) may also be teratogenic. Medications abused by patients (laxatives, diuretics, diet pills) may also have effects on the developing fetus. Tables 24.2 and 24.3 list the common medications used or abused, and their possible teratogenic risks or effects.

Treatment of the Pregnant Patient with an Eating Disorder

With patients who are in treatment, it is wise to counsel them to defer pregnancy until there is a full recovery from the eating disorder. However, for a patient with an active eating disorder who becomes pregnant, initial consultation with an obstetrician, psychiatrist, and geneticist regarding possible effects of the eating disorder and of various medications on the mother and fetus is appropriate. Knowledge abut the possible consequences of disturbed eating or misuse of drugs can facilitate the patient's decision to relinquish these behaviors during pregnancy.

A multidisciplinary team should include an

TABLE 24.3. Possible Teratogenic Effects of Nonprescription Drugs Abused by Eating Disorder Patients

Drug type	Brand name	Active ingredient(s)	Possible fetal effects
Diet pills	Acutrim	Phenylpropanolamine	?Clubfoot, inguinal hernia[a]
	Dexatrim	Phenylpropanolamine	
Diuretics	Aqua Ban	Caffeine	Withdrawal symptoms after birth,[b] low birth weight[c]
		Ammonium chloride	?Inguinal hernia, cataract, benign tumor[d]
Laxatives	Correctol	Phenolphthalein	None[d]
		Docusate	?Neonatal hypomagnesemia[e]
	Ex-Lax	Phenolphthalein	None[d]
	Senokot	Anthraquinone glucosides	None[d]
Purgative	Ipecac (brand and generic name)	Mixture of alkaloids	Probably none[a]

Note. The information in this table was obtained from the University of South Florida Teratogen Information Service.
[a]The data are from Heinonen, Sloan, and Shapiro (1977).
[b]The data are from Devoe, Youssif, Murray, and Arnaud (1993).
[c]The data are from Godel et al. (1992).
[d]The data are from Reproductive Toxicology Center (1988).
[e]The data are from Briggs (1994).

obstetrician specializing in high-risk pregnancies, a psychiatrist familiar with treating eating disorders, a nutritionist, and a neonatologist. Ramchandani and Whedon (1988) describe the difference in outcome for two pregnant bulimic patients, one of whom received adequate treatment and family support and one of whom did not. Management of the rare anorexia nervosa patient who becomes pregnant is very difficult. Hospitalization on a psychiatric unit, with frequent consultation by an obstetrician, is usually necessary. Pregnant anorexia nervosa patients usually require tube feeding and weeks to months in the hospital.

Psychoeducation can be a cornerstone in treatment, especially in facilitating appropriate weight gain. During the third trimester, there is an increased concern with change in body shape and weight gain; emphasizing that most of the weight gain in the third trimester is the baby can be helpful. (See Figure 24.2.)

Individual therapy can most usefully focus initially on assisting the patient in forming an emotional connection to the fetus and making the baby as real as possible. This may help the patient consume adequate nutrition and relinquish purging behaviors. Another issue is the meaning of the pregnancy in terms of the patient's own developmental process, which includes relinquishing girlhood and negotiating an altered relationship with her own parents, particularly her mother. Depending on the patient's marital circumstances, family therapy may focus on helping the patient solidify her relationship with her partner.

THYROID ABNORMALITIES

Primary thyroid disease may precipitate an eating disorder or complicate management of a preexisting eating disorder. Misuse of thyroid hormones or withholding appropriate antithyroid hormones may be used by patients with thyroid disease to promote weight loss or counteract binge eating. In addition, some patients without thyroid disease may abuse thyroid medications.

Diagnosis of Primary Thyroid Disease

Thyroid abnormalities may occur as consequences of semistarvation (Scanlon & Hall, 1989). Many anorexia nervosa patients have the

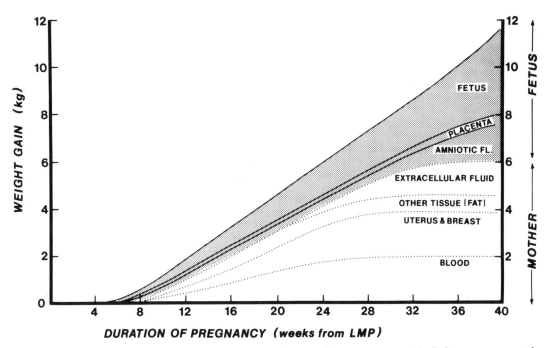

FIGURE 24.2. Pattern and components of average weight gain during pregnancy. Shaded areas represent the fetal components. LMP, last menstrual period. From Pitkin (1976, p. 489). Copyright 1976 by J. B. Lippincott Company. Reprinted by permission.

"sick euthyroid syndrome" (SES), characterized by low triiodotryronine (T_3), impaired peripheral conversion of thyroxine (T_4) to T_3, and increased formation of the inactive metabolite reverse T_3 (rT_3). This functionally decreases metabolism and conserves energy. T_3 uptake (T_3U) is indirectly proportional to thyroid-binding globulin (TBG) activity; when TBG is low, as in anorexia nervosa, the T_3U is high. Total T_4 can also be abnormal if there are TBG abnormalities. In a semistarved anorexia patient, low T_3 and elevated T_3U reflect SES (a metabolic adaptation to semistarvation) and a decrease in protein-binding capacity (another result of semistarvation), respectively (Warren, 1989). Neither abnormality should be treated. Typically, however, thyroid-stimulating hormone (TSH) is not elevated, and free T_4 is normal; abnormalities may indicate primary thyroid disease and should be further investigated.

The abnormalities of thyroid functioning in bulimia nervosa are less well understood, with two exceptions (Kigohara, Tamai, Kobayashi, & Nakagawa, 1988; Hudson & Hudson, 1984). First, rT_3 levels are not elevated. Second, the TSH response to thyroid-releasing hormone is blunted in about 20% of bulimics, but not delayed as in anorexia nervosa patients.

Iatrogenesis

The most common error is the use of thyroid medication to treat SES, which is actually a physiologically protective mechanism. Garfinkel and Garner (1982) found that 5% of patients with anorexia nervosa had been given thyroid hormones, presumably because of abnormal laboratory tests. Prescription of thyroid hormones in anorexics with SES may result in further weight loss. The treatment for SES is weight gain.

Misuse of Treatment for Thyroid Disease

Eating disorder patients may abuse thyroid medications to facilitate weight loss or counter binge eating. In many patients abuse is erratic, since the medication is not prescribed for the patients and is not readily available. Woodside, Walfish, Kaplan, and Kennedy (1991) and Rolla, El-Hajj, and Goldstein (1986) report two cases of patients with hyperthyroidism and co-existing eating disorders who were afraid of the weight gain that would ensue with appropriate

use of antithyroid medications. In my own practice, I have encountered two patients who have taken their mothers' thyroid medications and presented with clinical signs of hyperthyroidism, including weight loss. Both of these patients presented diagnostic challenges that required the combined clinical acumen of a psychiatrist (myself) and an endocrinologist to unravel.

Precipitation of an Eating Disorder

In vulnerable individuals, the onset of a primary thyroid disorder may precipitate an eating disorder. The weight gain that occurs in hypothyroidism, although typically only 5–15 pounds, may heighten fear of obesity and lead to dieting and other weight loss measures. The need for thyroid replacement hormones may provide a patient with a previously unavailable means of promoting weight loss. On the other hand, the weight loss that occurs with hyperthyroidism may be the factor that initiates an eating disorder.

Management Strategies

Patients who have both an eating disorder and primary thyroid disease usually require very close monitoring, and patients with anorexia nervosa usually require inpatient hospitalization. Among outpatients, parents may need to monitor the use of thyroid medications.

In individual psychotherapy, the same themes that are important in other eating disorder patients are also usually relevant. Typically, however, a patient who abuses thyroid medication or fails to take antithyroid medications will initially deny this behavior. Gentle confrontation in the context of a therapeutic relationship may permit the patient to acknowledge the abuse and formulate a plan to relinquish this behavior.

REFERENCES

Aitken, M. L., & Fiel, S. B. (1993). Cystic fibrosis. *Disease-A-Month, 39,* 1–52.

Alexander, F., Bacon, L., Wilson, G., Levey, H., & Levine, M. (1934). The influence of psychological factors upon gastrointestinal disturbances: A symposium. *Psychoanalytic Quarterly, 3,* 501–588.

Birk, R., & Spencer, M. L. (1989). The prevalence of anorexia nervosa, bulimia, and induced glycosuria in IDDM females. *Diabetes Educator, 15,* 336–341.

Briggs, G. G. (Ed.). (1994). *Drugs in pregnancy and lactation* (4th ed.). Baltimore: Williams & Wilkins.

Brinch, M., Isager, T., & Tolstrup, K. (1988). Anorexia nervosa and motherhood: Reproduction pattern and mothering behavior of 50 women. *Acta Psychiatrica Scandinavica, 77,* 611–617.

Cantwell, R., & Steel, M. (1996). Screening for eating disorders in diabetes mellitus. *Journal of Psychosomatic Research, 40,* 15–20.

Devoe, L. D., Youssif, A., Murray, C., & Arnaud, M. (1993). Maternal caffeine consumption and fetal behavior in normal third-trimester pregnancy. *American Journal of Obstetrics and Gynecology, 168,* 1105–1111.

Diabetes Control and Complications Trial Research Group. (1993). The effect of intensive treatment of diabetes on the development and progression of long-term complications in insulin-dependent diabetes mellitus. *New England Journal of Medicine, 329,* 977–986.

Drug Evaluations Manual. (1995). American Medical Association, pp. 43–44.

Drash, A. (1987). *Clinical care of the diabetic child.* Chicago: Year Book Medical.

Durie, P. R., & Pencharz, P. B. (1989). A natural approach to the nutritional care of patients with cystic fibrosis. *Journal of the Royal Society of Medicine, 82,* 11–20.

Fairburn, C. G., Peveler, R. C., Davies, B., Mann, J. I., & Mayou, R. A. (1991). Eating disorders in young adults with insulin dependent diabetes mellitus: A controlled study. *British Medical Journal, 303,* 17–20.

Fairburn, C. G., Stein, A., & Jones, R. (1992). Eating habits and eating disorders during pregnancy. *Psychosomatic Medicine, 54,* 665–672.

Garfinkel, P. E., & Garner, D. M. (1982). *Anorexia nervosa: A multidimensional perspective.* New York: Brunner/Mazel.

Garner, D. M., & Garfinkel, P. E. (1979). The Eating Attitudes Test: An index of the symptoms of anorexia nervosa. *Psychological Medicine, 9,* 273–279.

Garner, D. M., Olmsted, M. P., Bohr, Y., & Garfinkel, P. E. (1982). The Eating Attitudes Test: Psychometric features and clinical correlates. *Psychological Medicine, 12,* 871–878.

Godel, J. C., Johnson, K. E., Pabst, H. F., Froese, G. J., Hodges, P. E., & Joffres, M. R. (1992). Smoking and caffeine and alcohol intake during pregnancy in a Northern population: Effect on fetal growth. *Canadian Medical Association Journal, 147,* 181–187.

Gryboski, J. D. (1993). Eating disorders in inflammatory bowel disease. *American Journal of Gastroenterology, 88,* 293–296.

Gryboski, J. D., Katz, J., Sangree, M. H., & Herskoovic, T. (1968). Eleven adolescent girls with severe anorexia: Intestinal disease or anorexia nervosa? *Clinical Pediatrics, 7,* 684–690.

Heijerman, H. G. M. (1993). Chronic obstructive lung disease and respiratory muscle function: The role of nutrition and exercise training in cystic fibrosis. *Respiratory Medicine, 87,* 49–51.

Heinonen, O. P., Sloan, D., & Shapiro, S. C. (1977). *Birth defects and drugs in pregnancy.* Littleton, MA: Publishing Sciences Group.

Hilliard, J. R., & Hilliard, P. J. A. (1984). Bulimia, anorexia nervosa and diabetes: Deadly combinations. *Psychiatric Clinics of North America, 7,* 367–379.

Hudson, J. I., & Hudson, M. S. (1984). Endocrine dysfunction in anorexia nervosa and bulimia: Comparison with abnormalities in other psychiatric disorders and disturbances due to metabolic factors. *Psychiatric Developments, 4,* 237–272.

Hudson, J. I., Wentworth, S. M., Hudson, M. S., & Pope, H. G. (1985). Prevalence of anorexia nervosa and bulimia among young diabetic women. *Journal of Clinical Psychiatry, 46,* 88–89.

Hunt, J. V., Cooper, B. A., & Tooley, W. W. (1988). Very low birthweight infants at 8 and 11 years of age: Role of neonatal illness and family status. *Pediatrics, 82,* 596–603.

Johnson, M. R., Gershowitz, M., & Stabler, B. (1981). Maternal compliance and children's self-concept. *Journal of Developmental and Behavioral Pediatrics, 2,* 5–8.

Jones, E. (1938). *Papers in psychoanalysis.* Baltimore: Wood.

Kigohara, K., Tamai, H., Kobayashi, N., & Nakagawa, T. (1988). Hypothalamic–pituitary–thyroid axis abnormalities in bulimic patients. *American Journal of Clinical Nutrition, 47,* 805–809.

Lacey, H., & Smith, G. (1987). Bulimia nervosa: The impact of pregnancy on mother and baby. *British Journal of Psychiatry, 150,* 777–781.

Lawson, M. L., Rodin, G. M., Rydall, A. C., Olmsted, M. P., & Daneman, D. (1994). Eating disorders in young women with IDDM: The need for prevention. *Eating Disorders: The Journal of Treatment and Prevention, 2,* 261–272.

Lemberg, R., & Phillips, J. (1989). The impact of pregnancy on anorexia nervosa and bulimia. *International Journal of Eating Disorders, 8,* 285–295.

Lindner, R. (1955). *The fifty minute hour.* New York: Rinehart.

Meadows, G., & Treasure, J. (1989). Bulimia nervosa and Crohn's disease: Two case reports. *Acta Psychiatrica Scandinavica, 79,* 413–414.

Mitchell, J. E., Seim, H. C., Glotter, D., Soll, E. A., & Pyle, R. L. (1991). A retrospective study of pregnancy in bulimia nervosa. *International Journal of Eating Disorders, 10,* 209–214.

Namiri, S., Melman, K. N., & Yager, J. (1986). Pregnancy in restricter-type anorexia nervosa: A study of six women. *International Journal of Eating Disorders, 51,* 837–845.

Palla, B., & Litt, I. F. (1987). Medical complications of eating disorders in adolescents. *Pediatrics, 81,* 613–623.

Pearson, D. A., Pumariega, A. J., & Seilheimer, D. K. (1991). The development of psychiatric symptomatology in patients with cystic fibrosis. *Journal of the American Academy of Child and Adolescent Psychiatry, 30,* 290–297.

Peveler, R. C., & Fairburn, C. G. (1989). Anorexia nervosa in association with diabetes mellitus: A cognitive-behavioural approach to treatment. *Behaviour Research and Therapy, 27,* 95–99.

Peveler, R. C., & Fairburn, C. G. (1992). The treatment of bulimia nervosa in patients with diabetes mellitus. *International Journal of Eating Disorders, 11,* 45–53.

Pitkin, R. M. (1976). Nutritional support in obstetrics and gynecology. *Clinical Obstetrics and Gynecology, 19,* 489–513.

Powers, P. S., Malone, J. I., Coovert, D. L., & Schulman, R. G. (1990). Insulin-dependent diabetes mellitus and eating disorders: A prevalence study. *Comprehensive Psychiatry, 31,* 205–210.

Powers, P. S., Malone, J. I., & Duncan, J. A. (1983). Anorexia nervosa and diabetes mellitus. *Journal of Clinical Psychiatry, 44,* 133–135.

Price, W. A., Giannini, A. J., & Loiselle, R. H. (1986). Bulimia precipitated by pregnancy [Letter]. *Journal of Clinical Psychiatry, 47,* 275–276.

Pumariega, A. J., Pursell, J., Spock, A., & Jones, J. D. (1986). Eating disorders in adolescents with cystic fibrosis. *Journal of the American Academy of Child Psychiatry, 25,* 269–275.

Ramchandani, D., & Whedon, B. (1988). The effect of pregnancy on bulimia. *International Journal of Eating Disorders, 7,* 845–848.

Ramsey, B. Q., Farrell, P. M., Pencharz, P., & the Consensus Committee. (1992). Nutritional assessment and management in cystic fibrosis: A consensus report. *American Journal of Clinical Nutrition, 55,* 108–116.

Rand, C. S. W., Willis, D. C., & Kuldau, J. M. (1987). Pregnancy after anorexia nervosa. *International Journal of Eating Disorders, 6,* 671–674.

Reproductive Toxicology Center (Producer). (1988). *Reprotox database* [Machine-readable data file]. Washington, DC: Producer.

Rickards, H., Prendergast, M., & Booth, I. W. (1994). Psychiatric presentation of Crohn's disease. *British Journal of Psychiatry, 164,* 256–261.

Rodin, G. M., Craven, J. L., & Littlefield, C. (1991). Eating disorders and intentional insulin undertreatment in adolescent females with diabetes. *Psychosomatics, 32,* 171–176.

Rodin, G. M., Daneman, D., Johnson, L. E., Kenshole, A., & Garfinkel, P. E. (1985). Anorexia nervosa and bulimia in female adolescents with insulin dependent diabetes mellitus: A systematic study. *Journal of Psychiatric Research, 19,* 381–384.

Rolla, A. R., El-Hajj, G. A., & Goldstein, H. H. (1986). Untreated thyrotoxicosis as a manifestation of anorexia nervosa. *American Journal of Medicine, 81,* 163–165.

Rosenberg, I. H., Bengoa, J. M., & Sitrin, M. D. (1985). Nutritional aspects of inflammatory bowel disease. *Annual Review of Nutrition, 5,* 563–584.

Rydall, A., Rodin, G., Olmsted, M., Devenyi, R., & Daneman, D. (1994). A four year follow-up study of eating disorders and medical complications in young women with insulin-dependent diabetes mellitus. *Psychosomatic Medicine, 56,* 179. (Abstract)

Scanlon, M. F., & Hall, R. (1989). Thyroid stimulating hormone: Synthesis, control of release, and secretion. In L. J. DeGroot (Ed.), *Endocrinology* (pp. 337–383). Philadelphia: W.B. Saunders.

Seller, M. J. (1987). Nutritionally induced cognitive defects. *Proceedings of the Nutrition Society, 46,* 227–235.

Stancin, T., Link, D. L., & Reuter, J. M. (1989). Binge eating and purging in young women with IDDM. *Diabetes Care, 12,* 601–603.

Stark, L. J., Knapp, L. G., Bowen, A. M., Powers, S. W., Evans, S., Aussero, M. A., Mulvihill, M. M., & Hovell,

M. (1993). Increasing calorie consumption in children with cystic fibrosis: Replication with 2-year follow-up. *Journal of Applied Behavioral Analysis, 26,* 435–450.

Steel, J. M., Young, R. J., Lloyd, G. G., & Clarke, B. F. (1987). Clinically apparent eating disorders in young diabetic women: Associations with painful neuropathy and other complications. *British Medical Journal, 294,* 859–862.

Stein, A., & Fairburn, C. G. (1989). Children of mothers with bulimia nervosa. *British Medical Journal, 299,* 777–778.

Steiner, J., Rahimzadeh, P., & Lewiston, N. B. (1990). Psychopathology in cystic fibrosis and anorexia nervosa: A controlled comparison. *International Journal of Eating Disorders, 9,* 675–683.

Stewart, D. E., Raskin, J., Garfinkel, P. E., MacDonald, O. L., & Robinson, G. E. (1987). Anorexia nervosa, bulimia and pregnancy. *American Journal of Obstetrics and Gynecology, 157,* 1194–1198.

Treasure, J. L., & Russell, G. F. (1988). Intrauterine growth and neonatal weight gain in babies of women with anorexia nervosa. *British Medical Journal, 296,* 1038–1039.

Ward, A., Troop, N., Cachia, M., Watkins, P., & Treasure, J. (1995). Doubly disabled: diabetes in combination with an eating disorder. *Postgraduate Medical Journal, 71,* 546–550.

Warren, M. P. (1989). Anorexia nervosa. In L. J. DeGroot (Ed.), *Endocrinology* (pp. 2294–2302). Philadelphia: W.B. Saunders.

Weinfeld, R. H. (1977). Pregnancy associated with anorexia and starvation. *American Journal of Obstetrics and Gynecology, 129,* 698–699.

Westrate, J. A., & Deurenberg, P. (1989). Body composition in children: Proposal for a method for calculating body fat percentage from total body density or skinfold-thickness measurements. *American Journal of Clinical Nutrition, 50,* 1104–1115.

Willis, D. C., & Rand, C. S. W. (1988). Pregnancy in bulimic women. *Obstetrics and Gynecology, 71,* 708–710.

Wing, R. R., Norwalk, M. D., Marcus, M. D., Koeske, R., & Finefold, D. (1986). Subclinical eating disorders and glycemic control in adolescents with Type I diabetes. *Diabetes Care, 9,* 162–167.

Woodside, D. B., & Shekter-Wolfson, L. F. (1990). Parenting by parents with anorexia nervosa and bulimia nervosa. *International Journal of Eating Disorders, 9,* 303–309.

Woodside, D. B., Walfish, P., Kaplan, A. S., & Kennedy, S. H. (1991). Graves disease in a woman with thyroid hormone abuse, bulimia nervosa, and a history of anorexia nervosa. *International Journal of Eating Disorders, 10,* 111–115.

CHAPTER 25

Treatment of Patients with Personality Disorders

AMY BAKER DENNIS
RANDY A. SANSONE

Professionals are increasingly interested in effective treatment strategies for the significant minority of eating disorder patients with concomitant Axis II personality disorders. Many of these patients enter treatment with the same types of eating disorder pathology as non-personality-disordered patients. However, upon closer examination, these individuals often display serious characterological disturbances that can have a significant impact upon their ability to recover from their eating disorders. Although standardized treatments appear to be highly effective for approximately one-third to two-thirds of eating disorder patients, the remaining patients do not appear to respond well to conventional approaches. The majority of these nonresponders may be individuals with Axis II psychopathology. Therefore, individualized treatment plans for these patients must take their character structure into consideration.

The foundation of an individual's personality is established early in childhood and influenced by both constitutional and environmental factors. Personality traits evolve as a consequence of individual temperament and the family environment; which result in a distinctive way of viewing the world and the self, and of coping and relating to others. These traits consist of habits, attitudes, beliefs, and emotional responses that are enduring and not just prompted by stressful external events. Therefore, in the diagnosis of personality disorders, it is essential that the clinician distinguish between personality *traits* (ingrained and habitual patterns of psychological functioning) and personality *states* (reactions to stressful situations that tend to be transient or brief in duration, or that subside shortly after these conditions are removed) (Millon, 1981). If personality disturbance is identified in an eating disorder patient, the therapist's approach and treatment plan must accommodate the personality disorder.

This chapter begins with a brief review of the literature on the prevalence of personality disorders in patients with eating disorders, and highlights the clinical trends that this review suggests. The remainder of the chapter focuses on the personality disorders found most often in eating-disordered individuals. A description of each personality disorder and its relationship to eating disorders is followed by specific treatment issues.

THE PREVALENCE OF PERSONALITY DISORDERS IN THE EATING-DISORDERED POPULATION

Over the past decade, a fairly extensive literature has emerged on the prevalence of personality disorders in eating disorder patients. However, researchers have reported widely divergent findings. For example, the prevalence of personality disorders in bulimic subjects has been reported to range from 0% (Frankel et al., 1988) to 84.5% (Norman, Blais, & Herzog,

1986; Pope, Frankenburg, Hudson, Jonas, & Yurgelun-Todd, 1987; Reich, Nduaguba, & Yates, 1988; Wonderlich, Swift, Slotnick, & Goodman, 1990). Prevalence estimates of personality disorders in subjects with the restricting subtype of anorexia nervosa have also varied, with Garner, Marcus, Halmi, and Loranger (1989) reporting 31%, Normal et al. (1993) 77.8%, Wonderlich et al. (1990) 80%, and Piran, Lerner, Garfinkel, Kennedy, and Brouillette (1988) 86.7%. More recent studies have investigated the prevalence of character pathology in subjects with the binge-eating/purging subtype of anorexia nervosa and have reported estimates between 70% (Wonderlich et al., 1990) and 97.4% (Piran, Lerner, et al., 1988).

The inconsistencies found among these prevalence estimates may be attributed to the various instruments used to measure personality pathology, the differences between the clinical populations being investigated (e.g., inpatient vs. outpatient), vaguely defined eating disorder criteria, and small sample sizes. Despite these methodological limitations, several distinct and consistent themes have nevertheless emerged from the research literature on the prevalence of personality pathology in subjects with eating disorders.

1. *Cluster B's association with bulimia nervosa and anorexia nervosa, binge-eating/purging type.* When personality pathology is present, individuals suffering from bulimia nervosa or the binge-eating/purging type of anorexia nervosa are most likely to exhibit Cluster B personality pathology (particularly borderline or histrionic personality features) (Ames-Frankel et al., 1992; Dowson, 1992; Bossert-Zaudig, Zaudig, Junker, Weigand, & Krieg, 1993; Gwirtsman, Roy-Byrne, Yager, & Gerner, 1983; Levin & Hyler, 1986; McClelland, Mynors-Wallis, Fahy, & Treasure, 1991; Piran, Lerner, et al., 1988; Powers, Coovert, Brightwell, & Stevens, 1988; Rossiter, Agras, Telch, & Schneider, 1993; Steiger, Liquornik, Chapman, & Hussain, 1991; Wonderlich et al., 1990; Yates, Sieleni, Reich, & Brass, 1989; Zanarini et al., 1990).

2. *Borderline personality disorder's association with bulimia nervosa and anorexia nervosa, binge-eating/purging type.* In studies concurrently assessing for any Axis II diagnosis, a majority of researchers have reported that borderline personality is the predominant Axis II pathology associated with bulimia nervosa and the binge-eating/purging type of anorexia ner-

vosa (Ames-Frankel et al., 1992; Dowson, 1992; Gwirtsman et al., 1983; Herzog, Keller, Lavori, Kenny, & Sacks, 1992; Kennedy, McVey, & Katz, 1990; McClelland et al., 1991; Piran, Lerner, et al., 1988; Rossiter et al., 1993; Schmidt & Telch, 1990; Zanarini et al., 1990; Zerbe, Marsh, & Coyne, 1993).

Several studies have specifically focused on the prevalence of borderline personality disorder in bulimic subjects and binge-eating/purging anorexia subjects (Dennis, 1991; Gartner & Gartner, 1988; Gwirtsman et al., 1983; Levin & Hyler, 1986; Hudson, Pope, Jonas, & Yurgelun-Todd, 1983; Johnson, Tobin, & Enright, 1989; Kennedy et al., 1990; Piran, Lerner, et al., 1988; Sansone, Fine, Seuferer, & Bovenzi, 1989; Skodol et al., 1993; Sunday, Levey, & Halmi, 1993; Wonderlich et al., 1990; Yates et al., 1989). Prevalence rates have ranged from 1.9% (Pope et al., 1987) to 75% (Levendusky & Herring, 1989), with an average of 34%. This body of literature suggests that approximtely one in three bulimics or binge-eating/purging anorexics will have comorbid borderline pathology.

Of course, prevalence rates are significantly affected by the population sampled. In studies examining both bulimic inpatients and bulimic outpatients, a higher prevalence of borderline personality disorder was found in inpatients than in outpatients (Frankel et al., 1988; Levin & Hyler, 1986).

3. *Cluster C's association with anorexia nervosa.* In studies examining personality disorders in subjects with anorexia nervosa, primarily restrictors, researchers have reported a higher prevalence of Cluster C personality disorders (specifically, avoidant, obsessive–compulsive, or dependent personality disorders) compared to the other clusters (Dowson, 1992; Gartner et al., 1989; Herzog et al., 1992; McClelland et al., 1991; Norman et al., 1993; Piran, Lerner, et al., 1988; Skodol et al., 1993; Steiger et al., 1991; Wonderlich et al., 1990).

BORDERLINE PERSONALITY DISORDER

Description

Individuals with borderline personality disorder often appear superficially intact during brief social encounters, despite dramatic internal chaos. Borderline individuals have markedly low self-esteem, significant self-regulatory deficits, and great difficulty in maintaining stable interpersonal relationships. They also have significant problems in daily functioning, particularly in their social and work environments.

One of the most striking characteristics of borderline individuals is their extremely low self-esteem. They maintain the core belief that they are unequivocally "bad," and they attempt to mold and distort their world to reinforce this negative belief. Positive events, such as compliments, attention, affection, or praise from others, are often underexperienced because they are inconsistent with this negative self-perception. In fact, positive experiences can precipitate intense negative affective states, including anticipatory anxiety, panic attacks, suspiciousness, or even quasi-psychotic phenomena (e.g., paranoid ideation, rage reactions). Negative events, such as criticism, rejection, and verbal or physical punishment, are often experienced as ego-syntonic because they are perceived as being "deserved" and consistent with the individual's self-appraisal.

Borderline individuals have significant problems with maintaining ongoing, stable relationships with others. Close relationships tend to be chaotic, intense, and marked by the simultaneous fear of engulfment (should others become too close or intimate) and abandonment (should others go too far away). This inability to modulate interpersonal distance prevents the borderline individual from experiencing relationships in a satisfying way and promotes a sense of isolation, emptiness, and loneliness.

Still another prominent feature of borderline personality disorder is the inability to modulate affect. Clinically, this deficit may be manifested as overemotionality, extreme sensitivity, chronic dysphoria (e.g., anxiety, depression), hostility, or severe affective vacillation from rage to numbness (i.e., emotional lability).

Impulse difficulties, invariably present in patients with borderline personality disorder, are expressed in self-destructive behavior and self-regulatory problems. Self-destructive behaviors may include (but are not limited to) self-mutilation, such as cutting, burning, biting, or bruising body parts; suicide attempts; high-risk hobbies or behaviors; accident-proneness; and the sabotage of medical care. Self-regulation difficulties may manifest themselves as substance abuse/dependence, promiscuity, eating disorders, and excessive gambling or shopping.

Borderline personality disorder is heterogeneous in its clinical presentation. For example, it may coexist with a variety of Axis I diagnoses (e.g., eating disorders, affective disorders, anxiety disorders, substance abuse/dependence, dissociative disorders). In addition, borderline individuals vary in their level of functioning. Higher-functioning patients tend to have more reality-intact quasi-psychotic experiences (e.g., magical thinking, plausible fantasy), whereas lower-functioning patients may display more overt psychotic phenomena (e.g., fleeting hallucinations and/or delusions).

Relationship to Eating Disorders

As noted earlier, borderline personality disorder is relatively common in bulimic and binge-eating/purging anorexic patients. This is not surprising, because eating disorder behaviors serve a variety of adaptive functions for borderline patients. First, the pursuit of thinness often functions to enhance the patient's extremely low self-esteem. Second, these patients have a limited ability to self-soothe, and binge eating can serve as a self-soothing mechanism. Third, borderline patients have significant self-regulatory difficulties, and purging may function to help them regain a sense of self-control. Fourth, eating disorder behaviors (e.g., self-starvation, excessive exercising, laxative abuse, vomiting) are by nature self-destructive and can be utilized as a form of self-punishment. Finally, for some borderline patients, these behaviors can serve to numb them against intolerable emotional pain or help them to avoid decompensation.

Specific Treatment Issues

The borderline patient usually presents for treatment with the same drive for thinness and preoccupation with food, weight, and shape as other eating disorder patients exhibit. However, upon closer examination, the eating disorder symptoms are found to be part of a lifelong pattern of self-regulatory deficits and self-destructive behaviors. Treatment of the eating disorder symptoms should be addressed within the larger context of these behaviors and deficits.

The foundation for successful treatment of the borderline patient is intensive individual psychotherapy. We utilize a psychodynamic approach that is directive, confrontational, and interpretive, coupled with cognitive-behavioral techniques designed to improve self-esteem and contain self-destructive behaviors. Treatment focuses on the patient's character structure, with the reduction of the eating disorder symptoms as a simultaneous but secondary priority. The primary goals for individual psychotherapy are as follows: (1) the reparation of distortions in interpersonal relationships (e.g., the resolution of splitting), in order to increase the patient's ability to relate to others in a more realistic way; (2) the attainment of reasonable levels of self-regulation by confronting impulsive behaviors, including disordered eating behaviors; (3) the stabilization of mood and interpersonal boundaries; and (4) the enhancement of self-esteem. These goals are achieved through the promotion of self-regulation, the enhancement of evocative memory, the resolution of splitting, and the consolidation of object constancy.

We have previously outlined four clinical stages of treatment for the eating disorder patient with borderline personality disorder (Dennis & Sansone, 1991). Stage I ("Establishing the Therapeutic Milieu") entails establishing a consistent treatment environment, emphasizing the working relationship, limiting adjunctive treatments, structuring the integration of the family, maintaining a realistic treatment focus, managing projective identification, setting limits, and preparing for countertransference reactions.

The creation of a stable treatment environment in which a reparative relationship can take place is essential when working with these patients. Borderline patients appear to function best in an environment that is structured and predictable. For example, appointments should be scheduled each week at the same time, in the same office, with sessions beginning and ending on time. Facilitating a rhythm for time and space can provide these patients with a sense of safety and security.

The consolidation of a working therapeutic relationship is also critical with this subgroup of patients. Relationship building is often time-consuming and fraught with setbacks because of the patient's strong mistrust of others, recurrent splitting, and inability to regulate interpersonal distance. Relationship boundaries may be repeatedly challenged (e.g., constant phone calls to the office or home, frequent gift giving, inquiries about the therapist's private life, requests for special treatment), as these individuals have significant difficulty determining how close or how distant to be in interpersonal relationships. These potential boundary violations

may also represent "tests of caring." Therefore, the therapist should be aware of the constant need to realign interpersonal boundaries in a genuine and caring fashion. Caution should be exercised to avoid becoming either too close and indulgent or excessively distant and rejecting. The therapeutic relationship "should be one of trust and warmth, which allows closeness without fusion, separateness without abandonment, and confrontation without retaliation" (Dennis & Sansone, 1991, p. 138).

During the initial stage of treatment, adjunctive treatments (e.g., nutritional counseling, group therapy, support groups) as well as multiple therapeutic relationships are avoided, to decrease the potential for splitting and acting-out behaviors. However, family involvement in the therapeutic process may become necessary. Family sessions are designed to educate members about the symptoms and dynamics of the patient's behaviors, to process family events within the context of the patient's dynamics, to stress the importance of structure and consistency within the family setting, to define parental roles, and to promote nonjudgmental limit setting by parents.

As mentioned above, the primary goal for Stage I is the development of a viable therapeutic milieu and relationship. In order for the therapist to accomplish this task, he or she must maintain a realistic focus for the treatment process. For example, although the therapist can begin educating the patient on the social, behavioral, psychological, and physical complications of the eating disorder and monitoring food intake and compensatory behaviors during the relationship-building process, the elimination of the disordered eating behaviors is not the ultimate goal. Rather, the focus at this stage is helping the patient begin to globally explore issues of self-regulation, symptom management, and control.

From the onset of treatment, the therapist should be prepared to set firm, nonjudgmental, and concrete limits with the borderline patient. Limit setting is often required to clarify the boundaries of the therapeutic relationship, the therapist's ethical and legal responsibilities in crisis situations, the therapist's availability, acceptable behavior or language within the session, the consequences of acting-out or self-destructive behaviors, and so on. Oral or written contracts are helpful and can provide the patient with stability, predictability, structure, and a sense of control. Limits should be based on compassion and concern for the safety and welfare of the patient, and designed to preserve and protect the treatment relationship. They should not emerge solely in the midst of a crisis or in response to the therapist's anger.

Unfortunately, borderline patients can be challenging and frustrating to even the most skilled clinicians. Therefore, during Stage I, therapists should actively prepare to confront their countertransference reactions through either formal or informal supervision. Countertransference reactions are often forceful, raw, and primitive; they can range from panic, rage, or guilt to powerlessness, depression, or indifference. To manage these reactions, the therapist should first thoroughly educate themselves on the psychology of borderline patients and repeatedly relabel and reframe the patient's affect, behavior, and projections within the context of the borderline process. This will allow the therapist to remain neutral and not experience the patient's whirlwind of emotions as a personal attack. Second, therapists must recognize their personal limitations in treating these complex patients. An eating disorder patient with borderline personality requires a significant amount of dedication and time to treat. Their crises rarely occur between 8:00 A.M. and 5:00 P.M. on weekdays. By limiting the number of borderline patients in their caseloads at any given time, and ensuring that there are adequate backup services (e.g., inpatient programs, 24-hour emergency services, day hospital programs), therapists can improve their chances of successfully managing suicidal and/or self-destructive patients.

Stage II of treatment ("Stabilization of the Transference") consists of promoting reality testing, encouraging verbalization, staying in the "here and now," educating the patient, stabilizing symptoms, and managing self-destructive behaviors through the use of cognitive-behavioral and interpersonal restructuring techniques. With the therapeutic relationship firmly established in Stage I, Stage II utilizes that relationship to begin the process of changing behaviors and cognitions, with the goal of improving overall self-regulation.

To promote reality testing in the eating disorder patient with borderline personality disorder, the therapist should be genuine and model appropriate affect. Therapeutic neutrality does not work well with these patients; it can promote fantasizing and/or cause a predominantly negative transference. However, during episodes of acute crisis, decompensation, or self-destructive acting out, emotional neutrality is necessary and prevents the inadvertent reinforcement of these behaviors, which can occur if the therapist either overreacts or underreacts.

During Stage II, the treatment focuses directly on the management of self-destructive behaviors, including anorexic and bulimic symptomatology. Cognitive-behavioral and interpersonal restructuring techniques for the management of eating disorder symptoms, acting-out behaviors, and other self-destructive behaviors is extensively detailed elsewhere (Dennis & Sansone, 1989, 1991; Sansone & Johnson, 1995).

Once the therapeutic relationship is established and the transference is stabilized, the patient can begin to focus on "Resolving Internal Themes" (Stage III). This consists of a psychodynamic effort to promote object constancy through the strengthening of evocative memory (i.e., the ability to evoke the image of another when the other is absent), resolving splitting, dynamically managing self-destructive behaviors, and promoting global self-regulation.

In Stage III, the dynamic reasons for engaging in acting-out or self-destructive behaviors are explored with the goal of improving self-control. Poor impulse regulation serves a variety of purposes for these individuals, including self-soothing, self-numbing in the presence of escalating dysphoria, and/or punishing the negatively perceived self. For many individuals, physical pain (e.g., cutting, burning) is easier to manage than emotional pain. Finally, impulsive behaviors may help these individuals to reorganize themselves psychologically in the face of impending decompensation.

"Preparing for Termination" is the final phase of treatment (Stage IV). The decision to terminate treatment should be based on the patient's overall progress in the following areas: global self-regulation (i.e., the reasonable resolution of the eating disorder symptoms and other self-destructive behaviors, the stabilization of mood) and improved interpersonal relatedness through the realignment of interpersonal boundaries and the consolidation of object constancy (i.e., increased tolerance for aloneness, decreased dependence on others, enhanced capacity for self-soothing, resolution of splitting).

Psychotropic medications are only moderately useful in the treatment of eating-disordered borderline patients. Caution should be exercised in prescribing medication to these patients, for several reasons. First, borderline patients often respond inconsistently and unpredictablly to psychotropic medications. Second, medications may be helpful in managing target symptoms (e.g., depression, anxiety) for brief periods, but the long-term efficacy in this population is unknown. Third, many borderline patients do not take medications as prescribed, because of their highly impulsive and self-destructive nature. Clinicians must therefore weigh the risks of misuse, abuse, addiction, and/or overdose against the potential benefits when prescribing medications to this group of patients.

Although hospitalization should be avoided if at all possible, inpatient treatment may become necessary for metabolic stabilization, weight restoration, intractable binge eating and purging, concomitant substance abuse/dependence, highly lethal self-destructive behaviors (e.g., self-mutilation, suicide attempts), or psychiatric decompensation (e.g., psychotic episodes). Unfortunately, hospitalization can promote further regression, exacerbate splitting, and increase resistance to accepting personal responsibility for self-regulation. In most instances, the goals of inpatient treatment should be clearly defined and achievable within the short term (e.g., medical or psychiatric stabilization, normalization of eating patterns, disruption of the binge–purge cycle). The resolution of chronic suicidal ideation in a borderline patient is not a realistic short-term goal of hospitalization.

HISTRIONIC PERSONALITY DISORDER

Description

Histrionic personality disorder is characterized by a persistent need for attention, acceptance, and approval by others. To ensure that they always remain in the social spotlight, these individuals tend to be dramatic, exhibitionistic, and/or interpersonally seductive. Their extreme sensitivity to the moods and thoughts of others alerts them to potential criticism or rejection and helps them to manipulate others to avoid disapproval or abandonment. This manipulation may be manifested as overdependence, helplessness, exaggeration, fabrication, suicidal gestures, somatization, angry outbursts, tantrums, or provocative and seductive behaviors.

Histrionic individuals rapidly develop relationships that initially appear stimulating and satisfying. However, upon closer examination, these relationships are superficial and lack warmth, genuineness, integrity, and loyalty. Driven by their endless desire for stimulation and immediate gratification, histrionic individuals are easily bored, frequently frustrated, and continually disappointed. These individuals are highly susceptible to labile moods, depression, and dysphoria.

Unfortunately, the histrionic individual has little insight into their motivations, thoughts, or behaviors. Their external focus prevents them from utilizing inner resources, such as self-reflection, as a source of information. Individuals with histrionic personality disorder are easily distracted and appear demanding, immature, egocentric, erratic, and shallow. They rarely demonstrate an interest in academic or intellectual pursuits. However, many of these individuals are talented in the dramatic arts or other creative endeavors.

Relationship to Eating Disorders

Histrionic personality disorder is relatively common in individuals with eating disorders. The character structure of histrionic individuals is quite conducive to the development of an eating disorder. Their extreme external preoccupation with being socially acceptable and desirable may extend to an overconcern about weight, shape, and appearance, and lead them into chronic dieting. The eating disorder symptoms may also help these individuals to manage negative feelings and to alleviate boredom or chronic dysphoria.

Specific Treatment Issues

The development of a therapeutic relationship with a histrionic eating-disordered patient is accomplished relatively easily compared to patients with other personality disorders. Histrionic individuals possess both the social skills and the need for interpersonal connectedness that facilitates a therapeutic relationship. Because these individuals are excessively dependent on the approval of others, they will seek to elicit acceptance and attention from the therapist. A therapeutic alliance with such a patient usually develops quite rapidly, but the patient may lose interest in or terminate the treatment process if the therapist probes too deeply or pushes for symptom amelioration too quickly.

The primary goals for individual psychotherapy with a histrionic patient are to help the patient (1) decrease their dependence on others and work toward self-reliance; (2) develop the capacity to sustain healthier and deeper interpersonal relationships; (3) develop a more internal focus of awareness and self-evaluation; (4) enhance affective regulation; and (5) reduce the intense focus on appearance.

Normalizing eating patterns, breaking the binge–purge cycle, and restoring weight can be extremely threatening for histrionic individuals, because they have few internal skills and resources, and thus rely on their external appearance to draw attention and attract others. Cognitive restructuring around the meaning of weight, shape, and appearance, and helping these patients find other ways to determine self-worth, are essential to lasting recovery with this subgroup.

Group treatments may be beneficial in helping histrionic patients begin to relate to others in a more genuine and realistic fashion. However, these patients can be extremely competitive, particularly with attractive fellow patients of the same sex; which can result in excessive tension in the milieu or group setting. Histrionic patients may also be quickly dismissed by other patients, who perceive them as extremely superficial, not to be trusted, and uninterested in others. Indeed, the extreme external focus of these patients often precludes their capacity for psychological abstraction, meaningful feedback, or empathy with others. In some instances, fellow patients may end up shunning a severely histrionic patient.

Family therapy, like group treatment, may assist a histrionic patient in developing a healthier style of relating to others. Psychoeducational groups, nutritional counseling, and body image work may also be helpful. Psychotropic medications may be useful for the treatment of concomitant depression and/or anxiety.

AVOIDANT PERSONALITY DISORDER

Description

Avoidant personality disorder is characterized by the active but ambivalent detachment from social involvement with others. These individuals want to participate in relationships; they desire affection, attention, and an active social life. However, they deeply fear disapproval, ridicule, and rejection by others, and consequently lead isolated and unhappy lives. Individuals with avoidant personality struggle with low self-esteem, are hypersensitive to criticism, and experience extreme self-doubt that interferes with social and occupational functioning. They remain ever vigilant to social signs of disrespect, criticism, or abandonment, and fear social embarrassment, shame, and the confirmation of their inferiority.

Relationship to Eating Disorders

Avoidant personality disorder is more common in individuals with anorexia nervosa, especially the restricting subtype, than in those with bulimia nervosa. Eating disorder symptoms may serve several adaptive functions for individuals with avoidant personality disorder. First, significant weight loss may allow these individuals to "disappear" still further from their social environments, and may help them to feel less exposed or vulnerable to criticism or devaluation. Second, eating disorder behaviors can become substitutes for interpersonal relationships for the avoidant individual. These behaviors are predictable, are carried out in private, fill time, and are often comforting. Third, some avoidant individuals utilize eating disorder behaviors to put further distance between themselves and others. Exhaustive exercise, chronic vomiting, laxative abuse, and/or starvation may be utilized as methods to promote further self-alienation as well as self-degradation in these patients. Finally, for some individuals, the fantasized result of eating disorder behaviors (i.e., a new body) may offer renewed hope of social connectedness.

Specific Treatment Issues

Individual psychotherapy with avoidant eating-disordered patients is a lengthy and tedious process. From the outset, they are reluctant to seek help from therapists, who they fear will criticize them and/or expose their inadequacies. Therapy must progress slowly, with the initial emphasis on the development of a trusting and genuine relationship. As the therapeutic relationship is consolidated, therapy should focus on building an avoidant individual's self-esteem and self-worth by helping the patient discover strengths, abilities, and talents that may have been overlooked or devalued in childhood or adolescence. In the subsequent phases of the treatment, the emphasis shifts to (1) exploring the painful memories that led to the serious mistrust and fear of ridicule and rejection by others, and (2) reinitiating relationships with others. Through both cognitive and psychodynamic techniques, the therapist can begin to help the patient rework distorted attitudes and beliefs about the nature of relationships. The internal reworking of relationships will be reinforced by the patient's experience in the therapeutic relationship. However, for many of these patients, it is difficult to go beyond a relationship with the therapist.

Milieu and group treatments are not appropriate until an avoidant patient has consolidated a relationship with the therapist. These treatment environments can often tax and overwhelm avoidant individuals. Initiating a time-limited group treatment prior to milieu treatment is often more prudent and can reduce some of the internal stress precipitated by social demands. Group treatments can provide an initial forum for avoidant patients to learn new social skills and to recognize their ability to participate in relationships without rejection or humiliation. It is advantageous if the individual therapist is also the group therapist.

Psychotropic medication may be of moderate benefit to avoidant individuals who are suffering from mood and/or anxiety disorders. Responses are typically tempered by the presence of the personality disorder (comorbid condition). However, activating antidepressants such as fluoxetine (Prozac) may be of particular benefit in promoting social alertness; likewise, sedating antidepressants such as amitriptyline (Elavil) may lead to a retreat from others.

Family intervention is useful in terms of collecting information about a patient's early relationships with family members and peers. This information may be particularly useful in foreshadowing the type of transference–countertransference issues that may arise in the treatment, as well as in understanding the patient's reactions to others.

Expressive experiences, such as art therapy, can be useful in tapping into the deeper social and interpersonal themes of these individuals. Expressive experiences may initially be used in individual psychotherapy and expanded into a group format when the patient becomes more socially tolerant. The same recommendation is applicable to psychoeducational experiences and other types of adjunctive treatments. In integrating any type of intervention into the treatment of avoidant individuals, the most important guide for therapists is to monitor the patient's tolerance, particularly in regards to the social demands of dealing with others.

DEPENDENT PERSONALITY DISORDER

Description

Dependent personality disorder is characterized by a pervasive sense of inferiority, submissiveness, helplessness, and self-effacing behavior, coupled with an overwhelming fear of abandonment. Dependent individuals believe that they are unable to make competent decisions or effectively manage their personal lives. As a result, they attach themselves to individuals who will provide them with structure, guidance, and direction. By denying their individuality, subordinating their needs and desires, and being forever self-sacrificing in relationships, persons with dependent personality disorder avoid isolation, rejection, and abandonment.

Dependent individuals are passive participants in life. They tend to magnify their own weaknesses; to belittle their abilities, skills, and appearance; and to assume personal responsibility for any problems in their relationships. On the other hand, they provide consistent caring and support, and are compliant, generous, humble, and completely loyal to the individuals they are dependent upon. Their conciliatory, self-sacrificing attitude and inability to function independently may even lead them to passively accept verbal, sexual, or physical abuse.

Dependent individuals are prone to abandonment depression and isolation anxiety. If their efforts to remain attached to a person are thwarted, they urgently seek a new relationship, often settling for a less than desirable partner. By attaching themselves to individuals they perceive as powerful, all-knowing, and protective, dependent individuals can avoid assuming responsibilities, making decisions, or engaging in the competitive struggles of life.

Relationship to Eating Disorders

Dependent personality disorder is fairly common among patients with eating disorders, especially anorexia nervosa (Ames-Frankel et al., 1992; Gartner et al., 1989; Kennedy et al., 1990; Norman et al., 1993; Wonderlich et al., 1990;

Yager, Landsverk, Edelstein, & Hyler, 1989; Yates et al., 1989). The adaptive function of anorexia nervosa for dependent individuals may be to prevent separation from caregivers, avoid social/educational/occupational maturation, and eliminate the possibility of future independent functioning. The extreme physical debilitation of anorexia nervosa virtually guarantees that they will not have to separate from those they are dependent upon. To a lesser degree, bulimic symptoms may function in the same manner.

Specific Treatment Issues

Individual psychotherapy is the cornerstone of treatment with dependent eating-disordered patients. The therapeutic relationship often evolves quite rapidly, as such patients are eager to attach themselves to a therapist they perceive as strong, competent, and equipped to solve their problems. Accordingly, the therapist must be extremely careful to balance the therapeutic alliance and avoid a dominant–submissive relationship. The therapist can promote balance by (1) avoiding the repeated rescue of the patient; (2) avoiding the covert establishment of an overly dependent therapeutic relationship; (3) minimizing directives; and (4) encouraging the patient to make decisions independently.

As the therapeutic relationship progresses, the treatment goals will include: (1) the development of a sense of self-confidence and self-esteem; (2) the promotion of independent thinking, personal competence, and autonomous behavior; (3) the enhancement of self-awareness through the verbalization of feelings, desires, and needs; (4) the resolution of maturity fears that may be maintaining the eating disorder behaviors; and (5) the development of tolerance for the anxiety associated with growth and self-reliance.

Milieu and group treatments can be useful for dependent patients as "social laboratories" in which to reaffirm interpersonal dynamics, secure peer feedback on their dependent behaviors, and practice new behaviors. However, these interventions are often accompanied by predictable dynamics. Dependent individuals tend to become overly attached to staff members. These attachments may manifest themselves as frequent requests for one-on-one time, attempts to socialize with staff members during off-hours, misinterpretation of attempts to set limits as rejections, and attempts to elicit caring responses from the staff. Dependent pa-

tients also tend to form intense attachments with fellow patients and they may emotionally collapse as comrades are discharged from the milieu. At times, fellow patients may openly resist the dependent individual's attempts to cling and be guided, which can create tension in the milieu.

Psychotropic medications can be useful in the treatment of comorbid mood and anxiety disorders, although the comorbid presence of a personality disorder tends to temper the response. Family intervention can assist a patient in moving toward separation and independent functioning. Social skills training and assertiveness training can help dependent patients develop a sense of "I" versus "you." Finally, expressive therapies (e.g., art therapy) may facilitate these patients' identification of fears in relationships and within themselves.

OBSESSIVE–COMPULSIVE PERSONALITY DISORDER

Description

Obsessive–compulsive personality disorder is characterized by rigidity, stubbornness, perfectionism, excessive devotion to work, the devaluing of pleasurable or recreational activities, and the measuring of self-worth according to culturally defined productivity. The obsessive–compulsive individual is controlled by perceived rules, regulations, and authority figures. These individuals are preoccupied with being perceived as industrious, self-disciplined, and responsible. Unfortunately, in their strivings for organization, efficiency, and perfection, they are typically distracted by trivial details, inefficient with time management, and prone to procrastination. They often appear inflexible, stingy, overly conscientious, moralistic, and self-righteous. Their interpersonal relationships are dominated by logic and convention, and lack warmth and empathy.

Relationship to Eating Disorders

Obsessive–compulsive personality disorder is most commonly found in individuals with the restricting type of anorexia nervosa (Norman et al., 1993; Skodol et al., 1993; Wonderlich et al., 1990). For these individuals, the adaptive functions of the eating disorder may include (1) an opportunity to rebel and oppose authority figures, which can be personally justified in the context of achievement (i.e., weight loss); (2) the chance to retreat into a predictable world of numbers, measurements, regulations, and rules that never change; and (3) protection and withdrawal from the relationship demands of adolescence and early adulthood.

Specific Treatment Issues

As with most eating disorder patients with personality disorders, the first therapeutic task is the consolidation of the therapeutic relationship. Obsessive–compulsive patients resist a therapeutic relationship because they often view psychotherapy as potentially dangerous and disruptive to their well-organized and predictable world. Therapists must initially "join" these patients on their own cognitive plane, remaining respectful of their fears of expressing and experiencing emotions. As an example, exercise and eating rituals represent safety and stability to these individuals; cognitive-behavioral techniques can be initiated to alter these patterns, but change needs to be integrated gradually.

As the therapeutic relationship consolidates, the therapist must gradually shift from a cognitive interface to an emotional interface with the patient. The initiation of emotional experiencing (i.e., the identification, labeling, and expression of feelings) is often accompanied by a subjective feeling of being "out of control." It is critical that the therapist proceed cautiously and at a pace that the patient can tolerate.

As emotional experience becomes increasingly tolerated, the therapist must gradually progress to the arena of interpersonal relationships. Herein lie a host of complicated paradoxes for these individuals, such as autonomy versus healthy interdependence and giving to others versus allowing one's own needs to be met. Obsessive–compulsive individuals need to be "walked through" the fundamental emotional aspects of a relationship, and they require sufficient time to learn to tolerate the unfamiliar feelings and ambiguities inherent in all relationships. During this phase of the treatment, these individuals require a tremendous amount of support, reassurance, and psychoeducation.

In milieu and group settings, obsessive–compulsive individuals generally integrate well if they can quickly reestablish routines and tolerate the frequent disruptions in these environ-

ments. However, these individuals run the risk of being recruited by the staff to lead environmental cleanups, monitor other patients, and assist with program tasks. These types of activities are generally countertherapeutic, as they reinforce the very dynamics that the individual therapist is attempting to challenge and resolve.

Group psychotherapy can be helpful if these patients make a commitment to utilize the group to explore their personal issues. Group treatment may be complicated by the patient's tendency to intellectualize, avoid feelings, and appear "above all this." The therapist must remember that this particular style is an adaptive response to the stress of the group experience and needs to be sensitively managed. In addition, obsessive–compulsive patients understandably underrate the importance of their issues, compared with the crises of the Cluster B patients.

As for other interventions, family therapy can help members to relinquish their excessive need for perfectionism and practice more emotionally expressive communication. The Selective Serotonin Reuptake Inhibitors, such as sertraline (Zoloft), fluoxetine (Prozac), and paroxetine (Paxil), may be particularly helpful in reducing excessive worry and rumination. Self-expressive experiences provide an opportunity for these individuals to "practice" emotional expression without the pressure of a relationship. Cognitive-behavioral techniques may help to interrupt worry and rumination.

THE REMAINING PERSONALITY DISORDERS

Cluster A Disorders

Paranoid, schizoid, and schizotypal personality disorders are infrequently encountered in patients with eating disorders. The Cluster A disorders are characterized by social detachment, odd and eccentric patterns of thought or behavior, and a tenuous hold on reality. Under stress, individuals with these disorders may experience brief psychotic episodes.

We believe that Cluster A personality disorders are rare in patients with eating disorders because these individuals evolve outside the mainstream culture. Eating disorders develop within a distinct sociocultural context and are rarely found in cultures that do not place excessive value on appearance, body shape, and weight. Individuals with Cluster A personality disorders appear to maintain their own inner reality, apart from the values and beliefs of the broader culture. Therefore, psychiatric disorders that are in part culturally determined will be rare among this personality cluster.

Antisocial Personality Disorder

Antisocial personality disorder is also uncommon in patients with eating disorders. Again, antisocial individuals are at odds with the values of the broader culture and exist within their own system of "morality," which is governed by immediate personal gratification and the hedonistic pursuit of excitement or pleasure. They tend to prey actively upon other individuals, rather than to attempt to change themselves in order to be accepted by others (or the culture). Therefore, like individuals with the Cluster A personality disorders, antisocial individuals are not likely to succumb to disorders that are in part culturally determined.

However, some eating disorder patients, particularly those diagnosed with borderline personality disorder, may display prominent antisocial features. The presence of antisocial features requires some modifications in treatment approach. In working with these patients, the initial and ongoing treatment issue is honesty. This issue should be candidly addressed at treatment entry, in order to determine the patient's willingness or readiness to enter into intensive psychotherapy treatment. Therapists must be concrete and specific about their expectations regarding honesty, and dishonest behavior must be repeatedly challenged.

Patients with antisocial features can be a significant concern in group and milieu settings. They may quickly become the focal point of group treatments and can be readily scapegoated by other patients and staff members. In unstable milieus, these individuals often function as emotional lightning rods. When considering a milieu or group treatment for a patient with antisocial features, the therapist must carefully weigh the risks against the benefits.

Narcissistic Personality Disorder

Narcissistic personality disorder is also relatively uncommon in patients with eating disorders. These individuals tend to focus exclusively on their own internal desires and needs, to the exclusion of others' feelings. External cultural values or expectations concerning weight, shape, and appearance are promptly dismissed by narcissistic individuals because they do not gratify their inner needs ("What's important is what I need, not what you expect").

Although narcissistic personality disorder is uncommon in eating disorder patients, some individuals, particularly those with histrionic personality disorder, display narcissistic features. Individuals with narcissistic features have difficulty developing a working therapeutic alliance and tend to relate to the therapist in a self-aggrandizing fashion, interacting and responding for the purpose of gratifying their own needs. Their constant need for reinforcement and admiration, and ongoing demands for special attention, can rapidly exhaust a therapist. These patients resist even minor confrontations and may terminate treatment if challenged prematurely.

CONCLUSION

Throughout this chapter, we have attempted to emphasize the significant role of personality disorders in the treatment of individuals with eating disorders. We do not believe that effective treatment of these individuals can occur unless therapists recognize and attend to the personality disorders. Indeed, treatment at times will primarily focus on a personality disorder rather than an eating disorder. Interventions aimed at a personality disorder may be complicated by the presence of mixed personality features. On the other hand, some aspects of the personality pathology may gradually recede as the biological stress of the eating disorder (i.e., severe malnutrition, weight loss, recalcitrant vomiting) subsides.

Treatment of these patients is difficult, takes longer than treatment of patients who do not have personality disorders, and often requires a great deal of expertise at the individual psychotherapy level. Although some of these comorbid patients have reasonably good outcomes with an extended treatment, many do not. The general prognostic indicator is an individual's ability to develop a reasonably healthy attachment to a therapist, which is a difficult and compromising position for many patients (e.g., those with paranoid, antisocial, schizoid, schizotypal, and narcissistic personality disorders). One of the most challenging areas for future research will be the long-term treatment course and outcome for this subgroup of complex eating disorder patients.

REFERENCES

Ames-Frankel, J., Devlin, M. J., Walsh, B. T., Strasser, T. J., Sadik, C., Oldham, J. M., & Roose, S. P. (1992). Personality disorder diagnoses in patients with bulimia nervosa: Clinical correlates and changes with treatment. *Journal of Clinical Psychiatry, 53,* 90–96.

Bossert-Zaudig, S., Zaudig, M., Junker, M., Wiegand, M., & Krieg, J. C. (1993). Psychiatric comorbidity of bulimia nervosa inpatients: Relationship to clinical variables and treatment outcome. *European Psychiatry, 8,* 15–23.

Dennis, A. B. (1991). *Restricting behavior and borderline personality disorder in the formation of patient subgroups in bulimia nervosa.* Unpublished doctoral dissertation, Ohio State University.

Dennis, A. B., & Sansone, R. A. (1989). Treating the bulimic patient with borderline personality disorder. In W. Johnson (Ed.), *Advances in eating disorders* (Vol. 2, pp. 237–265). Greenwich, CT: JAI Press.

Dennis, A. B., & Sansone, R. A. (1991). The clinical stages of treatment for eating disorder patients with borderline personality disorder. In C. L. Johnson (Ed.), *Psychodynamic treatment of anorexia nervosa and bulimia* (pp. 126–164). New York: Guilford Press.

Dowson, J. H. (1992). Associations between self-induced vomiting and personality disorder in patients with a history of anorexia nervosa. *Acta Psychiatrica Scandinavica, 86,* 399–404.

Frankel, J. S., Sadik, C., Dantzic, S., Charles, E., Roose, S. P., & Walsh, B. T. (1988, May). *The systematic study of personality disorders in bulimic patients.* Paper presented at the annual meeting of the American Psychiatric Association, Montreal.

Gartner, A. F., & Gartner, J. (1988). Borderline pathology in post-incest adolescents: Diagnostic and theoretical considerations. *Bulletin of the Menninger Clinic, 52,* 101–113.

Gartner, A. F., Marcus, R. N., Halmi, K., & Loranger, A. W. (1989). DSM-III-R personality disorders in patients with eating disorders. *American Journal of Psychiatry, 146,* 1585–1591.

Gwirtsman, H. E., Roy-Byrne, P., Yager, J., & Gerner, R. H. (1983). Neuroendocrine abnormalities in bulimia. *American Journal of Psychiatry, 140,* 559–563.

Herzog, D. B., Keller, M. B., Lavori, P. W., Kenny, G. M., & Sacks, N. R. (1992). The prevalence of personality disorders in 210 women with eating disorders. *Journal of Clinical Psychiatry, 53,* 147–152.

Hudson, J. I., Pope, H. G., Jonas, J. M., & Yurgelun-Todd, D. (1983). Family history study of anorexia nervosa and bulimia. *British Journal of Psychiatry, 142,* 133–138.

Johnson, C., Tobin, D., & Enright, A. (1989). Prevalence and clinical characteristics of borderline patients in an eating-disordered population. *Journal of Clinical Psychiatry, 50,* 9–15.

Kennedy, S. H., McVey, G., & Katz, R. (1990). Personality disorders in anorexia nervosa and bulimia nervosa. *Journal of Psychiatric Research, 24,* 259–269.

Levendusky, P. H,. & Herring, J. (1989). *Therapeutic contract program for treatment of severe eating disorders.* Paper presented at the 97th Annual Convention of the American Psychological Association, New Orleans.

Levin, A. P., & Hyler, S. E. (1986). DSM-III personality diagnosis in bulimia. *Comprehensive Psychiatry, 27,* 47–53.

McClelland, L., Mynors-Wallis, L., Fahy, T., & Treasure, J. (1991). Sexual abuse, disordered personality and eating disorders. *British Journal of Psychiatry, 158,* 63–68.

Millon, T. (1981). *Disorders of personality: DSM-III, Axis II.* New York: Wiley.

Norman, D., Blais, M., & Herzog, D. (1993). Personality characteristics of eating disordered patients as identified by the Millon Clinical Multiaxial Inventory. *Journal of Personality Disorders, 7,* 1–9.

Piran, N., Lerner, P., Garfinkel, P. E., Kennedy, S. H., & Brouillette, C. (1988). Personality disorders in anorexic patients. *International Journal of Eating Disorders, 7,* 589–599.

Pope, H. G., Frankenburg, F. R., Hudson, J. I., Jonas, J. M., & Yurgelun-Todd, D. (1987). Is bulimia associated with borderline personality disorder? A controlled study. *Journal of Clinical Psychiatry, 48,* 181–184.

Powers, P. S., Coovert, D. L., Brightwell, D. R., & Stevens, B. A. (1988). Other psychiatric disorders among bulimic patients. *Comprehensive Psychiatry, 29,* 503–508.

Reich, J., Nduaguba, M., & Yates, W. (1988). Age and sex distribution of DSM-III personality clusters in a community population. *Comprehensive Psychiatry, 29,* 298–303.

Rossiter, E. M., Agras, W. S., Telch, C. F., & Schneider, J. A. (1993). Cluster B personality disorder characteristics predict outcome in the treatment of bulimia nervosa. *International Journal of Eating Disorders, 13,* 349–357.

Sansone, R. A., Fine, M. A., Seuferer, S., & Bovenzi, J. (1989). The prevalence of borderline personality symptomatology among women with eating disorders. *Journal of Clinical Psychology, 45,* 603–610.

Sansone, R. A., & Johnson, C. (1995). Treating the eating disorder patient with borderline personality disorder: Theory and technique. In J. Barber & P. Crits-Christoph (Eds.), *Dynamic therapies for psychiatric disorders (Axis I)* (pp. 230–266). New York: Basic Books.

Schmidt, N. B., & Telch, M. J. (1990). Prevalence of personality disorders among bulimics, nonbulimic binge eaters, and normal controls. *Journal of Psychopathology and Behavioral Assessment, 12,* 169–185.

Skodol, A. E., Oldham, J. M., Hyler, S. E., Kellman, H. D., Dodge, N., & Davies, M. (1993). Comorbidity of DSM-III-R eating disorders and personality disorders. *International Journal of Eating Disorders, 4,* 403–416.

Steiger, H., Liquornik, K., Chapman, J., & Hussain, N. (1991). Personality and family disturbances in eating-disorder patients: Comparison of "restricters" and "bingers" to normal controls. *International Journal of Eating Disorders, 10,* 501–512.

Sunday, S. R., Levey, C. M., & Halmi, K. A. (1993). Effects of depression and borderline personality traits on psychological state and eating disorder symptomatology. *Comprehensive Psychiatry, 34,* 70–74.

Wonderlich, S. A., Swift, W. J., Slotnick, H. B., & Goodman, S. (1990). DSM-III-R personality disorders in eating-disorder subtypes. *International Journal of Eating Disorders, 9,* 607–616.

Yager, J., Landsverk, J., Edelstein, C. K., & Hyler, S. E.

(1989). Screening for Axis II personality disorders in women with bulimic eating disorders. *Psychosomatics, 30,* 255–262.

Yates, W. R., Sieleni, B., Reich, J., & Brass, C. (1989). Co-morbidity of bulimia nervosa and personality disorder. *Journal of Clinical Psychiatry, 50,* 57–59.

Zanarini, M. C., Frankenburg, F. R., Pope, H. G., Hudson, J. I., Yurgelun-Todd, D., & Cicchetti, C. J. (1990). Axis II comorbidity of normal-weight bulimia. *Comprehensive Psychiatry, 30,* 20–24.

Zerbe, K. J., Marsh, S. R., & Coyne, L. (1993). Comorbidity in an inpatient eating disordered population: Clinical characteristics and treatment implications. *The Psychiatric Hospital, 24,* 3–8.

CHAPTER 26

Addressing Treatment Refusal in Anorexia Nervosa: Clinical, Ethical, and Legal Considerations

ELLIOT M. GOLDNER
C. LAIRD BIRMINGHAM
VICTORIA SMYE

A dilemma exists in the treatment of anorexia nervosa: What is one to do when a patient is seriously ill and refusing to accept treatment? Anorexia nervosa is a condition that diminishes life quality and is potentially lethal. Naturally, those interested in the welfare of an individual struggling with anorexia nervosa will wish to ensure that assistance is provided, particularly at a time when there is a crisis or a high risk of deterioration and death. Yet many individuals with anorexia nervosa protest against treatment initiatives and actively refuse treatment. How does one determine whether it is appropriate to comply with a person's refusal to accept treatment? When, if ever, should treatment such as feeding, medication, or psychotherapy be imposed? The problem of treatment refusal in anorexia nervosa presents a conundrum as perplexing as the paradox of Epimenides:[1] If anorexia nervosa is a dangerous condition characterized by the irrational belief that a person's weight must be driven down, can a person holding such a belief make a critical decision whether to accept weight-increasing treatment?

In this chapter, we address clinical, ethical, and legal considerations relating to treatment refusal in anorexia nervosa, and provide recommendations for a practical approach. In addition, we advance the notion that the treatment approach taken by health care providers may influence the degree of refusal encountered. Finally, we draw upon various clinical sources and our own experience to provide suggestions that we believe will prevent or diminish the appearance of treatment refusal in anorexia nervosa.

THE NATURE OF TREATMENT REFUSAL IN ANOREXIA NERVOSA

Refusal of treatment is common in anorexia nervosa. As a consequence, initial assessment and treatment are often delayed for months or years. Because treatment is often undertaken reluctantly in response to the pleas or demands of others, it is not unusual for patients to drop out (Scheuble & Dixon, 1987). Individuals with anorexia nervosa are more reluctant to accept those components of treatment that support increased food intake, weight gain, and reduced physical activity. Other treatment components, such as individual psychotherapy and family therapy, are less often refused. Some patients will overtly accept treatment but subvert unwanted components; for example, a person will enter a hospital inpatient program but secretly throw out food, or use hidden laxatives despite agreements to undergo laxative withdrawal. Others will flatly refuse all forms of treatment intervention and may employ legal means to support their refusal.

When treatment is imposed, some patients actively resist. Forced feeding can be difficult. Patients may refuse all food or supplements, remove feeding tubes or intravenous lines, and actually fight the efforts of nurses, physicians, or other treatment staff members. Chemical and physical restraints may be used, in conjunction with feeding tubes or parenteral nutrition; however, these interventions have accompanying risks (e.g., aspiration, rupture of the gastrointestinal tract, and septicemia).

For both the patient and the staff, the negative emotional consequences of using force or restraint may be profound. Imposed treatment in a hospital can persist over days or weeks, on a 24-hour basis; in such a case, the hospital ward comes to resemble a battle zone. The individual with anorexia nervosa is likely to be in extreme emotional distress, and dissension can develop among staff members. Moreover, a wake of trauma often follows imposed treatment. For patients, negative attitudes toward treatment become entrenched and intensify their sense of isolation. Staff members often experience burnout and confusion about the ethics of treatment imposition, leading to job dissatisfaction. Aversive experiences with imposed treatment may contribute to negative attitudes on the part of the hospital staff toward patients with anorexia nervosa (Garner, 1985; Tinker & Ramer, 1983).

Many who initially refuse treatment follow a different course from that described above. Even though it may be imposed, treatment comes to be accepted and valued. Patients may describe relief at having others assume the decision-making role. Their feelings of shame or guilt, which may otherwise accompany food intake, are diminished when treatment is imposed by an outside authority; thus, renourishment becomes less difficult to accept. Some individuals later identify treatment refusal as an element of the disorder and consider imposed treatment to have been life-saving.

Thus, the course of treatment refusal and imposed treatment in anorexia nervosa can be varied and unpredictable. In addition, clinicians are often confused about the laws and regulations related to imposing treatment.

AUTONOMY AND THE RIGHT TO REFUSE TREATMENT

Currently, the legal codes of most nations establish the right to refuse medical treatment, even if refusal is likely to cause or hasten an individual's death.[2] Infringement of this right may be considered a form of assault or battery. Such legal principles uphold the moral values of autonomy and personal freedom. If a patient is deemed to be incompetent as the result of a mental disorder, the right to refuse treatment may be denied, and decision-making authority may be legally shifted to others (Applebaum & Grisso, 1988). Minors may also be denied the right to refuse medical treatment.

Over recent years, the right of individuals with mental illness to refuse various treatments, particularly antipsychotic medications and electroconvulsive treatment, has been fiercely debated (Blackburn, 1990; Perlin, 1993; Slovenko, 1992). In a paper entitled "Limiting the Therapeutic Orgy," Plotkin (1978) criticized the unbridled power of health care professionals to impose treatments against the will of involuntarily committed patients. Applebaum and Gutheil (1979) countered such arguments and charged legal practitioners with winning nothing for their clients other than the "right to rot." The ongoing dispute has caused considerable dismay, as evinced in a commentary by a law professor in the United States (Slovenko, 1992):

> Over two decades of litigation and regulation on the right of the mentally ill to refuse treatment have left psychiatrists bewildered as to the state of the law. . . . The end result has benefited no one—the individual, the profession, or society. (p. 407)

Clinicians often resent the intrusion of cumbersome legal procedures into their practices, and puzzle at legislation that may detain patients in a hospital through commitment or "sectioning" but may preclude the initiation of treatment. The increasing requirement of clinicians to testify at hearings and clinical review panels, and the growing risk of civil litigation against health professionals, have caused some practitioners to lament the involvement of the legal system in this matter. Despite Perlin's (1993) characterization of this debate as a *"turf battle"* between patients' rights lawyers and clinicians" (p. 177), we hope that a healthy balance of the right to privacy with the right to receive optimal treatment will emerge.

Jurisdictions vary widely in the procedures and models used for overriding the right of patients to refuse treatment (Blackburn, 1990). Altmark, Sigal, and Gelkopf (1995) reported a situation in Israel where a district psychiatrist issued a commitment order for the hospitalization of a woman with anorexia nervosa who was refusing treatment. Implementation of the order was delayed until the woman's appeal was heard by the district psychiatric commission. It was decided by the commission that the patient was not immediately dangerous to herself, and, on that basis, the commission canceled the commitment.

Few disputes over treatment refusal by individuals with anorexia nervosa have reached the courts. However, decisions have been made by British courts in at least two cases. A 16-year-old girl (*In re W*, 1992) with anorexia nervosa, who was in the care of the local authority following the death of her parents, was refusing to consent to be transferred to a London specialist in anorexia nervosa. The court denied her right to refuse the transfer, and the decision was later upheld by the Court of Appeal. In a second British court case, a 37-year-old woman (*In re F*, 1994) in treatment under the Mental Health Act refused feeding, despite her critical medical condition as a result of anorexia nervosa. The judge held that forced feeding if needed would be medical treatment for the respondent's mental disorder.

In most cases involving individuals with anorexia nervosa, determination of the right to refuse treatment hinges on four elements: (1) the potential risk of the condition; (2) the likely benefit of treatment; (3) the likely harm of the treatment; and (4) the competence of the individual to make a reasonable decision about the preceding elements. We discuss each of these below.

Estimating Risk

When the condition of anorexia nervosa puts an individual at high risk for imminent death or disability, the urgent need for treatment is increased, and imposed treatment is more likely to be supported. When treatment is refused by a person with anorexia nervosa, a careful assessment of the health risks in the particular situation is warranted.

Premature death from anorexia nervosa most often results either from medical complications of the condition or from suicide (Hsu, 1991). Those who specialize in medical aspects of treatment report that it is difficult to estimate the precise risk and timing of medical deterioration and death from anorexia nervosa (Birmingham, 1989). The following signs and symptoms can signal medical instability and should prompt immediate medical attention (Goldner & Birmingham, 1994):

- Rapid weight loss (e.g., >15 pounds [7 kg] in 4 weeks)
- Seizures
- Syncopal episodes
- Organic brain syndrome
- Bradycardia (heart rate less than 40 beats per minute)
- Frequent exercise-induced chest pain
- Dysrhythmias
- Renal dysfunction or low urine output (<400 cc per day)
- Volume depletion
- Tetany
- Rapidly diminishing exercise tolerance

Although a medical professional can fairly easily identify an emergency situation in progress, there are few definitive indicators of *impending* crisis. Death from anorexia nervosa is often the result of a sudden, unheralded cardiac event (Isner, Roberts, Heymsfield, & Yager, 1985). Furthermore, when emaciation is severe, the patient may be unable to perceive accurately or describe his or her physical state, and therefore the reliability of symptoms related in the clinical history will be low. Laboratory measures (e.g., low potassium and magnesium levels), electrocardiogram findings (e.g., lengthened QT interval), and other investigations provide additional indicators. Ultimately, the burden of proof falls on the medical practitioner, who must use his or her best clinical judgment to estimate the severity of risk.

Between one-third and one-half of premature deaths of individuals with anorexia nervosa are suicides (Hsu, 1991; Theander, 1985). An estimate of risk should include a careful assessment of mood and risk factors for suicide.

Beneficence

"Beneficence," the intent to benefit a patient, is a principle central to health care ethics (Pellegrino & Thomasma, 1988). In considering whether imposed treatment is justifiable, it is important to estimate benefit as accurately as possible.

Many patients with anorexia nervosa recover, and there is an indication from a randomized, controlled study that the general type of treatment received is a factor in outcome: Patients receiving treatment in programs specializing in anorexia nervosa are likely to have better outcomes than those who receive treatment in nonspecialist programs (Crisp et al., 1991). In a review of uncontrolled treatment studies, Hsu (1991) estimated that approximately 75% of anorexic patients had improved after 4 years of treatment. However, data are not yet available to help estimate outcomes associated with specific interventions (e.g., refeeding) or with interventions in which treatment has been imposed.

Because there is wide variability in outcomes, with few prognostic indicators, clinicians cannot reliably predict the results of treatment. Although a patient's response to prior treatment attempts may provide some useful information, the changing course and evolution of the disorder and the multiple factors involved in treatment make it difficult to predict treatment response exactly. In estimations of outcome, quality-of-life measures are also considered important; however, the subjective nature of such estimates makes it notoriously difficult for any surrogate to make a decision about acceptable or unacceptable quality of life.

Although individuals with chronic anorexia nervosa have a guarded long-term prognosis (Patton, 1988), the short-term results of refeeding with medical and psychiatric treatment are generally good and are likely to lead to an improved quality of life. For those in acute crisis because of medical complications or depression, treatment can be life-saving.

The question of beneficence is perhaps most poignant in relation to individuals with chronic anorexia nervosa. At times, such individuals feel that treatment is futile, and clinicians have described feeling "infected" with pessimism (Hebert & Weingarten, 1991a, 1991b). Dresser (1984), in describing the position of individuals with chronic anorexia nervosa, states that they are "faced with the alternatives of painful life-prolonging treatment which is unlikely to restore health, but instead merely continues a life of debatable quality, and nontreatment and probably death" (p. 359). Dresser goes on to allege that "the anorexic whose condition persists

for a lengthy time despite numerous treatment efforts has demonstrated that coercive treatment furnished her no benefit" (p. 360). In a situation reported in Canada, the estimation that treatment would be futile appeared to influence a decision not to provide treatment to a 22-year-old woman in medical crisis because of anorexia nervosa; the decision led to her death (Hebert & Weingarten, 1991a). Sadly, the limited availability of specialist treatment appears to have influenced the determination of futility in this case (Leichner, 1991; Hebert & Weingarten, 1991b). O'Neill, Crowther, and Sampson (1994) reported the case of a 24-year-old patient with anorexia nervosa who died in Britain. The patient was considered "incurable" (p. 38) by her care-givers and was admitted to a terminal care facility where she received regular morphine injections and died within 8 days. Ramsay and Treasure (1996) sent a copy of this case report to the founding members of the Royal College of Psychiatrists' special interest group on eating disorders and, using a quantitative method, found that respondents did not consider the patient to have been incurable.

The powerful emotional impact of severe anorexia nervosa upon patients, families, and caregivers can influence judgments of the potential benefit of treatment. It can be difficult to maintain a balance between extremes of overexuberant intervention and therapeutic nihilism. Most individuals with anorexia nervosa, including those with chronic and severe illness, will benefit from appropriate treatment. In providing support for patients, particularly when the response to repeated intensive treatment has been poor, distinctive approaches may be warranted.

Nonmaleficence

The intent to avoid harm to a patient, "nonmaleficence," is another central principle of health care ethics. When one is considering imposed treatment for an individual with anorexia nervosa, it is important to evaluate the physical risks of all interventions, the negative psychological effects that may result from specific treatment components, and the negative effects of imposing treatment against the person's wishes. Patients refusing treatment often state that they do so to avoid aspects of treatment they consider noxious. These include (1) intrusive or aggressive refeeding methods; (2) unnecessary restriction of activity, social contacts, and other behaviors; and (3) insensitive or angry comments from staff members or other patients.

Although all methods of weight restoration are likely to be experienced as noxious by individuals with anorexia nervosa, some methods may be more likely to induce anxiety or discomfort. It is important to appreciate the intense anxiety experienced with weight increase, and the accompanying discomforts of abdominal fullness, bloating, and changes in body perception. There is no universally agreed-upon method of weight restoration, and not all patients will benefit from the same approach (Goldner & Birmingham, 1994). Imposed tube feeding and behavior modification methods have been criticized (Garner, 1985; Bruch, 1974); however, since these methods of weight restoration require less direct patient contact, they may be implemented in some hospitals or clinics because of limited staff availability.[3]

It is not unusual for patients to decry the prison-like atmosphere that can develop when their physical activity, bathroom use, and food intake are constantly monitored and directed. In support of this perception, Parker, Balzer, and Wyrick (1977) found that staff members were apt to embrace a "totalitarian ideology" when the staff controlled behavioral reinforcements.

Patients report that health professionals can appear insensitive and angry in their dealings with people with anorexia nervosa. These descriptions are buttressed by some clinicians' concerns that punitive methods and pejorative labeling are directed toward anorexic patients (Brotman, Stern, & Herzog, 1984; Morgan, 1977; Tinker & Ramer, 1983; Vandereycken, 1993). Often misconceptions about anorexia nervosa, countertransferential anger, and the hopelessness of caregivers lead to negative interactions with patients. Caregivers (whether health care professionals, family members, or others) often hold a strong belief that what is blocking recovery is the absence of cooperation from the person with anorexia nervosa. In particular, caregivers often believe that the lack of recovery is a result of complacency with the illness, the desire to manipulate others for secondary gain, or passive–aggressive behavior. These beliefs often increase in response to treatment difficulties. Ultimately, such assumptions and beliefs create a covert blaming of the patient, erode any vestiges of therapeutic alliance, and intensify the patient's negative self-appraisal.

Following any of these three types of negative treatment experience, individuals with anorexia nervosa may become more severely ill and are likely to avoid further contact with health professionals. Imposed treatment may result in anger, diminished self-esteem, and avoidance of further treatment. Many clinicians and treatment programs have addressed these concerns by minimizing the use of aggressive refeeding methods, maximizing patients' freedom and autonomy, and attending to patient–staff communication. Anxiety and discomfort have been reduced by providing choices about methods of weight restoration and other aspects of treatment. Specific suggestions are provided later in this chapter.

Competence to Consent to Treatment

A determination of "competence," a legal concept denoting one's mental capacity for decision making, is the crux of any decision about a person's ability to consent to or refuse treatment. Applebaum and Grisso (1988) suggest that marked inability to perform the following tasks may indicate incompetence: (1) communicating choices; (2) understanding relevant information; (3) appreciating the situation and its consequences; and (4) manipulating information rationally.

It is rare for anorexic patients to experience pervasive disturbance in mental function. General reasoning ability, calculation, memory, overall judgment, and other functions are usually intact. The thought disturbance present in anorexia nervosa is narrowly circumscribed to areas related to body weight and nutrition. Defined as "overvalued ideas" (beliefs that, like delusions, are persistently and tenaciously held despite contradictory evidence), these cognitive disturbances are considered by some to be the core phenomenological disturbances of the disorder (Cooper & Fairburn, 1992) and are thought to generate the manifold features of anorexia nervosa.

Evaluation of an anorexic patient's general intellectual ability will be unlikely to identify incapacity. The question of competence for individuals with anorexia nervosa typically centers on their specific ability to make rational decisions about nutrition, refeeding, and other medical treatments. In a discussion of the ethics of forced feeding, Kluge (1991) states:

Anorexic patients may understand full well what they are told and may be volitionally competent on occasion. However when they attach a value to what they are told that not only differs from the value given by the average person but is also neurotic, this lends a global incompetence to their decisions on such issues as eating, food and body image. (p. 1124)

Thus, a proper evaluation of competence in anorexic patients requires factual information regarding their ability to take rational steps to preserve health and life. Individuals with anorexia nervosa may sincerely declare the intent to resume eating; yet, when faced with food intake, they may find that the overwhelming anxiety and thought disturbance associated with anorexia nervosa paralyze the ability to preserve life.

Most clinicians have described the condition of anorexia nervosa as one that can disable a person from making a free and rational choice about the condition itself and about treatment. Tiller, Schmidt, and Treasure (1993) state:

> While commencing a diet may have been a conscious choice, when illness supervenes patients become trapped in weight-reducing behaviour. The desire, when emaciated, to avoid treatment leading to weight gain is not comparable to a decision to refuse medical intervention; rather it is a psychiatric symptom. (p. 679)

Fost (1984) shares this view and explains his justification of imposed treatment as follows:

> The justification, in my view, for interfering with the anorexic behavior, particularly when death is imminent, is precisely because the behavior does not result from free choice and, in fact, is likely to result in an outcome that is contrary to the real desires of the patient. (p. 366)

Not all clinicians, however, share this view. Robertson (1992) opposes the imposition of treatment and questions the assertion that medical or psychiatric treatments will be of benefit. In a critique of medical discourse on anorexia nervosa, the condition, which she prefers to call "self-starvation," is described as a choice made by women oppressed by patriarchal society:

> The question of how anorexia nervosa creates meaning for women is one over which medicine and feminism have differed. Simply put, the for-

mer has anorexia as a type of psychiatric illness, while the latter most often sees behavior as a symptom of women's oppression in a patriarchy. . . . Anorexia nervosa is simply one of many choices that women can make to express themselves within a dominant gender order where women's power is unequal to men's. (p. xiii)

Robertson (1992) is concerned that women are "totalized" by the label of anorexia nervosa, and feels that medicalization of their condition is counterproductive. Although such poststructuralist ideas may prove to be valuable in mapping better approaches to therapy, there is a danger of constructing a polemic that "totalizes" medical diagnosis and treatment as always harmful. In addition, there is no support for the notion that individuals diagnosed as anorexic are social or political activists who are consciously starving to death in a manner comparable to suffragettes or political prisoners. Tiller et al. (1993) warn that such "misconceptions and reasoning errors can trivialise the seriousness of the disorder and interfere with effective treatment" (p. 679).

Clearly, one's position on issues of competence and treatment refusal in anorexia nervosa is influenced by conceptualizations of the problem, which can be construed as having political and social valence. Table 26.1 lists ideas and values that either support or oppose imposed treatment of a person with anorexia nervosa. Although there may be general support for imposing treatment when an anorexic individual is in a life-threatening crisis, there is little agree-

TABLE 26.1. Opposing Ideas and Principles Underlying the Treatment Refusal Dilemma

Ideas in favor of imposed treatment	Ideas against imposed treatment
Patients' lives and health should be protected; death and suffering should be prevented.	Patients are entitled to personal autonomy (freedom to choose their fate).
Anorexia nervosa is a mental disorder that impairs judgment about treatment.	Anorexia nervosa is a sociopolitical phenomenon.
Imposed treatment will bring about recovery or improvement.	Imposed treatment will not lead to improvement and may cause harm.

ment when the immediate risk to life is lower. Furthermore, there is no consensus as to when to end imposed treatment. Such decisions are best served by a careful evaluation of risks and benefits, and are likely to be influenced by the ideas and values described in Table 26.1.

CONCLUSIONS AND PRACTICAL RECOMMENDATIONS

The problem of treatment refusal in anorexia nervosa requires difficult clinical, ethical, and legal decisions. The condition can interfere with a person's competence to make decisions about treatment. Both the risks and the benefits of treatment imposition must be carefully examined.

Below, we review the recommendations for addressing treatment refusal previously advanced by Goldner (1989), and provide an expanded discussion of each. We contend that clinicians can substantially prevent or diminish treatment refusal through attention to specific aspects of the treatment approach.

1. *Seek to engage in a sincere and voluntary alliance.* A strong therapeutic alliance will often be the most useful tool in preventing or diminishing treatment refusal, but clinicians often have difficulty assessing the therapeutic alliance and overestimate the strength of the alliance with anorexic patients who later refuse treatment (Gallop, Kennedy, & Stern, 1994). Warmth, consistency, and availability to the patient and family will promote an alliance. Also, it is important to express clearly the wish to be helpful. The demonstration of an interest in broad areas and qualities of a patient's life helps to show a sincere wish to understand his or her complexities and unique qualities.

One method that supports a strong therapeutic alliance is "externalizing the problem discourse" (White & Epston, 1990). This method is described within a framework of narrative ideas and is consistent with some feminist and poststructuralist approaches to psychotherapy. In this approach, anorexia nervosa is portrayed as a problem that is external to the person and encroaches on his or her quality of life. Hence, "the problem" is the problem, not the individual who struggles with the problem. This method removes blame from a patient and allows the clinician to engage with the person in an alliance against anorexia nervosa. Language

is used to support externalization, as in these examples: "It seems that anorexia nervosa is keeping you a prisoner and making the choice for treatment difficult," and "If anorexia nervosa continues to have its way with you, I am concerned that it will take you, and therefore I am determined to help you fight against it."

Acknowledgment of the patient's suffering and distress can also help to build an alliance. It is helpful to recognize the efforts of the patient frequently and to acknowledge his or her strength in fighting such a difficult problem.

2. *Identify the reasons for refusal.* Individuals who have not been exposed to treatment may fear the unknown and may be frightened of psychiatric or medical interventions in general. Other patients are fearful of repeating the negative experiences they have encountered in previous treatment interventions; they can feel confused and trapped. Individuals who struggle with anorexia nervosa tend to be shy, anxious, and conflict-avoidant (Strober, 1980), and are often uncomfortable voicing their concerns. Consequently, it may be difficult for members of the treatment staff to fully identify and understand such a person's subjective reasons for refusal. To better understand and diminish refusal, clinicians can be helpful by (a) assuming an active style of interaction, in which possible concerns and reasons for refusal are proposed, and the patient is invited to agree or disagree; (b) demonstrating an understanding of the thoughts and feelings common to individuals struggling with an eating disorder; and (c) sharing the wisdom expressed by other patients struggling with similar problems. The following is an example of an empathic question that may help to demonstrate an understanding and response to a patient's concerns: "I'm not sure that you are feeling this way, but many people, when beginning this part of their treatment, have told me they were frightened of gaining weight too quickly. Is this your experience, or is it different for you?"

Treatment is often refused because of specific concerns, such as the fear of tube feeding or involuntary committal. In some situations, patients refuse treatment because of severe depression or cognitive impairment. Such information is essential in developing an effective treatment approach. Most commonly, treatment refusal is driven primarily by the cognitive disturbances or overvalued ideas characteristic of anorexia nervosa (e.g., the irrational fear of weight gain) and by accompanying anxiety.

Treatment methods that address these central thoughts and fears, such as cognitive restructuring, reframing, psychoeducation, and distraction techniques, may help to diminish or prevent treatment refusal. In some situations, antianxiety agents (e.g., benzodiazepines) or medications with antiobsessive actions (e.g., selective serotonin reuptake inhibitors) may be useful treatment adjuncts.

3. *Provide careful explanations of treatment recommendations.* Prior to treatment, we undertake a preliminary intervention that we call "pre-care." In such sessions, we provide information, answer questions, and anticipate specific concerns. Pre-care can prevent and diminish treatment refusal. Because treatment is sometimes initiated following a crisis, with little opportunity for advance preparation, pre-care may need to be done on the day of admission; however, it is our experience that it is worthwhile. Pre-care can also include a visit to a treatment unit; a meeting with staff members; an overview of the program; and identification of an individual's expectations of treatment, including his or her short- and long-term goals and perceived needs regarding support from the staff. In cases where the presence of anxiety, concentration difficulties, and preoccupation with shape and weight diminish patients' ability to comprehend or retain information, it is helpful for staff members to repeat explanations and reassurances about treatment.

4. *Be prepared for negotiation.* It is likely that patients will wish to negotiate certain aspects of the treatment plan. Indeed, they often have good ideas about what might be useful to them. The treatment team should create an atmosphere in which a healthy process of negotiation can be readily undertaken. It is helpful to frame negotiation in the context of promotion of a patient's health and safety; modifying the treatment plan is possible, as long as the modifications are likely to support recovery. Individuals with anorexia nervosa are likely to respond positively to a clinician who is approachable, flexible, and comfortable with conflict. Lazare, Eisenthal, and Frank (1979) have emphasized the importance of negotiation in psychiatric practice and have listed effective strategies aimed at enhancing the power of both parties. Important element of negotiations include a clear appreciation of the other person's wishes and preferences, and an attempt to help achieve them when feasible.

5. *Promote autonomy.* It is important to re-spect the patient's autonomy to the greatest extent possible. Although the condition of anorexia nervosa may disable a person in certain areas of decision making, he or she will be competent to make many decisions relating to treatment and recovery. Treatment plans should minimize the use of intrusive interventions, such as involuntary commitment, tube feeding, and behavior modification. Wherever possible, outpatient programming should be used in place of inpatient treatment. Day programs and residential treatment can offer a level of intensive treatment usually associated with inpatient units, while diminishing the "role extrusion" that occurs when individuals undergo lengthy inpatient stays.

6. *Weigh the risks versus benefits of treatment imposition.* A careful analysis of the potential risks and benefits of imposed treatment is necessary. A realistic appraisal of the probable outcome of treatment versus no treatment will help guide the clinician to a rational plan; however, it is difficult to predict treatment outcome accurately in anorexia nervosa.

When treatment decisions are perplexing, the methodology known as "clinical decision analysis" can be valuable. In this method, a figure is drawn with the possible consequences of the decision to be made emanating from the primary decision itself. Once the figure is drawn, the probabilities of each of the possible consequences are estimated from experience or the literature, as is the relative worth or utility[4] of the outcomes. Each of these numbers is then added to the appropriate part of the figure. Clinical decision analysis allows for a visual and mathematical assessment of a question (Fletcher, Fletcher, & Wagner, 1988; Sox, Blatt, Higgins, & Marton, 1988; Weinstein & Fineberg, 1980).

A thorough explanation of clinical decision analysis is beyond the scope of this chapter, but Figure 26.1 provides an example. Here, the decision whether to impose feeding or not might result in either improvement or no improvement, and subsequently in death or chronicity in either case. The probabilities of the outcomes are specified below the line leading to the possible outcome, and at the end of each arm the utility or value of that outcome is listed. For example, if the probability of improving is 20% with forced feeding but only 1% without, the chance of death is 3% with no improvement in both arms, and the utilities are 0 for death, 1 for recovery, and .2 for chronicity with forced

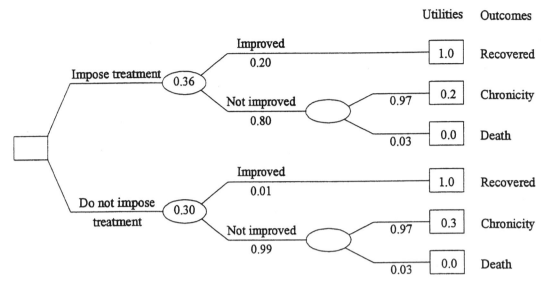

FIGURE 26.1. Example of the use of clinical decision analysis in deciding whether to impose treatment on a patient with anorexia nervosa.

feeding but .3 for chronicity without forced feeding. The preferred arm in this example is forced feeding, with a value of .36 as compared to .30 for no forced feeding. The decision regarding which choice is the best is therefore made by mathematically assessing each arm. Commercially available clinical decision analysis programs for Macintosh and IBM computers (e.g., Sonnenberg & Pauker, 1988) also allow for evaluation of ranges of probabilities and utilities (sensitivity analysis).

Perhaps the main benefit of clinical decision analysis is that it forces discussion of individual probabilities and utilities, as well as repeated mathematical evaluation over the entire range of probabilities and utilities thought to be possible. Treatment imposition should be considered only when the benefits of intervention outweigh the benefits of nonintervention and the risks associated with treatment.

7. *Avoid battles and scare tactics.* Sallas (1985) has discussed methods of diminishing the emergence of power struggles in the treatment of individuals with eating disorders. Power struggles generally result in an escalation of symptoms and an erosion of the therapeutic alliance. Patients who feel frightened or trapped respond in various ways. Some engage in battles with the staff; angry outbursts, withdrawal, and other responses are common. It is important for staff members to use respectful language and to avoid threats and destructive criticism.

8. *Convey a balance of control versus noncontrol.* A balanced treatment approach acknowledges the need for flexibility and yet maintains a firm sense of realistic constraints. The clinician should invite the patient to assume as much control as he or she is able to accept without endangering recovery. Although a patient may feel compelled to retain control of treatment decisions, he or she may feel overwhelmed and incapable of managing certain situations and decisions.

9. *Ensure that methods of treatment are not inherently punitive.* Treatment methods should consistently support patient's self-esteem. Punitive methods will erode the treatment alliance, will damage patients' self-concept, and may retraumatize individuals who have been previously victimized. The use of punitive treatment methods has been attributed to misguided assumptions about etiology and to the powerful negative emotional reactions elicited in some clinicians by individuals with eating disorders (Bruch, 1974; Garner, 1985). A patient who is refusing treatment may engender feelings of helplessness, frustration, and anger in caregivers. Consultation with experienced clinicians is helpful in ensuring that treatment interventions are nonpunitive.

10. *Involve the family.* Families are frequently distraught when a family member battling with anorexia nervosa is refusing treatment. There is generally conflict between a pa-

tient and family members regarding the need for treatment and the type of treatment required. We have found a narrative approach to family intervention (White & Epston, 1990) helpful in defusing family conflict and diminishing treatment refusal. Engagement of the family in a realistic treatment plan generally increases therapeutic leverage. Individuals receiving treatment for anorexia nervosa may request that family members not be contacted. An adult's request not to have the family involved is generally respected; however, some individuals who have refused involvement of family members have later changed their minds. In situations where there is acute risk of death or disability, and a patient is receiving involuntary treatment, the family should be contacted even if it is against the patient's wishes.

11. *Obtain ethical and legal clarification and support.* It may be helpful to undertake a formal or informal ethical decision-making process when one is considering imposed treatment. Various models of ethical analysis exist (Beauchamp & Childress, 1989; Thompson & Thompson, 1985), and bioethicists are often available for consultation. Similarly, when legal means of treatment imposition are being considered, it is helpful to obtain advice and support from legal experts. In this manner, smooth implementation of treatment procedures can be achieved.

12. *Consider legal means of treatment imposition only when refusal is judged to constitute a serious risk.* Because of the potential risks, it is generally agreed that legal means of imposing treatment upon an individual with anorexia nervosa should be reserved for situations in which nonintervention constitutes a serious and imminent danger.

13. *Consider differential treatment in chronic anorexia nervosa.* Individuals who have struggled with anorexia nervosa for an extended period of time often require a different approach than do individuals who have had an illness of shorter duration (Hsu & Lieberman, 1982; Morley, 1993). Chronic illness may indicate a particularly resistant form of anorexia nervosa and it may be inappropriate to approach the treatment of a chronic anorexic patient with a zealous or aggressive plan of intervention. Yet, clinicians must avoid characterizing such situations as futile. Instead, treatment goals should be modified to reflect practical and attainable objectives. Smye and Geller (in press) have described a specialized program for

individuals with chronic anorexia nervosa in which the overarching goal is to improve quality of life in keeping with the patient's own priorities. The program operates as a hospital-community partnership and aims to: (a) stabilize the individual's physical, nutritional, and mental state at or above a minimal level; (b) minimize the use of inpatient services; (c) increase involvement in community-based activities (e.g., interpersonal, recreational, and occupational endeavors); (d) reduce distress in family members and significant others related to the patient's illness. A unique feature of this model is the focus on rehabilitation and reintegration of the individual into the community.

14. *Conceptualize refusal/resistance as an evolutionary process.* Individuals who initially refuse treatment may later come to accept it (Honig & Bentovim, 1996). Generally, a person's gradually increasing recognition of the negative impact of anorexia nervosa on his or her life is accompanied by a wish to recover and benefit from effective treatment. This evolution appears to be facilitated by the presence of supportive individuals who provide consistent and realistic appraisal to the anorexic patient. Family members, fellow patients, support and self-help groups, and residential facilities will often facilitate this process. In addition, renourishment may itself result in diminished treatment refusal because of the improvements it brings about in emotional and cognitive processes. It is important to time the use of intensive interventions carefully; a treatment that is refused at one point may be welcomed a short time later.

NOTES

1. Epimenides, a Cretan philosopher, demonstrates by means of the paradoxical statement "All Cretans are liars" that truth can be difficult to determine.

2. As an example, the Canadian courts recognized this principle in the case of *Mulloy v. HopSang* (1935) and on several subsequent occasions.

3. We wish to note that tube feeding is often not experienced as a noxious treatment component by patients with anorexia nervosa; tube feeding may even be requested by some patients—particularly those who are able to eat little or nothing, and those who find that the tube placement inhibits vomiting.

4. The utility or relative worth of an outcome is estimated by considering the potential risks and benefits, in the context of the values and wishes of the affected individuals.

REFERENCES

Altmark, D., Sigal, M., & Gelkopf, M. (1995). Partial insanity: When the judiciary and the psychiatric world collide. *Journal of Psychiatry and Related Sciences, 32,* 109–113.

Applebaum, P. S., & Grisso, T. (1988). Assessing patients' capacities to consent to treatment. *New England Journal of Medicine, 319*(25), 1635–1638.

Applebaum, P., & Gutheil, T. (1979). "Rotting with their rights on": Constitutional theory and clinical reality in drug refusal by psychiatric patients. *Bulletin of the American Academy of Psychiatry and Law, 7,* 306–315.

Beauchamp, T. L., & Childress, J. F. (1989). *Principles of biomedical ethics* (3rd ed.). New York: Oxford University Press.

Birmingham, C. L. (1989). Anorexia nervosa and bulimia: Medical complications and management. *British Columbia Medical Journal, 31*(3), 155–158.

Blackburn, C. (1990). The "therapeutic orgy" and the "right to rot" collide: The right to refuse antipsychotic drugs under state law. *Houston Law Review, 27,* 447–513.

Brotman, A. W., Stern, T. A., & Herzog, D. B. (1984). Emotional reactions of house officers to patients with anorexia nervosa, diabetes and obesity. *International Journal of Eating Disorders, 3,* 71–77.

Bruch, H. (1974). Perils of behavior modification in treatment of anorexia nervosa. *Journal of the American Medical Association, 230,* 1419–1422.

Cooper, M. J., & Fairburn, C. G. (1992). Selective processing of eating, shape, weight and shape related moods in patients with eating disorders and dieters. *British Journal of Clinical Psychology, 31*(3), 363–365.

Crisp, A. H., Norton, K., Gowers, S., Halek, C., Bowyer, C., Yeldham, D., Levett, G., & Bhat, A. (1991). A controlled study of the effect of therapies aimed at adolescent and family psychopathology in anorexia nervosa. *British Journal of Psychiatry, 159,* 325–333.

Dresser, R. (1984). Feeding the hunger artists: Legal issues in treating anorexia nervosa. *Wisconsin Law Review, 2,* 297–374.

Fletcher, H. R., Fletcher, S. W., & Wagner, E. H. (1988). *Clinical epidemiology* (2nd ed.). Baltimore: Williams & Wilkins.

Fost, N. (1984). Food for thought: Dresser on anorexia. *Wisconsin Law Review, 2,* 375–384.

Gallop, R., Kennedy, S. H., & Stern, D. (1994). Therapeutic alliance on an inpatient unit for eating disorders. *International Journal of Eating Disorders, 16,* 405–410.

Garner, D. M. (1985). Iatrogenesis in anorexia nervosa and bulimia nervosa. *International Journal of Eating Disorders, 4,* 701–726.

Goldner, E. M. (1989). Treatment refusal in anorexia nervosa. *International Journal of Eating Disorders, 8,* 297–306.

Goldner, E. M., & Birmingham, C. L. (1994). Anorexia nervosa: Methods of treatment. In L. Alexander-Mott & D. B. Lumsden (Eds.), *Understanding eating disorders: Anorexia nervosa, bulimia nervosa, and obesity* (pp. 135–157). Hove, England: Taylor & Francis.

Hamburg, P., Herzog, D. B., & Brotman, A. (1996). Treatment resistance in eating disorders: Psychodynamic and pharmacologic perspectives. In M. H. Pollack, W. Otto, & J. F. Rosenbaum (Eds.), *Challenges in clinical practice: Pharmocologic and psychosocial strategies.* New York: Guilford Press.

Hebert, P. C., & Weingarten, M. A. (1991a). The ethics of forced feeding in anorexia nervosa. *Canadian Medical Association Journal, 144,* 141–144.

Hebert, P. C., & Weingarten, M. A. (1991b). The ethics of forced feeding in anorexia nervosa. *Canadian Medical Association Journal, 144*(10), 1206–1208.

Honig, P., & Bentovim, M. (1996). Treating children with eating disorders—ethical and legal issues. *Clinical Child Psychology and Psychiatry, 1*(2), 287–294.

Hsu, L. K. G. (1991). Outcome studies in patients with eating disorders. In S. M. Mirin, J. T. Gossett, & M. C. Grob (Eds), *Psychiatric treatment advances in outcome research* (pp. 159–180). New York: American Psychiatric Press.

Hsu L. K. G., & Lieberman, A. (1982). Paradoxical intention in the treatment of chronic anorexia nervosa. *American Journal of Psychiatry, 139,* 650–653.

In re F, 1 F.L.R. 614 (1994), 2 F.C.R. 577 (1994).

In re W, 3 W.L.R. 592–608 (1992).

Isner, J. M., Roberts, W. C., Heymsfield, S. B., & Yager, J. (1985). Anorexia nervosa and sudden death. *Annals of Internal Medicine, 102,* 49–52.

Kluge, E.-H. (1991). The ethics of forced feeding in anorexia nervosa: A response to Hebert and Weingarten. *Canadian Medical Association Journal, 144*(9), 1121–1124.

Lazare, A., Eisenthal, S., & Frank, A. (1979). A negotiated approach to the clinical encounter: II. Conflict and negotiation. In A. Lazare, (Ed.), *Outpatient psychiatry: Diagnosis and treatment* (pp. 137–152). Baltimore: Williams & Wilkins.

Leichner, P. (1991). The ethics of forced feeding in anorexia nervosa. *Canadian Medical Association Journal, 144*(10), 1206.

Morgan, H. G. (1977). Fasting girls and our attitudes to them. *British Medical Journal, 2,* 1652–1655.

Morley, J. E. (1993). The strange case of an older woman who was cured by being allowed to refuse therapy. *Journal of the American Geriatrics Society, 41,* 1012–1013.

Mulloy v. HopSang, W.W.R. 714 (Alta.S.C. App. Div. 1935).

O'Neill, J., Crowther, T., & Sampson, G. (1994). Anorexia nervosa: Palliative care of terminal psychiatric disease. *American Journal of Hospice and Palliative Care, 11,* 36–38.

Parker, J. B., Balzer, D., & Wyrick, L. (1977). Anorexia nervosa: A combined therapeutic approach. *Southern Medical Journal, 7,* 448–452.

Patton, G. C. (1988). Mortality in eating disorders. *Psychological Medicine, 18,* 947–952.

Pellegrino, E. D., & Thomasma, D. C. (1988). *For the patient's good: The restoration of beneficence in health care.* New York: Oxford University Press.

Perlin, M. I. (1993). Decoding right to refuse treatment law. *International Journal of Law and Psychiatry, 16,* 151–177.

Plotkin, (1978). Limiting the therapeutic orgy: Mental patients' right to refuse treatment. *Northwestern University Law Review, 72,* 461–525.

Ramsay, R., & Treasure, J. (1996). Terminal care for anorexia nervosa (letter). *British Medical Journal, 312,* 182.

Robertson, M. (1992). *Starving in the silences: An exploration of anorexia nervosa.* New York: New York University Press.

Russell, J. (1995). Treating anorexia nervosa: Humbling for doctors. *British Medical Journal, 311,* 584.

Sallas, A. A. (1985). Treatment of eating disorders: Winning the war without having to do battle. *Journal of Psychiatric Research, 19,* 445–448.

Scheuble, K. J., & Dixon, K. N. (1987). Premature termination: A risk in eating disorder groups. *Group, 11*(2), 85–93.

Slovenko, R. (1992). The right of the mentally ill to refuse treatment revisited. *Journal of Psychiatry and Law, 28,* 407–534.

Smye, V., & Geller, J. (in press). Treatment of chronic anorexia nervosa: A community outreach program. Proceedings of the Third International Conference on Eating Disorders, April 15–17, 1997.

Sonnenberg, F. A., & Pauker, S. G. (1988). *Decision maker* [Computer program]. Boston: New England Medical Center.

Sox, H. C., Blatt, H. A., Higgins, M. C., & Marton, K. I. (1988). *Medical decision making.* Boston: Butterworths.

Strober, M. (1980). Personality and symptomatological features in young, nonchronic anorexia nervosa patients. *Journal of Psychosomatic Research, 24,* 353–359.

Theander, S. (1985). Outcome and prognosis in anorexia nervosa and bulimia. *Journal of Psychiatric Research, 19,* 493–508.

Thompson, J. E., & Thompson, H. O. (1985). *Bioethical decision-making for nurses.* Norwalk, CT: Appleton-Century-Crofts.

Tiller, J., Schmidt, U., & Treasure, J. (1993). Compulsory treatment for anorexia nervosa: Compassion or coercion? *British Journal of Psychiatry, 162,* 679–680.

Tinker, D. E., & Ramer, J. C. (1983). Anorexia nervosa: Staff subversion of therapy. *Journal of Adolescent Health Care, 4,* 35–39.

Vandereycken, W. (1993). Naughty girls and angry doctors: Eating disorder patients and their therapists. *International Review of Psychiatry, 5,* 13–18.

Weinstein, M. C., & Fineberg, H. V. (1980). *Clinical decision analysis.* Philadelphia: W.B. Saunders.

White, M., & Epston, D. (1990). *Narrative means to therapeutic ends.* New York: Norton.

CHAPTER 27

Group Psychotherapy

JANET POLIVY
INGRID FEDEROFF

Eating disorder patients have several characteristics that make them particularly well suited to benefit from group psychotherapy. Their feelings of uniqueness, interpersonal distrust, low self-esteem, and ineffectiveness, as well as their distorted views of nutrition and their bodies, are the sorts of problems likely to be amenable to group treatments. The group format provides consensual validation, interpersonal feedback, models of coping, information, and enhanced self-esteem and feelings of control through active participation in helping oneself and others. Since the early 1980s, when the first reports of successful group therapies with eating disorder patients appeared, group treatments have proliferated, and there have been numerous studies examining their effectiveness. We begin by describing some of the most common types of group therapy, and then summarize the major review studies. Next, we outline the conclusions of these studies about group therapy for eating disorders, and indicate areas needing further investigation. We end the chapter with some practical guidelines drawn from the literature on how to conduct groups with eating disorder patients.

Before discussing the state of the group therapy literature, we must point out that there has been a marked shift of emphasis in studies on the treatment of eating disorders from the 1970s and early 1980s to the middle and late 1980s and 1990s. Earlier reports focused primarily on the treatment of anorexia nervosa. In the 1970s, of course, bulimia nervosa (or simply bulimia) was seen as a mere variant of anorexia nervosa and was not yet classified as a separate and distinct disorder. Since achieving the status of a separate diagnostic entity, bulimia nervosa has come to dominate treatment reports. As will become evident, treatment studies since the early 1980s have focused almost exclusively on bulimic patients. This is particularly true of group therapy studies, and some authors actually now recommend excluding anorexic patients from groups for bulimic patients. This is in marked contrast to the earliest reports of group therapy for eating disorders, which often included anorexic and bulimic patients in the same groups (e.g., Polivy, 1981; Polivy & Garfinkel, 1984). We discuss this further when we talk about patient selection criteria, but the review that follows is thus probably more relevant to the treatment of bulimic patients than to that of eating disorder patients in general, though it may well be that the conclusions would be unchanged if anorexic patients were included.

TYPICAL GROUP THERAPIES FOR EATING DISORDERS

We begin our discussion of the group therapy studies in the literature by describing the types of group therapy that are generally offered to eating disorder patients. A number of descriptive and experimental papers outlining the procedures used in eating disorder groups have been published in the last 15 years. Many types of group therapies are currently available for treating eating disorders, including psychodynamic/interpersonal, cognitive-behavioral, behavioral, psychoeducational, addiction-oriented, intensive short-term, single-issue (e.g., body image), and self-help approaches. We describe each of these approaches in turn.

Psychodynamic Therapy

Psychodynamic therapy for eating disorders focuses on centering, cultivating, and nurturing the self (Goodsitt, 1985; Bruch, 1982). Eating disorder patients tend to exhibit an intense focus on controlling their food intake and weight; this serves to contain their anxiety, to provide them with a sense of identity, to help them cope with underlying feelings of inadequacy and ineffectiveness, and to fill in the gaps in their sense of self. The goal of psychodynamic therapy is to foster an emotional experience that corrects underlying deficits in self-regulation, identity, autonomy, and self-esteem (Harper-Guiffre, Mackenzie, & Sivitilli, 1992). Psychodynamic group treatment primarily helps members to reexperience and reexamine problems relating to interpersonal relationships (Roy-Byrne, Lee-Benner, & Yager, 1984; Stevens & Salisbury, 1984).

This approach lends itself better to a longer-term treatment strategy—6 months or more, up to several years (Barth & Wurtman, 1986; Hendren, Atkins, Sumner, & Barber, 1987; Inbody & Ellis, 1985; Reiss & Rutan, 1992). It is also better suited to focusing on the more psychological and interpersonal issues than on management of the symptoms of eating, weight, and physical health (Harper-Guiffre et al., 1992). In fact, although many authors advocate the importance of a psychodynamic perspective, it is not unusual to combine this approach with other therapeutic strategies. Psychodynamic approaches have been used in conjunction with behavioral, cognitive, and educational components (Lacey, 1983; Sykes, Currie, & Gross, 1987; Yellowlees, 1988; Shisslak, Crago, Schnaps, & Swain, 1986; Stevens & Salisbury, 1984; Brisman & Siegel, 1985; Laube, 1990.

Cognitive-Behavioral Therapy

Cognitive-behavioral therapy (CBT) was the first specific approach for the treatment of bulimia nervosa to be described in detail and supported by clinical data (Fairburn, 1988). This approach attempts to change patients' system of beliefs about themselves and their environment through a semistructured, problem-oriented method, focusing directly on the patients' dysfunctional beliefs and values concerning their shape and weight (Fairburn, 1985). Key features of this treatment include helping patients identify circumstances that lead to a loss of control; obtaining specific changes in eating patterns; and reconsidering distorted beliefs associated with eating, weight, and body shape. There are three phases in treatment. The first stage focuses on establishing some control over eating, using mostly behavioral techniques; the second stage of treatment is more cognitive, stressing the identification and modification of dysfunctional thoughts, beliefs, and values; the third phase focuses on the maintenance of change.

This semistructured program has lent itself to empirical investigation of its efficacy in the treatment of eating disorders (Fairburn, 1988). In addition, a cognitive-behavioral manual has been developed to guide clinicians (Fairburn, Marcus, & Wilson, 1993). Most of the treatment studies using this technique have been conducted with bulimic patients. Fairburn (1985) lists some concerns over its usefulness in treating anorexia nervosa; he suggests that CBT may not be an appropriate treatment for severely emaciated anorexics or for those who have little motivation to change. Although Fairburn's work has generally involved individual treatment rather than group treatment, other researchers have used this type of treatment in a group format and found it to be an effective treatment strategy (e.g., Dedman, Numa, & Wakeling, 1988; Kirkley, Schneider, Agras, & Bachman, 1985; Freeman & Munro, 1988; Schneider & Agras, 1985; Lee & Rush, 1986; Kettlewell, Mizes, & Wasylyshyn, 1992; Stuber & Strober, 1987; Merril, Mines, & Starkey, 1987). Positive outcomes include reducing binge–purge frequency and decreasing levels of anxiety, depression, and the intensity of the dysfunctional attitudes concerning shape and weight (Fairburn, 1981; Wilson, 1987). Group interventions utilizing a cognitive-behavioral approach have been found to be more effective than waiting-list controls in reducing bulimic symptoms (Lee & Rush, 1986; Huon & Brown, 1985; Fairburn, Agras, & Wilson, 1992; Wolf & Crowther, 1992; Wilfley et al., 1993). Moreover, comparative studies have generally indicated that the outcome for cognitive-behavioral treatments is as favorable as that of any other treatments to which they are compared (Kirkley et al., 1985; Mitchell et al., 1989; Wilfley et al., 1993; Wolf & Crowther, 1992).

Behavioral Approaches

Behavioral approaches focus on disturbed eating symptoms, and utilize such techniques as self-monitoring, relaxation, stress management, nutritional management, and development of strategies to modify stimulus conditions. Behavioral group treatment has proved to be effective in decreasing binge frequency (Laessle & Pirke, 1987), though it has not been found to be more effective than group CBT (Wolf & Crowther, 1992).

A specific behavioral paradigm, exposure plus response prevention (ERP), is based on an anxiety reduction model of bulimia nervosa. This model rests on the assumption that vomiting fuels binge eating by alleviating the anxiety produced by bingeing; vomiting is thus an escape response that is reinforced by subsequent reduction in anxiety about weight and shape (Rosen & Leitenberg, 1985). It is proposed that if patients are exposed to eating normal foods while not being allowed to vomit afterwards, they will discover that anxiety will be reduced without recourse to vomiting. Therapy consists of exposure to and consumption of forbidden foods and prevention of subsequent vomiting. ERP has been found to be effective in reducing bulimic symptoms (Rosen & Leitenberg, 1982). Exposure plus response prevention treatment conducted in a behavioral group context was effective in reducing bingeing and vomiting and lowering binge-eating scores and symptoms of depression (Gray & Hoage, 1990). Franko (1993) has described a modification of ERP that includes a group meal within the context of group CBT. The group meal is an opportunity for bulimic patients to experience the beneficial effects of anxiety reduction in a group therapy setting. However, no data were presented concerning outcome.

When ERP was compared to CBT, there were no differences in effectiveness (Leitenberg, Rosen, Gross, Nudelman, & Vara, 1988). Fairburn (1988) suggests, however, that ERP adds little to CBT treatment, as well as having several problems. He points out that there is no standard ERP procedure; the optimal form of ERP is unclear; ERP demands more therapist time; and patients report ERP to be aversive. These criticisms may explain why few therapists seem to advocate ERP at present.

Psychoeducational Groups

Psychoeducational material related to starvation effects, physical complications of disordered eating behaviors, the biology of weight regulation, the consequences of dieting, proper nutrition, and the social context of eating disorders has proved effective in reducing symptomatic eating behavior and improving psychological functioning (Connors, Johnson, & Stuckey, 1984; Berry & Abramowitz, 1989). After participation in a group psychoeducation program that consisted of five 90-minute meetings, 21% of patients were symptom-free (Davis, Olmsted, & Rockert, 1990). In addition, there were clinically significant changes in dysfunctional attitudes and psychological distress. A report comparing group psychoeducation to cognitive psychotherapy found evidence of different therapeutic factors at work in the two modes of treatment (Olmsted, Davis, & Rockert, 1991). Compared to the cognitive therapy, the psychoeducation group had smaller benefits (as would be expected, since the cognitive treatment was longer in duration and employed specific therapeutic techniques), but a significant number of patients benefited from the less intense therapy.

A different psychoeducational approach (Wolchik, Weiss, & Katzman, 1986) offers a 7-week program focusing primarily on decreasing depression and improving self-esteem, assertion, and body image. In comparison to no-treatment controls, the bulimic women receiving this psychoeducation treatment showed significant improvement in self-reported depression, self-esteem, and number of binges per month.

The Addiction Model

One study found that participation in Overeaters Anonymous, a group that views eating disorders as addictive, was helpful in maintaining abstinence from overeating (Malenbaum, Herzog, Eisenthal, & Wyshak, 1988). An addiction orientation considers eating disorders to be variants of substance use disorders, and proposes the existence of an "addictive personality" (e.g., Brisman & Siegel, 1985; Vandereycken, 1990). The patient's relationship with food is viewed as an addiction. Brisman and Siegel (1985) describe a treatment strategy conducted in a group setting based on this addiction model.

Mitchell et al. (1985) have described a combined treatment coupling an addiction-oriented approach based on the Alcoholics Anonymous (AA) model and a behavioral psychological approach. Like standard addiction therapy, this treatment demands abstinence (from binge eating, as opposed to alcohol consumption) upon beginning the program, with a direct focus on the problem binge-eating behavior. The assumption is that other problems will resolve or become more controllable once the eating is corrected. Like AA, this is an intensive approach that relies to some extent on group pressure and confrontation to reinforce abstinence and compliance with the program.

On the other hand, the addiction model of eating disorders has been criticized (Wilson, 1991). Evidence shows a greater-than-expected rate of substance use disorders in eating disorder patients, and vice versa, but methodological problems make this finding hard to interpret. Wilson concludes that there is no evidence of an "addictive personality" in eating disorder patients. Moreover, he points out that the addiction model does not address the core clinical issues for eating disorder patients (e.g., the role of dietary restraint, abnormal attitudes about importance of body shape) and fails to account for psychobiological connections between dieting and eating disorders. Treatments for substance use disorders tend to promote abstinence, which for eating disorder patients would be encouraging dieting; this in itself undermines addiction-oriented therapy for eating disorders. The psychopathology underlying eating disorders (which goes beyond mere dieting and pursuit of thinness) is ignored by an addiction model. Finally, the addiction model also promotes a uniformity myth about eating disorders, ignoring differences among the various eating disorders. Criticisms such as these appear to have been accepted by the therapeutic community, and addiction models of treatment are not widely advocated.

Intensive Short-Term Therapies

Intensive short-term group psychotherapy, employing a variety of therapeutic approaches (either alone or in conjunction with individual psychotherapy), have emerged as effective alternatives to weekly group treatment in reducing bulimic symptomatology (Baell & Wertheim, 1992; Fernandez & Latimer, 1990; Frommer, Ames, Gibson, & Davis, 1987; Johnson, Conners, & Stuckey, 1983; Kirkley et al., 1985; Lee & Rush, 1986; Pyle, Mitchell, Eckert, Hatsukami, & Goff, 1984; Schneider & Agras, 1985; Stevens & Salisbury, 1984; Yates & Sambrailo, 1984). The length and duration of these groups differ widely. Treatments range from one or two meetings a week for 90–120 minutes, to more intensive marathon weekend workshops or treatment retreats lasting several weeks (Boskind-White & White, 1983; Bohanske & Lemberg, 1987; Brisman & Siegel, 1985; Gendron, Lemberg, Allender, & Bohanske, 1992; Mitchell et al., 1985; Wilson & Fairburn, 1993; Wooley & Lewis, 1987; Wooley & Kearney-Cooke, 1986).

It has been reported, for example, that marathon weekend retreats create therapeutic intensity and maximize the development of trust, cohesion, and peer support. Improvements in self-esteem, bulimic symptoms, and dysfunctional eating attitudes were found afterwards (Bohanske & Lemberg, 1987; Gendron, Lemberg, Allender, & Bohanske, 1992). Somewhat longer (but still short-term) intensive treatments, involving six to eight bulimic women living together in a hotel apartment for 24 days and receiving 8 hours of therapy each day, have been described as well (Wooley & Lewis, 1987; Wooley & Wooley, 1985). Similarly, Wooley and Kearney-Cooke (1986) reported positive results for an intensive therapy package lasting 6–8 hours a day for 3–5 weeks, and combining group, individual, and family therapies for bulimics' body image dissatisfaction and binge eating.

Mitchell et al. (1985) have described an intensive program for treating bulimic patients, which consists of 2 months of evening sessions. For the first week, patients are in therapy for 3 hours every evening (Monday through Friday), and then the frequency and duration of sessions are both decreased gradually over the 2 months to twice-weekly meetings for 90 minutes each. Patients are required to abstain from binge eating, and the therapy consists of a combination of lectures, group therapy, and support (often from recovered patients, who can volunteer to serve as role models for recovery).

A day hospital program offers another type of intensive treatment in a group setting. Patients attend the program in the hospital each weekday for 8 hours a day, and return home at night and for weekends (Piran, Kaplan, et al., 1989). The program in the day hospital setting generally includes a variety of therapeutic strategies within group contexts. A study found that this program was effective in promoting weight gain and maintained or improved clinical psychopathology (compared to inpatient discharge scores) in both anorexic and bulimic patients (Piran, Langdon, Kaplan, & Garfinkel, 1989).

Comparisons of these intensive treatments are complicated by the different durations of the programs, as well as the heterogeneous aims of the groups. Some concentrate on symptom relief, while others deal with broader issues such as self-esteem, depression, role conflicts, identity, assertion, body image, life skills, stress and anger management, and communication skills. We could find no studies that have investigated the optimal length, duration, content, or intensity for short-term group therapy for eating disorders.

Body Image Therapy and Other Single-Issue Approaches

Vandereycken and colleagues (Vandereycken, Probst, & Van Bellinghen, 1992; Vandereycken, Depreitere, & Probst, 1987, p. 403) focus on how eating disorder patients experience their bodies. They have developed a mode of group therapy ("body experience therapy") in order to help eating disorder patients "[re]build a realistic self concept and a positive body experience." Similarly, Rosen and his colleagues have developed a group treatment targeting disturbances in body image. Without any attention to eating or exercising, they have found improvements not only in how the body is perceived and evaluated, but also elevations in self-esteem, decreased levels of psychological symptoms, restraint, guilt/concern about eating, and reductions in bingeing (Rosen, Cado, Silberg, Srebnik, & Wendt, 1990; Rosen, Reiter, & Orosan, 1995).

Other treatments targeting a single aspect of eating disorders, such as assertiveness training, nutrition counseling, or relaxation training, have been recommended (e.g., Piran, Kaplan, et al., 1989). It has also been suggested that sexual abuse and accompanying feelings of powerlessness can be contributing factors in the development of an eating disorder and may require specific, focused treatment (Kearney-Cooke, 1988).

Self-Help Groups

Self-help groups offer eating disorder patients the opportunity to exchange information and experiences with others who have undergone similar problems. They also provide a source of information about eating disorders and available treatments. More importantly, they are alternatives to professionally managed treatments that can provide support to help these individuals manage their eating. The support offered by these groups serves to remediate dysfunction by offering comfort, acceptance, encouragement, and help, and by providing continual resources for developing and maintaining personal effectiveness. Differences from therapy groups are that there is generally no cost or charge to members; the groups meet in a nontherapy setting and are facilitated by nonprofessionals; and attendance is usually not mandatory, so membership fluctuates and may be less cohesive than that of professionally led therapy groups (Enright, Butterfield, & Berkowitz, 1985). Such groups are commonly used as adjuncts to professional treatments, and vary widely in philosophy and structure (Larocca, 1983; Enright et al., 1985).

REVIEWS OF GROUP THERAPY STUDIES

We begin our analysis of studies of the sorts of group therapies described above with reviews published in 1987, as they are able to include reasonable numbers of previously published studies. One such review of the literature on group therapy for bulimic patients (Oesterheld, McKenna, & Gould, 1987) pointed out some serious methodological problems with the studies that appeared prior to that time. A lack of uniform criteria made it difficult to be sure that patient populations were comparable or even representative of the disorder in question, and possible sampling biases attendant on comparing patients from general psychiatric clinics with those from specialized eating disorder programs may have exacerbated this sort of problem. Moreover, most of the earliest reports of the use of group therapy programs for eating disorder patients utilized small numbers of patients and were not actually experimental studies of group effectiveness. There were no control groups, no random assignment of subjects, no statistical comparisons of treatments, and no uniform measures of outcome or change. Although a few studies from the mid-1980s began to include these factors, there were not yet enough to evaluate. Finally, many group treatments were used in conjunction with individual, family, drug, and other therapeutic efforts, making it impossible to distinguish the particular contribution of the group treatment to change or improvement in the patients. The goals of treatment also differed markedly among the various groups: Some focused on symptom management and removal, whereas others attempted to produce self-understanding, insight, and emotional growth. Obviously, such contrasting purposes of the therapeutic endeavor would involve rather inconsistent methods' being used to achieve these outcomes. Oesterheld and colleagues thus found the comparison of group therapies a difficult enterprise. It was hard to compare and evaluate treatment results across studies when the outcome measures depended on the initial assumptions about what needs to be changed, and these varied with the orientations of the investigators.

Certain aspects of these group treatment studies did produce some consensus though (Oesterheld et al., 1987). The need for an active role for both therapy group leaders and members was emphasized in most accounts. Leaders were reported as teaching, guiding, giving external control to members, imparting information, and providing reality testing. Members were expected to observe their own behavior; to identify and communicate their emotional reactions, as well as to connect them with behaviors such as bingeing; and to set realistic goals for changing themselves with the help of the other group members. Most groups combined elements of cognitive-behavioral, psychoeducational, exploratory, and supportive techniques. Many used adjunct activities such as food diaries recording intake of food, the context of eating, and associated thoughts and feelings; identification and restructuring of distorted beliefs; individualized weekly goal setting and group feedback; and assertiveness and relaxation training.

Again, it was very difficult to compare and evaluate treatment results in such different studies (Oesterheld et al., 1987). The first problem was defining successful outcome. In this patient population, reduction in the number of episodes of bingeing and purging would be a reasonable outcome measure; this was the usual one reported, with posttreatment percentage of reduction in binge–purge episodes as the most common index of efficacy. This ranged from 52% to 97% reduction, and clustered around 70%. There was, however, a serious lack of long-term follow-up data (covering 1 year or more). Another problem is that reduction of symptoms was calculated only for those participants who completed a group, not those who started it; thus, dropouts (who were likely to be treatment failures) were ignored. This clearly biased the data in a favorable direction. Moreover, means were generally used to present the data; this could obscure wide individual variations or skews caused by an outlier. Finally, symptom improvement might be impressive, but a lot of pathological behavior could still remain. This made it unclear whether patients could be considered "cured," or how "improved" to consider them (Oesterheld et al., 1987).

Garner, Fairburn, and Davis (1987) reviewed 19 published therapy studies, of which 13 were of group therapies, in an attempt to determine whether any specific treatment technique (CBT, in particular) was more effective than other techniques. With respect to posttreatment frequency of binge-eating and vomiting episodes, most of the studied treatments had both statistically and clinically significant effects. There were no clear advantages to any given type of therapy, however, and group treatment seemed to be as effective as individual methods. The concerns Garner et al. raised about comparability of treatments (in terms of style and content); theoretical differences relating to etiology and to which aspects of the patient the primary focus of treatment efforts should be directed toward changing; diagnostic criteria; dropout rates; patient recruitment sources and screening procedures; treatment duration; and follow-up investigation were similar to those raised by Oesterheld et al. (1987). Garner and colleagues reiterated the importance of reporting attrition rates and treating the dropouts as treatment failures when evaluating treatment effectiveness. They also advocated a closer analysis of dropouts, to determine whether they differ fundamentally from patients who remain in therapy, and whether the dropouts might require a different sort of therapeutic approach. Garner et al. (1987) also suggested that uniform and converging measures of psychopathology and of bingeing and vomiting be adopted to allow comparability of studies. They suggested that therapists not be involved in data collection, but leave that to unbiased research technicians blind to the conditions of the study. Although few studies actually compared group and individual therapies, this review concluded that individual treatment appeared to be somewhat more effective at containing attrition rates and alleviating symptoms. Such a conclusion may be warranted eventually, but seems premature in terms of the small number of studies that had made direct comparisons at that time.

Controlled studies of individual and group therapy were reviewed by Fairburn (1988). He examined waiting-list control designs, placebo control designs, and comparative studies, though group and individual therapies were not considered separately. In general, treatment groups were more effective than controls. Fairburn pointed out that different types of therapy had many similarities, including cognitive restructuring, education, self-monitoring, and introduction of avoided foods into patients' diets. Again, no advantage for any particular type of therapy was detected.

Cox and Merkel (1989) reviewed 32 studies of individual and group therapy for bulimic patients, published between 1976 and 1986. Utilizing 14 criteria for quality and methodological rigor, they classified the studies into three categories, with three studies rates as high-quality, 17 as medium-quality, and 12 as low-quality. Behavioral and cognitive-behavioral treatments were the most commonly employed techniques, though some psychodynamic, experiential, and eclectic therapy studies were reported. Using abstinence from bulimic behaviors as the criterion for successful treatment, Cox and Merkel found that group therapy produced a 40.4% abstinence rate for completers, and individual therapy produced a 47.4% rate. These dropped to 37.6% and 41.5%, respectively, at follow-up. However, it appears that more patients dropped out of group therapy (26.1%) than individual therapy (7.5%). The authors noted, though, that most of the studies being evaluated in their review were not rated as high-quality research enterprises; they concluded that there was no compelling evidence that one treatment was more effective than another, and there was certainly no obvious way for an individual consumer to determine which treatment to select. On a positive note, all of the treatments did seem to help, and the overall conclusion was that any of the treatment modalities studied was likely to be at least somewhat efficacious.

Cox and Merkel (1989) did recommend improvements for future studies of therapy for bulimic patients. In particular, they suggested excluding patients who meet criteria for other disorders, such as anorexia nervosa, affective disorders, and/or substance abuse; controlling for duration of bulimic symptoms, age of onset, and frequency of symptomatic behaviors; using experienced therapists; incorporating multiple assessments and assessment times; using multiple observers and measures other than self-report; including at least a 6-month follow-up; and always including a control group.

A review of group therapy for bulimic patients (Zimpfer, 1990) concluded on the basis of 31 studies published between 1981 and 1989 that group treatments were universally described as successful according to the criteria chosen by the authors (at the least, binge–purge behavior was significantly reduced or eliminated among the group members). However, variability in treatment response and the problems of dropouts and relapses remained to be addressed satisfactorily. Earlier criticisms of group therapy studies still appeared to be true; the heterogeneity of participants in different studies, the many and varied methods of patient appraisal, differences in entry criteria for different studies, and the variety of settings used for treatment made comparisons across studies very difficult to carry out. In addition, small sample sizes limited the generalizability of most of the findings, and the use of inappropriate statistics reduced the credibility of many studies. In general, insufficient data were also provided on the orientation and skills of the therapists used in the studies (Zimpfer, 1990). On the positive side, Zimpfer noted some improvements: the reporting of more genuine experiments, more frequent comparisons of treatments (rather than mere pre–post designs), and more follow-ups of 6 months or more.

Rosenvinge (1990) also reviewed the literature on group therapy for bulimic patients between 1984 and 1989. He discussed the stages of the group therapy process and the use of inpatient versus outpatient groups, mixed groups, and open versus closed groups. He concluded that whatever type of group was used, approximately 40% of bulimic patients were more or less abstinent from bingeing and purging when therapy was terminated. He compared cognitive-behavioral groups with other approaches (particularly behavioral and nondirective groups) and found no evidence of superiority of one strategy over another. In addition, though groups were effective, they were not found to be any more effective than other therapeutic modalities. Methodological shortcomings of the literature noted in this review included the failure to use more than one therapist in a study; lack of distinctions between treatment effects and spontaneous remissions or nonspecific treatment effects; and inadequate follow-up length. Future researchers were advised to improve patient inclusion and exclusion criteria; to specify recruitment procedures, symptom severity, and duration of the disorder; to assess and report other psychopathology; to define outcome criteria (behavioral and psychological) operationally, and to use both subjective and objective measures before and after treatment and at follow-up; to avoid concurrent treatments; to include adequate control groups; and to incorporate dropouts in the results, so as to prevent a positive bias in the findings.

One study used meta-analysis to examine the literature systematically (Fettes & Peters, 1992). Forty outcome studies of group therapy for bulimic patients were coded on the basis of treatment, design, and subject variables, and meta-analyzed to determine the magnitude of the effect of group treatment. In addition, the authors attempted to identify the factors accounting for variations in attrition or outcome among different studies. They examined effect sizes representing pre- to posttherapy changes in bulimic symptoms. Self-reported measures of bulimic symptoms were the only consistent dependent variables across studies, so these were used to assess outcome. The average effect size for group treatment was +0.75 at posttreatment, suggesting moderate efficacy. Studies that reported 1-year follow-up data generally found the improvement to be maintained over this period. A greater number of hours of treatment per week was associated with larger posttherapy effect sizes, as was the addition of other treatment components such as individual therapy (although this complicated somewhat the determination of the efficacy of group therapy per se). The authors cautioned that although adding other treatment components may increase the number of patients who benefit from therapy, it is not likely to be cost-effective to administer multiple treatments across the board in the hopes of improving success rates for some patients. They advocated identifying characteristics of treatment responders and nonresponders, and then determining systematically whether adding alternative therapeutic measures elevates success rates in nonresponders. As in earlier investigations, treatment type did not predict outcome, nor was dropout rate associated reliably with any variable. The authors requested more complete reporting of dropouts in future investigations, as inaccurate treatment of these subjects can bias the interpretation of the results of the study. They also called for multiple outcome measures (in particular, for the addition of measures not reliant upon patients' self-reports), for better reporting of methodology in group therapy studies, and for longer follow-ups.

CONCLUSIONS FROM THE LITERATURE

This overview indicates that consensus exists on several dimensions, including the apparent efficacy of group therapy for bulimic patients. All studies have seemed to find that groups are effective treatments, and there has appeared to be no significant advantage to individual treatment where such comparisons are made. For either individual or group treatments, the posttherapy abstinence rate has tended to be about 40%. No particular type of therapeutic approach (such as cognitive-behavioral, behavioral, interpersonal, or psychodynamic) has produced consistently better or worse outcomes than any other. Nonspecific factors related to group process (such as those identified as curative factors of groups by Yalom, 1975), rather than any particular therapeutic style, have been frequently mentioned as important contributors to the success of group therapy. It seems safe to conclude that groups are a cost-effective and useful means of offering treatment to eating-disordered patients. There may be some patients who would actually do better in a group than an individual setting, or others who are less likely to benefit from a group than individual therapy, but this sort of fine-tuned identification of patient characteristics relating to successful or unsuccessful treatment has not yet been accomplished and awaits future developments.

A common thread also appears in the review papers with respect to methods for improving research in this area. Several areas of concern have been repeatedly indicated. All of the papers have mentioned a need for better subject definition and diagnostic criteria for potential patients' inclusion and exclusion in a given study. At present, inclusion–exclusion standards and symptomatology among those who are included are too variable across studies to allow for reliable comparisons.

Similarly, more uniform outcome criteria and measures are required; most reviewers have warned investigators not to rely solely on self-report measures or to use only abstinence from binge eating as the criterion of successful outcome. There are no accepted, universally agreed-upon definitions of what constitutes a binge or other symptoms, so the question of when a patient is truly abstinent or even significantly improved remains controversial. Again, the variability in assessments of therapeutic effectiveness hinders cross-study comparisons. Moreover, most studies measure outcome in terms of reduction of eating symptomatology, but pay less attention to improvement in psychological disturbance. For example, Davis et al. (1990) found that more change was reported in specific eating pathology than in personality and associated psychopathology after psychoeducational group treatment. Outcome measures should ideally assess both eating and psychological symptomatology, to ensure that improvement after therapy encompasses both.

Other problems exist as well. Treatments need to be described more fully, and patients participating in subsidiary treatments should be excluded from investigations of group therapy's effectiveness. Control group comparisons are a necessity, and ethical ways of studying patients waiting for active therapies must be developed. Dropouts from therapy present a particular problem for interpretation of results; those who leave treatment early have to be dealt with more systematically, and must always be included in final data reports. One study focused directly on addressing this problem (Riebel, 1990), but the literature in general does not yet reflect much attention to these treatment failures. Psychopathology other than bulimic symptoms (or eating disorder symptoms) in patients selected for study needs to be assessed and described at all stages of treatment. Finally, follow-ups lasting longer than 6 months are needed; short-term results may not hold up under the pressures of a return to unaided coping. Clearly, much work remains to be done in investigating the effectiveness of group therapy for eating disorders.

Some aspects of the use of group therapy have received very little systematic attention in the literature. As mentioned earlier, the question of patient characteristics that predict enhanced or reduced responsiveness to either group or individual therapy, or to one or another school of treatment, needs to be addressed. One study (Maddocks & Kaplan, 1991) did examine demographic variables, weight history, specific symptomatology, mood status, and pretreatment social adjustment ratings to find predictors of good versus poor response to group treatment. Depression and eating disorder symptomatology were the best predictors of outcome in this study, as well as in a study of psychoeducational groups (Davis, Olmsted, & Rockert, 1992). The relative benefits of focusing group therapy on eating symptoms, as opposed to concentrating on underlying psychological deficits, could be a fruitful area of inquiry. Moreover, the mechanisms by which group therapy exerts its beneficial influence have yet to be delineated. All this requires further investigation.

In conclusion, a decade and a half of work utilizing therapy groups to treat eating disorders indicates that groups are useful as more than single-focused (i.e., focused on unitary issues such as assertiveness training) adjuncts to some other individual therapy aimed at a whole disorder. Much work remains to be done to determine how groups can best contribute to the alleviation of eating disorders, and of what kinds of patients are most likely to benefit from group treatment, but more recently published studies (e.g., Agras et al., 1992; Crosby et al., 1993; Davis et al., 1992; Wilfley et al., 1993; Wolf & Crowther, 1992) are attempting to answer these sorts of questions and to rectify the shortcomings of the existing literature.

PRACTICAL GUIDELINES FOR CONDUCTING GROUP THERAPY

The variety of group therapy treatments reviewed above may seem daunting, but there are a number of common issues regarding the format of therapy groups. In this section, we review some practical guidelines for conducting group therapy for the eating disorders.

The first consideration is the selection of group members. A patient's suitability for group therapy depends upon a number of factors, including the patient's capacity and motivation for change, interpersonal skills, and prior therapy experience; the presence of comorbid psychiatric disorders; and the type of group therapy being considered (Dixon, 1986; Mitchell, 1990). Careful patient assessment and screening are recommended (Davis, 1988; Davis et al., 1990; Dixon, 1986; Mackenzie & Harper-Guiffre, 1992). Patients with little capacity or motivation for change are poor candidates for any therapy, but may be actively disruptive in a group setting. Those with poor social skills may benefit particularly from group treatment, but if they are too shy to speak in front of others, this could be counterproductive. Other characteristics thought to make patients poor candidates for participation in group therapy include the presence of coexisting psychiatric disorders such as substance abuse/dependence, severe depression, or personality disorders; medical crisis or high risk for suicide; or aggressive, hostile, or socially deviant or bizarre behaviors (other than eating behaviors) (Dixon, 1986; Frommer et al., 1987; Lee & Rush, 1986; Mackenzie & Harper-Guiffre, 1992; Davis & Olmsted, 1992; Piazza & Steiner-Adair, 1986; Toseland & Rivas, 1984; Yalom, 1975). Screening patients and preparing them for group therapy seem to reduce dropout rates and to improve the overall quality of the group. For example, Lacey (1983) got good results when he required that prospective patients, prior to participation in an insight-oriented group therapy, contract to attend all sessions, maintain their current weight, and eat a prescribed diet for the duration of the therapy. Participation in a short (time-limited) group has been found to be useful preparation for longer-term group therapy (Barth & Wurtman, 1986; Reiss & Rutan, 1992).

Group size and composition are dependent on the type and purpose of the group. Psychoeducational groups are more amenable to a larger group size and a heterogeneous eating disorder patient population. Group size in these can range from as few as 5 to more than 12 participants, usually meeting on a weekly basis for 6–12 weeks (Connor-Greene, 1987; Davis & Olmsted, 1992; Wolchik et al., 1986). The lecture-and-discussion format allows patients to learn about eating disorders and strategies for self-care, and offers a less threatening introduction to the treatment process than a therapy group may. Furthermore, psychoeducational groups are useful for individuals who have difficulty engaging in the therapeutic process, such as those with borderline personality features, and can prepare them for more intensive psychotherapy (Davis & Olmsted, 1992). However, psychoeducational groups are not generally recommended for anorexia nervosa patients, who are better served by more intensive psychotherapy.

When the format of the group is interactional rather than didactic, the size and homogeneity of the group become more important. A higher degree of patient participation (self-disclosure, discussion of beliefs and feelings) is more easily achieved in a smaller group. A range of 5 to a maximum of 10 members is optimal for interpersonal learning and participation (Mackenzie & Harper-Guiffre, 1992). Anorexic patients may function better in a smaller group, with membership limited to 4 or 5; this reduces the necessity for patients to vie for group time, and it maximizes patient interaction (Hall, 1985; Polivy, 1981).

Opinion is mixed regarding the preference for homogeneous or mixed groups of anorexia nervosa and bulimia nervosa patients. Short-term group therapies have been developed primarily to treat bulimia nervosa, and a homogeneous group has the advantage of a common presenting problem and group goals. However, a concern has been raised regarding the composition of bulimic groups. Mild bingers exposed to severe bulimics may develop greater severity of symptoms, raising the question of whether groups for bulimic patients should be homogeneous in symptom severity (Frommer et al., 1987). Research in university sororities indicates that symptoms tend to be emulated and a group norm gets established (Crandall, 1988), and this may well apply to therapy groups. Moreover, a mixture of anorexic and bulimic patients in a group may exacerbate feelings of envy and competition, with the bulimics viewing the anorexics as more "successful" and the anorexics considering themselves to have less of a problem than the bulimics (Mackenzie & Harper-Guiffre, 1992). Bulimics may prefer to discuss their feelings of shame and embarrassment about their symptoms with others who share similar problems (Roy-Byrne et al., 1984). Bulimics have also reported feeling intimidated by very thin anorexics, and this can magnify the bulimics' self-disgust (Enright et al., 1985). Other authors, however, report including both anorexics and bulimics (including males) in inpatient and outpatient groups, with no adverse effects on the group or on individual members (Edmands, 1986; Hendren et al., 1987; Inbody & Ellis, 1985; Piazza & Steiner-Adair, 1986; Polivy, 1981). One report of long-term psychotherapy noted that bulimic patients appeared to require fewer sessions than anorexics (Hendren et al., 1987).

Some investigators (Andersen, Morse, &

Santmyer, 1985; Hall, 1985) suggest that groups specifically for patients with anorexia nervosa are a useful therapeutic tool. The uniformity of patient concerns creates an atmosphere of trust and understanding. There are, however, potential drawbacks to exclusively anorexic groups, including concern that the patients will imitate and reinforce one another's pathology and teach other members new weight loss techniques. In addition, anorexics are often withdrawn and anxious, and have great difficulty identifying and expressing their feelings; this can make group therapy difficult for them (Hall, 1985; Polivy, 1981; Vandereycken & Meermann, 1984).

The age of group members may be another important consideration in composing a group. High school students are struggling with adolescent issues, whereas college-age and older women are dealing with career, marital, and life satisfaction issues (Hendren et al., 1987; Piazza & Steiner-Adair, 1986; Polivy, 1981).

The decision to operate an open or a closed group depends on a combination of practical and theoretical issues. Inpatient and day hospital groups are open, with members leaving as they are discharged and new patients joining as they are admitted to the hospital. Support and self-help groups generally have an open, more flexible format, with members attending as they feel the need. Short-term therapy groups are more often closed groups with specific starting and ending dates; participants agree to attend a specific number of sessions over a period of time. The advantage of such a closed group is that members can work together in deeper interactions (Mackenzie & Harper-Guiffre, 1992).

Group therapy is often conducted by cotherapists. Female pairs and male–female pairs are common. A male and female therapist team is particularly useful in recreating the nuclear family (Bohanske & Lemberg, 1987; Boskind-White & White, 1983; Edmands, 1986; Lacey, 1983; Mackenzie & Harper-Guiffre, 1992; Polivy & Garfinkel, 1984) and in reworking parent-related transference issues (Asner, 1990; Roy-Byrne et al., 1984; Weinstein & Richman, 1984). Some concerns have been expressed about the possibility that a male therapist may inhibit female patients' discussions of sexuality and body image (Hall, 1985; Polivy & Garfinkel, 1984). Sometimes a recovering patient is a coleader in conjunction with a professional therapist (Edmands, 1986), although this

occurs more often in support and self-help groups (Enright et al., 1985; Johnson & Connors, 1987; Larocca, 1983).

It is often useful for group therapy leaders to receive clinical supervision. This enables them to stay in touch with their reactions and countertransferences to group members and events, and maintains constructive functioning with the patients. It can be useful for group leaders to examine their own personal issues and beliefs about weight and body image (Mackenzie & Harper-Guiffre, 1992). Support group leaders can also benefit from supervision from clinical staff (Johnson & Conners, 1987).

The unique benefits of group therapy, such as instillation of hope, universality, altruism, group cohesion, and interpersonal learning (Yalom, 1975), are augmented in eating disorder patients by reductions in the social isolation and alienation they often experience. Patients can learn much-needed interpersonal skills through their group interactions, and can practice newfound beliefs and skills in the safe, structured environment of the group. However, it is important to monitor whether participants are overidentifying with other group members (Polivy & Garfinkel, 1984). There is a risk that patients will form a strong "anorexic," "bulimic," or "eating-disordered" identity. More disturbed individuals may undermine any movement toward health by other members, though it is worth considering the possibility that a mixture of healthier and less healthy patients will give the less healthy ones hope and inspiration that they too can recover from their eating disorder. Other concerns are (1) that patients may teach symptoms to one another; and (2) that some patients may become extremely dependent on others, and the others may not be prepared to support this (Piazza & Steiner-Adair, 1986; Polivy, 1981). For this reason, and to prevent some members from feeling excluded, socializing by members outside of the group is discouraged in some therapy groups (Mackenzie & Harper-Guiffre, 1992; Polivy, 1981). Support groups are more likely to offer socialization and friendships, and may well encourage members to contact one another outside the group.

These are some of the considerations in conducting group therapy with eating disorder patients. Obviously, a brief chapter such as this cannot attempt to be exhaustive. The literature reviewed herein can point the interested reader to more in-depth analysis and discussion. What should be clear, though, is that group treatment is a viable and cost-effective approach for alleviating eating disorders.

REFERENCES

Agras, W. S., Rossiter, E. M., Arnow, B., Schneider, J. A., Telch, C. F., Raeburn, S. D., Bruce, B., Perl, M., & Koran, L. M. (1992). Pharmacologic and cognitive-behavioral treatment for bulimia nervosa: A controlled comparison. *American Journal of Psychiatry, 149,* 82–87.

Andersen, A. E., Morse, C., & Santmyer, K. (1985). Inpatient treatment for anorexia nervosa. In D. M. Garner & P. E. Garfinkel (Eds.), *Handbook of psychotherapy for anorexia nervosa and bulimia* (pp. 311–343). New York: Guilford Press.

Asner, J. (1990). Reworking the myth of personal incompetence: Group psychotherapy for bulimia nervosa. *Psychiatric Annals, 20,* 395–397.

Baell, W. K., & Wertheim, E. H. (1992). Predictors of outcome in the treatment of bulimia nervosa. *British Journal of Clinical Psychology, 31,* 330–332.

Barth, D., & Wurtman, V. (1986). Group therapy with bulimic women: A self-psychological approach. *International Journal of Eating Disorders, 5,* 735–745.

Berry, D. M., & Abramowitz, S. I. (1989). Educative support groups and subliminal psychodynamic activation for bulimic college women. *International Journal of Eating Disorders, 8,* 75–85.

Bohanske, J., & Lemberg, R. (1987). An intensive group process–retreat model for the treatment of bulimia. *Group, 11,* 228–237.

Boskind-White, M., & White, W. C. (1983). *Bulimarexia: The binge/purge cycle.* New York: Norton.

Brisman, J., & Siegel, M. (1985). The bulimia workshop: A unique integration of group treatment approaches. *International Journal of Group Psychotherapy, 35,* 585–601.

Bruch, H. (1982). Anorexia nervosa: Therapy and theory. *American Journal of Psychiatry, 139,* 1531–1538.

Connor-Greene, P. A. (1987). An educational group treatment program for bulimia. *Journal of American College Health, 35,* 229–231.

Connors, M. E., Johnson, C. L., & Stuckey, M. K. (1984). Treatment of bulimia with brief psychoeducational group therapy. *American Journal of Psychiatry, 141,* 1512–1516.

Cox, G. L., & Merkel, W. T. (1989). A qualitative review of psychosocial treatments for bulimia. *Journal of Nervous and Mental Disease, 177,* 77–84.

Crandall, C. (1988). Social contagion of binge eating. *Journal of Personality and Social Psychology, 4,* 588–598.

Crosby, R. D., Mitchell, J. E., Raymond, N., Specker, S., Nugent, S. M., & Pyle, R. L. (1993). Survival analysis of response to group psychotherapy in bulimia nervosa. *International Journal of Eating Disorders, 13,* 359–368.

Davis, R. (1988). Clinical assessment of the eating disorders. In P. E. Garfinkel (Ed.), *Current update: Anorexia nervosa and bulimia nervosa* (pp. 11–18). Kalamazoo, MI: Upjohn.

Davis, R., & Olmsted, M. P. (1992). Cognitive-behavioral group treatment for bulimia nervosa: Integrating group psychoeducation and psychotherapy. In H. Harper-Guiffre & K. R. Mackenzie (Eds.), *Group psychotherapy for eating disorders.* Washington, DC: American Psychiatric Press.

Davis, R., Olmsted, M. P., & Rockert, W. (1990). Brief group psychoeducation for bulimia nervosa: Assessing the clinical significance of change. *Journal of Consulting & Clinical Psychology, 58,* 882–885.

Davis, R., Olmsted, M. P., & Rockert, W. (1992). Brief group psychoeducation for bulimia nervosa: II. Prediction of clinical outcome. *International Journal of Eating Disorders, 11,* 205–211.

Dedman, P. A., Numa, S. F., & Wakeling, A. (1988). A cognitive-behavioral group approach for the treatment of bulimia nervosa: A preliminary study. *Journal of Psychosomatic Research, 32,* 285–290.

Dixon, K. N. (1986). Group therapy for bulimia. *Adolescent Psychiatry, 3,* 391–404.

Edmands, M. S. (1986). Overcoming eating disorders. *Journal of Psychosocial Nursing and Mental Health Services, 24,* 19–25.

Enright, A. B., Butterfield, P., & Berkowitz, B. (1985). Self-help and support groups in the management of eating disorders. In D. M. Garner & P. E. Garfinkel (Eds.), *Handbook of psychotherapy for anorexia nervosa and bulimia* (pp. 491–512). New York: Guilford Press.

Fairburn, C. G. (1981). A cognitive-behavioral approach to the management of bulimia. *Psychological Medicine, 141,* 631–633.

Fairburn, C. G. (1985). Cognitive-behavioral treatment for bulimia. In D. M. Garner & P. E. Garfinkel (Eds.), *Handbook of psychotherapy for anorexia nervosa and bulimia* (pp. 160–192). New York: Guilford Press.

Fairburn, C. G. (1988). The current status of the psychological treatments for bulimia nervosa. *Journal of Psychosomatic Research, 32,* 635–645.

Fairburn, C. G., Agras, W. S., & Wilson, G. T. (1992). The research on the treatment of bulimia nervosa: Practical and theoretical implications. In G. H. Anderson & S. H. Kennedy (Eds.), *The biology of feast and famine: Relevance to eating disorders* (pp. 318–340). San Diego: Academic Press.

Fairburn, C. G., Marcus, M. D., & Wilson, G. T. (1993). Cognitive-behavioral therapy for binge eating and bulimia nervosa: A comprehensive treatment manual. In C. G. Fairburn & G. T. Wilson (Eds.), *Binge eating: Nature, assessment, and treatment* (pp. 361–404). New York: Guilford Press.

Fernandez, D., & Latimer, P. (1990). A group treatment program for bulimia nervosa. *Group, 14,* 241–245.

Fettes, P. A., & Peters, J. M. (1992). A meta-analysis of group treatments for bulimia nervosa. *International Journal of Eating Disorders, 11,* 97–110.

Franko, D. L. (1993). The use of a group meal in the brief therapy of bulimia nervosa. *International Journal of Group Psychotherapy, 43,* 237–242.

Freeman, C. P. L., & Munro, J. K. M. (1988). Drug and group treatments for bulimia/bulimia nervosa. *Journal of Psychosomatic Research, 32,* 647–660.

Frommer, M. S., Ames, J. R., Gibson, J. W., & Davis, W. N. (1987). Patterns of symptom change in the short-term group treatment of bulimia. *International Journal of Eating Disorders, 6,* 469–476.

Garner, D. M., Fairburn, C. G., & Davis, R. (1987). Cognitive-behavioral treatment of bulimia nervosa: A critical appraisal. *Behavior Modification, 11,* 398–431.

Gendron, M., Lemberg, R., Allender, J., & Bohanske, J. (1992). Effectiveness of the intensive group process retreat model in the treatment of bulimia. *Group, 16,* 69–78.

Goodsitt, A. (1985). Self psychology and the treatment of

anorexia nervosa. In D. M. Garner & P. E. Garfinkel (Eds.), *Handbook of psychotherapy for anorexia nervosa and bulimia* (pp. 55–82). New York: Guilford Press.

Gray, J. J., & Hoage, C. M. (1990). Bulimia nervosa: Group behavior therapy with exposure plus response prevention. *Psychological Reports, 66,* 667–674.

Hall, A. (1985). Group psychotherapy for anorexia nervosa. In D. M. Garner & P. E. Garfinkel (Eds.), *Handbook of psychotherapy for anorexia nervosa and bulimia* (pp. 213–239). New York: Guilford Press.

Harper-Guiffre, H., Mackenzie, K. R., & Sivitilli, D. (1992). Interpersonal group psychotherapy. In H. Harper-Guiffre & K. R. Mackenzie (Eds.), *Group psychotherapy for eating disorders.* Washington, DC: American Psychiatric Press.

Hendren, R. L., Atkins, D. M., Sumner, C. R., & Barber, J. K. (1987). Model for the group treatment of eating disorders. *International Journal of Group Therapy, 37,* 589–602.

Huon, G. F., & Brown, L. B. (1985). Evaluating a group treatment for bulimia. *Journal of Psychiatric Research, 19,* 479–483.

Inbody, D. R., & Ellis, J. J. (1985). Group therapy with anorexic and bulimic patients: Implications for therapeutic intervention. *American Journal of Psychotherapy, 39,* 411–420.

Johnson, C., & Connors, M. (1987). *The etiology and treatment of bulimia nervosa: A biopsychosocial perspective.* New York: Basic Books.

Johnson, C., Connors, M., & Stuckey, M. (1983). Short-term group treatment of bulimia. *International Journal of Eating Disorders, 2,* 199–208.

Kearney-Cooke, A. (1988). Group treatment of sexual abuse among women with eating disorders. *Women and Therapy, 7,* 5–21.

Kettlewell, P. W., Mizes, J. S., & Wasylyshyn, N. A. (1992). A cognitive-behavioral group treatment of bulimia. *Behavior Therapy, 23,* 657–670.

Kirkley, B., Schneider, J. A., Agras, W. S., & Bachman, J. A. (1985). Comparison of two group treatments for bulimia. *Journal of Consulting and Clinical Psychology, 53,* 43–48.

Lacey, H. (1983). Bulimia nervosa, binge eating, and psychogenic vomiting: A controlled treatment study and long term outcome. *British Medical Journal, 286,* 1609–1613.

Laessle, R. G., & Pirke, K. M. (1987). A structured behaviorally oriented group treatment for bulimia nervosa. *Psychotherapy and Psychosomatics, 48,* 141–145.

Larocca, F. E. F. (1983). The relevance of self-help in the management of anorexia and bulimia. In *Research medica* (pp. 16–19). St. Louis: St. John's Mercy Medical Center.

Laube, J. J. (1990). Why group therapy for bulimia? *International Journal of Group Psychotherapy, 40,* 169–187.

Lee, N. F., & Rush, A. J. (1986). Cognitive-behavioral group therapy for bulimia. *International Journal of Eating Disorders, 5,* 599–615.

Leitenberg, H., Rosen, J. C., Gross, J., Nudelman, S., & Vara, L. (1988). Exposure plus response-prevention treatment of bulimia nervosa. *Journal of Consulting and Clinical Psychology, 56,* 535–541.

Mackenzie, K. R., & Harper-Guiffre, H. (1992). Developing a healthy relationship with your body. In H. Harper-Guiffre & K. R. Mackenzie (Eds.), *Group psychotherapy for eating disorders* (pp. 329–333). Washington, DC: American Psychiatric Press.

Maddocks, S. E., & Kaplan, A. S. (1991). The prediction of treatment response in bulimia nervosa: A study of patient variables. *British Journal of Psychiatry, 159,* 846–849.

Malenbaum, R., Herzog, D., Eisenthal, S., & Wyshak, G. (1988). Overeaters Anonymous: Impact on bulimia. *International Journal of Eating Disorders, 7,* 139–143.

Merril, C. A., Mines, R. A., & Starkey, R. (1987). The premature dropout in the group treatment of bulimia. *International Journal of Eating Disorders, 6,* 293–300.

Mitchell, J. E. (1990). *Bulimia nervosa.* Minneapolis: University of Minnesota Press.

Mitchell, J. E., Hatsukami, D., Goff, G., Pyle, R. L., Eckert, E. D., & Davis, L. E. (1985). Intensive outpatient group treatment for bulimia. In D. M. Garner & P. E. Garfinkel (Eds.), *Handbook of psychotherapy for anorexia nervosa and bulimia* (pp. 240–253). New York: Guilford Press.

Mitchell, J. E., Pyle, R. L., Hatsukami, D., Goff, G., Glotter, D., & Harper, J. (1989). A 2–5 year follow-up study of patients treated for bulimia. *International Journal of Eating Disorders, 8,* 157–165.

Oesterheld, J. R., McKenna, M. S., & Gould, N. B. (1987). Group psychotherapy of bulimia: A critical review. *International Journal of Group Psychotherapy, 37,* 163–184.

Piazza, E. A., & Steiner-Adair, C. (1986). Recent trends in group therapy for anorexia nervosa and bulimia. In F. E. F. Larocca (Ed.), *Eating disorders: Effective care and treatment* (pp. 25–51). New York: Wiley.

Piran, N., Kaplan, A., Kerr, A., Shekter-Wolfson, L., Winocur, J., Gold, E., & Garfinkel, P. E. (1989). A day hospital program for anorexia nervosa and bulimia. *International Journal of Eating Disorders, 8,* 511–521.

Piran, N., Langdon, L., Kaplan, A., & Garfinkel, P. E. (1989). Evaluation of a day hospital program for eating disorders. *International Journal of Eating Disorders, 8,* 523–532.

Polivy, J. (1981). On the induction of emotion in the laboratory: Discrete moods or multiple affect states? *Journal of Personality and Social Psychology, 41,* 803–817.

Polivy, J., & Garfinkel, P. E. (1984). Group treatments for specific medical disorders: Anorexia nervosa. In H. B. Roback (Ed.), *Helping patients and their families cope with medical problems* (pp. 60–78). San Francisco: Jossey-Bass.

Pyle, R. L., Mitchell, J. E., Eckert, E., Hatsukami, D. K., & Goff, G. M. (1984). The interruption of bulimic behaviors: A review of three treatment programs. *Psychiatric Clinics of North America, 7,* 275–286.

Reiss, H., & Rutan, J. S. (1992). Group therapy for eating disorders: A step-wise approach. *Group, 16,* 79–83.

Riebel, L. K. (1990). The dropout problem in outpatient psychotherapy groups for bulimics and compulsive eaters. *Psychotherapy, 27,* 404–410.

Rosen, J. C., Cado, S., Silberg, S., Srebnik, D., & Wendt, S. (1990). Cognitive behavior therapy with and without size perception training for women with body image disturbance. *Behavior Therapy, 21,* 481–498.

Rosen, J. C., & Leitenberg, H. (1982). Bulimia nervosa: Treatment with exposure and response prevention. *Behavior Therapy, 13,* 117–124.

Rosen, J. C., & Leitenberg, H. (1985). Exposure plus response prevention treatment of bulimia nervosa. In D. M. Garner & P. E. Garfinkel (Eds.), *Handbook of psychotherapy for anorexia nervosa and bulimia* (pp. 193–209). New York: Guilford Press.

Rosen, J. C., Reiter, J., & Orosan, P. (1995). Cognitive behavioral body image therapy for body dysmorphic disorder. *Journal of Consulting and Clinical Psychology, 63,* 263–270.

Rosenvinge, J. H. (1990). Group therapy for anorexic and bulimic patients. *Acta Psychiatrica Scandinavica, 82*(Suppl. 361), 38–43.

Roy-Byrne, P., Lee-Benner, K., & Yager, J. (1984). Group therapy for bulimia. *International Journal of Eating Disorders, 3,* 97–116.

Schneider, J. A., & Agras, W. S. (1985). A cognitive behavioral group treatment of bulimia. *British Journal of Psychiatry, 146,* 66–69.

Shisslak, C. M., Crago, M., Schnaps, L., & Swain, B. (1986). Interactional group therapy for anorexic and bulimic women. *Psychotherapy, 23,* 598–606.

Stevens, E. V., & Salisbury, J. (1984). Group therapy for bulimic adults. *American Journal of Orthopsychiatry, 54,* 156–161.

Stuber, M., & Strober, M. (1987). Group therapy in the treatment of adolescents with bulimia: Some preliminary observations. *International Journal of Eating Disorders, 6,* 125–131.

Sykes, D. K., Currie, K. O., & Gross, M. (1987). The use of group therapy in the treatment of bulimia. *International Journal of Psychosomatics, 43,* 7–10.

Toseland, R., & Rivas, R. (1984). *An introduction to group practice.* New York: Macmillan.

Vandereycken, W. (1990). The relevance of body-image disturbance for the treatment of bulimia. In M. M. Fichter (Ed.), *Bulimia nervosa: Basic research, diagnosis and treatment* (pp. 320–330). New York: Wiley.

Vandereycken, W., Depreitere, L., & Probst, M. (1987). Body-oriented therapy for anorexia nervosa patients. *American Journal of Psychotherapy, 41,* 252–259.

Vandereycken, W., & Meerman, R. (1984). *Anorexia nervosa.* Berlin: de Gruyter.

Vandereycken, W., Probst, M., & Van Bellinghen, M. (1992). Treating the distorted body experience of anorexia nervosa patients. *Journal of Adolescent Health, 13,* 403–405.

Weinstein, H., & Richman, A. (1984). The group treatment of bulimia. *Journal of American College Health, 32,* 209–215.

Wilfley, D. E., Agras, W. S., Telch, C. F., Rossiter, E. M., Schneider, J. A., Cole, A. G., Sifford, L., & Raeburn, S. D. (1993). Group cognitive-behavioral therapy and group interpersonal psychotherapy for the nonpurging bulimic individual: A controlled comparison. *Journal of Consulting and Clinical Psychology, 61,* 296–305.

Wilson, G. T. (1987). Cognitive-behavioral treatment of bulimia nervosa. *Annals of Behavioral Medicine, 9,* 12–17.

Wilson, G. T. (1991). The addiction model of eating disorders: A critical analysis. *Advances in Behavior Research and Therapy, 13,* 27–72.

Wilson, G. T., & Fairburn, C. G. (1993). Cognitive treatments for eating disorders. *Journal of Consulting and Clinical Psychology, 61,* 261–269.

Wolchik, S. A., Weiss, L., & Katzman, M. A. (1986). An empirically validated short-term psychoeducational group treatment program for bulimia. *International Journal of Eating Disorders, 5,* 21–34.

Wolf, E. M., & Crowther, J. H. (1992). An evaluation of behavioral and cognitive-behavioral group interventions for the treatment of bulimia nervosa in women. *International Journal of Eating Disorders, 11,* 3–15.

Wooley, S. C., & Kearney-Cooke, A. (1986). Intensive treatment of bulimia and body image disturbance. In K. Brownell & J. Foreyt (Eds.), *Handbook of eating disorders: Physiology, psychology, and the treatment of obesity, anorexia, and bulimia* (pp. 476–502). New York: Basic Books.

Wooley, S. C., & Lewis, K. G. (1987). Multi-family therapy within an intensive treatment program for bulimia. In J. E. Harkaway (Ed.), *The family therapy collections.* Rockville, MD: Aspen.

Yalom, I. (1975). *The theory and practice of group psychotherapy.* New York: Basic Books.

Yates, A., & Sambrailo, F. (1984). Bulimia nervosa: A descriptive and therapeutic study. *American Journal of Orthopsychiatry, 54,* 156–161.

Yellowlees, P. (1988). Group psychotherapy in anorexia nervosa. *International Journal of Eating Disorders, 7*(5), 649–655.

Zimpfer, D. G. (1990). Group work for bulimia: A review of outcomes. *Journal for Specialists in Group Work, 15,* 239–251.

CHAPTER 28

Prepubertal Eating Disorders

BRYAN LASK
RACHEL BRYANT-WAUGH

In this chapter, we define the eating disorders seen in prepubertal children and discuss their management, paying particular attention to the differences in treatment of children and adults. It is important to distinguish between prepubertal eating disorders and the feeding difficulties and problems of early childhood. The latter are common in the preschool years and cover a wide spectrum of phenomena of variable clinical significance, ranging from variations of normal behavior (such as mild faddiness) to conditions of major developmental significance (such as failure to thrive) (Cooper & Stein, 1992). They have very little in common with the eating disorders of childhood, adolescence, and adult life. In contrast, the prepubertal eating disorders are rare before about 8 years of age, appear to have a far more complex pathogenesis and a generally more serious course, and have more in common with adolescent- and adult-onset eating disorders.

TYPES OF PREPUBERTAL EATING DISORDERS

There are a number of different eating disorders in prepubertal children, all of which share a common central theme—avoidance of food. Some of these disorders have not yet achieved formal diagnostic status, but their existence has been recognized and reported.

1. Anorexia nervosa in prepubertal children has been well documented (Jacobs & Isaacs, 1986; Fosson, Knibbs, Bryant-Waugh, & Lask, 1987; Higgs, Goodyer, & Birch, 1989; Gowers, Crisp, Joughin, & Bhat, 1991; Lask & Bryant-Waugh, 1993). In general, the symptoms are similar to those of the older population, including such core features as distorted body image (e.g., thinking oneself fat when underweight) and morbid fear of weight gain. Amenorrhea is of course always primary. There is a higher prevalence of boys (25%) than might be expected from the gender distribution in adolescents and adults (Lask & Bryant-Waugh, 1993).

2. In food avoidance emotional disorder (Higgs et al., 1989), food avoidance is a prominent symptom, but there is a failure to meet the full criteria for anorexia nervosa. Other affective symptoms are common, including anxiety, phobias, school avoidance, obsessionality, and depression. This may be a partial syndrome of anorexia nervosa, with a better prognosis.

3. Selective eating (Lask & Bryant-Waugh, 1993) is a term that has been applied to a condition in which children eat only a very narrow range of foods, even as few as three or four. These foods are often carbohydrate-based, and the diet does appear generally to be inadequate. However, such children tend to thrive physically and grow normally, although they do often have problems in social functioning.

4. Pervasive refusal syndrome (Lask, Britten, Kroll, Magagna, & Tranter, 1991) is a life-threatening condition, manifested by a profound and pervasive refusal to eat, drink, walk, talk, or engage in any form of self-care. The initial presentation is often that of anorexia ner-

vosa, but when attempts are made to commence refeeding, there is a dramatic intensification of symptoms. Pervasive refusal is most likely to be an extreme form of the avoidance behavior seen in post-traumatic stress disorder.

5. Bulimia nervosa is, so far as we can tell, very rare in prepubertal children, and we have seen very few such children in our own clinic. Our impression is that at present, this is a condition that normally occurs during or after puberty. Schmidt, Hodes, and Treasure (1992) reported 23 cases of early-onset bulimia nervosa (i.e., onset at age 15 or below), with a mean age of onset of 13.9 (± 1.4), and a range of 11 to 15. No mention was made of prepubertal bulimia nervosa, and all the girls had already commenced menstruation at the onset of the eating disorder.

Further information about the pathogenesis, demography, and course of these conditions is available elsewhere (e.g., Lask & Bryant-Waugh, 1993; Bryant-Waugh & Lask, 1995a, 1995b). Other childhood feeding problems (e.g., pica, rumination disorder, and failure to thrive) have been excluded because they are not eating disorders (e.g., Skuse, 1994). The remainder of this chapter is devoted to the assessment and treatment of prepubertal eating disorders.

ASSESSMENT AND TREATMENT

The treatment of prepubertal eating disorders differs from that of the older population; and it requires different skills and knowledge. Children are far more prone to severe physical complications, and there is a high incidence of persisting morbidity (Bryant-Waugh, Knibbs, Fosson, Kaminski, & Lask, 1988). A rapidly initiated, intensive, and comprehensive treatment program is required, and it should be conducted by child-oriented professionals. Eating disorder specialists without an awareness of developmental considerations or experience in working with children should consider referral to pediatrically trained colleagues.

The main components of a comprehensive program are as follows:

1. Conducting a multidisciplinary assessment.
2. Providing information and education.
3. Ensuring that adults are in charge.

4. Deciding about the need for hospitalization.
5. Determining a target weight range.
6. Implementing a refeeding program.
7. Providing parental counseling and family therapy.
8. Providing individual therapy.
9. Considering the need for medication.
10. Providing schooling.

Conducting a Multidisciplinary Assessment

Any child referred to our clinic undergoes a multidisciplinary assessment. On arrival, each child is seen by a pediatrician for a general evaluation and formal measurement of weight, height, and skinfold thickness. Any physical investigations considered necessary are arranged; all girls have a pelvic ultrasound scan to assess ovarian and uterine maturity, and all children have a bone age assessment.

The child is then seen with her family for a detailed review of the development of the disorder, current situation, and family functioning.[1] Next, the child is seen individually for a more detailed exploration of mental state and possible contributing factors, including any history of abuse or other forms of trauma. Such exploration requires considerable skill and patience.

It is always useful to make an assessment of how much insight the child has into her condition. We usually say something along these lines: "I can see that you don't think there is anything wrong with you and that you believe everyone is making a ridiculous fuss, but I wonder if there is just a very small part of you that can tell that something is not quite right, even if it's only a tiny bit of you." Most children are able to acknowledge that there is indeed a bit of them that is frightened or saddened by what is happening. We label this bit "the healthy or well part of you," and use it later.

Once these assessments have been completed, the team meets to discuss its findings. The consultant then meets with the child and family to discuss the findings.

Providing Information and Education

The parents need a clear statement about their child's disorder and its implications, the treatment required, the likely course of the condition, and its prognosis. We have found that parents are far more receptive to our recommendations if these are conveyed following a detailed assessment such as that described above, and if the parents are encouraged to ask questions and discuss the situation in as much detail as they wish. We have also found it helpful to provide a detailed handout that describes the specific eating disorder, and complements the information already given orally. Families are always invited to return later for further discussion, and most parents are only too eager to do so.

Ensuring That Adults Are in Charge

Many children with eating disorders are both physically and psychologically very ill; yet they are allowed to continue to decide what and how much they will eat, whether or not they should go to school, and how much exercise they should have. Unless adults take control, the interaction among these children's determination to retain control, their lack of insight, and the life-threatening nature of some eating disorders can prove fatal. It is therefore essential that when a child's health is threatened, the adults take charge of the child's eating until she is on the way to recovery. Adults should not attempt to take control over *all* aspects of the child's life, as this is neither necessary nor helpful; rather, they should restrict such measures to matters of health and safety. (Nor is it always necessary to take such firm command if the eating disorder is of the more benign variety, such as selective eating or food avoidance emotional disorder.)

A clear statement about the need for adult control of the child's eating is made as part of the provision of information and education, and the potential consequences of failing to take charge are spelled out. We try to convey this not as a battle between the child and adults, but rather a battle between the illness and everyone else, including the child. We use the analogy of teamwork, with all of us being on the same side fighting the illness. Not uncommonly during this process, a child freely and forcefully expresses antagonism to our advice by shouting, crying, threatening, or pleading. This is a helpful intervention on the child's part, as it demonstrates to the parents the very point the therapist is making about the need for the adults to help the child win the battle against the illness.

After such forceful advice is given to the par-

ents, it is important to acknowledge the child's fears and concerns. This is best done by addressing the child directly and making a sympathetic statement about her plight, including recognition of the child's anger and fright. We remind the child that the battle is inside her, between the illness and "the healthy part." It is likely that the child will angrily reject such an approach, but it should always be offered, and she should be reminded that the illness is winning the battle at present. Many children will say when they have recovered that although they hated us and what we were saying at the time, they knew it was right and felt a sense of relief that someone seemed to understand their fears and conflicts.

Deciding about the Need for Hospitalization

Hospitalization is rarely indicated for selective eating or food avoidance emotional disorder, but it is often required for anorexia nervosa and is mandatory for pervasive refusal syndrome. Hospitalization is indicated in any of the following circumstances:

1. The child's percentage of weight for height by age (Tanner–Whitehouse standards; Tanner, Whitehouse, & Takaishi, 1966) has fallen below 70% (see "Determining a Target Weight Range," below).
2. The child is dehydrated.
3. There are signs of circulatory failure, such as (a) bradycardia; (b) an increase of more than 20 beats per minute between supine and erect pulse rate; (c) systolic blood pressure of less than 80 mm Hg; (d) a drop of more than 30 mm Hg between supine and erect blood pressure; or (e) poor peripheral circulation, with inadequate pedal pulses or discoloration of the feet and hands (acrocyanosis).
4. There is persistent vomiting.
5. The illness is complicated by marked depression or other major psychiatric disturbance.

Once the decision to hospitalize a child is made, she should ideally be admitted to a child psychiatric unit that has experience in managing prepubertal eating disorders. If such a unit is not available, then a pediatric unit should be used, with care shared between the pediatric and psychiatric team. Every effort must be made to avoid admitting children to units that do not normally provide care for them.

Determining a Target Weight Range

A number of factors need to be taken into consideration when one is determining an appropriate weight for a child. First, weight must be considered in the context of the child's age and height, rather than in isolation; this necessitates the use of the Tanner–Whitehouse standards (Tanner et al., 1966), in which 100% represents average and less than 80% indicates wasting. Second, children with anorexia nervosa will be terrified by any target that is above average. However, pelvic ultrasound scanning indicates that ovarian and uterine maturity is less likely to be achieved in girls who are below 96% weight for height (Lai, De Bruyn, Lask, Bryant-Waugh, & Hankins, 1994). Setting a range rather than a specific target gives such girls some limited sense of control, which helps them to tolerate better the overall loss of control. Taking into account all these considerations, we encourage children to maintain weight within the range of 96–100%.

Implementation of a Refeeding Program

A refeeding program is indicated when there is dehydration, weight loss, or electrolyte disturbance. In general, selective eaters do not require a refeeding program, and children with food avoidance emotional disorder often start eating normally again once the underlying problems have been recognized and treated. However, children with anorexia nervosa and pervasive refusal syndrome invariably require some form of refeeding program.

The urgency of refeeding is determined by the severity or rapidity of weight loss, dehydration, or electrolyte disturbance. Marked dehydration or electrolyte disturbance requires immediate attention, and the assistance of a pediatrician should always be sought. If the child agrees to eat and drink adequate amounts over the next 24 hours, then artificial feeding can be withheld, but otherwise it should be implemented rapidly. The favored route is by nasogastric tube, although some pediatricians prefer intravenous feeding. The child is told that such measures will continue until they are no longer necessary, and that any calories taken by mouth will be deducted from the total amount of artificially administered foods. Although the use of nasogastric feeds is highly controversial in adult patients, in pediatrics tubes are used more commonly, and in severely emaciated children there may be no other preferable alternative. For a discussion of the ethical issues of nasogastric tube feeding, see Elton, Honig, Bentovim, and Simons (1995).

When artificial feeding is no longer required, then oral feedings can gradually be reintroduced. It is often easier for children to tolerate smaller portions initially; it is therefore wiser to commence with a relatively low calorie intake, but with the intention of increasing total daily intake to the required amount within a few days. The exact calorie requirement will be determined by age, weight, height, and amount of weight loss. In general, however, it is likely to be between 2,000 and 3,000 calories for children in the age range of 8 to 14. It can be helpful to have the advice of a dietitian in determining exact calorie needs and how these may best be provided. Many children find solid foods difficult to tolerate in the early stages of refeeding, and calorie-strengthened (or "top-up") drinks make an acceptable supplement to small amounts of solid foods.

Refeeding is a particularly stressful process for all concerned, whether it is undertaken in the hospital or at home. Children who are being refed need constant reassurance that they will not become fat, and that they will be able to regain normal control of their appetite and intake as they get better. Glendinning and Phillips (1993) have provided a most helpful and detailed account of the practicalities. Success is dependent upon a combination of sympathy, understanding, tolerance, firmness and determination, all in the context of everyone working together.

Children with anorexia nervosa are often skilled at concealing their techniques for avoiding weight gain. Hiding food, exercising, vomiting, and laxative abuse are all common. Some parents are convinced that their children do not do such things until they actually discover them so doing. It is best to assume that such activities are occurring and will continue to occur during refeeding. In this way they are more likely to be guarded against, and their ultimate and inevitable discovery is less traumatic for all concerned.

Providing Parental Counseling and Family Therapy

Parental counseling and family therapy constitute the *sine qua non* of the management of

480 SPECIAL TOPICS IN TREATMENT

prepubertal eating disorders. They are the only treatments to have been shown on empirical testing to be effective for early-onset anorexia nervosa (Russell, Szmukler, Dare, & Eisler, 1987).

The essence of these treatments is the focus on the family rather than the individual. The primary goals are the restoration of effective parenting and satisfactory family functioning. Characteristically, the family is in turmoil and despair. Excessive attention is paid to the sick child, to the detriment of other family members; generational boundaries are breached; conflict is rife; and consistency and cooperation are minimal. Alternatively, the family may have adapted to and accommodated the child's problematic eating habits to avoid conflict. It is often unclear whether such dysfunction has predated the eating disorder, but from a management viewpoint this is not particularly relevant, as it has to be tackled in any case. Indeed, it is rare for a child with an eating disorder to make a sustained recovery without there being a concomitant improvement in family functioning.

The Four Cs

Although there are many different schools of family therapy, there is no evidence that any one is superior to another in the treatment of prepubertal eating disorders. However, it is our clinical experience that parental counseling plays a crucial part. The key areas are the four Cs—cohesion, consistency, communication, and conflict resolution. The lack of each of these in the parental management of the eating disorder often contributes to the maintenance of the problem.

Cohesion. For their child to recover, the parents need to work together cohesively as a team—adopting a consistent approach to management, communicating openly and directly with each other and their child, and identifying and resolving conflicts. A useful means of enhancing cohesion is asking each parent in turn to suggest to the other parent things he or she could do differently that might be more helpful. By a process of discussion and negotiation, parents can be helped to reach agreement about how best to handle the problem. This approach is more likely to work than one based on didactic advice, which may not be acceptable to either

parent. Our experience is that it matters less what the parents do, and more that they are able to work cohesively to help their child eat.

Consistency. Consistency over time is also essential. The use of one approach today, a different one tomorrow, and yet another the day after is very unlikely to be helpful. Parents are therefore helped to persevere through the inevitable early difficulties, on the grounds that persistence usually works.

Communication. Dysfunctional modes of communication are common in many families, and those with eating disorders are no exception (Lask & Bryant-Waugh, 1993). Communication may be excessive, with much interrupting and overlapping and with little silence, so that the opportunity to be heard or to reply is limited. In contrast, communication may be inhibited, with limited responses and long silences. Noncongruent communications are those in which there is a lack of congruence between the verbal and nonverbal content, with subsequent confusion, misunderstanding, and frustration. Children with anorexia nervosa and their families often have difficulty communicating negative feelings, such as anger or sadness, and other symptoms or behaviors displace these feelings; this "displaced communication" again causes confusion and misunderstandings. Finally, communication may be deviant. For example, one person may speak on behalf of the whole family; someone repeatedly reports what another is supposedly thinking or feeling; or communication is either generally vague and woolly, or too complex and unwieldy to follow.

Communication needs to be clear, open, and direct, with all family members speaking for themselves, and each person being allowed the chance to respond when appropriate. Elsewhere, we have described in detail some techniques for helping parents and families to overcome dysfunctional communication styles (Lask & Bryant-Waugh, 1993, pp. 216–218). These can be implemented in parental or family meetings, rehearsed, and practiced at home.

Conflict Resolution. Parental counseling can be conducted with or without the children present. The advantage of the children's presence is that any involvement of the children in the parental subsystem (i.e., triangulation) rapidly becomes evident and can be dealt with at the time by the therapist, who can help the parents impose clear boundaries between themselves and the children. It is only when the personal aspects of the parental relationship are being discussed that it is inappropriate for the children to be present. It is important to emphasize here that there is a major difference between parental counseling and marital counseling: The former focuses on parenting, and the latter on the marital relationship. Marital counseling should not be embarked upon without the expressed agreement of both partners.

The restoration of appropriate interpersonal boundaries is an integral part of the work with many such families. Sometimes this follows automatically as the parental subsystem is reinforced during parental counseling. However, the therapist should ensure that all family members have an age-appropriate degree of autonomy and an opportunity to express their own thoughts and feelings.

The use of toys, drawings, games, family trees, and experiential techniques all also have a part to play in work with families. These are described more fully elsewhere (Lask & Bryant-Waugh, 1993, pp. 211–219).

Providing Individual Therapy

In this section, we give brief consideration to two forms of individual therapy—psychodynamic and cognitive.

Psychodynamic Psychotherapy

The psychodynamic approach has been one of the more commonly used methods of treatment for prepubertal anorexia nervosa, despite a lack of evidence for its effectiveness. Furthermore, it has often been used in isolation. The parents may not have received any counseling, and the child may not have been under the care of a child psychiatrist or pediatrician.

Magagna (1993) has described in detail the process of therapy with this age group. She sees the task as one of helping these children develop sufficient patience and trust to allow them to experience empathic nurturing, and thus to feel understood and loved:

In this way the child with eating difficulties may find a way of developing sufficient concern for the internal parental figures, siblings and the therapist to mitigate her [sic] rage about unmet needs. The development of a capacity for love and tolerance of the parents for their shortcomings enhances the capacity to bear separation from the parents in a mature way. Successful therapy involves the child taking responsibility for mothering herself, being concerned about the feelings of others and forgiving the parents. (Magagna, 1993, p. 191)

Magagna describes an effective therapeutic framework for individual psychodynamic psychotherapy as one that incorporates (1) an assessment of family strengths and weaknesses, (2) an individual assessment to ascertain the underlying individual pathology, (3) the continuing involvement of a medical practitioner, (4) ongoing parental or family work, and (5) the option of hospitalizing a child if necessary.

Cognitive Therapy

Cognitive approaches to the management of prepubertal anorexia nervosa form a powerful set of techniques that can be used in conjunction with a variety of other therapies, with either individuals, families, or groups (Turk, 1993). The same applies to the other prepubertal eating disorders. The therapy is aimed at altering maladaptive cognitions such as "I am grossly overweight," "If I eat even a small amount, I will become overweight," "I am useless," or "I am only a nice person if I am thin."

Turk (1993) states that cognitive approaches are best combined with direct (behavioral) efforts to alter eating behaviors, and that in severely emaciated children it is wise to restore physical health to some extent before commencing cognitive therapy. Age and intellectual level are less important considerations for suitability than the ability to entertain alternative ways of viewing situations. The therapist does not act to persuade a child or family that their views are illogical or inconsistent with reality; the skill is to assist the child and family in discovering this for themselves. Turk (1993) describes in detail the practicalities of the cognitive approaches, and concludes that when "enduring changes [are created] in modes of thinking and appraising situations and occurrences, the likelihood of relapse is reduced, and patients and their families are provided with a new set of techniques which can be applied to a wide variety of problems long after therapy has ended" (p. 189).

Considering the Need for Medication

There is little indication for the use of medication in this age group. Antidepressants may sometimes be of value if a child has psychomotor retardation, extreme feelings of guilt and worthlessness, and marked biological changes (e.g., insomnia and diurnal mood variation). However, they should be prescribed with caution because of their potential for cardiotoxicity, particularly in children of low weight. Their use should be reserved for children whose depression does not resolve, or who fail to gain weight, despite a comprehensive approach to their management. It is wise to obtain an electrocardiogram before commencing treatment. Tricyclics such as amitriptyline have yet to be superseded and should be used initially in low doses, which should be gradually increased until blood levels are in the therapeutic range. If effective, they should be continued for at least 4 months after improvement has been noted. The newer selective serotonin reuptake inhibitors have not been evaluated in children, but their lower side effect profile makes them an attractive alternative.

Anxiolytics should be used only rarely. Very occasionally, a child who becomes truly panic-stricken prior to eating may benefit from their judicious use, but they should not be prescribed on a routine basis.

Vitamin and mineral supplementation has no proven value. Constipation is best treated by adequate diet rather than with laxatives.

Providing Schooling

Schooling is an integral part of everyday life in childhood. Tate (1993) has commented that success at school is generally associated with good behavior and academic achievement, regular and punctual attendance, compliance, good manners, and diligence. By such measures, the majority of children with anorexia nervosa would be perceived by their teachers as excellent pupils, given their tendency to conscientiousness and perfectionism. It is hardly surprising, therefore, that such children are eager to continue their schoolwork despite severe ill health. In contrast, pervasive refusers avoid school quite early in their illness, and children

with food avoidance emotional disorder may manifest symptoms of school phobia.

The decision of whether or not a child with an eating disorder should continue to attend school can only be made on the basis of individual circumstances. Some will undoubtedly be too ill to do so; others may have their illness perpetuated by school-based or self-imposed pressures, or by the lack of supervision at exercise periods or mealtimes. Careful discussion with the child, the parents, and the school staff should precede any decision. Even when not attending school, many children will wish to continue their schoolwork or will worry about falling behind. A continuing liaison with the school staff and the parents is required to ensure that the correct balance is achieved between the conflicting demands of health and education.

CONCLUSIONS

The successful management of prepubertal eating disorders is dependent upon the comprehensive assessment and treatment of both children and their families. Management should not be undertaken by those who are not familiar with the developmental and systemic issues so pertinent to the care of children.

The different eating disorders require different treatments. For example, the treatment of food avoidance emotional disorder needs to be focused on the associated affective disorder as well as the eating difficulties. Selective eating is the least serious of the conditions, as it is not usually associated with weight loss or other physical symptoms, and it tends to run a benign course. The main issues in treatment are to help parents tolerate their anxieties so that these do not create other problems, and to help children overcome the social impairment associated with their very limited diet.

Both anorexia nervosa and pervasive refusal syndrome are life-threatening conditions requiring a comprehensive, intensive, and skilled approach to their management. They tend to run a stormy course and have a relatively poor prognosis. Only about two-thirds of children with anorexia nervosa make a full and sustained recovery; very few pervasive refusers make a full recovery, and these usually need to be placed away from home.

In our experience, complete recovery from

prepubertal eating disorders is associated with two crucial factors: (1) The parents are able to develop a cohesive relationship with each other and with us; and (2) the children go through a stage of overt negativism and assertiveness, which the parents and the therapy team must tolerate (Lask & Bryant-Waugh, 1993, pp. 134–135). The latter, though unpleasant, is important. Unless this stage of recovery is fully completed, most children either regress or experience an early relapse.

We look forward to further advancements in the understanding and treatment of prepubertal eating disorders. Meanwhile, we are left to ponder the implicit message of one child with anorexia nervosa: "Watch me, Mum. I can dice with death, and there's nothing you can do about it." We hope that this chapter has given an adequate reply.

NOTE

1. For ease of reading, the authors have used she, rather than (s)he or she/he and her rather than his/her, unless specifically referring to boys.

REFERENCES

Bryant-Waugh, R., & Lask, B. (1995a). Eating disorders in childhood and adolescence: Annotation. *Journal of Child Psychology and Psychiatry, 36,* 191–202.

Bryant-Waugh, R., & Lask, B. (1995b). Eating disorders: An overview. *Journal of Family Therapy, 17,* 13–30.

Bryant-Waugh, R., Knibbs, J., Fosson, A., Kaminski, Z., & Lask, B. (1988). Long-term follow-up of patients with early onset anorexia nervosa. *Archives of Disease in Childhood, 63,* 5–9.

Cooper, P., & Stein, A. (1992). *Feeding problems and eating disorders in children and adolescents.* Reading, England: Harwood Academic.

Elton, A., Honig, P., Bentovim, A., & Simons, J. (1995). Withholding consent to lifesaving treatment: Three cases. *British Medical Journal, 310,* 373–377.

Fosson, A., Knibbs, J., Bryant-Waugh, R., & Lask, B. (1987). Early onset anorexia nervosa. *Archives of Disease in Childhood, 62,* 114–118.

Glendinning, L., & Phillips, M. (1993). Nursing management. In B. Lask & R. Bryant-Waugh (Eds.), *Childhood onset anorexia nervosa and related eating disorders.* Hove, England: Erlbaum.

Gowers, S., Crisp, A., Joughin, N., & Bhat, A. (1991). Premenarchial anorexia nervosa. *Journal of Child Psychology and Psychiatry, 32,* 515–524.

Higgs, J., Goodyer, I., & Birch, J. (1989). Anorexia nervosa and food avoidance emotional disorder. *Archives of Disease in Childhood, 64,* 345–351.

Jacobs, B., & Isaacs, S. (1986). Pre-pubertal anorexia nervosa: A retrospective controlled study. *Journal of Child Psychology and Psychiatry, 27,* 237–250.

Lai, K., De Bruyn, R., Lask, B., Bryant-Waugh, R., & Hankins, M. (1994). Use of pelvic ultrasound to monitor ovarian and uterine maturity in childhood onset anorexia nervosa. *Archives of Disease in Childhood, 71,* 228–231.

Lask, B., Britten, C., Kroll, L., Magagna, J., & Tranter, M. (1991). Pervasive refusal in children. *Archives of Disease in Childhood, 66,* 866–869.

Lask, B., & Bryant-Waugh, R. (Eds.). (1993). *Childhood onset anorexia nervosa and related eating disorders.* Hove, England: Erlbaum.

Magagna, J. (1993). Individual psychodynamic psychotherapy. In B. Lask & R. Bryant-Waugh (Eds.), *Childhood onset anorexia nervosa and related eating disorders.* Hove, England: Erlbaum.

Russell, G., Szmukler, G., Dare, C., & Eisler, I. (1987). Evaluation of family therapy for anorexia nervosa and bulimia nervosa. *Archives of General Psychiatry, 44,* 1047–1056.

Schmidt, U., Hodes, M., & Treasure, J. (1992). Early onset bulimia nervosa: Who is at risk? A retrospective case–control study. *Psychological Medicine, 22,* 623–628.

Skuse, D. (1994). Feeding and sleeping disorders. In M. Rutter, E. Taylor, & L. Herson (Eds.), *Child and adolescent psychiatry* (3rd ed.). Oxford: Blackwell Scientific.

Tanner, J., Whitehouse, R., & Takaishi, M. (1966). Standards from birth to maturity for height, weight, height velocity and weight velocity: British children (1965, Parts 1 & 2). *Archives of Disease in Childhood, 48,* 454–471, 613–615.

Tate, A. (1993). Schooling. In B. Lask & R. Bryant-Waugh (Eds.), *Childhood onset anorexia nervosa and related eating disorders.* Hove, England: Erlbaum.

Turk, J. (1993). Cognitive approaches. In B. Lask & R. Bryant-Waugh (Eds.), *Childhood onset anorexia nervosa and related eating disorders.* Hove, England: Erlbaum.

CHAPTER 29

Adapting Treatment for Patients with Binge-Eating Disorder

MARSHA D. MARCUS

Binge-eating disorder (BED) is a syndrome of persistent and frequent binge eating that is not accompanied by the regular compensatory behaviors required for a diagnosis of bulimia nervosa. The diagnosis of BED has been included in the *Diagnostic and Statistical Manual of Mental Disorders,* fourth edition (DSM-IV; American Psychiatric Association, 1994) as an example of an eating disorder not otherwise specified, and in an appendix as a proposed diagnostic category requiring further study. "Binge eating" in BED is defined exactly as it is in bulimia nervosa—that is, as the ingestion of a large amount of food under the circumstances, along with a sense of loss of control over what, when, or how much one is eating.

Given the overlap between bulimia nervosa and BED, it is unsurprising that initial attempts to understand and treat BED have derived directly from the work in bulimia nervosa. Evidence to date has shown that treatments that are efficacious in the treatment of bulimia nervosa—specifically, cognitive-behavioral therapy, interpersonal psychotherapy, and antidepressant treatment—are also useful in treating BED (Smith, Marcus, & Eldredge, 1994). We now know, however, that there are clinically relevant differences between bulimia nervosa and BED; thus, treatment for BED must be adapted to the particular needs of the patients with this disorder. This chapter focuses on factors that discriminate BED and bulimia nervosa, and discusses treatment modifications indicated

by clinical experience and the growing body of research on BED.

CHARACTERISTICS OF BINGE-EATING DISORDER

Absence of Regular Compensatory Behavior

By definition, patients with BED do not regularly compensate for binge episodes with regular purge behaviors, strict dieting or fasting, or overexercise. Compensatory behaviors are not uncommon among BED patients (Marcus, 1993), but they do not occur with the regularity seen in bulimia nervosa. The relative absence of compensatory behaviors often makes it difficult to separate binge-eating episodes from non-binge-eating episodes. For example, many BED patients report eating a regular meal, and starting to binge only at the point of taking second helpings or dessert. Similarly, BED patients often report day-long binges, stating that once control is lost, an episode can continue until bedtime. Thus researchers in the field have generally agreed that it is more accurate to report the number of days of binge eating, rather than the number of episodes, as in bulimia nervosa (Marcus, Smith, Santelli, & Kaye, 1992; Rossiter, Agras, Telch, & Bruce, 1992).

More important, however, is that eating behavior in BED can be hard to characterize, and it often appears that BED patients have a general inability to regulate eating behavior both within *and* between binge episodes. In fact, research data from laboratory studies have confirmed that BED patients eat more than weight-matched individuals without binge-eating problems do, both at meals and during episodes of overeating (Guss, Kissileff, Walsh, & Devlin, 1994; Yanovski et al., 1992). It also appears that the meal durations of obese individuals with BED are significantly longer than those of obese non-BED subjects (Goldfein, Walsh, LaChaussee, Kissileff, & Devlin, 1993). Thus individuals with BED, when compared to equally overweight individuals with no binge problems, display a pattern of chaotic eating with high levels of consumption at and between meals. The implication of these data is that in order to normalize eating in BED, it is necessary to both ameliorate binge eating and modify eating between episodes.

Relationship between BED and Obesity

Most patients with BED are overweight, and there is a robust association between BED and obesity. The fact that bulimia nervosa is primarily a disorder of normal-weight individuals, whereas most BED patients are overweight, has numerous implications. For example, BED patients typically have sought treatment for obesity, rather than eating disorder treatment. As many as 30% of patients who receive obesity treatment at university-based clinics meet criteria for BED (Spitzer et al., 1992, 1993). In contrast, findings from community-based research have indicated that only about 2% of the general population and 8% of obese individuals have BED (Bruce & Agras, 1992). Moreover, the prevalence of serious problems with binge eating increases with level of obesity (Telch, Agras, & Rossiter, 1988). It is therefore critical for clinicians treating BED patients to be aware of research findings that relate to obesity as well as eating disorders. The etiology of obesity is unknown, but undoubtedly multifactorial, with biological, social, and behavioral factors all playing a role (Brownell & Wadden, 1992). There is little doubt, though, that sustained periods of binge eating may lead to substantial weight gain in BED patients, and therefore contribute to the development or maintenance of obesity.

Eating Disorder Psychopathology in BED

Patients with BED report levels of eating, shape, and weight concerns comparable to those of patients with bulimia nervosa (Marcus et al., 1992). They also report markedly less control over eating, more fear of weight gain, more preoccupation with food and weight, and greater body dissatisfaction than equally overweight individuals without binge-eating problems (Wilson, Nonas, & Rosenblum, 1993). Furthermore, BED patients have an intense desire to lose weight, and continually struggle to gain control over their weight and eating (Marcus, Wing, & Hopkins, 1988). Consistent with the ongoing battle to control weight, BED patients report unrealistically high dieting standards coupled with low self-efficacy for dieting (Gormally, Black, Daston, & Rardin, 1982).

In contrast to bulimia nervosa patients, however, BED patients have not reported elevated levels of dietary restraint—that is, actual restriction of calorie intake (Marcus et al., 1992). Despite high dieting standards, they do not generally succeed in limiting their calorie intake. Also in distinction to bulimia nervosa, BED is not characterized by overvalued ideas about the importance of thinness. Most BED patients feel comfortable with the notion of average to above-average body weight, but report intense feelings of body dissatisfaction, self-consciousness, and body disparagement (Marcus, 1993). In summary, it appears that there is considerable overlap in the eating disorder psychopathology of bulimia nervosa and BED; however, BED patients often do not succeed in restricting food intake, and do not report overvalued ideas about shape and weight.

Relationship between BED and Dieting Behavior

The data showing that BED patients report levels of eating, shape, and weight concerns comparable to those reported by bulimia nervosa patients, and significantly more preoccupation with body and weight, episodes of dieting, and weight fluctuations than obese patients with no binge-eating problems (Marcus et al., 1992), are in marked contrast with the evidence that BED patients do not report elevated levels of dietary restraint or restrict their food intake between binge episodes. Clinical evidence indicates that many BED patients alternate between periods of undercontrol over eating, and periods of dieting or satisfactory control over eating. Thus it is important to consider that the relationship between dieting and eating-disorder symptoms may be different in BED than in bulimia nervosa.

Dieting virtually always precedes binge eating in bulimia nervosa, but available evidence has indicated that as many as 50% of BED patients report the onset of binge episodes *before* any effort to diet or lose weight (Mussell et al., 1995; Wilson et al., 1993). Furthermore, considerable recent evidence has documented that in contrast to previous speculation, calorie restriction and weight loss does not exacerbate binge eating in BED patients (Agras et al., 1994; LaPorte, 1992; Marcus, Wing, & Fairburn, 1995; Telch & Agras, 1993; Wadden, Foster, & Letizia, 1992). Although it is axiomatic that dieting is harmful for normal-weight women with bulimia nervosa, this does not appear to be the case in BED (Marcus et al., 1995), and participation in weight control programs appears to improve binge eating and mood in these individuals (Marcus et al., 1995). Moreover, weight regain in BED patients does not appear to be associated with worsening of mood or binge eating (Marcus et al., 1995).

Why would dieting improve binge eating in BED when it is associated with the worsening of binge behavior in patients with bulimia nervosa? Although careful prospective research is needed to answer this question fully, it appears that BED may be best conceptualized as a syndrome of general dyscontrol over eating with associated eating disorder symptomatology in individuals who are vulnerable to obesity and/or mood problems. Dieting, then, may represent an effort to regain control over eating in individuals with BED.

BED and Depression

BED is associated with significant psychiatric comorbidity (deZwaan et al., 1994; Specker, deZwaan, Raymond, & Mitchell, 1994; Yanovski, Nelson, Dubbert, & Spitzer, 1993)—in particular, mood disorders (Marcus, Wing, Ewing, Kern, Gooding, & McDermott, 1990; Yanovski et al., 1993). Several studies have shown that 50% or more of BED patients have a lifetime history of major depressive disorder and high levels of depressive symptomatology (Antony, Johnson, Carr-Nangle, & Abel, 1994). There is a complex and interesting relationship among

mood, eating, and weight in BED patients. Changes in eating and weight, and changes in activity level, are among the diagnostic criteria for major depressive disorder (American Psychiatric Association, 1994). Although individuals typically lose weight during depressive episodes, weight gain is also common, with as many as 40% of individuals reporting weight gain during an episode of depression (Weissenburger, Rush, Gilles, & Stunkard, 1986).

There is evidence that obese individuals may be especially likely to report weight gain and decreases in activity when depressed (Stunkard, Fernstrom, Price, Frank, & Kupfer, 1990). Indeed, the weight gained during episodes of depression can be considerable; for example, in the Weissenburger et al. (1986) study, the average weight gain during a depressive episode was more than 17 pounds. The tendency to gain or lose weight during depression is consistent across episodes (Stunkard, Fernstrom, et al., 1990), and since depression is often recurrent, it is not hard to see that the weight gain associated with mood disorder can contribute to obesity or an eating disorder.

It is also important to recognize that both obesity and binge eating may contribute to depressive symptomatology (Wadden & Stunkard, 1985). Obesity is associated with serious stigmatization in Western society, and many observers have noted that daily coping with the effects of such prejudice may be depressogenic. Furthermore, the sense of being out of control over eating that is seen in both BED and bulimia nervosa is extremely aversive, and it may cause or exacerbate depressive symptomatology. For example, we (Marcus, Wing, Ewing, Kern, Gooding, & McDermott, 1990) reported that severity of depression among individuals with BED was strongly associated with frequency of binge eating. In summary, mood, weight, and binge-eating problems may interact to reinforce a pattern of continual struggle to control eating, lose weight, and maintain mood.

TREATMENT OF BINGE-EATING DISORDER

Initial evidence has indicated that cognitive-behavioral therapy (CBT; Marcus et al., 1995; Smith, Marcus, & Kaye, 1992; Telch, Agras, Rossiter, Wilfley, & Kenardy, 1990), interpersonal psychotherapy (IPT; Wilfley et al., 1993), and antidepressant treatment (McCann &

Agras, 1990) have utility in the treatment of BED. The best-studied treatment to date is CBT, and initial modifications of CBT for BED have been reported and manualized (Fairburn, Marcus, & Wilson, 1993). In contrast to CBT, neither IPT nor antidepressant treatment is symptom-focused, and therefore neither requires modifications specific to BED. Thus, the adaptations of CBT for BED incorporate the current knowledge of BED described above; these are further described below, followed by brief comments about the use of IPT, antidepressants, and other treatments for BED.

Modifications of CBT for BED

The CBT program for BED that has been developed at the University of Pittsburgh was based directly on Fairburn's well-studied treatment for bulimia nervosa (Fairburn, 1985; Fairburn et al., 1993). Therefore, the implementation of modifications described herein assumes familiarity with Fairburn's treatment program (see Wilson, Fairburn, & Agras, Chapter 6, this volume). In light of the differences between BED and bulimia nervosa, it is important to consider why CBT is effective in treating BED as well as bulimia nervosa. CBT for bulimia nervosa is based on the premise that chronic dieting in an effort to control weight promotes and maintains binge-eating behavior (Fairburn, 1985; Fairburn et al., 1993); thus, treatment focuses on decreasing dietary restraint, and on modifying maladaptive thoughts, beliefs, and values related to eating, shape, and weight. The focus in BED is comparable, as the cognitions relating to dietary restraint are similar (cognitions specific to BED are discussed below). However, the behavior of BED patients is frequently not in line with their values and beliefs. Thus, CBT for BED targets the tendencies both to overrestrict and to underrestrict; in other words, it focuses on overall moderation of food intake.

CBT as adapted for BED is somewhat longer than CBT for bulimia nervosa (22 sessions in 24 weeks), but the structure is identical. That is, treatment consists of three phases, is conducted individually, and makes use of empirically validated behavioral and cognitive strategies. Several investigators have reported the results of CBT programs conducted with groups (Smith et al., 1992; Telch et al., 1990; Wilfley et al., 1993), and economic or other considerations may dictate the use of groups in certain set-

tings. In our clinic, however, we have found that the treatment is most effectively delivered in the one-on-one context (Marcus et al., 1995).

The goals of Stage 1 of treatment (eight sessions) are the adoption of a plan of regular eating (i.e., a plan for *when* eating occurs), and the minimization or elimination of binge episodes. The goals of Stage 2 (eight sessions) are: the overall moderation of food intake without the adoption of rigid or inflexible rules, and the identification and modification of maladaptive thoughts and beliefs that perpetuate the eating problem. In Stage 3 (six sessions), the goals are the consolidation of progress and relapse prevention training.

Treatment Rationale

As in CBT for bulimia nervosa, patients are told that the primary goal of treatment is the normalization of eating. In the treatment of BED, however, most patients have two problems—binge eating and obesity. Therefore, patients have difficulties in moderating food intake; that is, they tend to have both binge episodes *and* uncontrolled eating, in combination with maladaptive beliefs about dieting, shape, and weight. Thus, like bulimia nervosa patients, they may have forbidden foods and stringent beliefs about restricting (Marcus, Wing, & Lamparski, 1985), but they often do not succeed in actually restricting intake. Accordingly, BED patients are instructed that normalization of eating involves learning to say no to food (i.e., to binge eating, overeating, and chaotic eating), as well as learning to say yes to food (i.e., to healthy and moderate consumption of all foods).

Patients are told that individuals with BED often feel that food is both their best friend and their worst enemy, and that the goal of treatment is to normalize both the binge behavior and such maladaptive beliefs about food. It is critically important to emphasize, however, that patients should not necessarily expect weight loss. Although some patients may lose weight with sustained abstinence from binge eating (Agras et al., 1995; Smith et al., 1992), several investigations have shown that elimination of binge episodes does not, *on average*, lead to weight loss (Telch et al., 1990; Marcus et al., 1995). Patients are informed that a weight loss program can be considered after treatment for the binge-eating problem. To reiterate, the goals of treatment are the normalization of eating and the promotion of a healthy pattern of eating and exercise.

Therapeutic Stance

It would be difficult to overemphasize the importance of understanding the consequences of obesity for individuals with BED. Overweight individuals, particularly women, are repeatedly faced with discrimination and scorn for a perceived personal flaw—failure to control their eating and weight (Weiner, 1993). That the determination of body size is not a simple matter of personal discipline is clear (Brownell & Wadden, 1992). Patients with BED, however, are all too aware that they actually do overeat, and are likely to have incorporated a particularly harsh version of the societal values and beliefs that do them such harm. That is, they negatively evaluate themselves for a self-perceived inability to moderate food intake and weight.

Therefore, shame is a prominent theme in work with BED patients. As discussed here, "shame" refers to an admixture of feelings outlined by Gilbert, Pehl, and Allan (1994) that includes self-consciousness, anger, helplessness, feelings of inferiority, and fear of negative evaluation, and in which body concerns play a central role. Recent work (Andrews, 1995) has documented an association between bodily shame and chronic depression, which suggests that shame may play a part in the complex relationship between binge eating and mood. Thus, an awareness of the presence of shame is important for treatment, since there is likely to be a tendency both to conceal binge eating, and to fear negative evaluation from the therapist.

It is therefore necessary for clinicians working with BED patients to examine their own preconceptions or prejudices about obesity and binge eating, in order to maximize their ability to maintain an empathic stance. Next, it is important to remember that CBT is a symptom-focused approach; thus, it is critical to retain a matter-of-fact insistence on the behavioral tasks, despite the fact that patients often resist them. This resistance provides an opportunity for a therapist to recognize the pain and shame associated with the binge behavior, and to point out that acknowledging and accepting the difficult feelings may help to resolve the problem. In summary, an empathic but matter-of-fact attitude on the part of the treating clinician is central to work with a BED patient.

Education about Obesity

Although BED patients readily concede that considerable distress is associated with their binge eating, most continue to want to lose weight and have persistent concerns about obesity. In addition to respectfully acknowledging these concerns, it is important to provide some information about obesity. Patients are told that there are multiple causes of obesity, and that genetic factors, environmental variables, and behavior contribute in varying degrees to cause overweight in specific individuals (Bouchard, 1991; Fabsitz, Sholinsky, & Carmelli, 1994; Stunkard, Harris, Pedersen, & McClearn, 1990). Clinicians should emphasize that obesity is not a simple matter of overeating, but they need not minimize the importance of behavioral factors. Approximately one-third of U.S. adults are overweight, and the prevalence of overweight has been steadily increasing (Kuczmarski, Flegal, Campbell, & Johnson, 1994). Despite the fact that biological factors play a critical role in the determination of body size, dietary and exercise factors are probably responsible for increases in the prevalence of overweight (Kuczmarski et al., 1994).

It is important, however, to point out that there is considerable evidence that weight lost through dieting is frequently regained (most patients have had numerous experiences with this), and that sustained weight change involves a permanent modification of eating and exercise patterns (National Institutes of Health Technology Assessment Conference Panel, 1992). It is also important for BED patients to understand that although obesity is associated with increased risks for heart disease, diabetes, and other diseases, it is not necessary to achieve large weight losses to improve risk factors. There is substantial evidence that sustained weight losses of about 10% of initial body weight can lead to significant improvements in modifiable risk factors, such as lipids and blood sugar levels (Atkinson, 1993). Most patients readily understand that their problems with binge eating must be resolved in order for them to make such permanent changes in lifestyle. Thus, we stress that individuals can consider a weight loss program after eating is normalized.

The Role of Exercise

In contrast to bulimia nervosa patients, who often use exercise as a compensatory behavior and overexercise consistently, individuals with BED tend to be inactive (Marcus, 1993). Patients are advised that exercise is an important part of their treatment. First, exercise is an excellent example of an activity that is incompatible with binge eating. Second, regular exercise is an effective tool for stress management. Finally, increased energy expenditure in the form of exercise is a critical component of long-term weight management (Grilo, 1994). Accordingly, patients are instructed to begin a program of regular exercise based on walking or biking. Weekly stepwise goals for exercise are set, starting slowly (e.g., 15 minutes of walking on 3 days of the week), and increasing until individuals are exercising an average of 45 minutes on 5 days of the week. Patients are also encouraged to increase daily activity (e.g., using stairs instead of elevators), and are reinforced for moves toward a more active lifestyle. These recommendations for physical activity are consistent with those made by the Centers for Disease Control and Prevention and the American College of Sports Medicine (Pate et al., 1995).

Is There a Role for Calorie Counting?

Although calorie counting in general is discouraged, we have found that it can be a useful tool for demonstrating the parameters of "normal" eating. Specifically, overweight BED patients frequently have little awareness of the amounts of food they consume either in meals or during binge episodes. Although "normal" intake varies considerably among individuals, we project that the average 200-pound woman eats approximately 2,400 calories a day to maintain a steady weight (12 calories per pound per day). Counting the calories reported on several days in the patients' self-monitoring record can be extremely useful in helping individuals learn what they are currently eating, and especially how many calories are ingested in episodes of binge eating. Patients are encouraged to moderate overall intake in a range between 1,500 and 2,500 calories a day; that is, they are encouraged not to over- or under-restrict.

Nutrition Information

Therapists should introduce the basic principles of good nutrition. Specifically, patients are encouraged to decrease total fat (Hill, Drougas, & Peters, 1993) and to increase complex carbohy-

drates and fiber (Wotecki & Thomas, 1992). It should be emphasized that such changes are consistent recommendations for *all* U.S. adults, in order to promote health and reduce risks for such illnesses as diabetes and cardiovascular disease. A therapist can use a patient's self-monitoring diary to make specific recommendations for dietary changes, taking into account the personal preferences of the individual. Patients should be reminded that the occasional intake of desserts or fattening foods is not inconsistent with a healthy diet or more normal weight.

Normalization of Eating

CBT for BED proceeds exactly as it does for bulimia nervosa—that is, the adoption of regular meals, with a concomitant focus on minimizing binge episodes. It is important, however, for clinicians to be aware that the thought of doing without food (i.e., being hungry or unable to self-soothe with food) can be extremely anxiety-provoking for BED patients (Nagler & Androff, 1990). Thus, it may be helpful to discuss the possibility that anxiety or distress may be associated with regaining control over eating. Patients are told that individuals with BED tend to rely on food to modulate a variety of uncomfortable feelings, and that their therapists will work with them to learn alternate ways of coping with discomfort. Unfortunately, however, other strategies (e.g., exercise, relaxation, talking to friends) do not work as reliably or quickly as does food to modulate aversive levels of self-consciousness (Heatherton & Baumeister, 1991), affective lability, or negative mood, and BED patients can be quite resistant to practicing them. It is important for therapists to convey both that alternate strategies will eventually be useful, and that, to a certain extent, uncomfortable affect need not be allayed—merely experienced.

Modification of Thoughts, Beliefs, and Values Associated with BED

As in the treatment of bulimia nervosa, patients are told that maladaptive thoughts about dieting, shape, and weight play a critical role in maintaining eating problems. In BED, however, it is often the contrast between patients' maladaptive thoughts and stringent beliefs (e.g., "I should never eat more than 1,200 calories a day") and actual eating behavior (e.g., daily intake in excess of 2,500 calories) that contributes to their feelings of shame and hopelessness and that perpetuates disordered eating.

Predictably, the disordered thoughts and beliefs about eating reported by individuals with BED frequently relate to societal stereotypes about obesity. Typical beliefs are that fat people lack discipline (are slobs, are lazy, are disgusting, etc.), that fat people don't deserve to eat, or that overweight people are disgusting. It is not hard to see that such thoughts are painful and self-defeating, and may contribute to negative mood and the cycle of disordered eating. It is important to make these prejudicial notions explicit, and to work assiduously to help patients to modify them. BED patients also report dysfunctional beliefs about normal-weight individuals, such as that thin people don't have to watch what they eat, or that thin people never feel self-conscious. These maladaptive beliefs should also be addressed, and patients should be helped to adopt more realistic notions of the effects of body size.

BED patients often also report beliefs that specific foods are harmful for them (e.g., "Sugar is toxic to me"). Such beliefs may have been adopted from the lay press or learned in specific treatment programs that advocate the avoidance of refined flour and sugar, which are believed to be "addictive." (Overeaters Anonymous no longer supports a specific meal plan, but individual groups may still promote the notion that specific foods are toxic or addictive.) The notion that BED patients are helpless to deal with certain foods is contrary to a basic tenet of CBT—namely, that individuals are capable of managing their own eating and exercise behavior. Therefore, patients are told that there is little evidence for these beliefs (Wilson, 1991); they are encouraged to avoid all rigid food rules, and helped to work "forbidden foods" slowly back into their diets. If patients insist that they have learned to avoid certain foods that trigger binges, they can be assisted in reframing the decision not to eat a particular food as effective behavior management.

Acceptance of Larger-Than-Average Body Size

As noted previously, BED patients do not, on average, report overvalued ideas about thinness; they do, however, assess themselves harshly on the basis of weight and shape. "Body image disparagement," which refers to feelings of revulsion toward and loathing of one's own body, is almost universal among these patients. Negative societal attitudes toward obesity also promote body image disparagement. It is important for therapists not to suggest that patients must like their bodies if they do not. It is, however, extremely important for them to accept that although they are larger than they would like to be, self-contempt only increases the feelings of desperation that perpetuate binge eating.

Therapists can also help patients to recognize that a larger-than-average body can be both attractive and healthy (an ongoing emphasis on physical activity is helpful in promoting body acceptance). Overweight patients often defer buying clothes in the hope that they will lose weight. We encourage patients to dress attractively at their current size in order to promote feelings of self-confidence, to identify attractive large people (especially women) as positive role models, and to identify and enjoy positive aspects of their bodies. Finally, therapists should help patients to identify situations that they have avoided because of body size (e.g., going to parties or to the beach), and to focus on decreasing weight-related social anxiety.

Other Treatments for BED

Pharmacotherapy

Drug treatments for eating disorders are discussed elsewhere in this volume (see Garfinkel & Walsh, Chapter 20), but a comment about drug treatment for BED is in order. Initial studies have indicated that antidepressants (McCann & Agras, 1990) and the opiate blocker naloxone (Drewnowski, Krahn, Demitrack, Nairn, & Gosnell, 1995) may have utility in the clinical management of BED. Available evidence, however, has indicated that combination treatment—specifically, the tricyclic antidepressant desipramine, plus CBT or weight loss therapy—does not yield greater reductions in binge eating than CBT or weight loss therapy alone (Agras et al., 1994).

There are several reasons not to come to a firm conclusion about the utility of antidepressants in the treatment of BED. First, there is as yet little research in this area, and additional studies are needed. Second, antidepressant treatment may serve to enhance dietary restraint (Craighead & Agras, 1991) and to improve compliance with a weight loss program (Agras et al., 1994; Marcus, Wing, Ewing, Kern,

McDermott, & Gooding, 1990). For example, in the Agras et al. (1994) study, the addition of desipramine to CBT did not enhance changes in binge eating in BED patients, but at follow-up the desipramine-treated patients lost significantly more weight than those who did not receive medication. Finally, co-occurring depression in BED may benefit from antidepressant treatment, and aggressive treatment for depression may help break the cycle of negative mood, binge eating, and weight gain. Until there is more research available to guide clinical decision making, the risks and benefits of antidepressant treatment should be considered on a case-by-case basis.

Interpersonal Psychotherapy

IPT for eating disorders is based on the assumption that interpersonal factors such as role transitions (e.g., separation or divorce) or conflicts (e.g., disagreements with a spouse or partner) are central in maintaining the cycle of disordered eating. Wilfley et al. (1993) have reported that IPT delivered in a group format was as effective as CBT in reducing binge eating in BED patients, both at posttreatment and at a 1-year follow-up. Although further research is needed to confirm this finding, IPT may be a useful alternative for BED patients who do not want a symptom-focused treatment. Furthermore, a combination of CBT and IPT may be useful in treating BED. In a recent study, Agras et al. (1995) examined whether IPT would enhance the treatment outcome of nonresponders to CBT. Unfortunately, IPT did not lead to further improvement, but longer or individual treatment might yield better results.

Obesity Treatment

The issue of obesity treatment per se is a critical one for BED patients. Obesity is associated with increased risk for a variety of serious health problems. Moreover, health risks are significant at a body mass index greater than 27 and increase with the severity of obesity (Pi-Sunyer, 1994). The evidence noted above has clearly indicated that dieting does not exacerbate binge eating, and may in fact help patients to regain control over eating. In addition, recent reviews of the empirical evidence have concluded that concerns about the potentially deleterious effects of dieting (French & Jeffery, 1994) or weight cycling (National Task Force on the Prevention and Treatment of Obesity, 1994) should not deter obese individuals from weight control efforts.

We have recently compared CBT for binge eating and behavioral weight control in the treatment of BED (Marcus et al., 1995). The results indicated that both approaches are equally effective in ameliorating binge eating and associated eating disorder psychopathology in BED patients. It seems, therefore, that weight loss programs for BED patients may be indicated after careful consideration of the pros and cons of such an endeavor. It is important for individuals to evaluate the likelihood that they will be able to sustain lifelong changes in eating and exercise, as well as the consequences of weight regain for their sense of well-being. Importantly, however, we know that the painful symptoms of BED can be ameliorated without dieting, and that patients need not lose weight to enhance their psychosocial functioning significantly.

REFERENCES

Agras, W. S., Telch, C. F., Arnow, B., Eldredge, K., Detzer, M. J., Henderson, J., & Marnell, M. (1995). Does interpersonal therapy help patients with binge eating disorder who fail to respond to cognitive-behavioral therapy? *Journal of Consulting and Clinical Psychology, 63,* 356–360.

Agras, W. S., Telch, C. F., Arnow, B., Eldredge, K., Wilfley, D. E., Raeburn, S. D., Henderson, J., & Marnell, M. (1994). Weight loss, cognitive-behavioral, and desipramine treatments in binge eating disorder: An additive design. *Behavior Therapy, 25,* 225–238.

American Psychiatric Association. (1994). *Diagnostic and statistical manual of mental disorders* (4th ed.). Washington, DC: Author.

Andrews, B. (1995). Bodily shame as a mediator between abusive experiences and depression. *Journal of Abnormal Psychology, 104,* 277–285.

Antony, M. M., Johnson, W. G., Carr-Nangle, R. E., & Abel, J. L. (1994). Psychopathology correlates of binge eating and binge eating disorder. *Comprehensive Psychiatry, 35,* 386–392.

Atkinson, R. L. (1993). Proposed standards for judging the success of the treatment of obesity. *Annals of Internal Medicine, 119,* 677–680.

Bouchard, D. (1991). Current understanding of the etiology of obesity: Genetic and nongenetic factors. *American Journal of Clinical Nutrition, 53,* 1561S-1565S.

Brownell, K. D., & Wadden, T. A. (1992). Etiology and the treatment of obesity: Understanding a serious, prevalent, and refractory disorder. *Journal of Consulting and Clinical Psychology, 60,* 505–517.

Bruce, B., & Agras, W. S. (1992). Binge eating in females: A population-based investigation. *International Journal of Eating Disorders, 12,* 365–373.

Craighead, L. W., & Agras, W. S. (1991). Mechanisms of action in cognitive-behavioral and pharmacological interventions for obesity and bulimia nervosa. *Journal of Consulting and Clinical Psychology, 59,* 115–125.

deZwaan, M. D., Mitchell, J. E., Seim, H. C., Specker, S. M., Pyle, R. L., Raymond, N. C., & Crosby, R. B. (1994). Eating related and general psychopathology in obese females with binge eating disorder. *International Journal of Eating Disorders, 15,* 43–52.

Drewnowski, A., Krahn, D. D., Demitrack, M. A., Nairn, K., & Gosnell, B. A. (1995). Naloxone, an opiate blocker, reduces the consumption of sweet high-fat foods in obese and lean female binge eaters. *American Journal of Clinical Nutrition, 61,* 1206–1212.

Fabsitz, R. R., Sholinsky, P., & Carmelli, D. (1994). Genetic influences on adult weight gain and maximum body mass index in male twins. *American Journal of Epidemiology, 140,* 711–720.

Fairburn, C. G. (1985). Cognitive-behavioral treatment for bulimia. In D. M. Garner & P. E. Garfinkel (Eds.), *Handbook of psychotherapy for anorexia nervosa and bulimia* (pp. 160–192). New York: Guilford Press.

Fairburn, C. G., Marcus, M. D., & Wilson, G. T. (1993). Cognitive-behavioral treatment for binge eating and bulimia nervosa: A comprehensive treatment manual. In C. G. Fairburn & G. T. Wilson (Eds.), *Binge eating: Nature, assessment, and treatment* (pp. 361–404). New York: Guilford Press.

French, S. A., & Jeffery, R. W. (1994). Consequences of dieting to lose weight: Effects on physical and mental health. *Health Psychology, 13,* 195–212.

Gilbert, P., Pehl, J., & Allan, S. (1994). The phenomenology of shame and guilt: An empirical investigation. *British Journal of Medical Psychology, 67,* 23–26.

Goldfein, J. A., Walsh, B. T., LaChaussee, J. L., Kissileff, H. R., & Devlin, M. J. (1993). Eating behavior in binge eating disorder. *International Journal of Eating Disorders, 14,* 427–431.

Gormally, J., Black, S., Daston, S., & Rardin, D. (1982). The assessment of binge eating severity among obese persons. *Addictive Behaviors, 7,* 47–55.

Grilo, C. M. (1994). Physical activity and obesity. *Biomedicine and Pharmacotherapy, 48,* 127–136.

Guss, J. L., Kissileff, H. R., Walsh, B. T., & Devlin, M. J. (1994). Binge eating behavior in patients with eating disorders. *Obesity Research, 2,* 355–363.

Heatherton, T. F., & Baumeister, R. F. (1991). Binge eating as escape from self-awareness. *Psychological Bulletin, 110,* 86–108.

Hill, J. O., Drougas, H., & Peters, J. C. (1993). Obesity treatment: Can diet composition play a role? *Annals of Internal Medicine, 119,* 694–697.

Kuczmarski, R. J., Flegal, K. M., Campbell, S. M., & Johnson, C. L. (1994). Increasing prevalence of overweight among US adults: The National Health and Nutrition Examination Surveys, 1960–1991. *Journal of the American Medical Association, 272,* 205–211.

LaPorte, D. J. (1992). Treatment response in obese binge-eaters: Preliminary results using a very low calorie diet (VLCD) and behavior therapy. *Addictive Behaviors, 17,* 247–257.

Marcus, M. D. (1993). Binge eating in obesity. In C. G. Fairburn & G. T. Wilson (Eds.), *Binge eating: Nature, assessment, and treatment* (pp. 77–96). New York: Guilford Press.

Marcus, M. D., Smith, D., Santelli, R., & Kaye, W. (1992). Characterization of eating disordered behavior in obese binge eaters. *International Journal of Eating Disorders, 12,* 249–255.

Marcus, M. D., Wing, R. R., Ewing, L., Kern, E., Gooding, W., & McDermott, M. (1990). Psychiatric disorders among obese binge eaters. *International Journal of Eating Disorders, 9,* 69–77.

Marcus, M. D., Wing, R .R., Ewing, L., Kern, E., McDermott, M., & Gooding, W. (1990). A double blind, placebo-controlled trial of fluoxetine plus behavior modification in the treatment of obese binge-eaters and non-binge-eaters. *American Journal of Psychiatry, 147,* 876–881.

Marcus, M. D., Wing, R. R., & Fairburn, C. G. (1995). Cognitive treatment of binge eating versus behavioral weight control in the treatment of binge eating disorder. *Annals of Behavioral Medicine, 17,* S090.

Marcus, M. D., Wing, R. R., & Hopkins, J. (1988). Obese binge eaters: Affect, cognitions, and response to behavioral weight control. *Journal of Consulting and Clinical Psychology, 56,* 433–439.

Marcus, M. D., Wing, R. R., & Lamparski, D. M. (1985). Binge eating and dietary restraint in obese patients. *Addictive Behaviors, 10,* 163–168.

McCann, U. D., & Agras, W. S. (1990). Successful treatment of nonpurging bulimia nervosa with desipramine: A double blind, placebo-controlled study. *American Journal of Psychiatry, 147,* 1509–1513.

Mussell, M. P., Mitchell, J. E., Weller, C. L., Raymond, N. C., Crow, S. J., & Crosby, R. D. (1995). Onset of binge eating, dieting, obesity, and mood disorders among subjects seeking treatment for binge eating disorder. *International Journal of Eating Disorders, 17,* 395–410.

Nagler, W., & Androff, A. (1990). Investigating the impact of deconditioning anxiety on weight loss. *Psychological Reports, 66,* 595–600.

National Institute of Health Technology Assessment Conference Panel. (1992). Methods for voluntary weight loss and control. *Annals of Internal Medicine, 116,* 942–949.

National Task Force on the Prevention and Treatment of Obesity. (1994). Weight cycling. *Journal of the American Medical Association, 272,* 1196–1202.

Pate, R. R., Pratt, M., Blair, S. N., Haskell, W. L., Macera, C. A., Bouchard, C., Buchner, D., Ettinger, W., Heath, G. W., King, A. C., Kriska, A., Leon, A. S., Marcus, B. H., Morris, J., Paffenbarger, R. S., Patrick, K., Pollock, M. L., Rippe, J. M., Sallis, J., & Wilmore, J. H. (1995). Physical activity and public health: A recommendation from the Centers for Disease Control and Prevention and the American College of Sports Medicine. *Journal of the American Medical Association, 273,* 402–407.

Pi-Sunyer, F. X. (1994). The fattening of America. *Journal of the American Medical Association, 272,* 238–239.

Rossiter, E. M., Agras, W. S., Telch, C. F., & Bruce, B. (1992). The eating patterns of non-purging bulimic subjects. *International Journal of Eating Disorders, 11,* 111–120.

Smith, D. E., Marcus, M. D., & Eldredge, K. L. (1994). Binge eating syndromes: A review of assessment and treatment with an emphasis on clinical application. *Behavior Therapy, 25,* 635–658.

Smith, D. E., Marcus, M. D., & Kaye, W. (1992). Cognitive-behavioral treatment of obese binge eaters. *International Journal of Eating Disorders, 12,* 257–262.

Specker, S., deZwann, M. D., Raymond, N., & Mitchell, J. (1994). Psychopathology in subgroups of obese women with and without binge eating disorder. *Comprehensive Psychiatry, 35,* 185–190.

Spitzer, R. L., Devlin, M., Walsh, B. T., Hasin, D., Wing, R., Marcus, M. D., Stunkard, A., Wadden, T., Yanovski,

S. Agras, S., Mitchell, J., & Nonas, C. (1992). Binge eating disorder: A multisite field trial of the diagnostic criteria. *International Journal of Eating Disorders, 11,* 191–203.

Spitzer, R. L., Yanovski, S., Wadden, T., Wing, R., Marcus, M. D., Stunkard, A., Devlin, M., Mitchell, J., Hasin, D., & Horne, R. L. (1993). Binge eating disorder: Its further validation in a multisite study. *International Journal of Eating Disorders, 13,* 137–153.

Stunkard, A. J., Fernstrom, M., Price, A., Frank, E., & Kupfer, D. (1990). Direction of weight change in recurrent depression. *Archives of General Psychiatry, 47,* 857–860.

Stunkard, A. J., Harris, J. R., Pedersen, N. L., & McClearn, G. E. (1990). The body-mass index of twins who have been reared apart. *New England Journal of Medicine, 322,* 1483–1487.

Telch, C. F., & Agras, W. S. (1993). The effects of a very low calorie diet on binge eating. *Behavior Therapy, 24,* 177–193.

Telch, C. F., Agras, W. S., & Rossiter, E. M. (1988). Binge eating increases with increasing adiposity. *International Journal of Eating Disorders, 7,* 115–119.

Telch, C. F., Agras, W. S., Rossiter, E. M., Wilfley, D., & Kenardy, J. (1990). Group cognitive-behavioral treatment for the nonpurging bulimic: An initial evaluation. *Journal of Consulting and Clinical Psychology, 58,* 629–635.

Wadden, T. A., Foster, G. D., & Letizia, K. A. (1992). Response of obese binge eaters to treatment by behavioral therapy combined with very low calorie diet. *Journal of Consulting and Clinical Psychology, 60,* 808–811.

Wadden, T. A., & Stunkard, A. J. (1985). Social and psychological consequences of obesity. *Annals of Internal Medicine, 103,* 1062–1067.

Weiner, B. (1993). On sin versus sickness. *American Psychologist, 48,* 957–965.

Weissenburger, J., Rush, A. J., Gilles, D. E., & Stunkard, A. J. (1986). Weight change in depression. *Psychiatry Research, 17,* 275–283.

Wilfley, D. E., Agras, W. S., Telch, C. F., Rossiter, E. M., Schneider, J. A., Cole, A .G., Sifford, L., & Raeburn, S. D. (1993). Group cognitive-behavioral therapy and group interpersonal psychotherapy for the nonpurging bulimic individual: A controlled comparison. *Journal of Consulting and Clinical Psychology, 61,* 296–305.

Wilson, G. T. (1991). The addiction model of eating disorders: A critical analysis. *Advances in Behavior Research and Therapy, 13,* 27–72.

Wilson, G. T., Nonas, C. A., & Rosenblum, G. D. (1993). Assessment of binge eating in obese patients. *International Journal of Eating Disorders, 1,* 25–33.

Wotecki, C. E., & Thomas, P. R. (1992). *Eat for life: The Food and Nutrition Board's guide to reducing your risk of chronic disease.* Washington, DC: National Academy Press.

Yanovski, S. Z., Leet, M., Yanovski, J. A., Flood, M., Gold, P. W., Kissileff, H. R., & Walsh, B. T. (1992). Food selection and intake of obese women with binge-eating disorder. American Journal of Clinical Nutrition, 56, 975–980.

Yanovski, S. Z., Nelson, J. E., Dubbert, B. K., & Spitzer, R. L. (1993). Association of binge eating disorder and psychiatric comorbidity in obese subjects. *American Journal of Psychiatry, 150,* 1472–1479.

CHAPTER 30

Self-Help and Guided Self-Help for Binge-Eating Problems

CHRISTOPHER G. FAIRBURN
JACQUELINE C. CARTER

The literature and research on the treatment of eating disorders are almost exclusively concerned with specialist therapist-led interventions. Although such interventions are undeniably important, this perspective fails to acknowledge the potential for sufferers to help themselves. This is regrettable, since self-help, either on its own or in conjunction with professional input, has strengths that ought to be exploited. In this chapter, we discuss the place of self-help books in overcoming binge-eating problems (including bulimia nervosa).

THE POTENTIAL ADVANTAGES OF SELF-HELP

1. *Self-help is empowering.* In eating disorders, low self-esteem and feelings of ineffectiveness are common, and issues relating to loss of control are prominent. Psychotherapists such as Bruch (1973) have stressed the importance of enhancing these patients' sense of effectiveness—a perspective shared by cognitive-behavioral therapists (Garner & Bemis, 1982). Self-help is inherently empowering, since there can be no doubt about who is responsible for any changes it produces. The converse also applies, however, since those who do not benefit tend to blame themselves rather than the self-help program.

2. *From a health economics perspective, self-help is an attractive alternative to more conven-tional forms of treatment.* Nowadays there is widespread interest in the economics of health care provision and the need to reduce the cost of treatment. Self-help has the potential to be a cost-free way of helping some people who might otherwise enter the health care system. It can also reduce the cost of helping those who present for treatment: It may be used in non-specialist settings (e.g., by nurses in primary care), thereby eliminating the need for a secondary referral; and in specialist settings it can reduce the amount of therapist input required.

3. *Self-help can circumvent obstacles to seeking help.* It is often forgotten that most people with bulimia nervosa are not in treatment, and the same is likely to be true of those with other binge-eating problems. A study conducted in 1980 in Britain revealed that of 499 cases of bulimia nervosa, 98% were not in treatment (Fairburn & Cooper, 1982); in a separate interview-based study conducted a decade later, the figure was 89% (Fairburn, Welch, Norman, O'Connor, & Doll, 1996). Although some of the cases (14%) in the latter study had received treatment in the past, the great majority had never received any form of professional help. Similar findings have emerged from the United States. For example, Whitaker et al. (1990) surveyed a county-wide secondary school population and found that although bulimia as defined in the *Diagnostic and Statistical Manual of Mental Disorders,* third edition (DSM-III) was associated with a

high level of functional impairment, it was also associated with the lowest history of service contact (28%) of any of the disorders studied (major depression, panic disorder, generalized anxiety disorder, obsessive–compulsive disorder, dysthymic disorder, and anorexia nervosa). Therefore, a major issue in the treatment of binge-eating problems is how to get help to all those with such problems, rather than just the minority who present for help.

It is not clear why so many sufferers are not in treatment. Our work suggests that a number of factors operate (Fairburn, 1995), some of which may be circumvented by self-help interventions. For example, a desire to keep the problem secret appears to be a major obstacle to seeking help. Self-help books may be a possible way to overcome the eating problem without having to disclose it. There can be stigma associated with psychiatric treatment; self-help may make such treatment unnecessary. Other barriers to seeking help include concerns about the practical difficulties involved in treatment, including its cost. Self-help is convenient and involves little cost to the sufferer.

4. *Self-help is easy to disseminate.* In most countries, there is a shortage of expertise in the treatment of eating disorders. Specialist treatment facilities tend to be unevenly distributed and can only deal with a small proportion of the cases that exist. The use of self-help books, either independently or with guidance from a nonspecialist therapist, is one means of getting help to the large numbers of people who would otherwise have no access to sound information and advice. Of course, not all self-help books are of equal merit, and there is no means of regulating their standards.

THE SELF-HELP BOOKS AND THEIR USE

Many self-help books exist for those who binge-eat. They vary greatly in their orientation and the advice that they provide. They include books that have family-oriented, abuse-oriented, feminist, nutritional, or eclectic views on eating disorders and their treatment. Table 30.1 lists some of the books currently available.

Few of these books have been written by recognized authorities on binge-eating problems, and many contain factual errors and myths. Just two of the books are directly based on cognitive-behavioral therapy (Fairburn, 1995; Coop-

TABLE 30.1. Some of the Books Currently Available for Helping Those with Binge-Eating Problems

Arenson, G. (1989). *A substance called food.*

Beasley, J. D., & Knightly, S. (1994). *Food for recovery.*

Brandon, C. W. (1993). *Am I hungry . . . or am I hurting?*

Cooper, P. J. (1995). *Bulimia nervosa and binge eating: A guide to recovery.*

Fairburn, C. G. (1995). *Overcoming binge eating.*

French, B. (1987). *Coping with bulimia.*

Greeson, J. (1990). *It's not what you're eating, it's what's eating you.*

Hall, L., & Cohen, L. (1992). *Bulimia: A guide to recovery.*

Hazelden Foundation (1992). *Food for thought.*

Hirschmann, J. R., & Munter, C. H. (1988). *Overcoming overeating.*

Hollis, J. (1985). *Fat is a family affair.*

Kolodny, N. J. (1992). *When food's a foe.*

Marx, R. (1992). *It's not your fault.*

Roth, G. (1989). *A guide to ending compulsive eating*

Roth, G. (1993). *Breaking free from compulsive eating,*

Schmidt, U. H., & Treasure, J. L. (1993). *Getting better bit(e) by bit(e).*

er, 1995). This is surprising, since cognitive-behavioral therapy is well suited to presentation in a self-help format, and in clinical trials it has been shown to be the most effective treatment for these problems (Wilson & Fairburn, in press).

Self-help books can be used in a number of different ways (see Table 30.1). For example, they can be used by sufferers on their own ("pure self-help"). They can also be used in combination with guidance and support from a professional ("guided self-help"). One of the strengths of guided self-help is that the guidance can be provided by a nonspecialist therapist, thereby rendering the intervention suitable for use in primary care (Carter & Fairburn, 1995).

Self-help books can also be used in specialist settings, with the aim of either reducing the amount of professional input required or increasing the effectiveness of the intervention. We have been using a cognitive-behavioral self-help book (Fairburn, 1995) to facilitate conventional cognitive-behavioral therapy for bulimia nervosa (see Fairburn, Marcus, & Wilson, 1993; see also Wilson, Fairburn, & Agras, Chapter 6, this volume). We are also using this book in conjunction with interpersonal psychotherapy, an entirely different form of treatment (see Fairburn, Chapter 14, this volume), in the hope that we will enhance its effectiveness by allowing the therapist to focus on interpersonal issues while providing the patient with a means of directly addressing the eating disorder.

RESEARCH ON THE EFFECTIVENESS OF SELF-HELP BOOKS

We are aware of six studies of the effectiveness of written self-help material in the treatment of binge-eating problems. Huon (1985) evaluated an intervention that involved sending 90 subjects with DSM-III bulimia seven monthly installments from a self-help program. The subjects, who had responded to an article in a women's magazine, were randomly assigned to one of three conditions: self-help plus the offer of contact by mail or telephone with a "cured" sufferer; self-help plus the offer of contact with an "improved" sufferer; or self-help alone. The program had a cognitive-behavioral orientation, and outcome was principally measured in terms of the frequency of binge eating and vomiting at the end of the intervention and at 3- and 6-month follow-ups (assessed by self-report questionnaire). An additional comparison group was formed from 30 subsequent respondents who were willing to wait 13 months before receiving help.

Although the design of this study makes it difficult to interpret the findings, the results suggest that receiving the program was superior to not receiving it, with 32% of the participants being "symptom-free" at the 6-month follow-up as opposed to 7% of the additional comparison group. It also appears that those who were offered contact with a sufferer (whether "cured" or not) did better than those who were not. Remarkably, none of the 120 subjects dropped out over the 13 months of the study.

Schmidt and Treasure have conducted two studies of pure self-help, using patients from a tertiary referral center. In the first (Schmidt, Tiller, & Treasure, 1993), 19 patients with bulimia nervosa as defined in the *International Classification of Diseases,* 10th revision (ICD-10) (4 of whom also met diagnostic criteria for anorexia nervosa) and 9 patients with atypical bulimia nervosa were asked to follow a cognitive-behavioral handbook for 4 to 6 weeks. Two

patients dropped out. At reassessment at the end of the intervention, 15 patients (54%) reported that they had been free from binge eating and vomiting over the past week, as compared with 5 patients at the outset. There was no change in the scores on a variety of self-report questionnaires. No follow-up data were reported.

In a second study (Treasure et al., 1994), 110 patients with ICD-10 bulimia nervosa or atypical bulimia nervosa (some of whom were not binge-eating at baseline) were randomly assigned to a multicomponent self-help manual (Schmidt & Treasure, 1993), the first eight sessions of a cognitive-behavioral treatment, or a waiting-list control group. Twenty-nine patients (26%) dropped out, the proportions being equivalent across the three conditions. At reassessment after 8 weeks, 22% of those who had received the manual, 24% of those who had received some cognitive-behavioral treatment, and 11% of those on the waiting list reported having been free from bingeing, vomiting, and other weight control behavior over the past week. There was also evidence of more general improvement in eating habits and attitudes among those in the two active treatment conditions, but not among those in the waiting-list control group. Fourteen-month follow-up data were collected on just over half the self-help sample (some of whom had subsequently received some sessions of cognitive behavior therapy). Forty percent were reported as being free from all bulimic symptoms (Treasure et al., 1996).

Cooper and colleagues have evaluated the effects of guided self-help on two series of patients seen in a secondary referral center. In the first (Cooper, Coker, & Fleming, 1994), 18 patients with bulimia nervosa received supervision in the use of a cognitive-behavioral self-help manual (Cooper, 1993). The supervision was provided by a social worker who had no specialist training in the management of eating disorders. The modal number of sessions was eight, and they were between 20 and 30 minutes long. At reassessment after 4 to 6 months with the Eating Disorder Examination (Cooper & Fairburn, 1987; Fairburn & Cooper, 1993), half the patients had not binged or vomited over the past month, and there were 85% and 88% near reductions in the frequency of binge eating and vomiting, respectively. There was also evidence of a decrease in dietary restraint and of a reduction in concerns about body

TABLE 30.2. Some Applications of Self-Help Books in Different Settings

Setting	Form of Application
Community	Pure self-help
Primary care	Pure self-help
	Guided self-help from a nonspecialist therapist
Specialist settings	As an adjunct to cognitive-behavioral therapy to reduce the amount of therapist input
	As an adjunct to interpersonal psychotherapy to enhance its effectiveness

shape and weight. No follow-up data were reported.

Cooper, Coker, and Fleming (1996) have since reported their experience with a further series of 82 patients managed and assessed in the same way. Fifteen (18%) dropped out. Among the remainder, there was substantial and sustained improvement. At 4 to 6 months reassessment, there was a marked reduction in the frequency of binge eating and vomiting, and 22 patients (33% of those who did not drop out) had not binged or vomited over the past month. Once again, there was evidence of a lessening of dietary restraint and of a decrease in concerns about body shape and weight. These changes were maintained six months later.

In an attempt to reproduce the conditions under which self-interventions are most likely to be used, Carter and Fairburn have recently completed a controlled evaluation of "pure" self-help and "guided" self-help in the treatment of a community-based sample of individuals with binge eating disorder. The guided self-help therapists (who were non-specialists and received only minimal supervision) were asked to encourage patients to follow the cognitive behavioral self-help program in *Overcoming Binge Eating* (Fairburn, 1995). They met their patients on 6 to 8 occasions over 12 weeks, each session lasting no more than 25 minutes. This intervention was compared with pure self-help in which subjects were simply mailed a copy of the book and advised to follow the self-help program, and with a 12-week waiting list control condition. Both forms of self-help produced substantial change with over forty percent of patients ceasing to binge eat, improvements that were well maintained at six-month

follow-up. In contrast, there was little change among the subjects in the waiting list control condition. Overall, the results marginally favoured the guided self-help condition (Carter & Fairburn, 1996).

THE CURRENT STANDING OF SELF-HELP

It is not possible to make firm recommendations about the use of self-help books in the management of binge-eating problems. This is primarily because the studies have evaluated the effects of nonspecialist interventions on specialist patient samples. The one exception is the study by Carter and Fairburn (1996). This study obtained substantial change with both pure and guided cognitive-behavioral self-help. Before conclusions can be drawn, its findings will need replicating and extending to bulimia nervosa.

At least three questions have to be answered to determine the place of self-help books in the management of binge-eating problems:

1. *Are self-help books used on their own effective, and if so, with whom?* If pure self-help is sufficient for some sufferers, as it appears from the Carter and Fairburn study (1996), then it could serve as a form of secondary prevention (i.e., as a means of reducing the delay between the onset of the disorder and the receipt of help). It could also be used in primary care, thereby eliminating the need to involve a therapist (Carter & Fairburn, 1995). Further controlled evaluations of pure self-help interventions are needed in which relevant samples are studied (i.e., cases recruited directly from the community, or patients in primary care) and longer-term effects are assessed. As for the choice of self-help book to study, it seems only rational to use one of the two books that are direct translations of the cognitive-behavioral treatment approach (Fairburn, Marcus, & Wilson, 1993; see also Wilson et al., Chapter 6, this volume).

2. *For those who present for treatment, is guidance from a nonspecialist therapist effective, and if so, with whom?* It is important to determine whether some people with binge-eating problems can be helped in primary care. Our experience suggests that many can. For example, Waller et al. (1996) working in primary care, found that about half their patients with

bulimia nervosa responded to a brief cognitive-behavioral intervention administered by a non-specialist therapist.

Guided self-help is an alternative to brief cognitive-behavioral therapy. It has the advantage that the primary source of information and advice is the self-help program itself rather than the therapist, with the consequence that little or no therapist training is required.

3. *For those who require specialist help, do self-help books have a role, and if so, with whom?* In specialist settings, the main role of self-help books would seem to be as an adjunct to conventional forms of treatment, although guided self-help might be appropriate for less severe cases. As mentioned earlier, we have been using a cognitive-behavioral self-help book (Fairburn, 1995) in combination with cognitive-behavioral therapy as a means of reducing the amount of therapist input, and in combination with interpersonal psychotherapy as a means of increasing the therapy's effectiveness. Both approaches merit evaluation in controlled trials, conducted in secondary or tertiary referral centers.

Until we have answers to these questions, it will be impossible to realize the full potential of self-help books. Self-help is likely to have much to offer individuals with binge-eating problems, whether these individuals are undetected in the community or seeking professional treatment. Rigorous tests of the effectiveness of the various forms of self-help, conducted in settings appropriate to their eventual use, are needed.

ACKNOWLEDGMENTS

We are grateful to the Wellcome Trust for their support. CGF holds a Principal Fellowship award (046386) and JC holds a Prize Studentship award (038539). We are also grateful to Zafra Cooper and Deborah Waller for their helpful comments on the manuscript.

REFERENCES

Arenson, G. (1989). *A substance called food.* New York: McGraw-Hill.

Beasley, J. D., & Knightly, S. (1994). *Food for recovery.* New York: Crown.

Brandon, C. W. (1993). *Am I hungry . . . or am I hurting?* San Diego: Recovery.

Bruch, H. (1973). *Eating disorders: Obesity, anorexia nervosa and the person within.* New York: Basic Books.

Carter, J. C., & Fairburn, C. G. (1995). Treating binge eating problems in primary care. *Addictive Behavior, 20,* 765–772.

Carter, J. C., & Fairburn, C. G. (1996). Self-help and guided self-help in the treatment of binge eating disorder: A controlled study. In preparation.

Cooper, P. J. (1993). *Bulimia nervosa: A guide to recovery.* London: Robinson.

Cooper, P. J. (1995). *Bulimia nervosa and binge-eating: A guide to recovery.* London: Robinson.

Cooper, P. J., Coker, S., & Fleming, C. (1994). Self-help for bulimia nervosa: A preliminary report. *International Journal of Eating Disorders, 16,* 401–404.

Cooper, P. J., Coker, S., & Fleming, C. (1995). An evaluation of the efficacy of cognitive behavioural self-help for bulimia nervosa. *Journal of Psychosomatic Research, 40,* 281–287.

Cooper, Z., & Fairburn, C. G. (1987). The Eating Disorder Examination: A semi-structured interview for the assessment of the specific psychopathology of eating disorders. *International Journal of Eating Disorders, 6,* 1–8.

Fairburn, C. G. (1995). *Overcoming binge eating.* New York: Guilford Press.

Fairburn, C. G., Agras, W. S., & Wilson, G. T. (1992). The research on the treatment of bulimia nervosa: Practical and theoretical implications. In G. H. Anderson & S. H. Kennedy (Eds.), *The biology of feast and famine: Relevance to eating disorders* (pp. 317–340). San Diego: Academic Press.

Fairburn, C. G., & Cooper, P. J. (1982). Self-induced vomiting and bulimia nervosa: An undetected problem. *British Medical Journal, 284,* 1153–1155.

Fairburn, C. G., & Cooper, Z. (1993). The Eating Disorder Examination (12th edition). In C. G. Fairburn & G. T. Wilson (Eds.), *Binge eating: Nature, assessment, and treatment* (pp. 317–360). New York: Guilford Press.

Fairburn, C. G., Marcus, M. D., & Wilson, G. T. (1993). Cognitive-behavioral therapy for binge eating and bulimia nervosa: A comprehensive treatment manual. In C. G. Fairburn & G. T. Wilson (Eds.), *binge eating: Nature, assessment, and treatment* (pp. 361–404). New York: Guilford Press.

Fairburn, C. G., Welch, S. L., Norman, P. A., O'Connor, M. E., & Doll, H. A. (1996). Bias and bulimia nervosa: How typical are clinic cases? *American Journal of Psychiatry, 153,* 386–391.

French, B. (1987). *Coping with bulimia.* London: Thorsons.

Garner, D. M., & Bemis, K. M. (1982). A cognitive-behavioral approach to anorexia nervosa. *Cognitive Therapy and Research, 6,* 123–150.

Greeson, J. (1990). *It's not what you're eating, it's what's eating you.* New York: Pocket Books.

Hall, L., & Cohen, L. (1992). *Bulimia: A guide to recovery.* Carlsbad, CA: Gurze.

Hazelden Foundation. (1992). *Food for thought.* New York: Harper & Row.

Hirschmann, J. R., & Munter, C. H. (1988). *Overcoming overeating.* New York: Fawcett Columbine.

Hollis, J. (1985). *Fat is a family affair.* San Francisco: Hazelden/HarperCollins.

Huon, G. F. (1985). An initial validation of a self-help program for bulimia. *International Journal of Eating Disorders, 4,* 573–588.

Kolodny, N. J. (1992). *When food's a foe.* Boston: Little, Brown.

Marx, R. (1992). *It's not your fault.* New York: Plume.

Roth, G. (1989). *A guide to ending compulsive eating.* New York: Plume.

Roth, G. (1993). *Breaking free from compulsive eating.* New York: Plume.

Schmidt, U., Tiller, J., & Treasure, J. (1993). Self-treatment of bulimia nervosa: A pilot study. *International Journal of Eating Disorders, 13,* 273–277.

Schmidt, U. H., & Treasure, J. L. (1993). *Getting better bit(e) by bit(e).* Hove, England: Erlbaum.

Treasure, J., Schmidt, U., Troop, N., Tiller, J., Todd, G., Keilen, M., & Dodge, E. (1994). First step in managing bulimia nervosa: Controlled trial of therapeutic manual. *British Medical Journal, 308,* 686–689.

Treasure, J., Schmidt, U., Troop, N., Tiller, J., Todd, G., & Turnbull. (1996). Sequential treatment of bulimia nervosa incorporating a self-care manual. *British Journal of Psychiatry, 168,* 94–98.

Waller, D., Fairburn, C. G., McPherson, A., Kay, R., Lee, A., & Nowell, T. (1996). Treating bulimia nervosa in primary care: A pilot study. *International Journal of Eating Disorders, 19,* 99–103.

Whitaker, A., Johnson, J., Shaffer, D., Rapoport, J. L., Kalikow, K., Walsh, B. T., Davies, M., Braiman, S., & Dolinsky, A. (1990). Uncommon troubles in young people: Prevalence estimates of selected psychiatric disorders in a nonreferred adolescent population. *Archives of General Psychiatry, 47,* 487–496.

Wilson, G. T., & Fairburn, C. G. (1993). Cognitive treatments for eating disorders. *Journal of Consulting and Clinical Psychology, 61,* 261–269.

Author Index

Subject Index